H. J. Wieler · R. E. Coleman (Eds.) **PET in Clinical Oncology**

Helmut J. Wieler
R. Edward Coleman
Editors

PET in Clinical Oncology

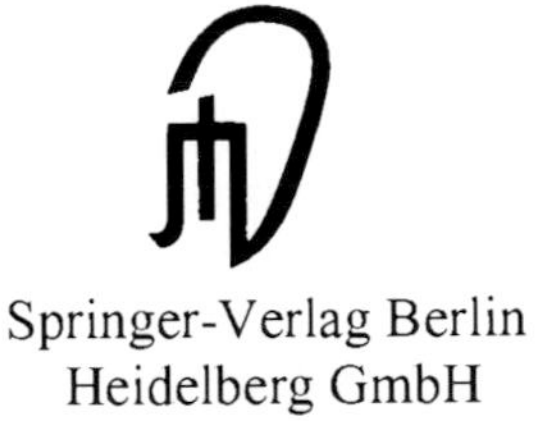

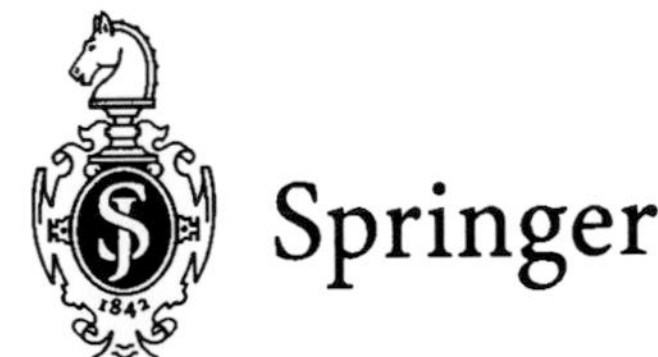

Springer-Verlag Berlin
Heidelberg GmbH

Prof. Dr. med. H.J. Wieler
Bundeswehrzentralkrankenhaus Koblenz
Abteilung XV – Nuklearmedizin
Rübenacher Straße 170
56072 Koblenz, Germany

R. Edward Coleman, M.D.
Professor of Radiology
Vice-Chairman, Department of Radiology
Director, Division of Nuclear Medicine
DUMC 3949, Room 1419, Duke North
Erwin Road, Durham, NC 27710, USA

ISBN 978-3-642-63329-4 ISBN 978-3-642-57703-1 (eBook)
DOI 10.1007/978-3-642-57703-1

Die Deutsche Bibliothek – CIP Cataloging-in-Publication-Data
A catalogue record for this publication is available from
Die Deutsche Bibliothek

Originally published by Steinkopff Verlag, Darmstadt in 2000
Softcover reprint of the hardcover 1st edition 2000

Medical Editor: Sabine Ibkendanz – English Editor: Mary K. Gossen
Production: Heinz J. Schäfer
Cover-Design: Erich Kirchner, Heidelberg
Typesetting: K+V Fotosatz, Beerfelden

Printed on acid-free paper

Foreword

In recent years the contribution of nuclear medicine to oncology has expanded and undergone significant change. With the advent of positron emission tomography (PET) cameras capable of producing whole-body scans in an hour or less with high image quality and linear spatial resolutions well below 1 cm, the use of this imaging technique for tumor staging has become a clinical reality.

Although a large repertoire of tracer substances has been used in oncology, mainly 2-[^{18}F]fluoro-2-deoxy-D-glucose (FDG) has been used to the extent that its role in clinical practice can be established. This tracer indicates glucose metabolism. This parameter has been demonstrated to be enhanced in many tumor types, thus allowing differentiation of malignant from benign disease, staging and grading malignant disease, differentiating recurrent disease from therapy-induced changes and monitoring response to therapy. The use of FDG and PET scanners for qualitative and quantitative evaluation of tumor metabolism is currently the fastest growing area in clinical PET.

This book intends to offer an overview of all different aspects of PET in clinical oncology.

The editors thank Brigitte Metternich for her valuable help in writing this book and Brigitte Mannheim, Annette Kreuter and Steven Wieler for secretarial assistance. We also thank Dave Edge and Doug Prager for their helpful suggestions.

Koblenz and Durham, Spring 2000

H. J. Wieler
R. E. Coleman

Contents

II. Clinical application

List of Contributors

Priv.-Doz. Dr. N. Avril
Nuklearmedizinische Klinik
und Poliklinik der TU München
Klinikum rechts der Isar
Ismaninger Str. 22
81675 München, Germany

Prof. Dr. M. Bähre
Abt. für Nuklearmedizin
Medizinische Universität
Ratzeburger Allee 160
23538 Lübeck, Germany

Prof. Dr. R. Bares
Radiologische Klinik
und Nuklearmedizin
Universität Tübingen
Röntgenweg 13
72076 Tübingen, Germany

Priv.-Doz. Dr. H. Bender
Klinikum und Poliklinik
für Nuklearmedizin
Universität Bonn
Sigmund-Freud-Str. 25
53127 Bonn, Germany

T. Beyer, Ph.D.
CTI PET Systems Inc.
810 Innovation Drive
Knoxville, TN 37932, USA

Dr. A. R. Börner
Klinik für Nuklearmedizin
Medizinische Hochschule Hannover
Carl-Neuberg-Str. 1
30625 Hannover, Germany

Priv.-Doz. Dr.
V. M. Bonkowsky
Hals-, Nasen-, Ohrenklinik
und Poliklinik
Klinikum rechts der Isar
Ismaninger Str. 22
81675 München, Germany

Dr. D. Brecht-Krauss
Abteilung Nuklearmedizin
Universität Ulm
Robert-Koch-Str. 8
89081 Ulm, Germany

Dr. J. Breul
Urologische Klinik
Klinikum rechts der Isar
Ismaninger Str. 22
81675 München, Germany

M. Charron, M.D. FRCP
Associate Professor of Radiology
Chief Nuclear Medicine
Children Hospital of Pittsburgh
University of Pittsburgh
3705 5th AVE
Pittsburgh, PA 15213, USA

R. E. Coleman, M.D.
Professor of Radiology
Vice-Chairman,
Department of Radiology Director,
Division of Nuclear Medicine
DUMC 3949, Room 1419,
Duke North
Erwin Road
Durham, NC 27710, USA

T. R. DeGrado, Ph.D.
Assistant Research Professor
PET Facility
Box 3949
Durham, NC 27710, USA

D. Delbeke, M.D., Ph.D.
Vanderbilt University
Department of Radiology
and Radiological Sciences
Section of Nuclear Medicine/PET
21st and Garland
Nashville, TN 37232-2675, USA

Dr. C. G. Diederichs
Abteilung Nuklearmedizin
Universität Ulm
Robert-Koch-Str. 8
89081 Ulm, Germany

Dr. A. Dimitrakopoulou-Strauss
Deutsches Krebsforschungszentrum
Im Neuenheimer Feld 280
69120 Heidelberg, Germany

Dr. B. Grünwald
Abteilung Gynäkologie
Universität Bonn
Sigmund-Freud-Str. 25
53127 Bonn, Germany

Prof. Dr. F. Grünwald
Nuklearmedizinische Klinik
Johann-Wolfgang-Goethe-
Universität
Theodor-Stern-Kai 7
60596 Frankfurt/M., Germany

Prof. Dr. U. Haberkorn
Abteilung Nuklearmedizin
Radiologische Universitätsklinik
Im Neuenheimer Feld 400
69120 Heidelberg

Dipl. Ing. W. Hamkens
Fa. PETNET GmbH
Am Wetterkreuz 21
91058 Erlangen, Germany

Priv.-Doz. Dr. Ing. H. Herzog
Institut für Medizin
Forschungszentrum Jülich
52425 Jülich, Germany

R. D. Hichwa, Ph.D.
PET Imaging Center
University of Iowa Hospitals
Iowa City, IA 52242, USA

Dr. M. Hofmann
Klinik für Nuklearmedizin
Medizinische Hochschule Hannover
Carl-Neuberg-Str. 1
30625 Hannover, Germany

P. E. Kinahan, Ph.D.
Associate Professor of Radiology
University of Pittsburgh
Medical Center
PET Facility B-938 PUH
200 Lothrop St.
Pittsburgh, PA 15213, USA

Dr. B. Klemenz
Abt. XV-Nuklearmedizin
Bundeswehrzentralkrankenhaus
Rübenacher Str. 170
56072 Koblenz, Germany

Prof. Dr. J. Kotzerke
Abteilung Nuklearmedizin
Universitätsklinikum
Robert-Koch-Str. 8
89081 Ulm, Germany

Priv.-Doz. Dr. B. J. Krause
Institut für Medizin
Forschungszentrum Jülich
52425 Jülich, Germany

Dr. J. Kretschko
Nuklearmedizinische Klinik
und Poliklinik
der TU München
Klinikum rechts der Isar
Ismaninger Str. 22
81675 München, Germany

Priv.-Doz. Dr. W. Kuhn
Frauenklinik
Klinikum rechts der Isar
Ismaninger Straße 22
81675 München, Germany

Dr. M. Kunkel
Klinik und Poliklinik für Mund-, Kiefer- und Gesichtschirurgie
Johannes-Gutenberg-Universität Mainz
Augustusplatz 2
55101 Mainz, Germany

Prof. Dr. T. Kuwert
Nuklearmedizinische Klinik und Poliklinik
Friedrich-Alexander-Universität Erlangen-Nürnberg
Krankenhausstraße 12
91054 Erlangen, Germany

S. M. Larson, M.D.
Medical Imaging Department
Memorial Hospital
1275 York Avenue
New York, NY 10021, USA

G. Lucignani, M.D.
Department of Nuclear Medicine
University of Milan
c/o H. S. Raffaele
20132 Milano, Italy

Dr. J. Marienhagen
Abteilung für Nuklearmedizin
Klinikum der Universität Regensburg
Franz-Josef-Strauß-Allee 11
93053 Regensburg, Germany

C. L. Melcher, Ph.D.
CTI PET Systems Inc.
810 Innovation Drive
Knoxville, TN 37932, USA

C. Meltzer, M.D.
Associate Professor of Radiology
Medical Director of PET
University of Pittsburgh
Medical Center
PET Facility B-938 PUH
200 Lothrop St.
Pittsburgh, PA 15213, USA

Dr. F. Moog
Klinik und Poliklinik für Nuklearmedizin
Klinikum Großhadern
Ludwig-Maximilians-Universität
Marchioninistr. 15
81377 München, Germany

Dr. V. Müller-Mattheis
Urologische Klinik
Heinrich-Heine-Universität
Moorenstr. 5
40225 Düsseldorf, Germany

R. Nutt, Ph.D.
CTI PET Systems Inc.
810 Innovation Drive
Knoxville, TN 37932, USA

Dr. M. Reinhardt
Gemeinschaftspraxis für Radiologie und Nuklearmedizin
Borkener Str. 136
46284 Dorsten, Germany

Priv.-Doz. Dr. P. Reuland
Praxis für Nuklearmedizin
Schwabentorplatz 6
79098 Freiburg, Germany

Prof. Dr. F. Rösch
Institut für Kernchemie
Johannes-Gutenberg-Universität Mainz
Fritz-Straßmann-Weg 2
55128 Mainz, Germany

Dr. E. Rota Kops
Institut für Medizin
Forschungszentrum Jülich
52425 Jülich, Germany

Priv.-Doz. Dr. K. Scheidhauer
Nuklearmedizinische Klinik und Poliklinik der TU München
Klinikum rechts der Isar
Ismaninger Str. 22
81675 München, Germany

Dr. H. Schirrmeister
Abteilung Nuklearmedizin
Universitätsklinikum Ulm
Robert-Koch-Str. 8
89081 Ulm, Germany

Dr. M. Schulte
Onkologische Ambulanz der Abt. für Unfall-, Hand- und Wiederherstellungschirurgie
Chirurgische Universitätsklinik
Steinhövelstr. 9
89075 Ulm, Germany

J.S. Schweitzer
Schlumberger-Doll Research
Old Quarry Rd.
Ridgefield, CT 06877-4108, USA

P.D. Shreve, M.D.
Internal Medicine Department
Internal MED/Nuclear MED,
B1G505 UH
University of Michigan
1500 E. Medical Center Drive
Ann Arbor, MI 48109, USA

Dr. H.J. Straehler-Pohl
HNO-Abteilung
Universitätsklinik Bonn
Sigmund-Freud-Str. 25
53127 Bonn, Germany

Prof. Dr. L.G. Strauss
Abteilung für onkologische
Diagnostik und Therapie
Deutsches Krebsforschungszentrum
Im Neuenheimer Feld 280
69120 Heidelberg, Germany

Dr. K.M. Taaleb
Dept. of Nuclear Medicine
Maadi Armed Forces Hospital
Kornish El-Nil-El Maadi
Cairo, Egypt

Prof. Dr. K. Tatsch
Klinik und Poliklinik
für Nuklearmedizin
Klinikum Großhadern
Ludwig-Maximilians-Universität
Marchioninistraße 15
81377 München, Germany

Dr. M.H. Thelen
Abteilung für Nuklearmedizin
Eberhard-Karls-Universität
Tübingen
Röntgenweg 13
72076 Tübingen, Germany

D.W. Townsend, Ph.D.
Professor of Radiology
University of Pittsburgh
Medical Center
PET Facility, B-938 PUH
200 Lothrop St.
Pittsburgh, PA 15213, USA

Dr. W. Weber
Nuklearmedizinische Klinik
und Poliklinik der TU München
Klinikum rechts der Isar
Ismaninger Str. 22
81675 München, Germany

Dr. H.-J. Wester
Nuklearmedizinische Klinik
und Poliklinik der TU München
Klinikum rechts der Isar
Ismaninger Str. 22
81675 München, Germany

Prof. Dr. H.J. Wieler
Abt. XV-Nuklearmedizin
Bundeswehrzentralkrankenhaus
Rübenacher Str. 170
56072 Koblenz, Germany

Dr. S.I. Ziegler
Nuklearmedizinische Klinik
und Poliklinik der TU München
Klinikum rechts der Isar
Ismaninger Str. 22
81675 München, Germany

1 Current status of PET in the United States

R.E. Coleman, H.J. Wieler

PET imaging is having a major impact in patient care. The increasing utilization of PET is related to several major factors: clinical data demonstrating the usefulness, reimbursement, availability of instrumentation and distribution of FDG. We are just beginning to see the "tip of the iceberg" in the clinical and research utilization of PET. PET is a molecular imaging technique, and PET imaging will be the major imaging modality of molecular medicine. The ability to label molecules with positron-emitting radionuclides and quantitatively determine their distribution will be important in disease characterization, drug discovery, drug therapy and gene therapy [8]. These uses will frequently begin with the mouse, which is the animal most widely used in drug development and in gene therapy. Systems such as the microPET permit high resolution (1–2 mm) of PET tracers in small animals including mice [2, 12]. These studies can then be performed in adult subjects to verify the results obtained in animals. The ethical drug industry is beginning to adapt this technology in their developmental efforts.

The advantages of PET have been known for many years. Attempts to develop the instrumentation for PET imaging were initially made in the 1960s by Anger, Brownell, Muehllehner and others, but the electronics were inadequate to handle the count rates, and the reconstruction algorithms were not available [3]. After the development of x-ray computed tomography and the use of filtered backprojection algorithms, Phelps and colleagues [10] at the Mallinckrodt Institute of Radiology in St. Louis, Missouri, were the first to obtain PET images. At that time, the instrument was called a positron emission transaxial tomograph (PETT). The initial tomograph consisted of a hexagonal array of sodium iodide detectors in a single ring. One slice with a resolution of approximately 1.5 cm required several minutes to acquire. That group demonstrated the ability of PET to quantify physiologic processes in vivo and its potential clinical applications [9].

This development of PET occurred in 1974, the same year that the initial image was produced using magnetic resonance imaging (MRI). MRI was rapidly developed by industry as an imaging technology and then was quickly accepted in clinical practice. PET has taken much longer to be incorporated into clinical practice. PET initially was considered an excellent, yet expensive, research modality. After the demonstration of the feasibility of performing PET imaging, limited interest in the technology was demonstrated by industry. However, improvements in the technology were taking place in both academic research centers and industry with limited resources. The tomographs were being built one at a time, only a few each year, and were very expensive for a nuclear medicine imaging system. In the 1970s, the purchase of a cyclotron for the production of the positron-emitting radionuclide was needed. The cyclotrons at that time were large, used vacuum tube technology, and required dedicated personnel for their operation and maintenance. For producing the radiopharmaceutical used in PET imaging, a radiochemist was needed. Thus, for a center to perform PET studies, which were only for research purposes at that time, an investment of 4–5 million US dollars was needed for the scanner, cyclotron, radiochemistry instrumentation and space. Furthermore, the annual personnel and support costs were approximately one million US dollars. Thus, PET was limited to a few academic research centers that could garner the support necessary to develop and maintain the facility. In the late 1970s, PET had the reputation of being an expensive and elegant research modality, but of limited clinical utility.

In 1979, Wolf and colleagues from Brookhaven National Laboratory synthesized 2[^{18}F]fluoro-2-deoxyglucose (FDG) [3]. The studies of its utilization in the early and mid-1980s were in the heart and brain [7]. The studies demonstrated the ability of FDG to detect ischemic, viable myocardium, grade the degree of malignancy of brain tumors, differentiate necrosis from recurrent brain tumor after therapy, identify the site of the seizure disorder in medically refractory partial complex seizure disorder, and differentiate the causes of dementia (i.e., to detect Alzheimer's disease prior to the clinical diagnosis being made) [1, 7, 11]. Several different groups reviewed the clinical applications of PET at that time and determined that the literature supported these indications.

In the late 1970s and early 1980s, the literature on the use of PET in oncology began to appear. The biochemical basis for its use had been well worked out; this glucose analog demonstrated the increased glucose utilization by cancer cells. Clinical studies were performed demonstrating the ability of FDG-PET to separate benign from malignant lesions, to stage the distribution of the malignancy, to determine the effects of therapy, and to detect recurrent disease [4]. The published results demonstrated a high accuracy for FDG-PET in characterizing indeterminate solitary pulmonary nodules, staging the mediastinum and whole body in patients with lung cancer, detecting recurrent colorectal cancer, staging lymphoma and detecting recurrent malignant melanoma. The FDG-PET scans were demonstrated to be cost-effective in these malignancies, to appropriately change patient management in 10–35% of patients, and to be more accurate than CT [4]. In January 1998, the Health Care Financing Administration (HCFA), which administers Medicare, began coverage of PET scans for two indications: evaluation of indeterminate solitary pulmonary nodules and staging lung cancer. A reimbursement amount of 1980 US dollars was established. After a "town hall" meeting at the HCFA in early 1999 during which the data for other indications of FDG-PET were presented, the HCFA added coverage policies for the following indications: recurrent colorectal cancer with a rising CEA value; recurrent malignant melanoma; and initial staging and restaging of lymphoma in place of gallium-67 citrate scanning. The reimbursement amount was set at 1980 US dollars for all indications. Because both camera-based and dedicated PET scanners were approved by the Food and Drug Administration (FDA) as PET scanners, these indications and reimbursement amounts were applicable to all PET imaging devices.

The number of instruments available for PET imaging has increased tremendously in the last few years [5]. Approximately 55 sites offered PET imaging in 1997, and now more than 300 sites have PET imaging capability (Fig. 1.1); the same situation happened in Germany (Fig. 1.2). The increase in sites has been primarily with the addition of camera-based PET instruments, but most of the clinical FDG-PET scans are still performed using dedicated PET scanners [5]. The private insurance carriers and health maintenance organizations have generally developed coverage policies similar to the HCFA coverage policies.

The Food and Drug Modernization Act (FDAMA) of 1997 changed the status of PET radiopharmaceuticals so that the HCFA could establish coverage policies. The FDA had previously determined that it had jurisdiction over clinically used PET radiopharmaceuticals, even if compounded and used locally by an institution [6]. Prior to FDAMA, a single New Drug Application (NDA) had been approved by the FDA for FDG at Methodist Medical Center in Peoria, Illinois. The FDAMA stated that PET radiopharmaceuticals had the equivalence of FDA approval for two years. During the 2-year period, the FDA was required to work with the PET community to develop guidelines for PET radiopharmaceutical production and approval. Furthermore, the FDA was to review currently used radiopharmaceuticals for approval. The FDA has worked effectively with the PET community for the past two years to develop guidelines for PET radiopharmaceutical production and guidelines for PET radiopharmaceutical approval. These guidelines are to be published in 2000. In addition, the FDA has provided an NDA for FDG, ^{18}F-sodium fluoride, [^{18}F]fluorodopa, [^{13}N]ammonia, and [^{15}O]water. The indications for FDG as written by the FDA provide broad utilization in oncology and usage for determination of myocardial viability. The indications for ^{13}N-ammonia are for a myocardial perfusion tracer to detect coronary artery disease. The indications for the other tracers are being determined at this time.

In 1997, a company (PETNet Pharmaceutical, Inc.) was formed for the production and distribution of FDG. This company has grown rapidly and presently has 19 sites, primarily in the metropolitan areas of the United States. The FDG is distributed primarily by ground transportation, but air transportation is used for distant sites. The company provides PET radiopharmaceuticals to sites within 2 h of the production facility. Several smaller companies are now producing and distributing FDG to limited geographic areas.

Because of the large amount of data documenting the clinically utility of PET, these changes in the policies of the FDA, improved coverage policies by

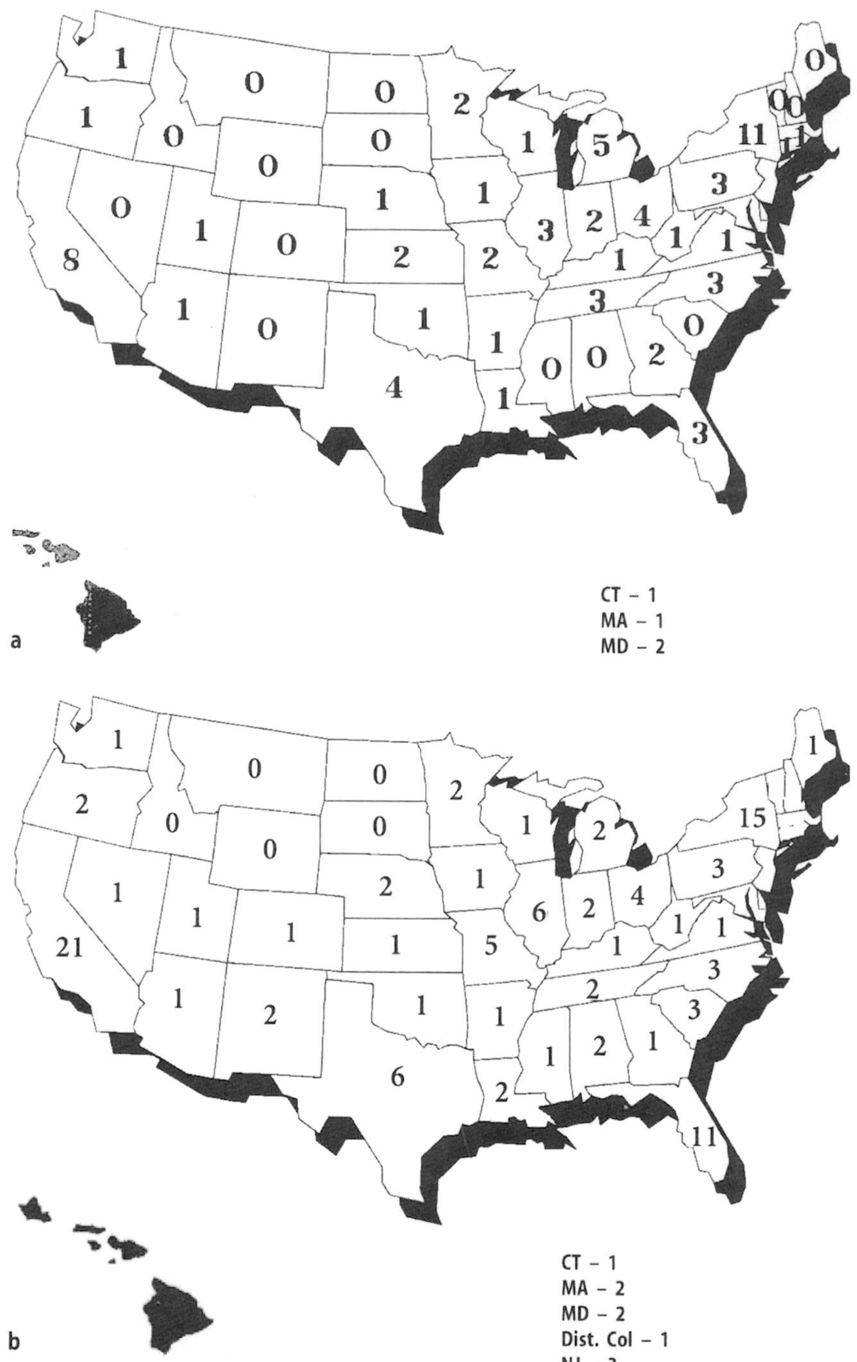

Fig. 1.1. Dedicated PET scanners (**a**) and coincidence PET scanners (**b**) in the United States in February 2000. (*CT* Connecticut, *MA* Massachusetts, *MD* Maryland, *Dist Col* District of Columbia, *NJ* New Jersey).

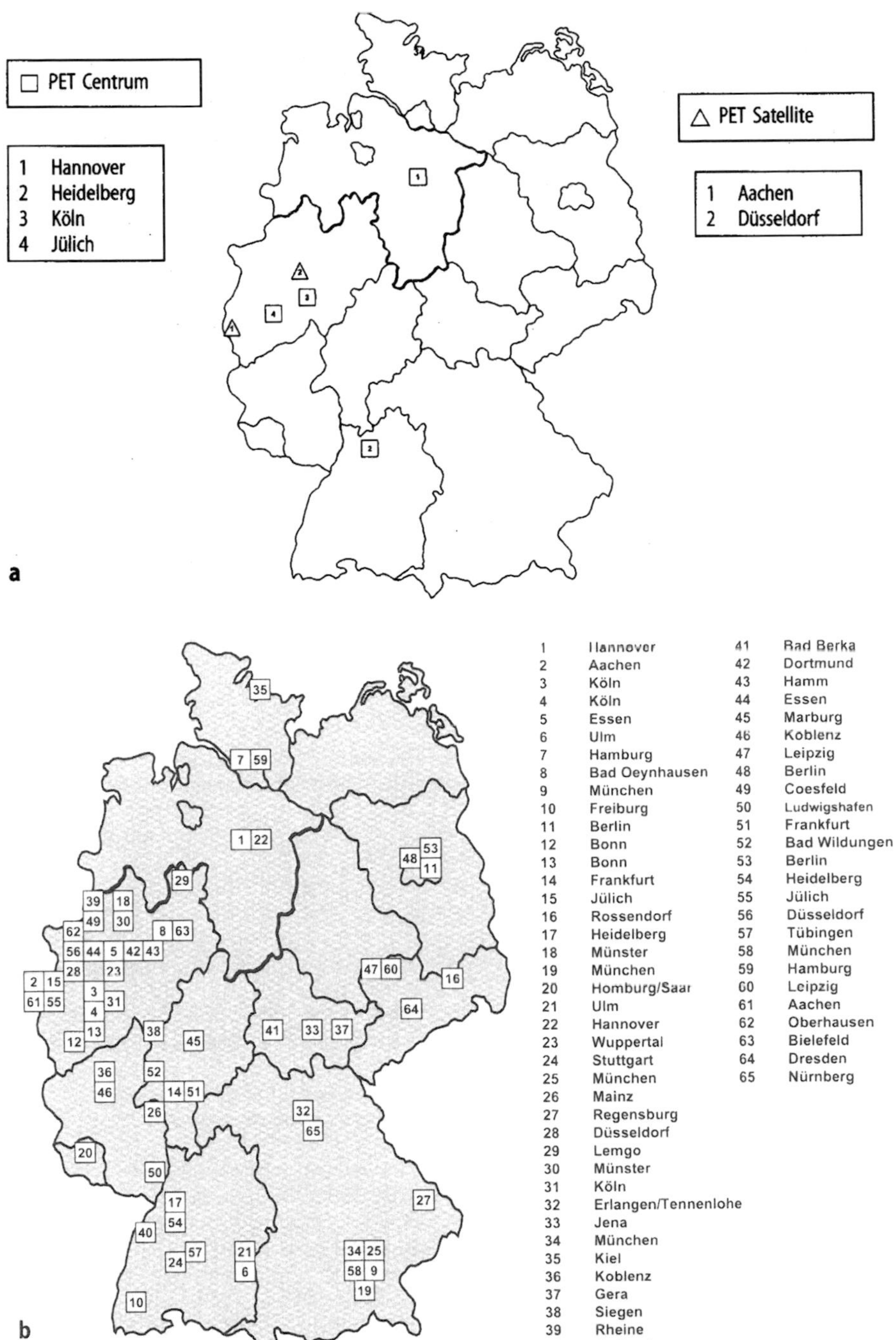

Fig. 1.2. PET installations in Germany in 1988 (**a**) and in October 1999 (**b**). Data from J. Murmann, Siemens AG, Erlangen, Germany.

the HCFA and private insurance carriers, improvements in instrumentation, and commercial distribution of FDG, the usage of FDG-PET is increasing rapidly in the United States. A concerted effort is being made to educate the public, patient advocacy groups, physicians, politicians, regulators, and third-party payers on the benefits of PET. Also, efforts are being made to increase the number of indications for which third-party payers have coverage policies.

The future for the application of PET in oncology in the United States and in Germany [13] is very promising. The clinical demand is increasing, availability is improving and coverage policies for increasing numbers of indications are occurring. In addition, the research studies now being performed in animals and patients are providing the foundation for further clinical applications of PET.

References

[1] Al-Aish M, Coleman RE, Larson SM, et al. (1990) Advances in clinical imaging using positron emission tomography. National Cancer Institute Workshop Statement. Arch Int Med 150:735–739

[2] Chatziioannou AF, Cherry SR, Shao Y, et al. (1999) Performance evaluation of micro-PET: a high-resolution lutetium oxyorthosilicate PET scanner for animal imaging. J Nucl Med 40(7):1164–1175

[3] Coleman RE (1997) Editorial: Camera-based PET: the best is yet to come. J Nucl Med 38(11):1796–1797

[4] Coleman RE (1998) Clinical PET in oncology. Clinical Positron Imaging 1:15–30

[5] Coleman RE, Tesar RD (2000) A perspective on clinical PET imaging. Clin Pos Imag 3:41–44

[6] Coleman RE, Robbins MS, Siegel BA (1992) The future of PET in clinical medicine and the impact of drug regulation. Semin Nucl Med 12:193–201

[7] Kuhl DE, Wagner HN, Alavi A, Coleman RE, Larson SM, Mintun MA, Siegel BA, Strudler PK (1988) Positron emission tomography (PET): Clinical status in the United States in 1987. J Nucl Med 29:1136–1143

[8] Phelps ME, Coleman RE (2000) Editorial: Nuclear medicine in the new millennium. J Nucl Med 41:1-4

[9] Phelps ME, Hoffman EJ, Coleman RE, Welch MJ, Raichle ME, Weiss ES, Sobel BE, Ter-Pogossian MM (1976) Tomographic images of blood pool and perfusion in brain and heart. J Nucl Med 17:603–612

[10] Phelps ME, Hoffman EJ, Mullani NA, Ter-Pogossian MM (1975) Application of annihilation coincidence detection to transaxial reconstruction tomography. J Nucl Med 16:210–224

[11] Report of the Therapeutics and Technology Assessment Subcommittee of the American Academy of Neurology (1991) (Panel members: Mazziotta J, Coleman RE, Di Chiro G, Foster N, Fox P, Frackowiak R, Gilman S, Martin W, Raichle M, Theodore W) Assessment: Positron emission tomography. Neurology 41:163–167

[12] Tornai MP, Jaszczak RJ, Turkington TG, Coleman RE (1999) Editorial: Small-animal PET: advent of a new era of PET research. J Nucl Med 40:1176–1179

[13] Wieler HJ (1999) PET in der klinischen Onkologie. Steinkopff Verlag, Darmstadt

2 Physics, quality control

S.I. Ziegler

2.1 Introduction

Positron emission tomography (PET) is a nuclear medical modality which provides quantitative tomographic images and allows one to noninvasively determine the time course of a radioactive substance in vivo. Positron emitters are used for labeling biochemical substances. After injection of the radioactive tracer, the radiation from the body is registered by external detectors and tomographic images of the tracer distribution in the body are reconstructed using mathematical algorithms. The measured intensity and time course of the activity concentration in tissue depend on the specific physiological process in which the tracer takes part. Developments in PET instrumentation aim at improving resolution and sensitivity, in order to obtain precise measurements with as little radioactivity as possible. The recent clinical success of PET promoted new developments in scanner technology, thus bringing conventional nuclear medicine and PET closer together [26].

2.2 Physics background

Proton-rich nuclei are instable and decay into stable nuclei by emission of a positron and a neutrino. Depending on the nuclide, the positron has a certain amount of kinetic energy which it loses to the surrounding tissue by ionization and excitation processes. Once the positron is slowed down, a positronium atom consisting of a positron and an electron is created. The positronium has a very short half-life, and the masses of the positron and its antiparticle electron are finally transferred into energy. For energy and momentum to be conserved, this annihilation results in two gamma rays which are emitted back-to-back and which have an energy of 511 keV each. Decay events are detected by coincidence registration of the gamma quanta. Thus, it is not the location of positron emission but the location of positron annihilation which is detected in PET. This physical effect results in an uncertainty in localization which can amount to as much as several millimeters. Since the positronium does not always decay at rest, the angle between the two gamma quanta can vary by up to $\pm 0.5^{\circ}$, adding to the physical limita-

Table 2.1. Frequently used positron emitters, radioactive half-life $T_{1/2}$, maximum positron energy E_{max}, and path length R_p in water within which 50% (95%) of the positrons are stopped (from [18]).

	$T_{1/2}$ (min)	E_{max} (MeV)	R_p (mm)
C-11	20.4	0.97	0.3 (1.6)
N-13	9.9	1.19	0.5 (2.1)
O-15	2.05	1.72	0.7 (3.3)
F-18	109.7	0.64	0.2 (0.9)

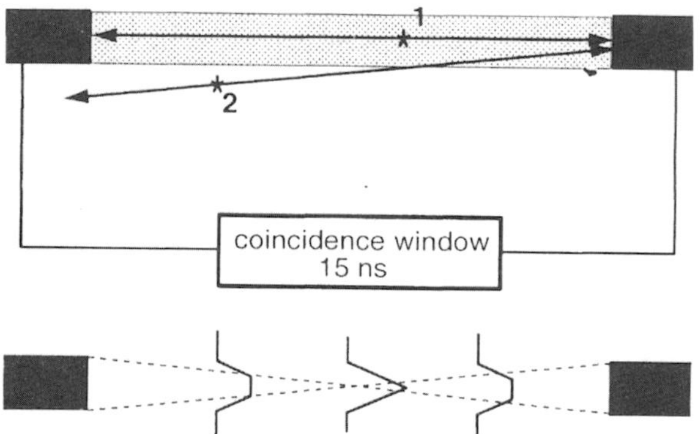

Fig. 2.1. Coincidence detector pair. Top: Collimation is accomplished through the measurement of only those events which are detected in both detectors simultaneously (event 1). The hatched area delineates the coincidence field-of-view of the detector pair. Event (2) can not be registered within the coincidence line. The intrinsic spatial resolution perpendicular to the detector axis corresponds to one half of the detector front face (bottom).

tion of spatial resolution. Table 2.1 summarizes the most commonly used positron emitters with their properties. Because of the short physical half-lives (minutes), it is necessary to produce them as close to the positron tomograph as possible. Cyclotrons are used to accelerate charged particles for nuclear reactions which result in positron emitters. Substances labeled with ^{18}F have the advantage of a physical half-life of almost two hours, allowing distribution of the tracer to distant centers, given that the infrastructure exists. In oncological PET, ^{18}F-labeled FDG has gained the highest significance.

Annihilation events are registered by coincidence detectors consisting of two opposing detector units. Only those events are counted that occur within the sensitive volume between the detectors and which emit gamma quanta along a line connecting the two detectors (Fig. 2.1), so that they can be detected within a very short time interval (coincidence window) in both detectors. The connecting line between the two detectors represents a coincidence line. Thus, there are no lead collimators needed, in contrast to single photon tomography (SPECT), but colinearity of the gamma quanta is exploited and used as "electronic collimation". Therefore, sensitivity is much higher than in SPECT (more than 100 times). Intrinsic resolution of a coincidence detector pair is defined by the size of the detectors and does not change much between the detectors (Fig. 2.1). It corresponds to one half of the detector front face. Furthermore, sensitivity is independent of source position between the detectors as long as the source covers the detector face [5]. The coincidence timing window is 15–20 ns in modern tomographs. Therefore, there is still a chance that two uncorrelated gamma rays are detected within the timing window. These random coincidences reduce the image contrast and developments in hard- and software aim at reducing this background.

The number of events measured in a coincidence line corresponds to the sum of all events along the direction of the coincidence pair through the object. In order to determine the activity distribution in the object, this integral information needs to be measured in many lines with different angles through the object. Therefore, detectors are arranged in a ring and coincidence events are logged for a number of opposing detector channels. As in SPECT acquisitions, radial as well as angular sampling must be provided for artifact-free reconstructions. The spatial distribution of the activity concentration within the field-of-view can be reconstructed from the measured projections using mathematical algorithms (see chapter 3).

2.3 Detectors for PET

Similar to conventional nuclear medicine, for the detection of annihilation quanta scintillation crystals, which are read out by photomultiplier tubes, are used. Photodiodes or avalanche photodiodes may replace the photomultiplier tubes in the future [28].

For efficient detection of high energy gamma rays in PET, scintillation materials need to fulfill special requirements: high density and atomic number are necessary for high photoabsorption at 511 keV. Besides improving localization accuracy in Anger-type detectors, high scintillation light yields results in good energy resolution and efficient discrimination of background events. Scintillators with a short light decay time have very good timing and count rate characteristics, which in turn allows the use of short coincidence timing windows for reduced random background.

The first positron tomographs consisted of individual thallium-doped sodium iodide (NaI:Tl) crystals coupled to photomultiplier tubes. This material, well known in nuclear medicine, has excellent characteristics for the detection of gamma rays with 140 keV energy; it is luminous and inexpensive. Unfortunately, its hygroscopic nature necessitates the encapsulation of the scintillation crystal. The biggest drawback with respect to positron imaging is its low detection probability for gamma rays with 511 keV (Table 2.2). A thicker crystal can make up for this, but the effect of crystal thickness on spatial resolution has to be considered [21].

BGO (bismuth germanate) is most commonly used in PET, since it has a high atomic number and therefore high detection efficiency. The light yield of BGO, on the other hand, is low and the decay time is long, limiting the coincidence timing window width. Recently, new scintillators were characterized

Table 2.2. Scintillation crystals which are in use for PET. *NaI:Tl* thallium-doped sodium iodide, *BGO* bismuth-germanate, *LSO:Ce* cerium-doped lutetium-oxyorthosilicate.

	NaI:Tl	BGO	LSO:Ce
Light yield (% NaI)	100	15	75
Wave length (nm)	410	480	420
Scintillation light decay time (ns)	230	300	40
Attenuation length at 140 keV (mm)	4.2	0.8	1.0
Attenuation length at 511 keV (mm)	30	11	12

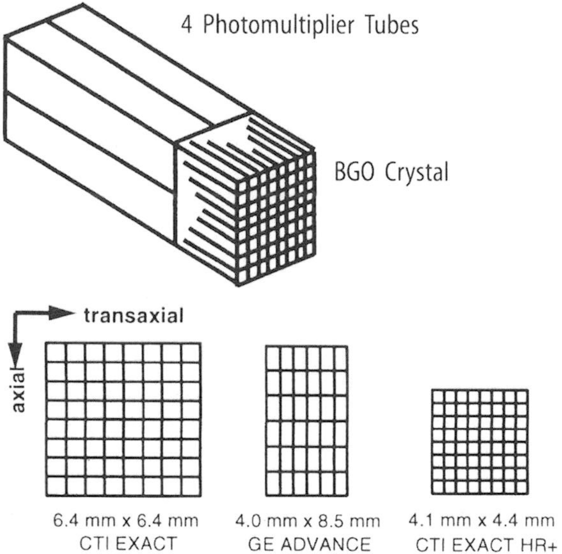

Fig. 2.2. BGO-Block detector, in which 4 photomultiplier tubes read out 64 scintillation crystals. The Anger principle is used for identification of the crystal. The size of the crystals defines the spatial resolution, examples of which are seen in the bottom row.

for the efficient and fast detection of 511 keV gamma rays. In 1992, cerium-doped lutetium-oxyorthosilicate (LSO) was developed [20, see chapter 8]. For PET application it is currently the most promising scintillator (Table 2.2). Small, high-resolution research tomographs for animal studies are already available with this material [8, 28]. A high-resolution PET scanner, dedicated to brain imaging, is being built with this crystal material [6, 29, 30]. Clinical tomographs with LSO-block detectors will show high sensitivity in combination with improved count rate performance and reduced random fraction.

Two different detector concepts are implemented in the current PET scanners. One is based on large area NaI-detectors which are read out like gamma cameras [22], the other concept uses block detectors [7]. Block detectors are BGO-blocks which are cut into small (e.g., 6 mm × 6 mm) subcrystals with light sharing between them for crystal identification by the Anger principle.

Thus, it is possible to pack small scintillation crystals in a dense matrix but use only a small number of photomultiplier tubes (e.g., 64 crystals read out by 4 photomultipliers). The size of the subcrystals defines the resulting spatial resolution (Fig. 2.2).

2.4 Positron tomographs

After the introduction of tomographic reconstruction in CT, coincidence techniques were used for emission tomography for the first time in the 1970s [27]. Since then, resolution and sensitivity have been improved [26]. Scatter and random fraction are equally important, because, for systems with the same spatial resolution, detectability of small tracer accumulations is degraded in the system with higher background counts.

With a ring tomograph, simultaneous measurement of the necessary projection data is possible. Good spatial sampling is accomplished by dense packing of detector modules. Tungsten septa between the detector slices were traditionally used in the 2D acquisition mode. This shielding reduces the accepted angle but keeps the scatter fraction low. For higher sensitivity, tomographs with retractable septa were developed [9]. The number of accepted angles is much higher in this 3D mode and dedicated reconstruction algorithms were developed (see chapter 3). Although sensitivity is increased (Table 2.3), more scattered and random events are detected, a fact which needs to be addressed in quantitative studies [3]. Shielding for reduction of single count rates in the detectors can improve the situation [14, 31]. It can be expected that the 3D mode will gain from shorter coincidence timing windows which will be possible with fast crystals (LSO).

Table 2.3. Characteristics of full ring tomographs (Siemens/CTI ECAT EXACT HR+ [4], GE Advance [13, 19], ADAC CPET [16]), a sector scanner (Siemens/CTI ECAT ART) and a coincidence camera (ADAC Vertex MCD [23]).

	EXACT HR+		Advance		ART	CPET	MCD[d]
	2D[a]	3D[b]	2D[a]	3D[c]			
Crystal material	BGO		BGO		BGO	NaI	NaI
Axial field-of-view (cm)	15.5	15.5	15.2	15.2	16.2	25	38
Resolution in the center:							
transaxial FWHM (mm)	4.3	4.4	4.5	4.5	5.7	4.2	5.0
axial FWHM (mm)	4.2	4.1	4.0	6.0	6.0	4.2	5.3
Sensitivity (cps/Bq/ml)[e]	5.7	27.7	5.7	27.6	7.5	10.8	3.2
Scatter fraction (%)[e]	17	33	9	36	37	28	32

[a] With tungsten septa (2D), lower energy threshold 350 keV
[b] Without tungsten septa (3D), lower energy threshold 350 keV
[c] Without tungsten septa (3D), lower energy threshold 300 keV
[d] Acquisition in 2 energy windows (511 keV, 310 keV) 30% width, detector separation: 62 cm
[e] Measured with a cylinder (20 cm diameter)

Due to the limited axial field-of-view (Table 2.3), whole-body acquisitions can only be accomplished by a sequence of several bed positions [11]. In order to keep the total scan time reasonably short, acquisition times per bed position need to stay in the range of several minutes. Measurements in the 3D mode yield higher counting statistics [10], but also higher background levels. Therefore, 3D acquisition is not yet in general use for whole-body PET.

Besides high resolution tomographs, there are several systems available which were developed for the purpose of cost-efficient imaging (Table 2.3). Application of the different tomographs needs to be decided according to their physical characteristics. Today the highest performance can be achieved with full ring BGO-block detector scanners [4, 13, 34]. With these systems it is possible to, for example, measure short-lived isotopes in dynamic sequences. Most of the published data were acquired using tomographs of this type.

A less expensive design is a scanner employing NaI instead of BGO. In order to efficiently detect coincidence events, the crystals in this scanner are thicker (25 mm). Systems with six large area NaI detectors are operated in 3D mode for increased system sensitivity [16, 17, 22]. Spatial resolution of these tomographs is very good; sensitivity and count rate performance limit the application to static or whole-body scans with ^{18}F-labeled FDG.

Another example for reduced system cost is a sector tomograph with fewer detector units than a full ring tomograph (Fig. 2.3). One of the commercial positron tomographs consists of only one third of the BGO block detectors, which cover 165° and are continuously rotated around the patient [2, 33]. This tomograph is also operated in 3D, resulting in a system sensitivity similar to a full ring tomograph in 2D mode.

Dual head coincidence cameras represent a further step in the direction of cost reduction, and provide two different imaging modes: SPECT (with collimators) and coincidence imaging (without a collimator) [25]. The NaI crystals in these cameras are thicker (5/8–6/8 inch) compared to conventional SPECT instrumentation. The thickness of the crystal can only be increased as long as the performance in single photon detection is not compromised.

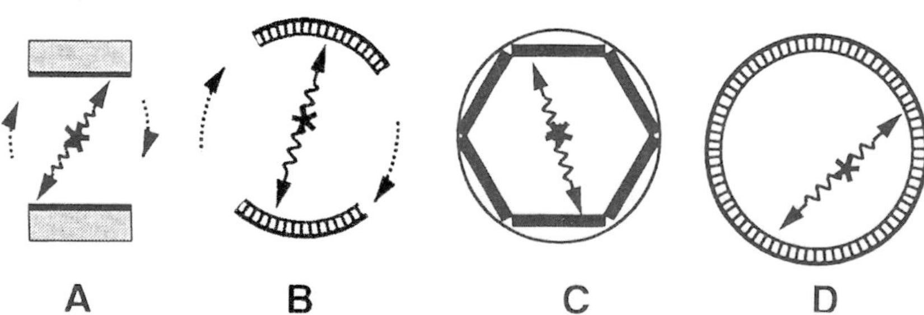

Fig. 2.3. Various types of positron tomographs: **A** rotating coincidence camera, **B** rotating sector tomograph, **C** ring with NaI detectors, and **D** ring with BGO blocks.

Since they need to be rotated and because of their lower intrinsic sensitivity, coincidence cameras require longer acquisition times than full ring tomographs. The spatial resolution of coincidence cameras is very good (5 mm), but low counting statistics and elevated background levels result in low contrast in the reconstructed image, as compared to ring tomographs. In the large area detectors a number of events originating from outside the coincidence field-of-view either direct or after scattering inside the patient's body are detected, increasing the detector rates and thus the chance for random events. This reduces the image contrast and several means to minimize this effect have been implemented (side shields, "septa", graded absorbers). The ratio of coincidence versus single events in a coincidence camera is 1 to 2%, depending on the crystal thickness. In order to register reasonable coincidence rates, single rates of more than 1 million counts per second need to be processed in a detector head. Fast electronics and pulse shaping are implemented in modern systems to overcome the problem of low sensitivity but nevertheless high count rates. Furthermore, digital camera head technology allows the use of different setups for coincidence or single photon mode, an option which was not available at the time of the first experimental coincidence cameras [1]. Recently, several schemes have been introduced for transmission measurement and attenuation correction in dual head coincidence cameras. While these techniques provide better delineation of anatomical structures and in combination with background correction algorithms enhance lesion detectability, other improvements in data processing and reconstruction will certainly further improve image quality.

A hybrid detector consisting of two layers with different crystal material has been proposed as a new approach for the detector front end in dual head coincidence cameras [12, 29]. The front layer, made of NaI, will be used for single photon detection, the second layer will be made of LSO, specially suited for coincidence detection. The pulse shape characteristics of the two layers are so different that they can easily be discriminated for event localization. Once the first clinical systems of this type are available, it will be seen as to how much SPECT and PET imaging will merge.

2.5 Quality control

Quality control in nuclear medicine is based on standardized measurements which are performed at regular intervals to detect any changes compared to the performance at the time of installation of the camera. During acceptance testing, data are collected under standard conditions [15, 24] which are used as reference values.

The differences in efficiency (geometric or intrinsic) of the various lines-of-response need to be corrected before reconstruction. Rotating Ge/Ga transmission rod sources (see chapter 3) are used to generate a measurement with high count statistics covering each line-of-response. In combination with the measurement of a homogeneously filled cylinder, a normalization file is created, similar to homogeneity matrices in SPECT systems. Every day, the relative sensitivity of coincidence lines is measured to detect deviations from the basic normalization data set. Automated procedures using the transmission sources in ring PET scanners offer a convenient way to do this [32]. In addition to the automated statistical comparison, visual inspection of the raw data may help in identifying weak detector channels.

System sensitivity is determined with a 20 cm diameter cylindrical phantom, homogeneously filled with ^{18}F. From these data, the calibration factor is calculated as cps/pixel in the reconstructed image per Bq/ml in the phantom. Since changes in system sensitivity can only be expected after major tuning of the electronics or after changes in the lower energy threshold, this procedure does not have to be performed frequently. One might decide to include it more often (e.g., every week), since it offers the opportunity to check the whole processing procedure from acquisition, through correction methods, to reconstruction and image display.

Currently, quality control procedures in PET are mainly tailored to the needs in full ring PET. Little experience is available for quality control measurements in coincidence cameras. For these systems, it may be necessary to specify model-specific quality control procedures, since the various implementations may be affected by different performance drifts. Nevertheless, the primary quality control of these cameras according to the requirements for SPECT mode is mandatory.

References

[1] Anger H (1963) Gamma-ray and positron scintillation camera. Nucleonics 21:10–56

[2] Bailey D, Young H, Bloomfield P, et al. (1997) ECAT ART – a continuously rotating PET camera: performance characteristics, initial clinical studies, and installation considerations in a nuclear medicine department. Eur J Nucl Med 24:6–15

[3] Bendriem B, Townsend D (1998) The theory and practice of 3D PET. Dordrecht, Kluwer Academic Publishers

[4] Brix G, Zaers J, Adam LE, et al. (1997) Performance evaluation of a whole-body PET scanner using the NEMA protocol. National Electrical Manufacturers Association. J Nucl Med 38(10):1614–1623

[5] Budinger T (1998) PET instrumentation: what are the limits? Semin Nucl Med 28:247–267

[6] Casey M, Eriksson L, Schmand M, et al. (1997) Investigation of LSO crystals for high resolution positron emission tomography. IEEE Trans Nucl Sci 44:1109–1113

[7] Casey M, Nutt R (1986) Multicrystal two dimensional BGO detector system for positron emission tomography. IEEE Trans Nucl Sci 33:460–463

[8] Chatziioannou A, Cherry S, Shao Y, et al. (1999) Performance evaluation of microPET: a high-resolution lutetium oxyorthosilicate PET scanner for animal imaging. J Nucl Med 40:1164–1175

[9] Cherry S, Dahlbom M, Hoffman E (1991) 3D PET using a conventional multislice tomograph without septa. J Comput Assist Tomogr 15:655–668

[10] Cherry S, Dahlbom M, Hoffman E (1992) High sensitivity, total body PET scanning using 3D data acquisition and reconstruction. IEEE Trans Nucl Sci 39:1088–1092

[11] Dahlbom M, Hoffman E, Hoh C, et al. (1992) Whole-body positron emission tomography: Part I. Methods and performance characteristics. J Nucl Med 33:1191–1199

[12] Dahlbom M, MacDonald L, Eriksson L, et al. (1997) Performance of a YSO/LSO detector block for use in a PET/SPECT system. IEEE Trans Nucl Sci 44:1114–1119
[13] DeGrado TR, Turkington TG, Williams JJ, et al. (1994) Performance characteristics of a whole-body PET scanner. J Nucl Med 35:1398–1406
[14] Ferreira N, Trebossen R, Bendriem B (1998) Assessment of 3-D PET quantitation: influence of out of the field of view radioactive sources and of attenuating media. IEEE Trans Nucl Sci 45:1670–1675
[15] Karp J, Daube-Witherspoon M, Hoffman E, et al. (1991) Performance standards in positron emission tomography. J Nucl Med 32:2342–2350
[16] Karp J, Muehllehner G, Geagan M, et al. (1998) Whole-body PET scanner using curve-plate NaI(Tl) detectors. J Nucl Med 39:50P
[17] Karp J, Muehllehner G, Mankoff D, et al. (1990) Continuous-slice PENN-PET: a positron tomograph with volume imaging capability. J Nucl Med 31:617–627
[18] Levin CS, Hoffman EJ (1999) Calculation of positron range and its effect on the fundamental limit of positron emission tomography system spatial resolution. Phys Med Biol 44(3):781–799
[19] Lewellen T, Kohlmyer S, Miyaoka R, et al. (1996) Investigation of the performance of the General Electric ADVANCE positron emission tomograph in 3D mode. IEEE Trans Nucl Sci 43:2199–2206
[20] Melcher CL, Schweitzer JS (1992) A promising new scintillator: cerium-doped lutetium oxyorthosilicate. Nucl Instr and Meth 314:212–214
[21] Muehllehner G (1979) Effect of crystal thickness on scintillation camera performance. J Nucl Med 20:992–993
[22] Muehllehner G, Karp J (1986) A positron camera using position-sensitive detectors: PENN-PET. J Nucl Med 27:90–98
[23] Nellemann P, Hines H, Braymer W, et al. (1995) Performance characteristics of a dual head SPECT scanner with PET capability. IEEE Medical Imaging Conference, San Francisco
[24] NEMA (1994) Performance measurements of positron emission tomographs NU 2-1994. National Electrical Manufacturers Association, Washington
[25] Patton JA, Turkington TG (1999) Coincidence imaging with a dual-head scintillation camera. J Nucl Med 40(3):432–441
[26] Phelps M, Cherry S (1998) The changing design of positron imaging systems. Clin Pos Imag 1:31–45
[27] Phelps M, Hoffman E, Mullani N, et al. (1975) Application of annihilation coincidence detection to transaxial reconstruction tomography. J Nucl Med 16:210–224
[28] Pichler B, Boening G, Lorenz E, et al. (1998) Studies with a prototype high resolution PET scanner based on LSO-APD module. IEEE Trans Nucl Sci 45:1298–1302
[29] Schmand M, Dahlbohm M, Eriksson L, et al. (1998) Performance of a LSO/NaI(Tl) phoswich detector for a combined PET/SPECT imaging system. J Nucl Med 39:9P
[30] Schmand M, Eriksson L, Casey M, et al. (1998) Detector design of a LSO based positron emission tomograph with depth of interaction capability for high resolution brain imaging. J Nucl Med 39:133P
[31] Sossi V, Barney J, Harrison R (1995) Effect of scatter from radioactivity outside of the field of view in 3-D PET. IEEE Trans Nucl Sci 42:1157–1161
[32] Spinks T, Jones T, Heather J, et al. (1989) Quality control procedures in positron tomography. Eur J Nucl Med 15:736–740
[33] Townsend D, Wensveen M, Byars L, et al. (1993) A rotating PET scanner using BGO block detectors: design, performance and applications. J Nucl Med 34:1367–1376
[34] Wienhard K, Eriksson L, Grootoonk S, et al. (1992) Performance evaluation of the positron scanner ECAT EXACT. J Comput Assist Tomogr 16:804–813

3 Image reconstruction, quantification and standard uptake value

H. Herzog, R.D. Hichwa

3.1 Introduction

One of the important characteristics of positron emission tomography (PET) is the ability to quantify metabolic function in vivo. To achieve this goal, radioactivity data (activity per volume) measured by PET is transformed into metabolic parameters of interest by using the simultaneously measured radioactivity in blood and an appropriate physiological or biochemical model of tracer uptake and distribution. PET data (sinograms) are often collected into specific time periods called frames. The PET system sums coincidence counts within a frame and reconstructs these data into images of radioactivity concentration using dedicated software. This chapter describes different methods for image reconstruction of PET data and presents further preprocessing procedures, such as attenuation and scatter correction, which are necessary for accurate determination of the measured radioactivity concentration.

In clinical practice, conversion to a quantitative parametric image from the reconstructed activity concentration is often not necessary since the primary PET data are highly correlated with the observed physiological function. A qualitative evaluation of PET data is nearly equivalent to studies that are performed with conventional planar or single photon tomographic scintigraphy (SPECT), but has the added advantage of positron emitting radiopharmaceuticals mimicking more closely true physiological uptake and distribution of the tracer. In order to examine and compare activity data, intra- and interindividually relative parameters have been introduced such as the standard uptake value (SUV). This semiquantitative tool for analyzing PET data is discussed at the end of this chapter.

3.2 Reconstruction of the radioactivity distribution

PET information is derived from the decay of proton-rich nuclei (positron emitters) that are formulated into biologically compatible molecules. These short-lived positron-emitting radioactive biomolecules are also called radiotracers or radiopharmaceuticals and are distributed within the patient's body after an injection. The decay proceeds as positron emission. After the positron's initial kinetic energy is lost, the positron annihilates with an electron and creates a pair of diametrically opposed 511 keV photons as described in detail in the preceding chapter. These photon pairs isotropically exit the body. Those that interact in the detectors that surround a portion of the body are recorded by the coincidence electronics and are registered as coincidence events. The exact location of the annihilation is not known, instead the event is attributed to a point along the ray subtended by the front faces of the detector pair. A projection value $P(r,\alpha)$ represents the sum of all photon pairs recorded within the measurement time interval along each possible ray (Fig. 3.1). A matrix containing all $P(r,\alpha)$ within one measurement plane is called a sinogram. In 2-dimensional (2D) PET, the sinograms contain data measured in planes perpendicular to the patient axis and in 3-dimensional (3D) PET, oblique planes are additionally collected. Eq. 3.1 describes the basic relationship between the measured projection data $P(r,\alpha)$ and the unknown distribution of radioactivity $A(x,y)$ within the body:

$$P(r,\alpha) = \int_{L(r,\alpha)} A(x,y)\, dl\,(r,\alpha) \cdot \exp(- \int_{L(r,\alpha)} \mu(x,y)\, dl\,(r,\alpha) \tag{3.1}$$

$$P(r,\alpha) = \int_{L(r,\alpha)} A(x,y)\, dl\,(r,\alpha) \cdot AF \tag{3.1a}$$

$$P^{corr}(r,\alpha) = P(r,\alpha)/AF = \int_{L(r,\alpha)} A(x,y)\, dl\,(r,\alpha) \tag{3.2}$$

The sinogram of events from the radioactivity distribution within the body comprise the emission data. Eq. 3.1 also takes into account photon attenua-

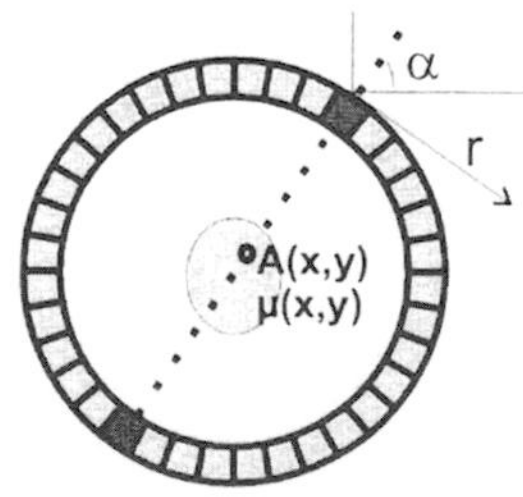

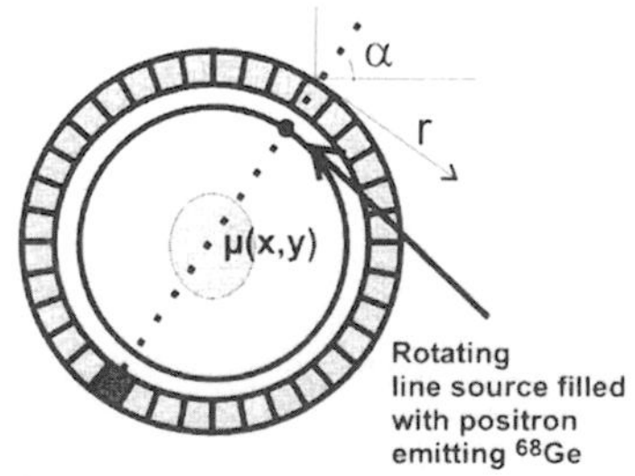

Fig. 3.1. Schemes demonstrating the emission measurement as well as the related transmission measurement.

tion within the patient's body. The exponential expression represents the attenuation factors (AF) from Eq. 3.1 a. μ(x,y) describes the distribution of attenuation coefficients.

The integral over the activity distribution, A(x, y), and the exponential expression containing μ(x,y) are two factors that can be determined in two successive steps, one following the other. The factor related to photon absorption is usually determined by a transmission measurement, which utilizes a positron-emitting radioactivity source (typically ^{68}Ge/^{68}Ga) that rotates around the patient within the field-of-view (FOV) of the detector geometry. During this procedure the detectors measure all photon coincidence events which are able to traverse the body and are not absorbed. A blank scan is identical to a transmission scan but the measurement is made without the patient in the detector FOV. The blank scan is performed daily or weekly and can also be utilized as a quality control check of the system response for each detector in the PET camera. The ratio of the transmission and the blank data yields the attenuation factors AF and is used to calculate the corrected projection data $P^{corr}(r,\alpha)$ (Eq. 3.2). When a line source is used, the transmission measurement may be performed even after tracer injection or simultaneously with the emission measurement.

The standard method to calculate the unknown activity distribution A(x, y) employs the technique of filtered backprojection (FBP) [26, 32]. According to the term backprojection the projection data recorded for a ray angle combination is distributed continuously along the ray into the x,y-plane. The superposition of all backprojected data for all ray angle combinations yields a blurred image of the true activity distribution. The data are sharpened by multiplying the projection information in the Fourier domain by a ramp filter which amplifies high rather than low frequency components of the Fourier spectrum. The resulting image is derived by performing an inverse Fourier transform of the filtered data and more accurately represents the actual activity distribution A(x, y). In practice the ramp filter must be modified as described below. The ramp filtering may be performed before the backprojection, if desirable from a software perspective. To make images in units of activity concentration (kBq/ml), the reconstructed count rate data are uniformly multiplied by a calibration factor that relates PET counts per pixel to a known activity per volume.

In many applications FBP is the reconstruction method of choice, especially with 2-[^{18}F]deoxy-D-glucose (FDG) imaging of brain or heart in which sufficient count statistics are present. Often, however, count rates are low or a region of interest (ROI) with low activity is near an organ with high activity (e.g., bladder). Under these circumstances radial artifacts are visible in the background and may even prohibit the evaluation of areas with high activity contrast. Such problems are frequent in PET oncology and results in stripes appearing in and across the image.

The artifacts caused by the FBP of low count data are avoided by using an alternative reconstruction method that calculates the activity image iteratively in an algebraic fashion. The method can be described either statistically or numerically. For iterative reconstruction, the relationship between projection and activity as given in Eq. 3.1 is written numerically as follows:

$$p_n = z_{mn} a_m \tag{3.3}$$

Here the projections p_n ($n = 1 \ldots N$) are related to the activity data a_m in M image pixels of the measured radioactivity distribution. The members of the matrix z_{mn} describe how those coincidence events emitted from an image pixel m with the activity value a_m contribute to a single data projection value p_n. If the matrix z_{mn} and the measured projection data are known, the unknown activity data a_m can theoretically be calculated using Eq. 3.4

$$a_m = z_{mn}^{-1} p_n \tag{3.4}$$

with z_{mn}^{-1} being the inverse matrix of z_{mn}. In general z_{mn}^{-1} can not be obtained, because z_{mn} is not symmetric. Even if this were to be true, a direct solution of a system consisting of an enormous number of equations is at least burdensome. It is much more appropriate to solve Eq. 3.3 by iterative methods. To begin, it is necessary to assume a starting image which is often a homogeneous distribution of activity with the mean being equivalent to the average projection data. Using Eq. 3.3, the theoretical projection data p_n are calculated and compared with the measured projection data. Based on this comparison the assumed activity data a_m are corrected. Using the updated values of a_m, theoretical projection data are calculated once more and again compared to the measured projection data. Then a_m is corrected a second time. This procedure is repeated until certain criteria which halt the process are fulfilled. The available iterative reconstruction methods differ with respect to the definition of the matrix z_{mn}, the ways for comparing the theoretical and measured projection data, and the methods for correcting the activity data. Common approaches for optimizing the convergence of the iteration utilize the root mean square error [4], the maximum likelihood [20, 22, 33] or more heuristic concepts [13, 29].

Among these methods the maximum-likelihood expectation-maximization (ML-EM) method is best adapted to the statistical nature of the underlying physical phenomena for detecting the annihilation photons from PET radionuclide decay, i.e., the Poisson distribution. Here z_{mn} represents the probability with which an activity event emitted in image pixel m is seen in projection p_m. The iterative formula for the ML-EM reconstruction is shown in Eq. 3.5.

$$a_m^{n+1} = a_m^n \Sigma z_{mn} \frac{p_n}{\Sigma z_{mn} a_m^n} \tag{3.5}$$

In general, the different iterative reconstruction methods do not produce artifacts observed with filtered backprojection. Iterative reconstruction is especially appropriate for PET applications in oncology which suffer from low count rates or from problems of high contrast due to nearby organs that contain high tracer concentration. The advantages of the iterative reconstruction approach were originally counterbalanced by very long computation times. Fast computers have diminished these problems considerably. Furthermore, the use of acceleration parameters [30] or the ordered subset method [14] results in a dramatically decreased computation time. The quantitative accuracy which is assured for the original ML-EM procedure should be examined for the accelerated procedures of the iterative reconstruction approach. It is necessary to mention that quantitation is not just the calibration of the reconstructed image in units of activity concentration but must also include the demonstration of linearity across the computational process. Even if absolute values of activity concentration are not necessary, the approach must be linear. As an example, a twofold increase of activity concentration in a certain tissue must be represented by a similar twofold increase in the pixel value of the reconstructed image.

Before proceeding with details of image quantification, a brief discussion of 3D reconstruction is warranted. The 3D acquisition of PET data has already been detailed in the preceding chapter.

For iterative reconstruction methods, the algorithms which are commonly used for the reconstruction of 2D data are modified to include the third dimension. There is a dramatic increase in the number of matrix members z_{mn} for 3D reconstructions which means a very high demand is placed on storage capacity and computing time. It is possible to perform the reconstruction with the help of highly parallel computers or workstation clusters. As with the 2D FBP, a 3D FBP requires less computation time compared to iterative procedures. Although Eq. 3.2 cannot exactly be solved for the case of 3D, several approaches for the 3D FBP have been developed [7, 19], are shown to be quantitatively accurate, and are successfully utilized with commercial PET systems.

It is possible to rebin the 3D data into 2D sinograms so that the data can be reconstructed with 2D algorithms. In the case of single slice rebinning the oblique projections are assembled into a 2D sinogram for the plane in which they cross the central axis [6]. The method of multislice rebinning distributes the oblique projections into the sinograms of those planes which are crossed by the oblique projection [23]. The same is achieved with the Fourier rebinning method (FORE) which additionally applies specific weights to the distribution of the oblique sinograms [8]. The 2D sinograms that result from the different rebinning approaches are reconstructed by conventional 2D filtered backprojection or by an iterative reconstruction method.

3.3 Factors that influence quantitative accuracy

3.3.1 Coincidence events and acquisition modes

This section introduces several phenomena and factors which influence the PET measurement and the ability to accurately quantify the radiotracer distribution.

The different reconstruction procedures presented thus far assume ideal data, i.e., the photon pairs measured by the coincidence detectors consist only of true coincidences which are not disturbed on their way from the point of emission within the human body to the detector. As shown in Fig. 3.2 there are additional events that consist of random, scattered, and absorbed coincidences which considerably influence the quantitative accuracy of the PET measurement.

A coincidence event requires that both photons from a positron annihilation be detected by the system electronics within approximately 10–12 ns. The actual time of flight of a photon traversing the detector ring is considerably less; however, the longer time of 10–12 ns is necessary to account for the signal delay within the detector modules and corresponding electronics. The prolongation of the coincidence time window results in an increased probability that two single photons that belong to two different annihilation events will be registered by opposing detectors. These false events are called random coincidences and cause a low frequency background signal.

Scattered coincidences occur if at least one partner of a photon pair undergoes Compton scattering and the scattered photon changes its direction. If the scattered photon and the unscattered photon remain within the PET camera field-of-view, a line of response (LOR) is assumed between the two opposing detectors that observe the pair of photons. The LOR assigned to the photon pair does not coincide with the correct location of the positron emission. In addition to the random coincidences, the scattered coincidences

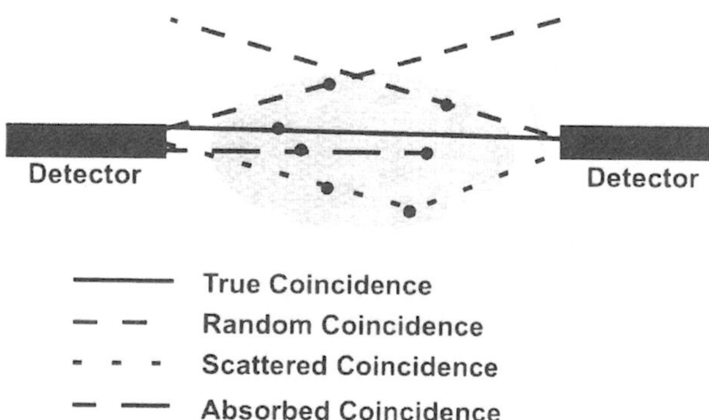

Fig. 3.2. Four different types of coincidences must be distinguished and taken into account to achieve proper quantitation.

cause a slowly varying spatially dependent background signal. It is possible that the number of scattered and random coincidences surpass the number of true coincidences. The absence of tungsten or lead septa between detector planes in a 3D PET system leads to a considerable increase of scattered and random coincidences. Furthermore, scattered and random photons from body regions outside the field-of-view combine to register LORs that are incorrect and indistinguishable from true events.

In the following, correction procedures are presented in the sequence in which they are commonly applied to PET data and preceed the final image reconstruction. As an intermediate step, some PET scanners make sinograms available after all corrections on raw data have been performed so that user-implemented iterative reconstruction algorithms may be applied.

3.3.2 Dead time correction

PET systems exhibit a dead time effect if the measured count rate is very high. The dead time is dependent on all photon events measured by the detectors and not just on the rate of coincidences. Radioactivity outside the FOV contributes to the system dead time losses. Dead time corrections require a calibration measurement to be performed which relates the counts that originate from a single photon emitting source with the events measured by the individual detector modules. For oncological FDG-PET the dead time correction is minimal since the activity within the field-of-view of the camera at the time of imaging is relatively low.

3.3.3 Correction for random coincidences

There are two procedures to correct for random coincidences. A hardware-based method uses a delayed coincidence time window that has the same time length as the original coincidence window. The time delay is often equal to several times the coincidence window width and begins at the onset of the first photon event that arrives at one of the detectors of the coincidence pair. All coincidences counted in the second (delayed) coincidence interval are regarded as being random. They are directly subtracted from the measured coincidences which are often called prompt coincidences. For the second method, a calculated correction is performed. In this case the single count rates S_i are measured for each detector. Knowing these rates and the coincidence time window τ, the random coincidences R are determined by [1, 12]

$$R = 2\,S_i S_j \tau \tag{3.6}$$

3.3.4 Correction for scattered coincidences

As already indicated, scattered coincidences considerably influence the accuracy of quantitative PET results. Using the 2D acquisition mode the rate of scattered coincidences is approximately 10–20% of the true coincidence count rate, whereas the scattered coincidence rate increases to 50% or more in the 3D acquisition mode. The 2D correction is generally performed according to the technique of Bergström et al. [2] and is based on point source images measured in a scattering medium (water) and compared with images acquired in air. A scattering function is derived and the scattered coincidences are subtracted from the random corrected (net true) coincidences. For the 3D PET different scatter correction methods are available. Some manufacturers model the scatter distribution with parabolic [16] or Gaussian functions [35] that assume scattered radiation is smoothly distributed. An alternative approach utilizes a physical model (Klein-Nishina formula) together with transmission data and a first pass reconstructed emission image [40]. Although the different methods produce reasonable images, problems may occur, especially if high activity concentrations are located just outside the field-of-view and are not fully taken into account by the scatter correction models. Furthermore, the Klein-Nishina approach requires that a transmission measurement be performed which is not the usual case in whole-body imaging for oncological PET.

3.3.5 Attenuation correction

The correction for absorbed coincidences has already been discussed above and mathematically detailed through Eqs. 3.1 and 3.2. The attenuation correction is essential if the PET measurement is to be quantitative, meaning the observed count rate is linear and varies on an absolute scale when compared to radioactivity concentration in tissue. If this correction is not performed, which is mostly the case, in order to shorten the acquisition time for whole-body studies, the PET results can only be judged qualitatively. Without attenuation correction the reconstructed PET images show distortions. Imaging a uniform distribution of activity without attenuation correction appears as an underestimation at the center of the object while an overestimation of the concentration appears at the exterior boundary of the object; hence the unattenuated image is nonlinear. This error is accentuated as the object size increases. Performing the attenuation correction requires considerable time, which is typically on the order of 25–50% of the acquisition time that is required for collecting emission data. Therefore, one must seek methods to shorten the transmission measurement in order to collect fully quantitative PET images.

A review of the literature suggests that a transmission measurement time of 10 min per bed position is widely accepted. Based upon our experience in whole-body measurements this time is only adequate when transmission sources of the recommended strength are used. After one half-life of ^{68}Ge (270 d) which is the typical nuclide used for transmission measurements, the count rate is reduced to one half of the original source and requires that the imaging time be doubled in order to collect equivalent image statistics. Several studies have shown that inadequate or poor statistical quality transmission measurements cause additional noise in the reconstructed PET images. The noise problem becomes even more severe when PET cameras with high resolution in the z-axis are used since the data are collected in thinner slices which place fewer count statistics in each slice. A measurement time of 20 min per bed position is adequate for weak ^{68}Ge sources in slim patients, but requires even longer transmission scans to be performed for obese patients.

In order to improve the quality of transmission data, especially of those with low statistics, they may be processed additionally. For this purpose, attenuation factors are not derived directly from the transmission measurement. Initially the transmission data are reconstructed which results in an attenuation coefficient map $\mu(x,y)$. The μ map is segmented into contiguous regions with a homogeneous absorption coefficient μ assigned to each region. The resulting μ maps are free of any statistical noise. The processed transmission image is forward projected to yield calculated attenuation factors AF that are also noise free. This method allows one to shorten the transmission scan time. Furthermore, it supplies reasonable low noise data for the Klein-Nishina approach of the 3D scatter correction.

Single photon emitters instead of positron emitters offer a second approach for improving the signal to noise ratio of transmission measurements [9, 17]. In this case more counts can be measured in a much shorter time. If the transmission measurement is performed with positron emitters, one photon is required for the transmission information (absorption through the patient) and the other photon of the annihilation pair is only used to define the line of response (Fig. 3.1). For single photon sources, similar lines of response are achieved by tracking the position of the transmission source and measuring the attenuation of photons traversing the patient by detectors opposite the source. Hence, positron emitters are no longer needed. The ideal single photon nuclide would have a similar photon energy to the annihilation photons, but possess a much longer half-life. ^{137}Cs is an excellent candidate with a photon energy of 622 keV and a half-life of 30.17 y, which would require that only one source be employed over the useful longevity of the PET scanner rather than purchasing ^{68}Ge sources at 6 month intervals. Due to the higher photon energy of ^{137}Cs, attenuation factors and absorption coefficients μ different from ^{68}Ge are measured, although the transmission image appears identical. To correct for the differences between attenuation coefficients the measured attenuation factors can be adjusted to the photon energy of 511 keV or the reconstructed transmission image segmented and the standard attenuation coefficients for the different tissues inserted. In this way the transmission time may be reduced to only 10 min for multiple bed positions (approximately 5).

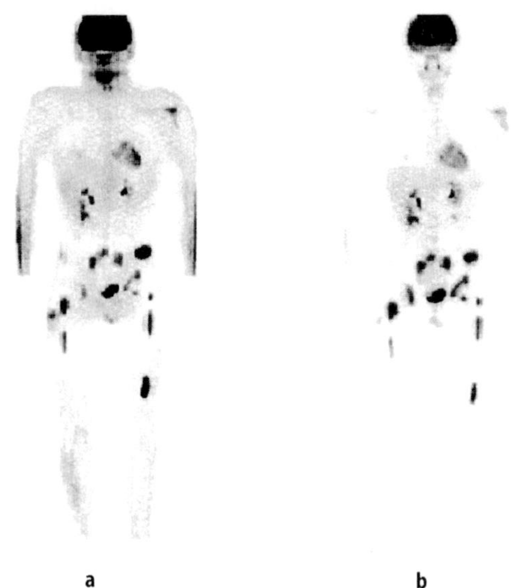

Fig. 3.3. FDG scans of a patient with multiple metastases. The whole-body images were calculated using the maximum projection method and were based on ML-EM reconstructed transversal tomograms without (**a**) and with (**b**) attenuation correction.

To shorten the total study time the transmission scan is often performed after tracer injection [5]. In this case transmission counts (T) are measured together with emission counts (E) which originate from the radiopharmaceutical distributed throughout the patient's body. Since the count rate of the T photons is much greater than that of the E photons, the contamination by the E photons in the T data is often neglected. An acceptable T:E ratio is approximately 20:1. Our research has shown that this results in a residual quantitation error of about 5 to 10% in the reconstructed activity [28].

3.3.6 Choice of filter for the FBP reconstruction

As discussed earlier, the ramp (high pass) filter is an integral part of the filtered backprojection reconstruction process and counterbalances the low pass characteristics of straight backprojection. A disadvantageous outcome of high pass filtering is the amplification of the statistical noise present in the measured count data. Therefore, the ramp filter is limited at low frequencies or multiplied by an appropriate window function which weakens the high pass characteristics of the ramp filter. Examples of useful functions are the Hann, Shepp-Logan, Hamming, Parzen, or the Butterworth window. Although the reduction of the high frequency statistical noise is welcome, as a byproduct of window filtering the image resolution worsens when compared to images created with a ramp filter. The decreased image resolution results in blurring of small details and a reduction of the image maxima (maximum counts per pixel or high concentration values in the image). Use of a frequency-limiting window has similar consequences to that observed from a PET camera with low intrinsic detector resolution. In both cases the partial volume effect increases. This effect causes an underestimation of the observed activity in areas close to structures with low count density, an overestimation near structures with high activity concentrations (see also the following chapter) and is especially relevant for small structures [11]. To reduce such errors in combination with an acceptable suppression of noise, the window function and its associated upper frequency limit should be selected carefully.

Knowledge about the partial volume effect is particularly important in whole-body FDG PET imaging. Metastases are often smaller than 1 cm in diameter and the count density or metabolic rate is typically underestimated due to the partial volume effect. A direct comparison between metastases of different sizes even in the same patient is difficult because the partial volume effect variably influences the boundary delineation of these structures. Similar problems are present in follow-up FDG studies that are performed to examine the efficacy of therapeutic treatment by combinations of radiation and chemotherapy in which metastases have become smaller. Therefore, use of a PET scanner with the highest intrinsic resolution along with techniques that elicit the best and most quantitative reconstruction is warranted.

Special characteristics of the iterative reconstruction process effect final image outcome. It is not necessary to select a specific filter for iterative reconstruction since the final image resolution approaches the scanner resolution. In practice, however, the resultant image resolution is dependent on the individual reconstruction algorithm applied and the specific implementation by the vendor. It is advised to confirm the resolution performance of the supplied software. As a general rule, resolution improves with the number of iterations. Some iterative reconstruction procedures, such as the ML-EM method, exhibit high frequency noise after many iterations, although convergence of the method is ultimately guaranteed. Postprocessing filtering has been proposed in an effort to reduce the noise component, but degrades image resolution and augments partial volume effects. As a consequence, the quantitative accuracy of the PET result is reduced.

3.4 Quantitative analysis of oncological FDG-PET

Strict implementation of the FDG method requires that quantitative determination of the rate of glucose consumption should be the final aim. This procedure was originally developed to measure cerebral glucose consumption [25, 27] and is based on autoradiographic studies by Sokoloff and coworkers in rats using [^{14}C]deoxyglucose [34]. The FDG method has been extended to applications in heart and tumors. Such approaches imply that the rate constants (k) and the lumped constant (LC) can be regarded as invariable. Whereas this is true for brain tissue of normal subjects and even in patients with brain disorders, this is not the case for myocardial and tumor tissue. Since tumors exhibit a variety of different histological characteristics, one cannot expect standard values of the rate constants and the LC to describe the uptake kinetics of FDG. In this situation individual rate constants may be determined with the help of a dynamic PET measurement which requires arterial or arterialized venous blood sampling simultaneous with the PET image measurement. The resulting time-activity curves can be evaluated by fitting the measured data to the dynamics of the FDG model so that the rate constants are obtained. The LC can be determined by a comparative measurement that uses FDG and radioactively labeled glucose. Such individualized measurements are, however, not practical in the clinical routine. Animal-based values of LC cannot be effectively transferred to studies in humans due to the differences in histological types of tumors. The dynamic approach to determine individual rate constants is not readily compatible with whole-body PET protocols. A dynamic measurement might be performed on one to three specific bed positions between the injection and the start of the whole-body PET measurements. The uptake time for rate constant determination is usually 40–60 min. Dynamic rate constant measurements require additional imaging time during which the PET camera is not available for imaging of other patients. Therefore, the dynamic analysis of PET data and the quantitative determination of the glucose consumption is for the most part limited to scientific investigations and not routine clinical practice [15, 38, 39].

3.5 Standard uptake value (SUV)

In order to obtain more than just qualitative findings in cancer studies with FDG, as well as with other tracers such as [^{11}C]methionine [24] or [^{18}F] fluorouracil [10], semiquantitative evaluations have been adopted. One widely applied method is the determination of the standard uptake value (SUV) [36, 41]. Expressions that include differential uptake ratio (DUR), differential absorption (activity) ratio (DAR), or dose uptake ratio (DUR) are synonymous. These parameters relate the value of activity concentration found in a certain tissue volume of interest to the injected activity per the patient's body weight. In this way interindividual differences and varying amounts of administered activity are taken into account. The amount of activity found in a region is, however, not always static and may change after tracer injection by increased uptake of the PET tracer or by washout of the tracer from the tissue. Recently, it was found that FDG uptake increased in breast cancer and metastatic sites for at least three hours after injection [3] (Fig. 3.4). In this case the SUV is time dependent and varies according to when the regional activity concentration was determined.

FDG uptake in tumor as well as normal tissue is influenced by factors such as the blood glucose level, which is considered as part of the FDG model

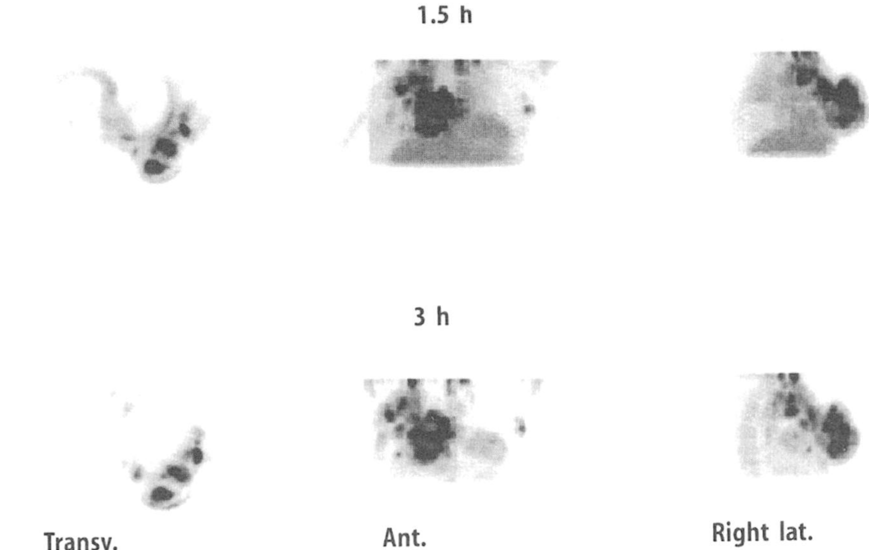

Fig. 3.4. FDG images of a patient with breast cancer and its metastases. The images recorded at 3 h exhibit an increased tumor to background contrast.

for calculating glucose consumption. The glucose level is rarely considered when calculating the SUV [21]. When investigating radiolabeled amino acids the SUV is dependent on the endogenous level of natural amino acids. Therefore, the specific PET protocol must be designed to control the substrate levels in blood by defining periods of fasting or other dietary manipulations prior to the PET measurement.

The tumor uptake of the tracer is not only dependent on the injected dose, but also on the tracer concentration within the blood pool. Measurements of radioactivity level in blood are not performed for determination of SUV; hence, other means to estimate the tracer concentration are necessary. The blood activity level is dependent upon the whole-body volume of distribution of the radiotracer. Body weight is also regarded as a measure that correlates with the distribution volume. Several studies have shown that the SUV may be dependent on the body weight, especially in obese patients [18, 42]. Therefore, alternative measures which show a better correlation with the distribution volume have been suggested such as the body surface area (BSA), the lean body mass (LBM) [18, 31, 42], or the revised definition of lean body mass [37]. Despite these potential differences in semi-quantitative evaluation of PET images, the standard SUV based on body weight is widely used for reporting of tumor uptake in oncological PET. The range of SUV varies between normal tissue and tumor sites. As expected, higher SUV numbers correspond to greater metabolic activity. The literature as detailed in the following chapters suggests that a SUV greater than 2.5 is indicative of metastatic disease for regions identified as suspected tumor sites. SUVs should be compared with those from regions in normal brain and heart tissues as well as regions defined as normal from tissues near the suspected oncological involvement. It is further suggested that each PET site create a database of normal and tumor SUV values since different image reconstruction and processing techniques may affect the specific numerical value of the SUV. Literature values for SUV should be regarded as guidelines and not absolute for determination of metastatic involvement.

3.6 Conclusion

Although one of the important characteristics of PET is its ability to quantify radioactive substrates in vivo, most of its clinical oncological applications are still performed as qualitative 2D studies. In order to shorten the study times and to decrease the costs associated with PET scanning, attenuation correction is typically not performed. Attenuation correction is likely to be adopted, if single photon transmission scanning and segmentation of transmission images, which both allow a shorter transmission time, become generally available. The 3D mode with its higher sensitivity offer a way to increase patient throughput since shorter emission scanning times are possible and lower doses of FDG are required. In this way, a quantitatively based diagnosis using relative parameters such as the SUV or more advanced functional analysis schemes may augment the acceptance of oncological PET even beyond the success that it has already been envisaged in recent years.

References

[1] Bergström M, Bohm C, Ericson K, Eriksson L, Litton J (1980) Corrections for attenuation, scattered radiation, and random coincidences in a ring detector positron emission transaxial tomograph. IEEE Trans Nucl Sci NS-27:435–444

[2] Bergström M, Eriksson L, Bohm C, Blomqvist G, Litton J (1983) Correction for scattered radiation in a ring detector positron camera by integral transformation of the projections. J Comput Assist Tomogr 7:42–50

[3] Börner AR, Weckesser M, Herzog H, Schmitz T, Audretsch W, Nitz U, Bender HG, Müller-Gärtner HW (1999) Optimal scan time for fluorine-18 deoxyglucose positron emission tomography in breast cancer. Eur J Nucl Med 26:226–230

[4] Budinger TF, Gullberg GT, Huesman RH (1979) Emission computed tomography. In: Herman GT (ed) Image Reconstruction from Projections. Springer, Berlin, pp 147–246

[5] Carson RE, Daube-Witherspoon ME, Green MV (1988) A method for postinjection PET transmission measurements with a rotating source. J Nucl Med 29:1558–1567

[6] Daube-Witherspoon ME, Muehllehner G (1987) Treatment of axial data in three-dimensional PET. J Nucl Med 28:1717–1724

[7] Defrise M, Townsend D, Clack R (1989) Three-dimensional image reconstruction from complete projections. Phys Med Biol 34:573–587

[8] Defrise M, Kinahan PE, Townsend DW, Michel C, Sihomana M, Newport DF (1997) Exact and approximate rebinning algorithms for 3-D PET data. IEEE Trans Med Imaging 16:145–158

[9] DeKemp RA, Nhamias C (1994) Attenuation correction in PET using single photon transmission measurement. Med Phys 21:771–778

[10] Dimitrakopoulou A, Strauss LG, Clorius JH, Ostertag H, Schlag P, Heim M, Oberdorfer F, Helus F, Haberkorn U, van Kaick G (1993) Studies with positron emission tomography after systemic administration of fluorine-18-uracil in patients with liver metastases from colorectal carcinoma. J Nucl Med 34:1075–1081

[11] Hoffman EJ, Huang SC, Phelps ME (1979) Quantification in positron emission computed tomography: I. Effect of object size. J Comput Assist Tomogr 299–308

[12] Hoffman EJ, Huang SC, Phelps ME, Kuhl DE (1981) Quantification in positron emission computed tomography: 4. effect of accidental coincidences. J Comput Assist Tomogr 5:391–400

[13] Holte S, Schmidlin P, Lindén A, Rosenqvist G, Eriksson L (1990) Iterative image reconstruction for positron emission tomography: a study of convergence and quantitation problems. IEEE Trans Nucl Sci NS-37:629–635

[14] Hudson HM, Larkin RS (1994) Accelerated image reconstruction using ordered subsets of projection data. IEEE Trans Med Imaging 20:100–108

[15] Hunter GJ, Hamberg LM, Alpert NM, Choi NC, Fischman AJ (1996) Simplified measurement of deoxyglucose utilization rate. J Nucl Med 37:950–955

[16] Karp JS, Muehllehner G, Mankoff DA, Ordonez CE, Ollinger JM, Daube-Witherspoon ME, Haigh AT, Beerbohm DJ (1990) Continuous-slice PENN-PET: a positron tomograph with volume imaging capability. J Nucl Med 31:617–627

[17] Karp JS, Muehllehner G, Qu H, Yan XH (1995) Singles transmission in volume-imaging PET with a ^{137}Cs source. Phys Med Biol 40:929–944

[18] Kim CK, Gupta NC (1996) Dependency of standardized uptake values of fluorine-18 fluorodeoxyglucose on body size: comparison of body surface area correction and lean body mass correction. Nucl Med Commun 17:890–894

[19] Kinahan PE, Rogers JG (1989) Analytic three-dimensional image reconstruction using all detected events. IEEE Trans Nucl Sci NS-36:964–968

[20] Lange K, Carson R (1984) EM reconstruction algorithms for emission and transmission tomography. J Comp Assist Tomogr 8:306–316

[21] Langen K-J, Braun U, Rota Kops E, Herzog H, Kuwert T, Nebeling B, Feinendegen LE (1993) The influence of plasma glucose levels on fluorine-18-fluorodeoxyglucose uptake in bronchial carcinomas. J Nucl Med 34:355–359

[22] Levitan E, Herman GT (1987) A maximum a posteriori probability expectation maximization algorithm for image reconstruction in emission tomography. IEEE Trans Med Imag MI-6:185–192

[23] Lewitt RM, Muehllehner G, Karp JS (1994) Three-dimensional reconstruction for PET by multi-slice rebinning and axial filtering. Phys Med Biol 39:321–340

[24] Lindholm P, Leskinen S, Lapela MJ (1998) Carbon-11-methionine uptake in squamous cell head and neck cancer. J Nucl Med 39:1393–1397

[25] Phelps ME, Huang SC, Hoffman EJ, Selin C, Sokoloff L, Kuhl DE (1979) Tomographic measurement of local cerebral glucose metabolic rate in humans with (F-18)2-fluoro-2-deoxy-D-glucose: validation of method. Ann Neurol 6:371–388

[26] Ramachandran GN, Lakshminaraynan AV (1971) Three-dimensional reconstruction from radiographs and electron micrographs: application of convolutions instead of Fourier transforms. Proc Natl Acad Sci 9:22–36

[27] Reivich M, Kuhl D, Wolf A, Greenberg J, Phelps M, Ido T, Casella V, Fowler J, Hoffman E, Alavi A, Som P, Sokoloff L (1979) The [^{18}F]fluorodeoxyglucose method for the measurement of local cerebral glucose utilization in man. Circ Res 44:127–139

[28] Rota Kops E, Herzog H, Schmid A, Holte S, Feinendegen LE (1990) Performance characteristics of an eight-ring whole-body PET scanner. J Assist Comput Tomogr 14:437– 445

[29] Schmidlin P (1972) Iterative separation of sections in tomographic scintigrams. Nucl Med 11:1–16

[30] Schmidlin P, Bellemann ME, Brix G (1997) Iterative reconstruction of PET images using a high-overrelaxation single-projection algorithm. Phys Med Biol 42:569–582

[31] Schomburg A, Bender H, Reichel C, Sommer T, Ruhlmann J, Kozak B, Biersack HJ (1996) Standardized uptake values of fluorine-18 fluorodeoxyglucose: the value of different normalization procedures. Eur J Nucl Med 23:571–574

[32] Shepp LA, Logan BF (1974) The Fourier reconstruction of a head section. IEEE Trans Nucl Sci NS-21:21–43

[33] Shepp LA, Vardi Y (1982) Maximum likelihood reconstruction for emission tomography. Trans Med Imag MI-1:113–122

[34] Sokoloff L, Reivich M, Kennedy C, DesRosiers MH, Patlak CS, Pettigrew KD, Sakurada O, Shinohara M (1977) The [^{14}C]deoxyglucose method for the measurement of focal cerebral glucose utilization: theory, procedure and normal values in the conscious and anesthetized albino rat. J Neurochem 28:897–916

[35] Stearns CW (1995) Scatter correction method for 3D PET using 2D fitted Gaussian functions. J Nucl Med 36:105P

[36] Strauss LG, Conti PS (1991) The applications of PET in clinical oncology. J Nucl Med 32:623–648

[37] Sugawara Y, Zasadny KR, Neuhoff AW, Wahl RL (1999) Reevaluation of the standardized uptake values for FDG: variations with body weight and methods for correction. Radiology 213:521–525

[38] Suhonen-Polvi H, Ruotsalainen U, Kinnala A, Bergman J, Haaparanta M, Teras M, Makela P, Solin O, Wegelius U (1995) FDG-PET in early infancy: simplified quantification methods to measure cerebral glucose utilization. J Nucl Med 36:1249–1254

[39] Takikawa S, Dhawan V, Spetsieris P, Robeson W, Chaly T, Dahl R, Margulleff D, Eidelberg D (1993) Noninvasive quantitative fluorodeoxyglucose PET studies with an estimated input function derived from a population-based arterial blood curve. Radiology 188:131–136

[40] Watson CC, Newport D, Casey ME (1996) A single scatter simulation technique for scatter correction in 3D PET. In: Grangeat P, Amans JL (eds) Proc 1995 Int Meeting Fully 3D-Image Reconstruction in Radiology and Nucl Med. Kluwer Academic Publ, Dordrecht, pp 215–219

[41] Woodard HQ, Gigler RE, Freed B, Russ G (1975) Expression of tissue isotope distribution. J Nucl Med 16:958–959

[42] Zasadny KR, Wahl RL (1993) Standardized uptake values of normal tissues at PET with 2- [fluorine-18]-fluoro-2-deoxy-D-glucose: variations with body weight and a method for correction. Radiology 189(3):847–850

4 Partial volume effects/corrections

E. Rota Kops, B.J. Krause

4.1 Introduction

Positron emission tomography (PET) allows the quantitative *in vivo* measurement of the regional uptake of radioactive tracers. The low spatial resolution of PET scanners is one of the limiting factors in the absolute quantification of, for example, blood flow and metabolism in small anatomic structures like the cerebral cortex. The direct consequence of the low spatial resolution is a partial loss of the signal in structures which are smaller than twice the resolution of the tomograph (i.e., the full width at half maximum (FWHM)). As a consequence, the affected structures cover only partly the point spread function (PSF) of the scanner [9–11]. The measured PET signal in this case represents a mean activity concentration, which is lower than the real activity concentration. In clinical use, the question often arises, as to whether a decrease in the PET signal corresponds to a lower tissue accumulation or is a consequence of a partial volume effect, or a combination of both.

In the beginning, the partial volume (PV) effect was thought to be caused by a decrease in the signal due to the limited axial (parallel to the axis of the tomograph) extent of an object compared to the axial PSF (the slice thickness). Later on, the partial overlap of the object with the transverse component of the PSF was included in the definition of the effect [13]. Furthermore, the limited spatial resolution causes a contamination of activity from neighboring tissues, the so-called *spillover* effect [7, 8, 11, 19]. However, the PV effect comprises both the loss of signal as well as the *spillover* effect.

4.2 Partial volume effect

After the reconstruction of a PET image, the measured activity concentration is proportional to the real concentration (kBq/cc) in the object. If the object is smaller than twice the PSF of the scanner (at least in one spatial dimension), this object only partly covers the sensitive solid angle of the detectors. In the reconstructed image, an underestimation or a decrease of the signal of the activity concentration occurs.

We have performed phantom studies and calculations with simulated data to characterize and correct the PV effect. The loss of signal, which is the

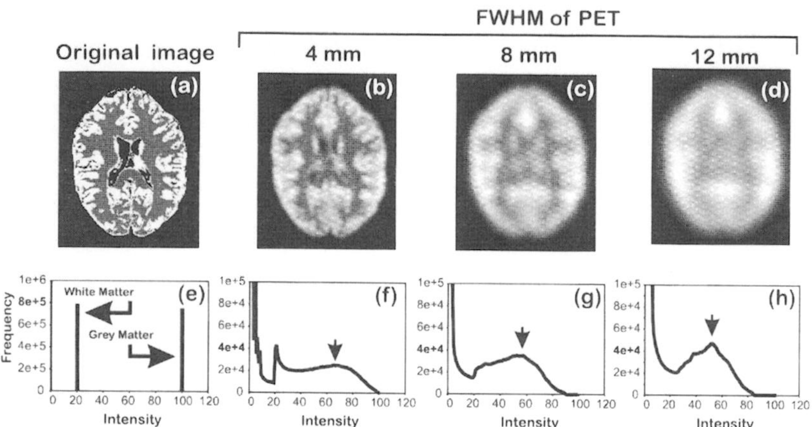

Fig. 4.1. a Simulated data set with predefined intensity values for grey matter (100), white matter (20), and CSF (0); **b–d** Influence of limited resolution of PET images after application of three different 3D filter kernels; **e–h** the corresponding histograms of the images **a–d** show the intensity distribution.

consequence of the limited spatial resolution, is shown in Fig. 4.1. A simulated brain data set was created (Fig. 4.1 a) in which all voxels of the grey matter (G) were set to a value of 100, the voxels of the white matter (W) to a value of 20, and those of the cerebral spinal fluid (CSF) to zero; the histogram in Fig. 4.1e shows the distribution of the intensity values. The zero value includes not only the CSF but also the background values, so that the numeric value of the zero values in the graph is very high. The simulated data set was blurred with a three dimensional Gaussian filter with FWHM of 4, 8, and 12 mm, respectively. Figs. 4.1 b–d show the visual effect of the filter on the images; the histograms in Figs. 4.1 f–h demonstrate how the intensity distribution changes as a function of the FWHM of the filter. With a filter of 4 mm FWHM (Fig. 4.1 f), the maximum value of G decreases by about 35% and is flattening to a intensity value of 65 (arrow). The *spillover* effect is also visible; there is no clear distinction between grey and white matter. The maxima of both grey and white matter are shifted towards each other in such a way that both brain tissue compartments can no longer be distinguished. In order to characterize the PV effect more fully, measurements were carried out with a GE/Scanditronix PC4096+ scanner [17]. This scanner has a resolution of 4.9 mm in the center of the FOV, while the resolution after reconstruction (image resolution) is 6.5 mm. The following experiment was performed to evaluate the underestimation of the activity concentration in the reconstructed image. A cylindrical phantom with a diameter of 20 cm was used, which contained 6 spheres (Fig. 4.2 a). The diameters of the spheres were 9.6, 12.1, 16.8, 21.3, 26.2, and 35.6 mm (spheres 3 through 6 had a diameter greater than twice the image resolution). They were filled with a ^{18}F solution with equal activity concentration. Fig. 4.2 b shows the reconstructed PET image of the phantom. The smaller the sphere diameter is, the lower the

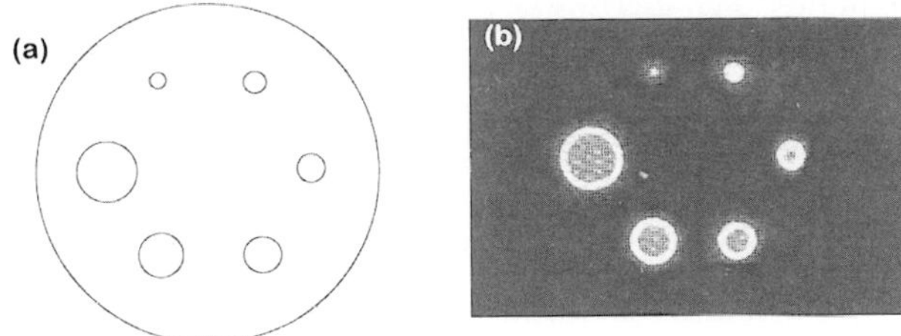

Fig. 4.2. a Cross section of the sphere phantom with 6 different spheres. **b** PET image of the sphere phantom. The spheres were filled with the same activity concentration.

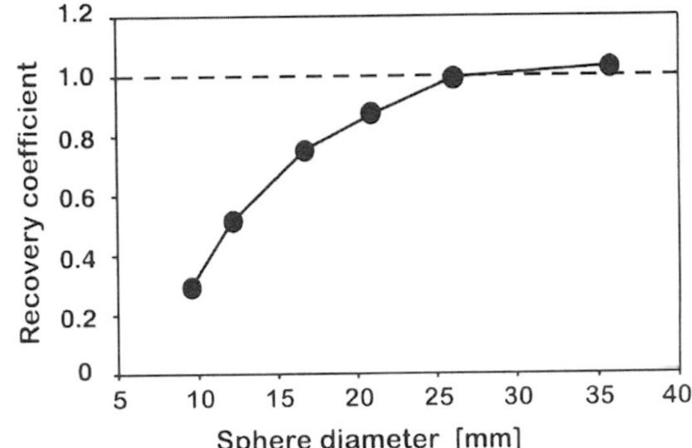

Fig. 4.3. *Recovery coefficient* as function of the sphere diameters.

activity concentration appears, although the spheres were filled with the same activity concentration. This is the consequence of the partial volume effect. The corresponding graph is shown in Fig. 4.3: the ratio of the measured activity concentration in the spheres and the real activity concentration is plotted as a function of the sphere diameter. This ratio is called the *recovery coefficient* (RC) and it is a measure of the influence of the PV effect on the qualitative, but especially the quantitative characterization of the signal.

On the image plane of a PET data set (i.e., on the transverse component of the PSF), each pixel can be described by a PSF; this means that each pixel or measured object always overlaps the center of the PSF. Conversely, in the axial dimension this might be different, if the axial component of the PSF is clearly larger than its transverse component and overlaps more than one detector (i.e., its extent is larger than the thickness of one slice). As a result, the overlap of the axial component of the PSF with the object is unknown and it may only overlap with parts of the PSF. However, this case concerns only the scanners with strongly non-isotropic detectors. The consequence of non-isotropic detectors is that the error caused by the PV effect not only depends on the size of the object, but also on its shape. The "shape" of an object is a complex variable which cannot be fully characterized with phantom measurements and simulations. Furthermore, spherical structures are less influenced by the partial volume effect than irregular structures. When the structure extends more in the axial dimension, the error can be minimized by summing up multiple slices. The spatial position of the object and its relation to neighboring radioactive or strongly absorbing structures represents a further source of error. Objects in an area of very different activity concentration are strongly more influenced by the PV effect than objects in an area with an activity concentration similar to their own.

4.3 Partial volume correction

Several techniques have been developed to correct PV effects. A variety of methods for PV correction are used in the context of neurological questions and are supported by CT or MR images with high spatial resolution. There are only a few cardiac or oncological applications.

The first methods which were developed corrected for the contamination of the brain signal, which was caused by the non-active cerebral spinal fluid [14, 21]. In a second stage, the influence of white matter on the quantitation of the grey matter activity concentration was included in the methodological development [16]. The latter method assumed a homogeneous distribution of the activity in the grey matter compartment. This method was further extended. First, the heterogeneous activity distribution was corrected by a region-of-interest (ROI) method [15] and, second, 3D data processing was introduced [5]. The PV correction in our group is based on fully 3D data processing [18] and additionally includes the implementation of an algorithm for precise classification of the tissue classes in the MR data [6]. Another method calculates a matrix of coefficients, which characterize the reciprocal contamination of tissue components. This matrix is used for PV correction [20]. Recently, another group proposed a neuronal network model to reduce the partial volume effect in the restoration of blood flow data [12].

In the following section, three PV correction methods are described. The first PV correction method was developed in our group and it is mainly used in neurological contexts (e.g., for brain tumors in oncology). The second and third methods are universally applicable and can also be used for PV correction in cardiology and oncology.

4.3.1 PV correction methods for brain

The PV correction is strongly influenced by the exact classification of the corresponding MR data. We use an algorithm that can separate up to eight different intensity classes on a voxel by voxel basis (including background) [6]. Therefore, not only grey matter, white matter and CSF can be classified, but also, for example, tumor tissue which shows different intensity values on the MR image than the neighboring tissue. T_1 (*single echo*) as well as T_2 and proton density (*double echo*) weighted MR images can be classified; with the help of Markov random fields it is possible to include neighborhood correlations and signal inhomogeneities. After classification of the MR data set, an accurate registration with the PET data set is performed. The 3D PV correction method [18] – expanded on a further intensity class for tumor tissue – can now be applied. The correction comprises of two steps: first, a MR data set is classified, and the grey matter compartment includes the tumor tissue compartment. The classified data are used to generate masks (X_{tissue}), which have the value 1 for all voxels of the given tissue and the value 0 for all other voxels. The PV corrected activity concentration values A_G^* for the grey matter can now be calculated according to the following equation:

$$A_G^* = [A_{meas} - (X_W A_W^* + X_{CSF} A_{CSF}^*) \otimes h] / X_G \otimes h \tag{4.1}$$

A_W^* and A_{CSF}^* are the estimated activity concentration values for white matter and cerebral spinal fluid; A_{meas} is the measured activity concentration in the PET scanner; h is a non-isotropic three dimensional filter kernel that corresponds to the PET scanner resolution; the symbol $\otimes$ indicates a convolution. Second, the PV correction of the tumor area is performed. A second classification of the original MR data set now separates the tumor tissue from the grey matter tissue. The final PV correction uses Eq. 4.2 which represents the extension of Eq. 4.1:

$$A_{tum}^* = [A_{meas} - (X_G A_G^* + X_W A_W^* + X_{CSF} A_{CSF}^*) \otimes h] / X_{tum} \otimes h\,. \tag{4.2}$$

The A_G^* value is estimated from a non-tumor area with the help of a ROI. A_{tum}^* is the PV corrected activity concentration in the tumor area.

In order to validate this method, phantom measurements were performed (cylindrical phantom; see chapter 4.2). The spheres were filled with the same activity concentration; Fig. 4.3 shows the corresponding RC curve. These data have been PV corrected with the presented method, where the sphere content was assumed to be grey matter. Fig. 4.4 again shows the RC curve (dots) as well as with the corrected values (asterisks).

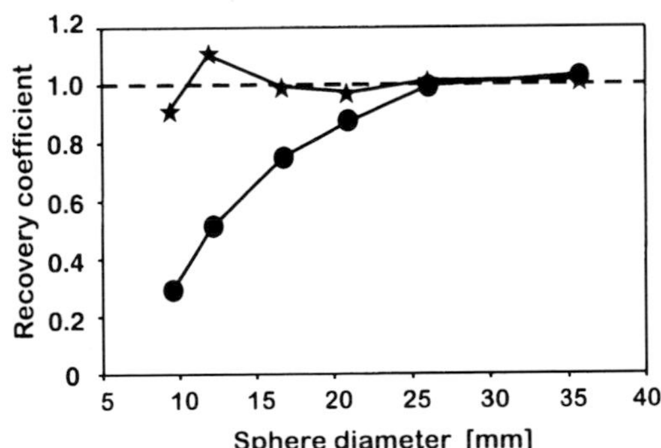

Fig. 4.4. *Recovery coefficient* as function of the sphere diameters: measured values (dots) and PV corrected values (asterisks).

4.3.2 PV correction methods for whole-body measurements

The method described above is based on anatomical information (CT or MR). The anatomical information is used to infer knowledge not only about the spatial position, but also about the extent of different tissue compartments after the registration of MR and PET images. However, in oncology, the anatomical (MR) and the metabolic landmarks (PET) are not always identical. Furthermore, the registration of MR images with the corresponding PET images is difficult, when handling oncological images from whole-body measurements. It is easier to apply methods that are independent from the high resolution anatomical information, i.e., they do not require a registration of MR and PET images.

4.3.2.1 PV correction with a *recovery coefficient*

The correction of the PV effect can be achieved through the calculation of the *recovery coefficient* as a function of the object extent. In order to be able to implement the method, phantom measurements have to be performed. Either a phantom as described above, or a cylindrical phantom with several tubes of different diameters can be used. However, using the latter, the PV effect in the axial direction cannot be corrected. In both cases the spheres/tubes are filled with a ^{18}F solution of equal activity concentration. The measurement must be repeated several times with the main volume of the phantom filled with different low activity concentrations every time (e.g., with a ratio between main volume and spheres/tubes concentration of 10 to 1, 5 to 1, etc.) in order to simulate different background activities. The parameters of standard patient measurements for acquisition and reconstruction should be also used for phantom data processing. A high resolution MR image of the phantom is helpful, but not necessary. Such a high resolution image helps to characterize the exact position of the spheres/tubes, in particular, in the case of small diameters. Circular ROIs are drawn on the MR images delineating the spheres/tubes. After registration with the PET images, these ROIs are transferred to the PET images so that the mean activity concentration within each ROI can be obtained. The ratios of these measured concentrations with the known real concentration are plotted as a function of the diameters, creating the RC curve for the scanner. An algorithm fitting this curve provides the mathematical tool to calculate the right RC for every diameter. However, this only represents an approximation and does not provide quantitative values. The reason for this is the difficulty of estimating tumor size based on scintigraphic images. Avril et al. [1] recently described a helpful method, which allows one to assess the tumor size. The MR images also contain information about size and the extent of the tumor after registration with the PET images. However, this does not apply to all kinds of tumors, where the MR images do not always characterize the actual tumor extent correctly.

4.3.2.2 A nonlinear spatially variant object-dependent system model

The method developed by Chen and colleagues [3] offers a generalized approach for the estimation of the PV effect in tumor imaging and receptor quantification. A mathematical model is described, which takes into account the PV effect correction as well as the scatter correction (see chapter 3.3.4) simultaneously. In contrast to other models, it is based on a spatially variant – i.e., object dependent – PSF of the system, which relates the object O (i.e., the non-scatter corrected reconstructed activity distribution) with the scatter and PV corrected final activity distribution O_{corr}:

$$O_{corr}(\vec{x}) = \int O(\vec{\alpha})PSF(\vec{x},\vec{\alpha})d\,\vec{\alpha} \tag{4.3}$$

$\vec{x}$ is a three dimensional vector representing each point in space; $\vec{\alpha}$ is a dummy variable of integration. O is reconstructed as described in chapter 3.2. The point spread function PSF comprises four terms which describe its Gaussian form, the scatter portion in active volume as well as in collimators and detectors. The authors use four different phantoms with different sizes and forms to derive the manifold parameters required for the calculation of the PSF. Because PSF depends on the object O, it is necessary to calculate it once for every reconstruction algorithm used (filtered backprojection or iterative reconstruction) and again for every different filter applied. First results using this method arc promising. A phantom containing spheroids (similar to Fig. 4.2a) was measured among others and the RC curve was obtained. The mean value for this RC is 1.03 ± 0.07 (compare with Fig. 4.4). In this article [3], the idea was that the PSF was object-dependent and related to different sphere positions or other target organs, to the object geometry as well as to the attenuation characteristics. However, measurements and calculations have shown [4] that the PSF changes depend on the different neighboring activity distributions despite equal geometry, position and attenuation characteristics. A modified version of Eq. 4.3 was derived [4] which provides a more exact estimate of the spheroid size and activity concentration compared to the more simple RC method. However, the scatter correction – taken into account in the former article – is now no longer applicable, but three so-called "adjusting factors" could be easily incorporated into the previous model to include the contrast dependence into the PSF.

4.4 Discussion

The partial volume correction has been increasingly used over the last few years in the quantification of PET brain studies, because the activity concentration in the grey matter is underestimated as consequence of its limited thickness. Methods allowing absolute quantification of the PET signals have been developed to quantify blood flow, metabolism, and receptor density. Several

PV correction models have been implemented on the basis of MR and CT images. In case of oncological and cardiological questions, PV correction methods are not commonly used. One reason for this is that there are problems with movement artifacts. Furthermore, the "gold standard" for the tumor extent still does not exist. The analysis of scintigraphic information in the framework of oncological diagnostics is mostly performed on a visual basis and may additionally include the regional value of the tracer uptake. The use of quantitative parameters probably offers a more objective and observer-independent criterion in diagnosis and therapy. In oncology, several methods to determine quantitative parameters have been proposed (chapter 3.5). With these methods, the tracer uptake is normalized to the injected activity and the body weight. However, up to now no generally accepted method for quantitative analysis exists. Additionally, regional uptake values in small lesions are affected by the PV effect.

The correction of the PV effect may play a relevant role in clinical diagnosis, in the follow-up, and in therapy monitoring for a higher accuracy and an exact analysis of quantitative parameters.

In case of neurooncology, the PV correction methods developed for PET brain studies, as explained in chapter 4.3.1, can be applied using anatomical information from high resolution morphological imaging (CT, MR). This method could be utilized for brain tumors, e.g., with application of radioactive labeled amino acids (e.g., [^{11}C]methionine), given that the tumor extent is exactly derived using MR or CT. However, this is often complicated in gliomas. This approach seems less promising in studies with [^{18}F]fluorodeoxyglucose (FDG), which is also accumulated in healthy tissue. The PV correction can be relevant, for example, to determine the uptake ratio in a small tumor after surgery in the case of suspected recurrence or therapy monitoring. However, there are implications of PV correction of uptake ratios in clinical oncology using [^{18}F]FDG PET: PV effects will occur in cases of tumors, recurrent disease, and lymph node metastasis, which are smaller than twice the resolution of the PET scanner, thus, the tracer uptake is underestimated due to the PV effect. The tumor size can be approximately determined from the analysis of axial [^{18}F]FDG image slices, where a spherical shape can be assumed for the calculations. The extent of malignant disease is often not exactly delineated with CT or MR. This problem has an important effect on the method presented in section 4.3.2.1. Since this method is based on phantom measurements, the values of the *recovery coefficient* are determined based on idealized geometrical bodies (e.g., spheres), which cannot be exactly transposed to an individual tumor form. Furthermore, it is assumed that within the spheres the activity concentration is homogeneous. This is not true for tumor tissue. A tumor may contain necrotic areas which show a change of the density or of the signal in MR images as compared with viable tumor tissue and, therefore, do not show a homogeneous uptake of [^{18}F]FDG. A further source of error arises from motion artifacts, which affect the assessment of the size and the regional tracer uptake. Below a size of about 1 cm the PET visualization of malignant disease is hardly possible.

The quantitative analysis of PET studies in oncological diagnosis is going to become more significant. It will be important to develop diagnostic tools that take into account a PV correction in order to increase diagnostic precision. These models will have to be validated from the clinical point of view and should provide semiquantitative and quantitative parameters for the judgment of lesions related to recurring, metastatic disease in oncology. An important approach was presented by Avril et al. [1], who examined the diagnostic precision of several semiquantitative and quantitative methods in the diagnosis of breast cancer. It could be shown that the precision is increasing with visual analysis, if additional quantitative parameters are used.

References

[1] Avril N, Bense S, Ziegler SI, Dose J, Weber W, Laubenbacher Ch, Römer W, Jänicke F, Schwaiger M (1997) Breast imaging with fluorine-18-FDG PET: quantitative image analysis. J Nucl Med 38:1186–1191

[2] Brooks RA, Chiro GD (1976) Principles of computer assisted tomography (CAT). Phys Med Biol 21:689–732

[3] Chen C-H, Muzic RF Jr, Nelson AD, Adler LP (1998) A nonlinear spatially variant object-dependent system model for prediction of partial volume effects and scatter in PET. IEEE Trans Med Imag 17:214–227

[4] Chen C-H, Muzic RF Jr, Nelson AD, Adler LP (1998) Simultaneous recovery of size and radioactivity concentration of small spheroids with PET data. J Nucl Med 40:118–130

[5] Frost JJ, Meltzer CC, Zubieta JK, Links JM, Brakeman P, Stumpf MJ, Kruger M (1996) MR-based correction of partial volume effects in brain PET imaging. In: Myers R, Cunningham V, Bailey D, Jones T (eds) Quantification of Brain Function Using PET. Academic Press, pp 152–157

[6] Held K, Rota Kops E, Krause BJ, Wells WM, Kikinis R, Müller-Gärtner HW (1997) Markov random field segmentation of brain MR images. IEEE Trans Med Imag 16:878–886

[7] Henze E, Huang SC, Ratib O, Hoffman E, Phelps ME, Schelbert HR (1983) Measurement of regional tissue and blood-pool radiotracer concentrations from serial tomographic images of the heart. J Nucl Med 24:987–996

[8] Herrero P, Markham J, Bergmann SR (1989) Quantitation of myocardial blood flow with $H_2{}^{15}O$ and positron emission tomography: assessment and error analysis of a mathematical approach. J Comput Assist Tomogr 5:862–873

[9] Hoffmann EJ, Huang SC, Phelps ME (1979) Quantitation in positron emission tomography: 1. Effect of object size. J Comput Assist Tomogr 3:299–308

[10] Hoffmann EJ, Huang SC, Plummer D, Phelps ME (1982) Quantitation in positron emission computed tomography: 6. Effect of nonuniform resolution. J Comput Assist Tomogr 5:987–999

[11] Kessler RM, Ellis JR, Eden M (1984) Analysis of emission tomographic scan data: limitations imposed by resolution and background. J Comput Assist Tomogr 3:514–522

[12] Kosugi Y, Sase M, Suganami Y, Momose T, Nishikawa J (1996) Dissolution of partial volume effect in PET by an inversion technique with the MR-embedded neural network model. In: Myers R, Cunningham V, Bailey D, Jones T (eds) Quantification of Brain Function Using PET. Academic Press, pp 166–169

[13] Mazziotta JC, Phelps ME, Plummer D, Kuhl DE (1981) Quantitation in positron emission tomography: 5. Physical-anatomical effects. J Comput Assist Tomogr 5:734–743

[14] Meltzer CC, Leal JP, Mayberg HS, Wagner HN, Frost JJ (1990) Correction of PET data for partial volume effects in human cerebral cortex by MR imaging. J Comput Assist Tomogr 14:561–570

[15] Meltzer CC, Zubieta JK, Links JM, Brakeman P, Stumpf MJ, Frost JJ (1996) MR-based correction of brain PET measurements for heterogeneous gray matter radioactivity distribution. J Cereb Blood Flow Metab 16:650–658

[16] Müller-Gärtner HW, Links JM, Leprince JL, Bryan RN, McVeigh E, Leal JP, Davatzikos C, Frost JJ (1992) Measurement of radiotracer concentration in brain gray matter using positron emission tomography: MR-based correction for partial volume effects. J Cereb Blood Flow Metab 12:571–583

[17] Rota Kops E, Herzog H, Schmid A, Holte S, Feinendegen LE (1990) Performance characteristics of an eight-ring whole body PET scanner. J Comput Assist Tomogr 14:437–445

[18] Rota Kops E, Krause BJ, Herzog H, Müller-Gärtner HW (1998) 3D-Partial volume correction and simulated PET studies. Eur J Nucl Med 25:900 (abstr)

[19] Rousset OG, Ma Y, Kamber M, Evans AC (1993) Three dimensional simulations of radiotracer uptake in deep nuclei of human brain. Comput Med Imaging Graphics 4/5:373–379

[20] Rousset OG, Ma Y, Evans AC (1998) Correction for partial volume effects in PET: principles and validation. J Nucl Med 39:904–911

[21] Videen TO, Perlmutter JS, Mintun MA, Raichle ME (1988) Regional correction of positron emission tomography data for the effects of cerebral atrophy. J Cereb Blood Flow Metab 8:662–670

5 Radiation safety in PET

J. Kretschko

5.1 Introduction

Positron emission tomography (PET) is an integral part of nuclear medicine diagnostics. In the future an increase in the application of this method in general health care can be expected. Compared with conventional nuclear medicine, a number of factors relating to radiation safety in PET have to be taken into account:

- The energy of the annihilation photons of 511 keV is much higher than the photon energy of radionuclides used in conventional nuclear medicine, especially ^{99m}Tc. As a result of the higher photon energy the attenuation is lower, and this must be considered in the calculation of necessary radiation shielding.
- Due to the short half-life of certain radionuclides commonly used in PET, it is necessary to produce and carry out the radiochemical preparation of these radionuclides at the location of their use. The radiochemical preparation, and also the application of the radionuclides involves working with relatively high levels of activity.
- During production of radionuclides with a cyclotron, fast neutrons can be produced in nuclear reactions as well as components of the equipment used can be activated. High-energy primary and secondary gamma radiation can be released in nuclear reactions.
- During procedures associated with the preparation of radioisotopes, volatile radioactive substances are produced, which lead to contamination of the air exhausted from the cyclotron room and also from the corresponding synthesis units of the radiochemical laboratory.
- Quantitative PET studies involve temporal blood sampling. This entails an additional radiation exposure to personnel.

These aspects of PET have to be taken into account in the constructional, technical, and organizational aspects of radiation safety.

5.2 Radiation protection of the patient

The administration of radioactive substances in nuclear medicine examinations is accompanied with radiation exposure to the patient. The level of exposure to the patient is dependent on the following factors:

- The activity administered.
- The physical properties of the radionuclide (physical half-life of radioactive decay, type and energy of the emitted radiation).
- The biokinetics of the radiopharmaceuticals used (local distribution factor, biological half-life).
- The mass of the respective organ and also on the age of the patient.

In general, radiation exposure to the patient is expressed quantitatively, as effective dose.

The effective dose can be determined in a simple manner by means of dose factors (f_D) and the applied activity (A_i) according to the following formula:

$$H_{eff} = f_D \cdot A_i \tag{5.1}$$

The numerical dose factors for certain PET pharmaceuticals are presented in the ICRP Publication 53, for different age groups (4, 10, 15 and > 18 years of age) [4]. The new weighting factors indicated in ICRP Publication 60 have not yet been taken into account within these values [5]. Johansson et al. have calculated the dose factors for many PET radiopharmaceuticals on the basis of the new weighting factors [6]. In Table 5.1, the dose factors for a number of PET radiopharmaceuticals calculated in accordance with the indications given in ICRP 53 and ICRP 60 are presented.

To reduce radiation exposure to the patient the following measures from the medical and physical point of view have to be taken into account:

- Precise indication including patient history, in particular where children, young persons and pregnant women are concerned.
- Optimization of the applied activity and instrumental settings in view of

Table 5.1. Dose factors for a number radiopharmaceuticals used in PET and conventional nuclear medicine expressed in mSv/MBq [4, 6].

Radiopharmaceutical	ICRP-53 Age				ICRP-60 Age
	1	10	15	>18	>18
$[^{11}C]CO_2$ (Inhalation 1 h)	6.0 E-03	2.0 E-03	1.3 E-03	1.1 E-03	1.0 E-03
$[^{13}N]NH_3$	1.5 E-02	4.9 E-03	3.2 E-03	2.7 E-03	2.0 E-03
$[^{18}F]FDG$	1.3 E-01	4.7 E-02	3.2 E-02	2.7 E-02	2.0 E-02
$[^{99m}Tc]MDP$	6.1 E-02	1.7 E-02	1.1 E-02	8.2 E-03	5.8 E-03
$[^{201}Tl]TlCl$	3.0 E 00	1.5 E 00	3.6 E-01	2.3 E-01	2.3 E-01

achieving optimal quality in imaging.

- Certainty that the positioning of the patient is correct and that the patient is willing to cooperate.
- Quality control of radiopharmaceuticals and nuclear medicine instruments.
- Frequent emptying of the bladder following the examination.

For the application of radioactive substances in clinical research, an authorization by the local radiation safety authority in accordance with the national radiation safety ordinance is required [14, 15]. Many PET examinations, in particular those involving new radiopharmaceuticals, are still in the research phase, therefore, attention to the legal regulations must be given. Within the framework of applications for authorization, the following items will, among others, be demanded by the authorization authorities:

- A precise description of the research project.
- Presentation of data concerning patient (age, sex, etc.) and volunteers who are to undergo examination.
- Determination of the effective dose for persons undergoing examination.

5.3 Radiation protection of personnel

Radiation exposure to personnel working in the field of nuclear medicine can be caused by either external radiation or incorporation of radioactive substances. External exposures will be caused mostly by photons or neutrons. Internal radiation exposure, however, will be caused essentially by positrons. The maximum energy and maximum range for positrons in water respectively in body tissue and air are listed in Table 5.2 [1, 16].

5.3.1 Ambient dose rate

The decisive factor for radiation exposure due to external irradiation is the actual ambient dose rate of photons and neutrons at the place of work.

Table 5.2. Maximum energy and maximum range in water and air of positrons of radionuclides commonly used in PET.

Radionuclide	E_{max}/MeV	R_{water}/mm	R_{air}/mm
^{18}F	0.635	2.15	1.66
^{11}C	0.970	3.80	2.94
^{13}N	1.200	5.00	3.87
^{15}O	1.740	8.00	6.19
^{68}Ga	1.900	9.00	6.96
^{82}Rb	3.150	15.50	11.99

5.3.1.1 Photons

The ambient dose rate for photon radiation is generally indicated as the photon equivalent dose rate (H). For radioactive point sources, this can be determined by means of dose rate constants (Γ_H) of the radionuclide considered, the activity of the radioactive source (A) and the distance from the source (r), in accordance with the formula:

$$H = \Gamma_H \cdot \frac{A}{r^2} \tag{5.2}$$

The half-life, the photon energy, and the dose rate constant for a number of radionuclides important in nuclear medicine applications are listed in Table 5.3 [2]. The dose rate constant for ^{18}F is lower compared with other positron emitters, since radioactive decay occurs partly in the form of electron capture. It can be noted that the dose rate constants for the radionuclides which are used in conventional nuclear medicine are significantly lower. To establish a PET center, a radiation protection plan must be presented. The calculation of the thickness of a given material necessary for shielding has to be carried out in relation to the energy of the annihilation radiation (511 keV). The basis for these calculations are the maximum permitted levels for the ambient dose rate in accordance to the given National Radiation Protection Ordinance (see Table 5.4 according to the German standards [2]). The absorption potential of shieldings made of different materials (F) and thus,

Table 5.3. Half-life, photon energy and dose rate constants for a number of PET nuclides compared with radionuclides used in conventional nuclear medicine applications [7].

Radionuclide	$T_{1/2}$	E_γ/keV	$\Gamma_H/\mu Sv\ m^2\ h^{-1}\ GBq^{-1}$
^{11}C	20.4 min	511	159
^{13}N	9.97 min	511	159
^{15}O	2.04 min	511	159
^{18}F	109.8 min	511	155
^{99m}Tc	6.01 h	140	16
^{123}I	13.2 h	159	44
^{131}I	8.02 d	360	59

Table 5.4. Maximum ambient dose rate (H_{max}) in controlled areas in accordance with DIN 6844-3 [2].

Protected areas	$H_{max}/\mu Sv\ h^{-1}$
Controlled areas	5.0
Monitored areas	2.5
Nuclear medicine measuring rooms	0.02
Measuring equipment locations	0.02
Working rooms beyond radiation operational areas	0.75
Living areas	0.18

at the same time, the required wall thickness can be determined from the imposed dose rate (H_{max}) and the activities handled in the areas concerned, on the basis of the following formula (see DIN 6844-3 [2]):

$$F = \frac{H}{H_{max}} = \frac{\Gamma_H \cdot A}{H_{max} \cdot r^2} \qquad (5.3)$$

The high energy photons produced by activation processes (n, γ), (p, γ) etc., during the production of the radionuclides with the cyclotron, are also to be taken into account in the calculations for the shielding. In the German standards, so-called DIN standards, only the attenuation level (F) for annihilation radiation is given. The attenuation levels for other photon energies must be calculated separately, or determined experimentally.

Kearfort et al. have calculated and measured exposure rates due to patient sources, pneumatic transport systems, and gas lines in a PET imaging facility [8].

5.3.1.2 Neutrons

As a result of activation processes with charged particles (protons, deuterons, α-particles), neutrons can be produced in the cyclotron unit. Special criteria are to be applied with respect to the shielding for neutrons. This applies particularly to particle accelerators which are not fitted with shielding. The presence of neutrons beyond the shielding at non-negligible dose rates is, however, also expected, where so-called self-shielding compact cyclotrons are used [12].

To calculate the necessary shielding, the potentially occurring flux and energy of the neutrons have to be considered. These are dependent on the operating characteristics of the particular cyclotron concerned (type of particle, energy level, current intensity, etc.). For the purposes of neutron shielding, building materials with some water content, such as normal concrete, are particularly suitable. In such cases, water can also be present in crystallized form. The effectiveness of shielding made of concrete can be increased using an additive limonite element ($2\ Fe_2O_3 \cdot 3\ H_2O$). The shielding effect is achieved here by means of elastic impact (absorption of recoil protons). The formulas for the calculation of shielding for fast neutrons are presented in the contribution of Junker and Fitschen [7].

5.3.1.3 The ambient dose rate in different areas of the PET center

The ambient dose rates (H_x) determined in the different operational areas of the PET center in Munich are presented in Table 5.5. It can be seen from this table that the highest dose rate is detected at the targets of the cyclotron when the shielding has been withdrawn. The dose rate in the patient mea-

Table 5.5. Ambient dose rate in different areas of the PET center in Munich

Measuring location	$A_{F\text{-}18}$/GBq	H_x/μSv h^{-1}
Cyclotron shielding (neutrons)	122	60
Cyclotron shielding (γ-radiation)	122	160
Targets without shielding	122	10 000
Cabinet (dose calibrator)	37	< 500
Cabinet ([^{18}F]FDG synthesis module)	37	< 2
Hot cells	37	1.2–13.4
Cyclotron operating room	–	< 0.1
Measuring distance to patient (10 cm)	–	< 300
Tomograph operating room	–	0.2

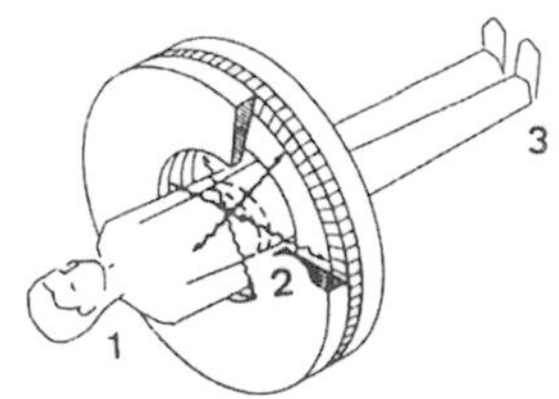

			Position				
			1		2		3
Radiopharmaceutical	A_i / MBq	t_{pi}/min	10 cm	100 cm	10 cm	100 cm	10 cm
^{18}F-FDG (Injection)	378	37	0.132	0.019	0.106	0.027	0.058
^{18}F-FDG (Infusion)	373	31	0.308	0.018	0.148	0.009	0.012
[^{13}N]NH_3	639	5	0.344	0.039	0.470	0.050	0.024
[^{15}O]water	370	0	0.216	0.019	0.243	0.022	0.022

Fig. 5.1. Ambient dose rate/applied activity determined at the PET center in Munich in different positions and distances expressed in μSv h^{-1} MBq^{-1}.

surement room is dependent on the individual examination. Fig. 5.1 shows the ambient dose rate for three different PET radiopharmaceuticals, at various locations in the patient measurement room. Procedures to reduce radiation exposures to personnel working at a PET center are described in contributions of Brown et al. [1] and Schober et al. [12, 13].

5.3.2 Occupational groups at the PET center

The personnel working at a PET center include various occupational groups who receive different levels of exposure according to their precise field of activity and their allocation to the different operational units of the PET center. The decisive factor is the ambient dose rate in each individual case and the type of occupational activity.

5.3.2.1 Physicists and technicians working in the area of the cyclotron

Using self-shielded cyclotrons, the ambient dose rate from both the neutrons produced here and photon radiation can be minimized. Where the shielding has been withdrawn, i.e., in the case of maintenance, care should be taken with respect to activated components of the equipment.

Measurements of activity after the end of bombardment are carried out automatically in an adequately shielded cabinet.

5.3.2.2 Radiochemists

The staff of the radiochemical laboratory is concerned with the preparation of the activated cyclotron products to produce the necessary radiopharmaceuticals and with the implementation of the required quality control measures, in accordance with the given national legal regulations on Medical Products (e.g., in Germany the "*Arzneimittelgesetz*" [11]).

Due to the short half-life of the cyclotron products used in nuclear medicine applications, relatively high initial activities of greater than 37 GBq are produced. For this reason, "hot cells", with lead walls of approx. 6 cm thickness fitted with appropriate mechanical handling equipment, are used by the radiochemists for synthesizing the radiopharmaceuticals. In order to reduce the level of radiation exposure to the personnel of the radiochemical laboratory, radiolabeling and synthesis modules with adequate shielding are used.

The laws relating to medical products require quality control assays for all radiolabeled substances to be used in medical applications. The percent purity of the radionuclides as well as the radiochemical, chemical and pharmaceutical purities of the products, are to be determined and listed. It is required that these assays be carried out in a separate room. This room must comply with all requirements under the law affecting pharmaceutical products and be equipped with the required instruments [3, 11].

5.3.2.3 Physicians, medical laboratory technicians and nursing staff

Medical laboratory technicians are responsible for the preparation of injections and, along with the nursing staff, for taking care of the patients in the PET camera room. The injection of radiopharmaceuticals is the responsibility of the physicians.

Due to the high levels of initial and applied activity, special safety measures are required with regard to the preparation of the injections and care of patients. In particular, the following safety measures are indicated:

- The transport of radioactive substances between the radiochemical laboratory and the treatment room must be carried out by means of a pneumatic transport system or otherwise in adequately shielded carrying containers.

- The preparation of the injections must be carried out behind adequate shielding walls.
- Suitable syringe shields with adequate protection against the high-energy annihilation radiation are at present not commercially available. For this reason, shielded infusion set-ups with integrated dose calibrators are recommended for the application of the PET radiopharmaceuticals.
- Mobile shielding walls made of lead can be used to provide shielding against radiation emitted by the patient during measurement.

The radiation exposure received by medical laboratory physicians and technicians for different working procedures are presented in Table 5.6. Radiation doses to positron emission tomography technologists during specific tasks have been measured and reported by McCormick and Miklos [10]. The radiation dose to physicians during specific medical applications and examinations is, per examination, at a level of 0.02–0.03 mSv for the whole body, and 0.20 – 0.40 mSv to the fingers (Junker et al. [7]). Values of the radiation exposure of personnel determined at the PET center in Munich in 1997 are shown in Table 5.7. These values represent the maximum and minimum values determined within the scope of the monthly determination of personal dose.

Table 5.6. Radiation exposure to physicians and technicians obtained in different working procedures as indicated by Linnemann et al. [9].

Working procedure	Number	Dose/Examination in μSv		
		Whole-body dose	Left hand	Right hand
Preparation of injections	44	1–7	387	173
Injection	45	3	27	170
Taking of blood samples	28	6	–	–
Positioning and caring of patients	15	2–16	–	–

Table 5.7. Whole-body doses determined in 1997 for the personnel of the PET center in Munich, expressed in mSv/a.

Occupational group	Film dosimeter	Finger dosimeter
Cyclotron physicist	0.8	8.0
Radiochemist	0.2–0.8	40–170
RMLT * (PET)	4.2–5.6	15–81
RMLT * (conventional)	1.2–6.4	2.4–81
Nursing staff (PET)	0.4–3.2	–
Maximum permissible dose	50	300

* Radio-medical laboratory technicians

5.4 Environmental protection

During operation of the cyclotron, radioactive substances can be produced in gas form, which can lead to the contamination of room air in the area surrounding the accelerator. During production of the cyclotron products, volatile and liquid radioactive waste substances are likewise formed. In addition, metabolites exhaled by the patient can result in a further contamination of air in the examination room. The uncontrolled discharge of liquid radioactive wastes into the public sewage system and the release of volatile radioactive substances can lead to radiation exposure in the environment. For this reason, legal limits for the discharge of radioactive substances in liquid and gaseous form into the environment are determined by the given National Radiation Protection Ordinance (in Germany: *Strahlenschutzverordnung, StrlSchV* [14, 15]). Environmental protection measures are essentially applied in the form of the installation of ventilation and retention equipment.

5.4.1 Ventilation equipment

The various control areas of the PET center are to be equipped with a special ventilation system which also continuously measures contamination in the exhaust air during ventilation. In order to prevent radioactive room air escaping into neighboring rooms, a reduced pressure level of around 5 Pa is maintained in both the cyclotron area and the radiochemical laboratory. For releases of activity into the environment with exhaust air, limits are specified in the Radiation Protection Ordinance [14, 15]. Levels of released volatile radioactive substances with exhaust air into the environment from the PET center are shown in Table 5.8. The measured values registered show that during the year 1997, the levels of activity released with exhaust air into the environment, represented merely 86.1% of the permitted activity.

Table 5.8. Release of radioactive gases into the environment.

Radionuclide	Limits		Measured values	
	c_A/Bq m^3	A_G/GBq	A_x/GBq	A_x/A_G
^{18}F	1000	66.4	4.00	0.060
^{11}C; ^{15}O	200	13.3	10.7	0.801
Total:				0.861

5.4.2 Retention installations

Radioactive liquids and radioactive gases may not be released into the environment in an uncontrolled fashion. Due to the relatively short half-lives of the radionuclides used, waste products in liquid form can easily be put into intermediate storage in suitable containers, until the permitted level of concentration is reached. Where a decay plant is available to a therapy ward, wastes from the PET center with short-lived radionuclides can be directed into the plant without reservation.

Radioactive gases, e.g., [^{11}C]CO_2, from limited areas such as "hot cells", can be filled into steel flasks by means of a compressor and be put in this form into intermediate storage, until decay has reached the necessary level (Fig. 5.2).

5.5 Conclusion

The radiation protection-relevant aspects of positron emission tomography must be taken into account. By comparison with conventional nuclear medicine applications, radiation protection in relation to PET requires the application of specified evaluation criteria. Radiation exposure to the patient and to personnel falls within the same order of magnitude as for conventional nuclear medicine applications. For environmental protection purposes, both ventilation and measuring equipment must be installed. During the planning

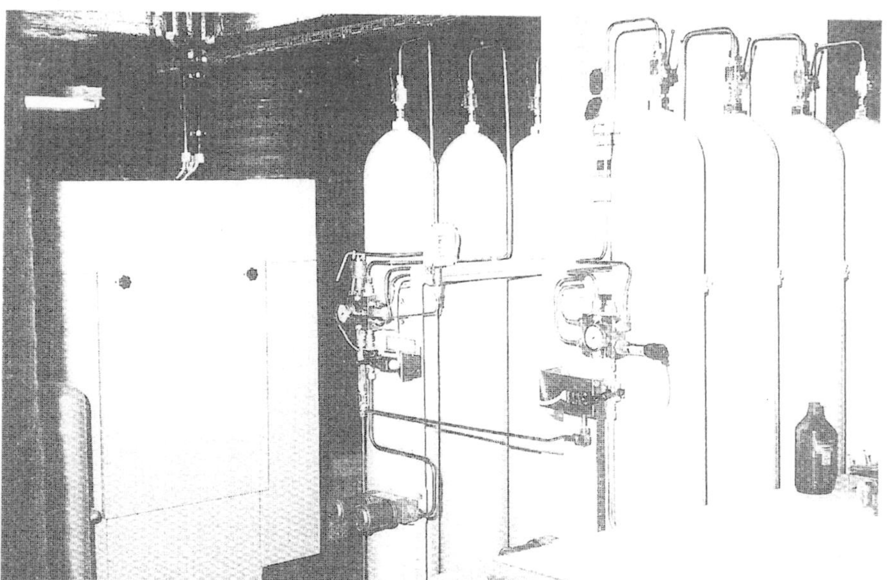

Fig. 5.2. Steel flasks used for storage of volatile radioactive wastes (e.g., [^{11}C]CO_2) at the PET center in Munich.

of PET centers, one should proceed, in principle, in both a generous and farsighted manner, since subsequent extension of the facilities of the center will not only lead to additional costs, but also to the occurrence of considerable problems in operation. The quality of radiation protection for PET applications can be further improved by means of suitable shielding facilities and the development of automated radiochemical and application processes which take place in shielded radiolabeling and synthesis units as well as injection systems.

References

[1] Brown TF, Yasillo J (1997) Radiation Safety Considerations for PET Centers. J Nucl Med Technol 25:98–102

[2] DIN 6844-3 (1989-09) Nuklearmedizinische Betriebe: Strahlenschutzberechnungen

[3] Feiden K (1995) Betriebsverordnung für pharmazeutische Unternehmer. Deutscher Apotheker Verlag, Stuttgart

[4] ICRP publication 53 (1993) Radiation Dose to Patient from Radiopharmaceuticals. Pergamon, Oxford

[5] ICRP publication 60 (1991) 1990 Recommendations of the International Commission on Radiological Protection. Pergamon, Oxford

[6] Johansson L, Mattson S, Nosslin B, Leide-Svegborn S (1992) Effective dose from radiopharmaceuticals. Eur J Nucl Med 19:933–938

[7] Junker D, Fitschen J (1988) Spezielle Probleme des Strahlenschutzes. In: Hundeshagen H (ed) Handbuch der medizinischen Radiologie, Nuklearmedizin. XV, Teil 18, Springer-Verlag, Heidelberg Berlin New York, pp 119–147

[8] Kearfott KJ, Carey JE, Clemenshaw MN, Faulkner DB (1992) Health Phys 63(5):581–589

[9] Linnemann H, Will E, Beuthen-Baumann B (1998) Strahlenbelastung des medizinischen Personals bei PET-Untersuchungen und Möglichkeiten zur Reduzierung. Posterpräsentation auf der Jahrestagung der Deutschen Gesellschaft für Medizinische Physik 1998, Dresden

[10] McCormick VA, Miklos A (1993) Radiation dose to positron emission tomography technologists during quantitative versus qualitative studies. J Nucl Med 34:769–772

[11] Pabel HJ (1991) Arzneimittelgesetz. Deutscher Apotheker Verlag, Stuttgart

[12] Schober O, Lottes G, Junker D (1990) Strahlenexposition bei der Positronen-Emissionstomographie (PET) mit Möglichkeiten der Reduktion der Strahlenexposition bei Patienten und Personal. In: Börner W, Holeczke F, Messerschmidt O (eds) Strahlenschutz in der nuklearmedizinischen Diagnostik. Gustav Fischer Verlag, Stuttgart New York, pp 133–148

[13] Schober O, Lottes G (1994) Positronen-Emissionstomographie und Strahlenexposition. Nuklearmedizin 33:174–177

[14] Veith H-M (1997) Strahlenschutzverordnung. Bundesanzeiger Verlags GmbH, Köln

[15] Verordnung über den Schutz vor Schäden durch ionisierende Strahlen (Strahlenschutzverordnung – StrlSchV) in der Fassung der Bekanntmachung vom 30. 06. 1989 (BGBl. I S. 1321, 1926)

[16] Wienhard K, Wagner R, Heiss W-D (1989) PET: Grundlagen und Anwendungen der Positronen-Emissions-Tomographie. Springer-Verlag, Berlin Heidelberg

6 FDG: biochemical concept and radiochemical synthesis

W. Hamkens, F. Rösch

2-[^{18}F]Fluoro-2-deoxy-D-glucose (FDG) is the most frequently used oncologic PET tracer and it has been *the* standard PET compound for more than ten years. The reason for this unequaled success lies in the coincidence of two main chemical concepts: a solid *bio*chemical concept of the compound's behavior with respect to the intercellular metabolism of carbohydrates, and the reliability of the *nuclear* chemical synthesis of this glucose tracer.

6.1 Biochemistry of glucose

The metabolism of free glucose (or polysaccharides like glycogen or starch, which consist of glucose units) results in the formation of adenosine triphosphate (ATP) with a gain in energy. This process is called glycolysis. Under anaerobic conditions, final products are lactic acid or ethanol. Under aerobic conditions, the metabolism takes similar steps but final products are acetaldehyde (via the intermediate pyruvic acid) and acetyl coenzyme A (cp. Fig. 6.1). Both reaction pathways take place in the cytosol.

First, a glucose molecule passes the membrane into the cell. There the enzymes *hexokinase* or *glucokinase* (i, Fig. 6.1) catalyze the phosphorylation to glucose-6-phosphate. Most cells use the enzyme hexokinase for phosphorylation since it is more common than glucokinase. Especially in muscles or brain, only hexokinase can be found, whereas glucokinase is common in hepatic tissue. Glucose-6-phosphate has an allosterically inhibiting effect on the hexokinase concentration. An increasing glucose uptake into the cell is thus dependent on the further metabolization of glucose-6-phosphate. The enzyme *glucose-6-phosphate isomerase* (ii) converts glucose-6-phosphate into fructose-6-phosphate. In this reaction of an aldose into a ketose, the carbonyl function is transferred from the C1-position to the C2-position of the ring.

The subsequent degradation of fructose-6-phosphate is induced by the analogous enzyme *fructose-6-phosphate kinase* (iii). The product is fructose-1,6-diphosphate, which can either exist in the cyclic or in the open-chain form. Through an aldose endo-reaction with the enzyme *fructose-1,6-diphosphate aldolase* (iv) one molecule of glyceraldehyde phosphate and dihydroxyacetone phosphate are formed. This is a cleavage of a C_6-body into two C_3

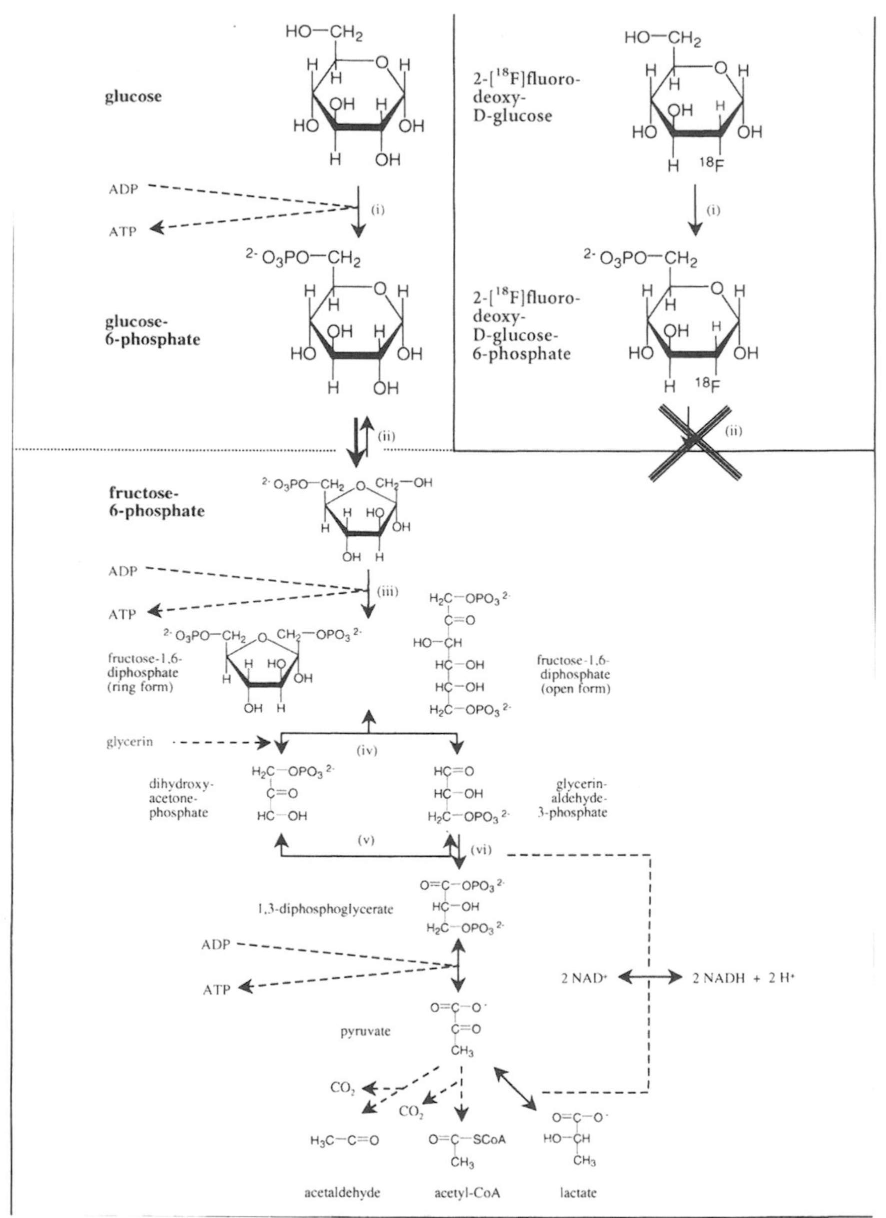

Fig. 6.1. Biochemical pathways of the metabolism of glucose and FDG (denotation of the essential enzymes v.i.)

units. Usually, dihydroxyacetone phosphate is nearly completely converted by *triose phosphate isomerase* (v) into glyceraldehyde phosphate. The enzyme *triose phosphate dehydrogenase* (vi) oxidizes glyceraldehyde phosphate by absorbing an inorganic phosphate to yield 1,3-diphosphate glycerate. Thus, a part of the oxidation energy is accumulated by the molecule. Only the energy-rich mixed acid anhydride of phosphoric acid and carboxylic acid can transfer the phosphate moiety that is bound to the carboxyl group to adenosine diphosphate (ADP); ATP is formed. The electrons that are released by the oxidation are taken up by NAD^+, which is reduced to NADH. In further steps of the glycolysis, the energy-rich phosphoenol pyruvate is produced, which can also transfer a phosphate group to an ADP molecule to form ATP. The reaction product is pyruvate.

Enzymes that are determining glycolysis are mainly fructose-1,6-diphosphate aldolase and the allosterically regulating phosphofructokinase. The latter is inhibited by a high concentration of ATP and activated by high concentrations of ADP or AMP. Thus, the amount of metabolized glucose is adapted to the energy state of the cell.

6.2 Biochemistry of 2-deoxyglucoses

Just like glucose itself, 2-deoxyglucoses are transported to the endothelium or cell membrane by the bloodstream. After the glucose carrier-induced transfer into the cell, the metabolism of the 2-deoxyglucoses follows the same route as for glucoses as long as the participating enzymes accept them as a substrate. This is the case for phosphorylation: 2-deoxyglucose-6-phosphates are formed. Thus, 2-deoxyglucoses become glucose analogues for the uptake into the cell and for the phosphorylation (cp Fig. 6.1).

Because the oxygen at the C2-position of the ring is missing, further metabolization processes cannot take place: 2-deoxyglucose-6-phosphates are not a substrate for the enzyme glucose-6-phosphate isomerase (ii). If glucose-6-phosphatase is present, it can only induce a dephosphorylation. Especially in the brain, this metabolism is irreversible because neither glucose-6-phosphate nor deoxyglucose-6-phosphate is dephosphorylated. The phosphorylated products of 2-deoxyglucoses remain in the cell.

Because of structural variations and different affinities of the enzymes, especially in certain tumor cells, there are gradual differences between the metabolism or tracer kinetics of 2-deoxyglucoses and glucose. Based on initial experiments by Gaitonde et al. (1965) [13] with ^{14}C-labeled glucose, the principal treatment of the kinetics and metabolism of glucose analogues is based on Sokoloff et al. (1977) [34]. This group autoradiographically quantified the behavior of ^{14}C-labeled 2-deoxyglucose in the brain of rats. The three-compartment model derived from these experiments with rats with respect to the irreversible metabolism of $[^{14}C]$-2-deoxyglucose on the one hand and analogous data of ^{14}C-labeled glucose on the other hand allow deviations in the quantification to be bridged mathematically with a "lumped constant". The handling is dependent on the presence or absence of glucose-6-phosphatase. Only in the latter case is a unidirectional phosphorylation taken as the basis of the assumption that all glucose analogues that are transported into the cell are phosphorylated and remain in the cell in that state. Details of the mathematical treatment are summarized in Gjedde [16]. Analogous quantifications have been performed with glucoses that were labeled with ^{14}C in different positions (C1, C2, C6) [3, 4, 18–20].

The application of ex vivo studies with ^{14}C-labeled glucose tracers in in vivo studies of the human glucose metabolism required the labeling of defined 2-deoxyglucose analogues with suitable photon emitters. For dynamic measurements, additional extensions of the mathematical concept were necessary to take into account not only the irreversible metabolism of glucose analogues [7, 16, 23] but also the actual dephosphorylation rate [11, 23].

The experiments with ^{14}C-labeled deoxyglucoses finally led to the development of the ^{18}F-labeled FDG for the application in positron emission tomography. The non-radioactive compound 2-fluoro-2-deoxy-D-glucose was first described in studies of the reactions of 1,6-dehydro-β-D-gluco-pyranose [26]. Decisive for this approach was the then popular research of fluorinated carbohydrates. They were prepared by the reaction of 1,6-2,3-dehydro-4-benzyl-β-D-gluco-pyranose with potassium hydrogen fluoride (KHF_2). After a reaction time of two hours, separation by column chromatography was performed, followed by acid hydrolysis over several hours. The synthesis gave yields of about 50%.

Systematic research of the cytotoxic properties of fluoro-deoxy-D-glucoses showed promising results especially for compounds fluorinated at the C2-position. Starting from this, a new synthetic strategies for the preparation of 2-[^{18}F]fluoro-2-deoxy-D-glucose (2-[^{18}F]FDG) and 2-fluoro-2-deoxy-D-mannose (2-[^{18}F]FDM) were developed [1]. The reaction of 3,4,6-tri-O-acetyl-D-glucal (TAG) with fluoro-oxy-trifluoromethane in chlorotrifluoromethane at $-80\,^{\circ}C$ including a subsequent hydrolysis with hydrochloric acid led to a yield of 2-[^{18}F]FDG and 2-[^{18}F]FDM of about 65% in a ratio of 4:1.

6.3 Radiochemistry of [^{18}F]FDG

The widespread use of 2-[^{18}F]FDG in clinical research and especially in clinical routine diagnostics of tumors would be unthinkable if a successful radiochemical synthesis of the tracer could not be added to the successful investigation of the 2-[^{18}F]FDG metabolism. However, it has a long way from the beginning to the currently used synthesis of FDG, which will be retraced here without claiming to be complete. The development of the ^{18}F-labeled compound FDG for the application in positron emission tomography required, on the one hand, an optimization of the radiochemical synthesis and, on the other hand, the availability of ^{18}F in sufficient activity and radiochemical purity as well as in a well-defined chemical state.

First productions of ^{18}F used particle-induced nuclear reactions in a cyclotron [8, 33]. After the discovery of nuclear fission and the building of the first nuclear reactors, interest in particle accelerators declined. In the early 1950s, initial efforts were made to produce ^{18}F with research reactors. The irradiation of ^{6}Li-enriched lithium oxygen compounds with neutrons results in the formation of tritium via the ^{6}Li(n,α) reaction. In a subsequent process, a nuclear reaction between the newly, in situ formed tritium and the oxygen of the original lithium compound can take place to yield ^{18}F via the ^{16}O(^{3}H,n)^{18}F reaction. The yields obtained with this method are very low. A two-hour bombardment in a 1 MW research reactor with a neutron flux of 10^{13}n/cm^{2}s yields around 1.5 GBq ($\approx$40 mCi) of ^{18}F [15]. Nonetheless, this way of producing ^{18}F was the basis for the synthesis of [^{18}F]FDG for some time.

The renaissance of cyclotrons allowed access of much higher activities [5]. Target nuclides such as ^{16}O, ^{18}O or ^{29}Ne are irradiated with accelerated particles like protons, deuterons, ^{3}He or ^{4}He [25, 28]. Depending on the target material, ^{18}F is obtained either as fluoride (F^-), as hydrogen fluoride (HF) or as elemental fluorine (F_2). The chemical state of the fluorine is decisive for the subsequent synthesis. Electrophilic additions are, for example, reactions of F_2 with carbon-carbon double bonds or reactions of HF with 1,2-dihydro-compounds. Nucleophilic substitutions require a good leaving group at the position that is to be labeled, which can be displaced by fluoride under suitable conditions.

The historical development of ^{18}F-producing nuclear reactions at cyclotrons also influenced the development of [^{18}F]FDG syntheses: beginning with electrophilic substitutions using fluorine prepared after the ^{20}Ne(d,α)^{18}F reaction, the first synthesis of [^{18}F]FDG with significant yields was described in 1978 [21]. The fluorine produced with the neon target was brought into contact with a solution of 3,4,6-tri-O-acetyl-D-glucal (TAG) in fluorotrichloromethane (freon 11) at –78 °C. After removal of the solvent, the residue contained the protected and labeled glucose and mannose in a ratio of 4:1 in a radiochemical yield of 25%. After a 30-min hydrolysis and subsequent separation via a system of cartridges, radiochemical yields of [^{18}F]FDG dropped to 8%.

Maintaining the principle of electrophilic addition, several approaches to optimize the [^{18}F]FDG synthesis were made in the following years. The aim was to increase the radiochemical yield and at the same time reduce the amount of FDM, the unwanted epimer that is simultaneously formed. Glucal or triacetylglucal (TAG) were used as precursors, solvents were water, acetylhypofluorite or freon. Labeling precursors were [^{18}F]F_2, Xe[^{18}F]F_2 or CH_3COO[^{18}F]F (acetylhypofluorite). The amounts of activity obtained were rather low compared to modern standards, because the ^{20}Ne(d,α)^{18}F nuclear reaction yields relatively low ^{18}F activities to begin with.

An electrophilic addition with a radiochemical purity for [^{18}F]FDG of 95% was achieved by Bida et al. (1984) [2]. Their conversion of TAG with acetylhypofluorite in $CFCl_3$ at room temperature yielded 50%.

An attempt at a nucleophilic substitution of [^{18}F]fluoride with a suitable precursor was first publicized by Levy et al. (1982) [24]. The ^{18}F from the neon target was isolated from the gas stream by silverwool coated with cesium fluoride. The conversion of CsH[^{18}F]F_2 with methyl-4,6-O-benzylidene-

3-O-methyl-2-O-trifluormethane-sulfonyl-β-D-manno-pyranose in DMF with subsequent acid hydrolysis produced a decay-corrected radiochemical yield of 10% after an overall reaction time of 180 min.

From 1980 onward, the $^{18}O(p,n)^{18}F$ nuclear reaction allowed research of nucleophilic substitutions with [^{18}F]fluoride [36]. The [^{18}F]F^- produced in the gas target was taken up with water, separated via an anion exchanger and eluted with tetraethyl ammonium hydroxide in acetonitrile. The resulting tetraethyl ammonium fluoride was finally converted with 4,6-benzylidene-1-β-methyl-manno-pyranoside-2,3-cyclosulfate.

The introduction of phase transfer catalysis into nucleophilic substitutions of 1,3,4,6-tetra-O-acetyl-2-O-trifluormethane-sulfonyl-β-D-manno-pyranose with [^{18}F]F^- produced in $H_2{}^{18}O$ water targets in dry acetonitrile led to a product of high radiochemical purity and high yield. This is considered as *the* breakthrough in the development of positron emission tomography. The development of this synthesis allowed for the supplying of an increasing number of PET scanners with a sufficient amount of [^{18}F]FDG. This phase transfer catalyzed nucleophilic substitution served as a basis for further attempts to increase radiochemical yields, to shorten reaction times and to simplify the synthetic strategy.

Besides the toxic Kryptofix®, tetrabutyl ammonium hydroxide can also be used as the phase transfer catalyst. Especially remarkable in this respect is the solid-phase reaction of Toorongian et al. (1990) [37], which has found entry into commercial [^{18}F]FDG synthesis modules.

As an alternative to acid hydrolysis which had already been used by Pacàk in 1969 [26] in his first synthesis of [^{18}F]FDG and which had been taken over into all subsequent synthetic strategies, Füchtner et al. (1995) [26] suggested an alkaline hydrolysis. This results in the cleavage of the protecting groups already at room temperature with shorter reaction times. Alkaline hydrolysis requires a strict control of both temperature and reaction time to prevent a loss of radiochemical yields by decomposition. With this synthesis, 2-[^{18}F]-fluoro-2-deoxy-D-mannose is formed to a minor extent (up to 5%).

6.4 Validated methods for synthesizing [^{18}F]FDG

The currently authorized methods are described in detail in the pharmacopoeia (European Pharmacopoeia 1999).

The only authorized practicable *electrophilic* synthesis of [^{18}F]FDG is the conversion of [^{18}F]acetylhypofluorite with TAG in $CFCl_3$ as proposed by Bida et al. in 1984 [2]. For preparing ^{18}F, a gas mixture of neon with 0.2% fluorine is irradiated. The target gas is passed through a cartridge with sodium acetate ($NaOAc \cdot 3H_2O$). The resulting [^{18}F]acetylhypofluorite is passed into a solution of the precursor containing 45–50 mg TAG in 20 ml $CFCl_3$. The reaction already takes place at room temperature while the gas stream is passed into the solution. The solvent is distilled off at 60 °C. After hydrolysis with 1 ml 1.0 N hydrochloric acid (10 min, 125 °C), the solution containing the product is taken up with 9 ml water and is passed through an ion retardation cartridge (AG11 A8). The separation of partially hydrolyzed compounds is performed with a C-18-SepPak cartridge. The solution is isotonically adjusted with 90 mg NaCl and sterile filtered. Besides 2-[^{18}F]FDG, this synthesis also yields about 5% of 2-[^{18}F]FDM.

The most frequently used method for preparing [^{18}F]FDG is the *nucleophilic* synthesis according to Hamacher et al. [17]. The synthesis starts with the separation of the [^{18}F]fluoride from the ^{18}O-water via an anion exchanger. The [^{18}F]F$^-$ is eluated into a sigradur reaction vessel with a K_2CO_3 solution. Acetonitrile and phase transfer catalyst are added. The solvents are evaporated at 85 °C with a helium gas stream to absolute absence of water. The [^{18}F]fluoride is only weakly bound to the remaining aminopolyether-complexed potassium carbonate. Due to the solubility of the aminopolyether complex in organic solvents, the [^{18}F]F$^-$ is available for nucleophilic substitutions of 1,3,4,6-tetra-O-acetyl-2-trifluormethane-sulfonyl-β-D-manno-pyranose in acetonitrile. The substitution of the trifluormethane-sulfonyl group by the [^{18}F]F$^-$ results in the intermediate 1,3,4,6-tetra-O-acetyl-2-[^{18}F]fluoro-β-D-manno-pyranose.

In order to separate the phase transfer catalyst, the reaction mixture was originally concentrated to a smaller volume, taken up with a surplus of water and passed through a SepPak-C-18 cartridge. The aminopolyether was eluted with 0.1 N hydrochloric acid and the protected sugar was transferred back into the reaction vessel with tetrahydrofuran (THF). After removal of the THF, the acid hydrolysis with 1 ml 1 N hydrochloric acid followed (15 min, 130 °C). The solution was diluted with water and passed through a column containing ion retarding resin (AG11 A8) and neutral aluminum oxide for neutralization. The aluminum oxide was used for separating [^{18}F]fluoride. The neutral solution was isotonically adjusted with NaCl and filtered sterilely. By using various solid-phase extraction cartridges, the separation of the phase transfer catalyst as described above can be eliminated.

The phase transfer-catalyzed nucleophilic substitution according to Toorongian et al. [37] is not performed in a reaction vessel but on specially prepared ion-exchange material. The phase transfer-catalyzing ion exchanger is prepared by addition of 4-(4-methyl-1-piperidino)pyridine to "Merrifield's Resin", an ion exchanger on the basis of polystyrene. Subsequently, the resin is transferred into the carbonate form. For the application of this method, an apparatus was developed that is run with a single-use cassette. The cassette contains all solvent and gas transfer pipelines, the ion exchange column and the vessel for hydrolysis. Before the cassette is attached to the apparatus, the vials with the solvents and the precursor are fixed into position. By attaching the cassette to the apparatus, the connection with the target water pipeline and those for the transport gas and the outlet air are made. In order to attain the reaction temperatures, the ion-exchange column and the vessel for hydrolysis are embedded in a heating block for the duration of the synthesis. First, the [^{18}F]F$^-$ is fixed on the ion exchanger at room temperature. Adhering water is displaced by dry acetonitrile. 1,3,4,6-tetra-O-acetyl-2-trifluormethane-sulfonyl-β-D-manno-pyranose (20 mg), dissolved in dry acetonitrile, is slowly passed through the ion exchanger that was heated to 85 °C. The reaction solution reaches the vessel for hydrolysis, where the acetonitrile is evaporated by heating in a gas stream. Subsequently, the hydrolysis with 2 ml 1.0 N hydrochloric acid takes place for 15 min at 130 °C. The solution is neutralized by addition of 10 ml of a sodium hydrogenphosphate solution. Finally, the solution is passed through a C-18-SepPak cartridge, an alumina-N-SepPak cartridge and a sterile filter into a sterile vessel. The advantage of this method lies in the easy handling of the single-use cassette. After a synthesis, the module is ready to be used again in a very short time without any cleaning process.

6.5 [^{18}F]FDG quality control

The aim of quality control is to supply a product that is physiologically absolutely safe. The European Pharmacopoeia 1997/99 lists the various syntheses, the characterizations and the respective methods of quality control for 2-[^{18}F]FDG. Also listed are the permissible concentrations of the constituents in milligram per dose. Quality control of [^{18}F]FDG can be divided into three sectors:

- analysis of the chemical composition
- determination of radiochemical data
- bacteriologic examination

The chemical composition is investigated with several chromatographic procedures: the determination of the glucose content is achieved by high-performance liquid chromatography (HPLC). The determination of the radiochemical purity is performed parallel to this. In the course of the synthesis, not only [^{18}F]FDG but also glucose and, depending on the synthetic method, 2-chloro-2-deoxy-D-glucose (2-ClDG) in the case of an acid hydrolysis and 2-[^{18}F]FDM in the case of an alkaline hydrolysis are formed. The analytic separation of those very similar compounds places high demands on the chromatographic technology. A very alkaline anion-exchange column on a polystyrene basis with 0.1 N NaOH as the mobile phase has proved successful. The various monosaccharides are then characterized using an RI detector (differential refractometer). A maximum of 10 mg per dose for [^{18}F]FDG and 2 mg per dose of 2-ClDG is allowed.

Besides the glucose derivatives, it is also necessary to test for any residue of the employed phase transfer catalyst. This is mostly performed by means of chromatographical methods, too. Thin layer chromatography is used for detecting potential residues of the aminopolyether (Kryptofix®). A defined volume of the product solution (e.g., 2 μl) is applied to a plate next to a spot of a reference solution containing the phase transfer catalyst in a concentration near the permissible limit of 2.2 mg per dose. The plate is then developed over a path of 8 cm using a mixture of 1 volume of ammonia and 9 volumes of methanol. After drying it for about 15 min in air, the plate is exposed to iodine vapor, which makes the aminopolyether spots visible. The intensity of the spots is a measure for the Kryptofix® concentration of the solution. This allows for the determination by visual comparison of the aminopolyether concentration of the product solution.

Tetraalkyl ammonium salt residues are examined by HPLC. An aliquot of the product solution is eluted with a mixture of 25% 0.05 N toluene sulfonic acid and 75% acetonitrile from an analytical RP-18 column. The presence of tetraalkyl ammonium salts is detected by a spectrophotometer set at 254 nm. Quantification is achieved by peak-size analysis. The UV detector is calibrated with standard solutions of the compound with concentrations around the admissible maximum of 2.75 mg per dose.

The solid-phase reaction according to Toorongian can lead to residues of 4-(4-methylpiperidino)pyridine in the product solution. They can be detected by an UV detector set at 263 nm. The absorption is dependent on the concentration and can be compared to a standard solution of this compound whose concentration is equivalent to the limit of 0.02 mg per dose.

Possible residues of solvents like methanol, ethanol and acetonitrile are detected through gas chromatography and quantified through peak-size analysis. Calibration is performed with standard solutions containing the respective solvent in a concentration near the permissible limit. The maximum amount of acetonitrile is 4.1 mg per dose.

Analogously to the chemical purity, the radiochemical purity of the product is determined via HPLC with a suitable activity detector. The calculated peak areas correspond to the percent composition of the total activity. $[^{18}F]$-fluoride, partial hydrolysates, 2-$[^{18}F]$FDG and 2-$[^{18}F]$FDM can be detected. $[^{18}F]$FDG and $[^{18}F]$FDM together must represent up more than 95% of the activity, the $[^{18}F]$FDM share of this being at most $1/10^{th}$. As an alternative to HPLC, the radiochemical purity can also be determined by thin layer chromatography on a silica plate with an eluent consisting of 95% acetonitrile and 5% water. The analysis is performed with a TLC scanner.

Because the amount of $[^{18}F]$FDG is below the detection level of the RI detectors used, the specific radioactivity must be exactly determined with special detection systems, e.g., an EC detector. Due to the minimum detection limit of the used RI detector being known, the volume activity is a minimum value for the specific activity (in MBq/mmol).

Radionuclidic purity can be determined by a determination of the half-life or by recording the gamma-ray spectrum.

According to the Pharmacopoeia, the absence of bacterial endotoxins is confirmed by controlling the temperature of rabbits which have had an i.v. injection of the solution to be tested. A permitted alternative to this method is the limulus-amoebocytes-lysate test (LAL). For testing the endotoxin concentration of the product solution, an extract of the blood cells of horseshoe crabs is used. This extract becomes turbid and coagulates if even a small amount of bacteriologic endotoxins is present, resulting in a change of the optical density. The rate of the turbidity development up to a threshold value is called reaction time. It is detected with a photodiode and it is proportional to the endotoxin concentration. The reaction time is compared to LAL-standard solutions of known endotoxin concentrations close to the maximal permissible value, which is 175 pg/ml.

The sterility of the product solution is affirmed if a suitable nutrient medium for bacteria and fungi shows no signs of microbial growth after an incubation period of seven days.

References

[1] Adamson J, Foster AB, Hall LD, Johnson RN, Hesse RH (1970) Fluorinated carbohydrates. Carbohyd Res 15:351–359

[2] Bida GT, Satyamurthy N, Barrio JR (1984) The synthesis of 2-[^{18}F]Fluoro-2-deoxy-D-glucose using glycals: a reexamination. J Nucl Med 25:1327–1334

[3] Blomqvist G, Bergström K, Bergstrom M, Elvin E, Eriksson L, Garmelius B, Lindberg B, Lilja A, Litton JE, Lundmark L, Lundqvist H, Malmberg P, Moström U, Nilsson L, Stone-Elander S, Widén L (1985) Models for ^{11}C-glucose. In: Greitz T, Ingvar DH, Widén L (eds) The Metabolism of the Brain Studied with Positron Emission Tomography. Raven Press, New York, pp 185–194

[4] Brøndsted HE, Gjedde A (1988) Measuring brain glucose phosphorylation with labeled glucose. Am J Physiol 254:E443–E448

[5] Clark JC, Silvester DJ (1966) A cyclotron method for the production of fluorine-18. Int J Appl Radiat Isot 17:151–154

[6] Conti PS, Liliern DL, Hawley K, Keppler J, Grafton ST, Bading JR (1996) PET and [^{18}F]-FDG in oncology: a clinical update. Nucl Med Biol 23:717–735

[7] Cunningham VJ, Cremer JE (1981) A method for the simultaneous estimation of regional rates of glucose influx and phosphorylation in rat brain using radio-labelled 2-deoxy-glucose. Brain Res 221:319–330

[8] Dubridge LA, Barnes SW, Buck JH (1937) Letters to the editor, proton induced radioactivity in oxygen. Phys Rev 51:995

[9] European Pharmacopoeia 3rd Edition (1997) Radiopharmaceutical Preparations. pp 1424–1433

[10] European Pharmacopoeia 3rd Edition, Supplement (1999). pp 515–518 (abstr)

[11] Evans AC (1987) A double integral form of the three-compartmental, four-rate-constant model for faster generation of parameter maps. J Cereb Blood Flow Metab 7 (Suppl 1):S453

[12] Füchtner F, Steinbach J, Mäding P, Johannsen B (1996) Basic hydrolysis of 2-[^{18}F] fluoro-1,3,4,6-tetra-O-acetyl-D-glucose in the preparation of 2-[^{18}F]Fluoro-2-deoxy-D-glucose. Appl Radiat Isot 47:61–66

[13] Gaitonde MK (1965) Rate of utilization of glucose and 'compartmentation' of α-oxoglutarate and glutamate in rat brain. Biochem J 95:803–810

[14] Gallagher BM, Fowler JS, Gutterson NI, MacGregor RR, Wan CN, Wolf AP (1978) Metabolic trapping as a principle of radiopharmaceutical design: some factors responsible for the biodistribution of [18-F] 2-deoxy-2-fluoro-D-glucose. J Nucl Med 19:1154–1161

[15] Gatley SJ, Shaughnessy WJ (1982) Production of ^{18}F-labeled compounds with ^{18}F^{-} produced with a 1-MW research reactor. Int J Appl Radiat Isot 33:1325–1330

[16] Gjedde A (1995) Glucose metabolism. In: Wagner HN, Szabo Z, Buchanan JW (eds) Principles of Nuclear Medicine, 2nd Edition. W. B. Saunders, Philadelphia

[17] Hamacher K, Coenen HH, Stöcklin G (1986) Efficient stereospecific synthesis of no-carrier added 2-[^{18}F]-fluoro-2-deoxy-D-glucose using aminopolyether supported nucleophilic substitution. J Nucl Med 27:235–238

[18] Hawkins R, Miller AL, Cremer JE, Veech RL (1974) Measurement of regional brain glucose utilization by rat brain in vivo. J Neurochem 23:917–923

[19] Hawkins R, Hass K, Ransohoff J (1979) Measurement of regional brain glucose utilization in vivo using [2-^{14}C]glucose. Stroke 10:690–703

[20] Hawkins R, Mans AM, Davis DW, Vina JR, Hubbard LS (1985) Cerebral glucose use measured with [^{14}C]glucose labeled in the 1, 2, or 6 position. Am J Physiol 248:C170–C176

[21] Ido T, Wan CN, Casella V, Fowler JS, Wolf AP (1978) Labeled 2-deoxy-D-glucose analogs. ^{18}F-labeled 2-deoxy-2-fluoro-D-glucose, 2-deoxy-2-fluoro-D-mannose and ^{14}C-2-deoxy-2-fluoro-D-glucose. J Label Comp Radiopharm 14:175–183

[22] Kuwabara H, Evans AC, Gjedde A (1990) Michaelis-Menten constraints improved cerebral glucose metabolism and regional lumped constant measurements with [^{18}F] fluorodeoxyglucose. J Cereb Blood Flow Metab 10:180–189

[23] Kuwabara H, Gjedde A (1991) Measurements of glucose phosphorylation with FDG and PET are not reduced by dephosphorylation of FDG-6-phosphate. J Nucl Med 32:692–698

[24] Levy S, Elmaleh DR, Livni E (1982) A new method using anhydrous [^{18}F]fluoride to radiolabel 2-[^{18}F]fluoro-2-deoxy-D-glucose. J Nucl Med 23:918–922

[25] Nickles RJ, Gatley SJ, Votaw JR, Kornguth ML (1986) Fluorine radiopharmaceuticals. Production of reactive fluorine-18. Appl Radiat Isot 37:649–661

[26] Pacàk J, Tocík Z, Cerný M (1969) Synthesis of 2-deoxy-2-fluoro-D-glucose. Chem Comm 77

[27] Phelps ME, Huang SC, Hoffman EJ, Selin C, Sokoloff L, Kuhl DE (1979) Tomographic measurement of local cerebral glucose metabolic rate in humans with 2-[^{18}F]fluoro-2-deoxy-D-glucose: validation of method. Ann Neurol 6:371–388

[28] Qaim SM, Clark JC, Crouzel C, Guillaume M, Helmeke HJ, Nebeling B, Pike VW, Stöcklin G (1993) PET radionuclide production. In: Stöcklin G, Pike VW (eds) Radiopharmaceuticals for Positron Emission Tomography. Methodological Aspects. Kluwer Academic Publishers, pp 1–46

[29] Reivich M, Kuhl D, Wolf A, Greenberg J, Phelps M, Ido T, Casella V, Folwer-Hoffman E, Alavi A, Som P, Sokoloff L (1979) The [^{18}F]fluoro-deoxyglucose method for the measurement of local cerebral glucose utilization of man. Circ Res 44:127–137

[30] Reivich M, Alavi A, Wolf A, Fowler J, Russell J, Arnett C, MacGregor RR, Shine CY, Atkins H, Anand A (1985) Glucose metabolic rate kinetic model parameter determination in humans: the lumped constants and rate constants for [^{18}F] fluorodeoxyglucose and [^{11}C]deoxyglucose. J Cereb Blood Flow Metab 5:179–192

[31] Rigo P, Paulus P, Kaschten BJ, Hustinx R, Bury T, Jerusalem G, Benoit T, Foidart-Willems J (1996) Oncological applications of positron emission tomography with fluorine-18 fluorodeoxyglucose. Eur J Nucl Med 23:1641–1674

[32] Schmidt KC, Lucignani G, Sokoloff L (1996) Fluorine-18-fluorodeoxyglucose PET to determine regional cerebral glucose utilisation: a re-examination. J Nucl Med 37:394–399

[33] Snell AH (1937) A new radioisotope of fluorine. Phys Rev 51:143

[34] Sokoloff L, Reivich M, Kennedy C, des Rosiers MH, Patlak CS, Pettigrew KD, Sakurada O, Shinohara M (1977) The [^{14}C]deoxyglucose method for the measurement of local cerebral glucose utilization: theory, procedure, and normal values in the conscious and anesthetized albino rat. J Neurochem 28:897–916

[35] Som P, Atkins HL, Bandoypadhyay D, Fowler JS, MacGregor RR, Matsui K, Oster ZH, Sacker DF, Shiue CY, Turner H, Wan CN, Zabinski SV (1980) A fluorinated glucose analog, 2-fluoro-2-deoxy-D-glucose (F-18): nontoxic tracer for rapid tumor detection. J Nucl Med 21:670–675

[36] Tewson JT (1983) Synthesis of no-carrier-added fluorine-18 2-fluoro-2-deoxy-D-glucose. J Nucl Med 24:718–721

[37] Toorongian SA, Mulholland GK, Jewett DM, Bachelor MA, Kilbourn MR (1990) Routine production of 2-deoxy-2-[^{18}F]fluoro-D-glucose by direct nucleophilic exchange on a quaternary 4-aminopyridinium resin. Nucl Med Biol 17:273–279

[38] Warburg O (1925) Über den Stoffwechsel der Carcinomzelle. Klin Wochenschr Berl 4:534–536

7 Current developments of ^{18}F-labeled PET tracers in oncology

F. Rösch, H.-J. Wester, T.R. DeGrado

7.1 Introduction

2-[^{18}F]Fluoro-2-deoxy-D-glucose (2-[^{18}F]FDG or FDG) is by far the most frequently used PET tracer in nuclear medical diagnostics. The high sensitivity of FDG PET to detect oncologic disease reflects an increased rate of glycolysis or/and glucose transport in most neoplasms relative to normal tissues. However, from a biochemical point of view FDG is not an ideal means of diagnosis because both normal and neoplastic cells metabolize glucose. As the metabolism of a tumor cell does not generally differ from that of a normal cell, other metabolic oncologic tracers also cannot be judged by exclusivity (i.e., accumulation solely in the tumor cell, no accumulation in normal cells) either. Furthermore, the metabolic rate, i.e., glucose consumption, is not a sensitive parameter in characteristically slow growing neoplasms, such as prostate cancer. Thus, tracers based on other biochemical concepts are valuable tools in nuclear medicinal diagnosis (for an overview see [120]). The development of the adequate selective tracers, which will allow deeper insight to tumor biochemistry from outside the human body using PET, is one of the most active areas in current radiopharmaceutical research.

This chapter will mainly focus on the following approaches:

• metabolism of carbohydrates:	glycolysis versus transport of glucose
• cell proliferation:	DNA building blocks
• amino acid transport and peptide synthesis:	amino acids
• receptors:	peptides and steroids
• cell oxygenation:	hypoxia tracers
• metabolism of bones:	tracers with affinity to hydroxylapatite

Due to the variety of approaches and tracers, this brief and inevitable incomplete survey of oncologic PET tracers will be confined to ^{18}F-labeled compounds and concepts with proven clinical relevance or outstanding potential except for 2-[^{18}F]FDG, for which the radiochemistry and radiopharmacology is described in chapter 6 in detail. In contrast to other "organic" PET isotopes such as ^{15}O, ^{13}N and ^{11}C, the physical half-life of fluorine-18 ($T_{1/2}$ = 109.7 min) is compatible to most of the biochemical pathways in tumor physiology and biochemistry. Furthermore, the feasibility of distributing ^{18}F-labeled tumor diagnostics within the frame of a satellite system makes these tracers also accessible for PET centers without an on-site cyclotron.

7.2 Analogs of 2-[^{18}F]fluoro-2-deoxy-D-glucose

Identical to glucose, 2-[^{18}F]fluoro-2-deoxy-D-glucose (2-[^{18}F]FDG) is actively transported through the cellular membrane by glucose transporter proteins (GLUT) and is subsequently phosphorylated to 2-[^{18}F]FDG-6-phosphate by the enzyme hexokinase. In contrast to glucose-6-phosphate, 2-[^{18}F]FDG-6-phosphate is not a substrate for phosphoglucose isomerase and does not take part in subsequent reactions of the glycolytic pathway. In parallel, 2-[^{18}F]FDG-6-phosphate cannot leave the cell, neither by transport nor by diffusion: it is metabolically trapped.

Today, the most widely used production route to 2-[^{18}F]FDG consists of kryptofix 2.2.2-mediated nucleophilic substitution (^{18}F for trifluoromethane sulfonate) on 1,3,4,6-tetra-O-acetyl-2-O-trifluoromethane sulfonyl-β-D-manno-pyranose in the presence of potassium carbonate [50]. Hydrolysis of the protected intermediate and chromatographic purification gives epimeric pure 2-[^{18}F]FDG in about 50% yield in about 50 min from end-of-bombardment, cf. chapter 6.

In brain, the glucose phosphorylation rate is mainly determined by hexokinase activity rather than glucose transport rate. In tumors, changes in transport rate via modulation of expression of the glucose transporters can influence the accumulation of 2-[^{18}F]FDG as well [18, 21, 59, 135, 136, 145]. In order to quantify the contribution of glucose transporters to the accumulation of 2-[^{18}F]FDG in tumors, tracers are needed which have no substrate

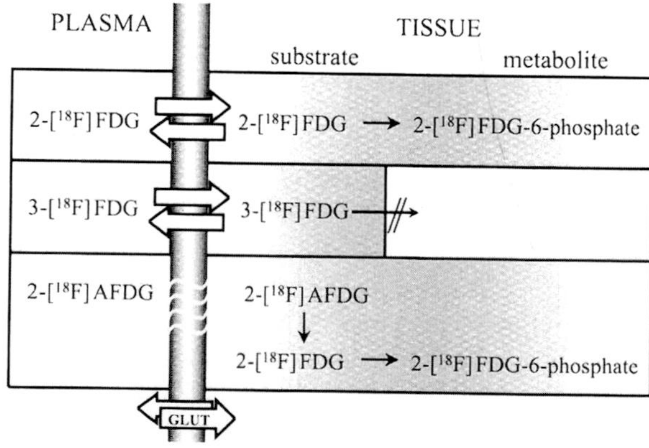

Fig. 7.1. Schematic metabolism of ^{18}F-labeled glucose analogs.

specificity for hexokinase or pass the cell membrane independently of glucose carriers and are phosphorylated analogously to glucose. A representative of the first concept which has been known for some time is 3-[^{18}F]FDG, which is transported into the cell but is not metabolized, similar to 3-O-[^{11}C]methyl-D-glucose. It undergoes subsequent backdiffusion from the cells to the plasma in a non-phosphorylated, i.e., chemically intact state [133]. For the second concept, tetra-acetylated 2-[^{18}F]FDG (1,3,4,6-tetra-acetyl-2-[^{18}F]fluoro-2-deoxy-D-glucose, 2-[^{18}F]AFDG) is a promising candidate [58, 133–137]. Due to its lipophilicity, 2-[^{18}F]AFDG passes through the membrane via diffusion. There it is hydrolyzed to 2-[^{18}F]FDG and subsequently accumulated in the cell like 2-[^{18}F]FDG itself (cf. Fig. 7.1). Because 2-[^{18}F]AFDG is an intermediate in the nucleophilic synthesis of 2-[^{18}F]FDG [50], the synthesis of 2-[^{18}F]AFDG can be performed with commercially available modules – radiochemical yields are above 60%.

7.3 Amino Acids

Amino acids play an important role in a variety of physiological processes, such as protein syntheses, neurotransmission and intercellular communication (for an overview see [86] and references therein). Since cell proliferation and the growth of the extracellular matrix and connective tissue is linked to increased amino acid utilization at neoplasmic foci, targeting of amino acid

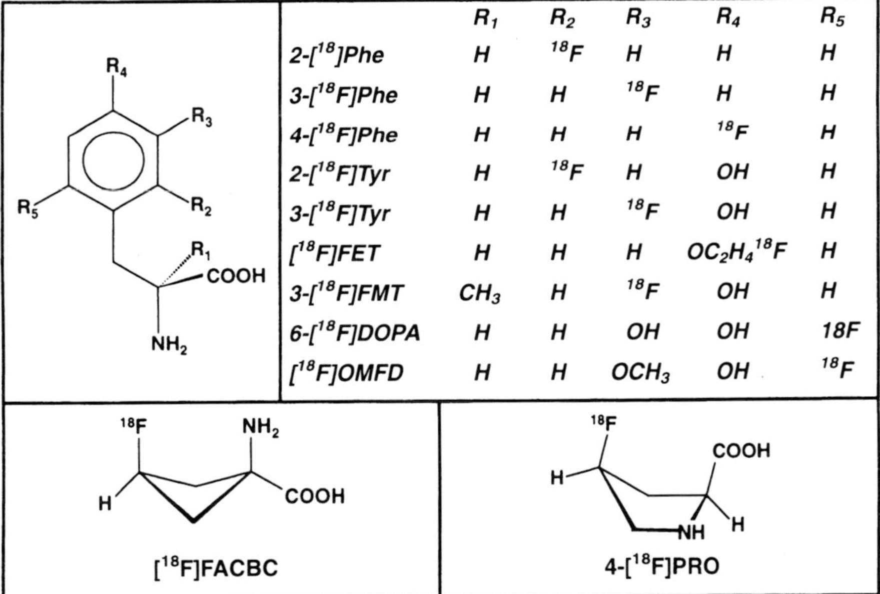

	R_1	R_2	R_3	R_4	R_5
2-[18]Phe	H	^{18}F	H	H	H
3-[^{18}F]Phe	H	H	^{18}F	H	H
4-[^{18}F]Phe	H	H	H	^{18}F	H
2-[^{18}F]Tyr	H	^{18}F	H	OH	H
3-[^{18}F]Tyr	H	H	^{18}F	OH	H
[^{18}F]FET	H	H	H	$OC_2H_4{}^{18}F$	H
3-[^{18}F]FMT	CH_3	H	^{18}F	OH	H
6-[^{18}F]DOPA	H	H	OH	OH	18F
[^{18}F]OMFD	H	H	OCH_3	OH	^{18}F

Fig. 7.2. ^{18}F-labeled amino acids proposed for measuring amino acid transport and protein synthesis rate in vivo.

transport and the measurement of regional protein synthesis rate (rPSR) are important biochemical concepts in the application of PET in oncology.

For this purpose a variety of ^{18}F-labeled amino acids were synthesized and evaluated (Fig. 7.2).

Due to their high brain uptake, predominantly tyrosine and phenylalanine were labeled with ^{18}F so far. L-2-[^{18}F]phenylalanine (L-2-[^{18}F]Phe) [10, 22, 23], the preferentially formed isomer in direct electrophilic fluorination of phenylalanine [24, 98] with about 20% radiochemical yield, takes part in protein synthesis but also undergoes partial metabolization [10, 22, 23, 100]. L-2-[^{18}F]Phe was evaluated as a tracer for neutral amino acid transport using two- and three-compartment models [64, 79, 80, 102]. The two other isomers, L-3-[^{18}F]Phe and L-4-[^{18}F]Phe are formed in the above mentioned reaction with radiochemical yields of 2–4%, depending on the use of [^{18}F]F_2 or CH_3COO[^{18}F]F [23, 24]. Due to the high toxicity ($LD_{50,mice}=5.9$ mg/kg) of L-3-[^{18}F]Phe [see 27 and references therein] and the high amount of carrier after electrophilic [^{18}F]-fluorination, no in vivo studies were carried out using this isomer. In contrast, the para- and ortho-isomers are well tolerated in vivo. Compared to Phe, the enzymatic hydroxylation of L-4-[^{18}F]Phe is slow [73]. However, its slow protein incorporation of only about 60% at 120 min postinjection and the formation of unidentified metabolites of L-4-[^{18}F]-Phe in considerable amounts [10, 7], which interferes kinetic modeling, are drawbacks of this tracer.

Compared to L-4-[^{18}F]Phe, L-3-[^{18}F]tyrosine (L-3-[^{18}F]Tyr) is incorporated into cerebral proteins to a somewhat higher extent [25]. Again, compared to the ortho-isomer, the meta-isomer exhibits significantly higher toxicity. Cerebral protein incorporation of L-2-[^{18}F]Tyr is fast and reaches >80% at 60 min [26]. In the brain, no metabolites were observed besides in the striatum, whereas peripherally L-2-[^{18}F]Tyr is partially defluorinated. Considering the high brain uptake, the high protein bound portion of L-2-[^{18}F]Tyr, its irreversibility with respect to the time scale of a PET study and the lack of significant amounts of metabolites in the brain, L-2-[^{18}F]Tyr fulfills all requirements for the quantitation of the regional protein synthesis rate in vivo.

While 2-[^{18}F]Phe is predominantly formed upon the electrophilic ^{18}F-fluorination of Phe using [^{18}F]F_2 or AcO[^{18}F], mainly the 3-isomer is formed in the case of tyrosine [22]. Acetylation of the phenol group increases fluorination of the 2-position. This approach leads to a radiochemical yield of about 10% in 2-[^{18}F]Tyr. 4-[^{18}F]Phe can be prepared by ^{18}F-fluorodemetallation with about 25% yield [23].

Production of no-carrier-added ^{18}F-fluorinated aromatic amino acids can be carried out via multistep synthesis [82]. To overcome the formation of the undesired D-enantiomers, asymmetric syntheses using a chiral inductor were developed. The enantiomeric excess obtained are up to >96%. Syntheses are completed in about 125 min with radiochemical yields of 11–17% [83] and up to a 25% radiochemical yield was observed using a chiral catalytic phase transfer alkylation procedure [83].

Because in vivo evaluation and kinetic modeling of the amino acid uptake in the tumor indicates that transport is the dominating accumulation process while the irreversible trapping is of minor importance [63, 86, 144], artificial amino acids not incorporated into proteins are also useful tracers in oncology. Among the artificial amino acids, O-(2-[^{18}F]fluoroethyl)-L-tyrosine ([^{18}F]FET) seems to be the most promising tracer [142]. While most fluorine-18-labeled amino acids are prepared via electrophilic, carrier-added synthesis with yields less than 20%, no carrier-added (nca) [^{18}F]FET can be produced with >40% radiochemical yield via nucleophilic ^{18}F-fluorination of bis-tosyloxyethane and subsequent alkylation of unprotected L-tyrosine or direct nucleophilic fluorination of a protected precursor and subsequent deprotection. The brain uptake of L-[^{18}F]FET, which is transported mainly by the amino acid transport system L [57], into mice brain was shown to be stereoselective, fast and reached levels of >2% ID/g 60 min postinjection [142]. Neither protein incorporation, nor metabolites were observed in plasma and tissue samples and no considerable in vivo defluorination was found (<1.7–2.2%ID/g in mice at all time points up to 120 min). L-[^{18}F]FET is predominantly cleared via the kidneys without considerable accumulation in peripheral organs and nontumor tissue. Preliminary human studies indicate that the uptake of L-[^{18}F]FET in recurrent brain tumors is closely correlated to the uptake of L-methyl-[^{11}C]methionine ([^{11}C]MET) [138]. Furthermore, preliminary in vivo studies in mice indicate that both [^{11}C]MET and [^{18}F]FDG are accumulated in stimulated lymph nodes and tumor-invaded lymph nodes, whereas L-[^{18}F]FET only accumulates in tumor-invaded lymph nodes [95]. Based on the present available data and the ease of synthesis, L-[^{18}F]FET is a promising tracer for imaging cerebral [138], and possibly peripheral tumors [65].

Another artificial amino acid, 3-[^{18}F]fluoro-α-methyl-tyrosine (3-[^{18}F]FMT), is produced via electrophilic fluorination with 10% radiochemical yield (based on [^{18}F]F_2) [61, 124]. The clearance from the circulation is fast but a considerable renal uptake of about 24%ID/g and 17%ID/g 30 and 60 min p.i., respectively, remarkably increases the radiation dose to the whole body (about 45 μSv/MBq 3-[^{18}F]FMT versus 24 μSv/MBq 2-[^{18}F]FDG). Metabolization was quantified with 22% in human plasma at 60 min postinjection and 13% in the urine [62]. Although the first human studies provided high contrast PET images [63], the suitability of this tracer may be limited by low syntheses yields, dosimetric considerations and metabolic instability.

6-[^{18}F]DOPA and one of its metabolites, 3-O-methyl-6-[^{18}F]DOPA [40], were also proposed as tumor imaging agents [56]. While only one study was reported with the former compound, the latter one is presently being evaluated.

Furthermore, two aliphatic amino acids have been labeled with fluorine-18: 1-amino-3-[^{18}F]fluorocyclobutane-1-carboxylic acid ([^{18}F]FACBC) for brain tumor imaging [117] and 4-[^{18}F]fluoroproline (4-[^{18}F]Pro) [51] as a potential marker of pathological nonregulated collagen synthesis [52, 72]. Both compounds are prepared via nucleophilic fluorination and subsequent acidic deprotection. [^{18}F]FACBC (12% radiochemical yield, 60 min) exhibits low brain uptake and is accumulated in a variety of organs including lung, kidney, spleen and liver. High tumor to brain ratios of 5.6 and 6.6 at 5 min and 60 min postinjection, respectively, are observed in rats bearing intracerebrally implanted gliosarcomas. [^{18}F]FACBC uptake in rat brain is found to be the lowest of all organs [117]. This suggests that [^{18}F]FACBC is selectively excluded from the brain by the blood-brain barrier (BBB), which will significantly affect the suitability of this tracer for imaging of brain tumors with an intact BBB.

Racemic 4-fluoroproline has been labeled [127] and proposed in diastereomeric pure form (4-[^{18}F]PRO) as a physiological marker of collagen synthesis [51]. Both isomers, cis- and trans-4-[^{18}F]PRO, exhibit high in vivo stability towards degradation and defluorination [54]. Speciation studies revealed protein incorporation only for cis-4-[^{18}F]PRO. Quantitative analysis of protein bound activity at 240 min p.i. indicated about 70% protein incorporation [143]. Preliminary studies in patients with clear cell renal cancer relevant-cis-4-[^{18}F]PRO accumulation was observed, but no or non-diagnostic 2-[^{18}F]FDG accumulation was detected [16]. Further studies are needed to evaluate this tracer for peripheral tumors [14, 15] and to elucidate the suitability of this tracer for differentiating amino acid transport from normal protein synthesis and collagen synthesis.

7.4 DNA building blocks

7.4.1 5-[^{18}F]Fluorouracil

An example for direct labeling of the pyrimidine moiety is [^{18}F]fluorouracil (5-[^{18}F]FU) (cf. Fig. 7.3). It also reveals the interest in the respective antimetabolites which are employed as chemotherapeutics (cytarabine, idoxuridine, 5-fluorouracil). 5-Fluorouracil is anabolically metabolized to 5-fluoro-2′-deoxyuridine-monophosphate, which blocks the *thymidylate synthetase*, an en-

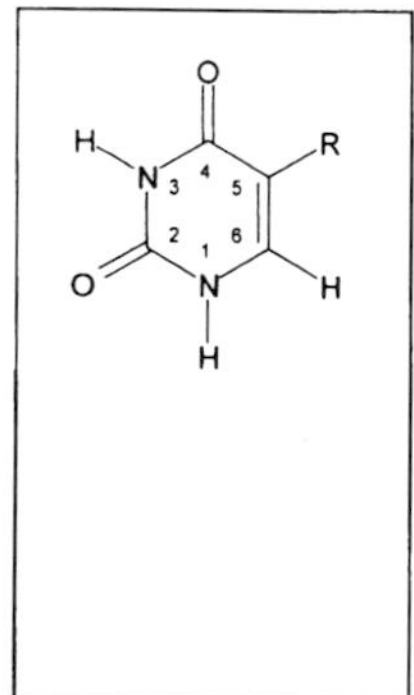

R = H: uracil
R = ^{18}F:
5-[^{18}F]fluorouracil

R = OH: thymidine
R = ^{18}F:
3′-deoxy-3-[^{18}F]fluorothymidine

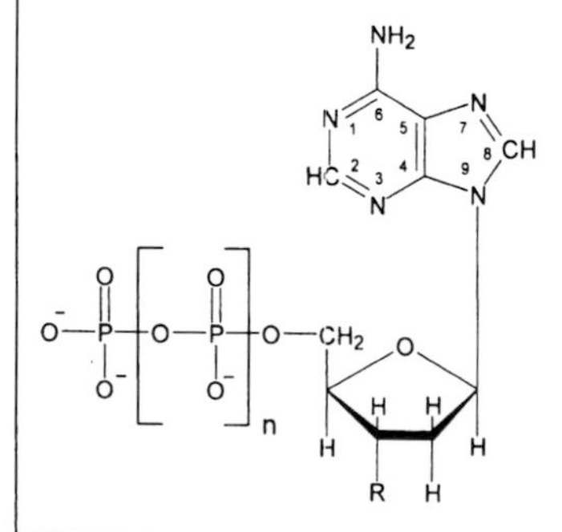

adenosine-5′-phosphate
(n = 0,1,2: mono-, di-, triphosphate)

Fig. 7.3. Examples of nucleic acids, nucleosides and nucleotides.

zyme necessary for methylating 2′-deoxyuridine-monophosphate to thymidine. This results in an inhibition of the thymidine synthesis and thus in a breakdown of DNA synthesis [17]. The corresponding PET tracer 5-[^{18}F]FU is catabolized in the liver to β-fluoroaniline and is accumulated in hepatic metastases of colorectal tumors. 5-[^{18}F]FU can nevertheless be used for controlling the efficacy of a chemotherapy with 5-fluorouracil [33–35]. Syntheses of 5-[^{18}F]FU have been established for some time [39, 130] and optimized more recently [19].

7.4.2 Nucleosides

The nucleosides adenosine, guanosine [75], cytidine, uridine [29] and thymidine are derived by coupling the respective nucleotide base with the sugar ribose or deoxyribose (cf. Fig. 7.3). An example for direct labeling of the pyrimidine moiety is 3′-deoxy-3′-[^{18}F]fluorothymidine ([^{18}F]FLT) (cf. Fig. 7.3). Following its uptake, [^{18}F]FLT is phosphorylated by *thymidine kinase 1* and accumulated in the cell. The accumulation effect is a measure for the cellular *thymidine kinase* activity, which is in turn directly correlated to the cell's proliferation. The presently used synthesis for [^{18}F]FLT yields only about 10% [46, 114, 115]. On the other hand, there have been successful PET studies conducted on human subjects with activities of less than 185 MBq [116], so that these low yields could possibly be accepted. However, a new synthetic approach has been developed with the advantage of high reproducibility. The radiochemical yields are still below 20%, but the labeling method can easily be performed. Batch yields of 1.6 GBq product ready for injection are obtained in routine production [89].

Acetylated 2′-[^{18}F]fluoro-2′-deoxyarabinose derivatives have been labeled as adenosine analogs and have been successfully tested on animals [67, 68]. Several other ^{18}F-labeled pro-drugs have been developed which are taken up into the cell via active carrier mechanisms and which are phosphorylated to yield nucleotides (normally the triphosphate). There are several interesting antimetabolites which have resulted from the development of new proliferation tracers for PET. These are incorporated into the DNA as nucleoside analogs and are employed as chemotherapeutics (cytarabine, fludarabine, cladribine, gemcitabine and others).

In gene therapy, transduction of neoplastic cells can lead to higher sensitivity towards specific antiviral agents. Thus, *herpes simplex virus thymidine kinase* (HSV-tk) catalyzes the phosphorylation of those nucleoside analogs which are usually pure substrates for thymidine kinase in normal cells. Apart from the localization, the quantification of the gene therapy's success, i.e., the amount of HSV-tk expression, is especially interesting for further therapeutic planning. Among the investigated ^{18}F-labeled HSV-tk substrates are 5-[^{18}F]fluorinated ribofuranosyl and -arabinofuranosyl derivatives of uracil [28, 44], [^{18}F]fluoroacyclovir (8-[^{18}F]fluoro-9-((2-hydroxy-ethoxy) methyl)-

guanine) [6], [^{18}F]fluoropenciclovir (9-(4-[^{18}F]fluoro-3-hydroxymethylbutyl)-guanine [3] or 8-[^{18}F]fluoro-9-[4-hydroxy-3-(hydroxymethyl)-1-butyl] guanine [41, 42]), and [^{18}F]fluoroganciclovir (9-(3-[^{18}F]fluoro-1-hydroxy-2-propoxy) methyl)guanine [92–94] or 8-[^{18}F]fluoro-9-[[2-hydroxy-1-(hydroxymethyl)ethoxy]methyl]guanine [5]). 9-(3-[^{18}F]fluoro-1-hydroxy-2-propoxy)-methyl)guanine is selectively phosphorylated by the viral kinase at 63% the rate of thymidine [94]. There is an approximately twofold higher accumulation of the penciclovir analogs relative to the ganciclovir analogs in HSV1-tk-transduced tissues [43]. The radiochemical yields of the [^{18}F]fluoroguanine derivatives are only about 10% [1, 2, 4, 92].

7.4.3 Nucleotides/oligonucleotides/nucleic acids

Esterification of a nucleoside's ribose-5′-hydroxyl function with phosphoric acid yields ribonucleoside monophosphates or nucleotides (cf. Fig. 7.3). Through esterification of the 5′-phosphate function of each monomer with the 3′-hydroxyl moiety of an adjacent monomer, polymers are formed. Smaller chains with up to 30 units are called oligonucleotides. Nucleic acids are the biopolymers made of nucleoside monophosphates. Ribonucleic acid (RNA) is formed of the 4 standard ribonucleoside monophosphates adenosine-5′-, cytidine-5′-, guanosine-5′- and uridine-5′-monophosphate. Deoxyribonucleic acid (DNA) is formed of the deoxyribonucleoside monophosphates of adenine, cytosine, guanine and thymine. 5′-deoxy-5′-[^{18}F]fluorothymidine was conceived as a biochemical analogue to thymidine-5′-monophosphate, which inhibits *thymidine-5′-monophosphate kinase* and thus DNA synthesis as well [131].

Above all, "antisense oligonucleotides" are interesting in oncology for their duplex formation with specific t-RNA regions [36, 37 and others]. At present, radiochemical approaches for labeling complete oligonucleotides in 5′-position [55] are being investigated. Other approaches include [^{18}F]-fluorinated nucleoside components as terminal (e.g., 5′-deoxy-5′-[^{18}F]fluorothymidine [105, 132]) or as intermediate structural units (e.g., via 4-(2-[^{18}F]fluoroethylamino derivatives [31] or via 3′-[^{18}F]fluoro-3′ derivatives [47]).

7.5 Peptides/steroids

Another often used biochemical concept in targeting pathophysiological processes is based on receptor-ligand interactions. For oncological studies, the majority of investigations were focused on the development of synthetic analogues of endogenous peptide hormones. Thus, a variety of radioiodinated and radiometal-labeled peptides were evaluated, and promising results were observed [119]. However, due to the time-consuming multistep ^{18}F-labeling chemistry of peptides the often observed tracer transfer from SPECT to PET and vice versa is somewhat inhibited. In addition, the physical half-life of ^{18}F of 109.7 min somewhat restricts its use for peptide labeling and is too short compared to the pharmacokinetics of many peptides. Labeled antibodies or antibody fragments employed in immunologic diagnostics and therapy exhibit even longer pharmacokinetics. In these cases, positron emitters with a longer half-life would be interesting.

^{18}F-labeling of peptides has to be carried out via prosthetic groups (for a survey compare [119]), which are prepared nearly exclusively by multistep procedures [140]. Thus, for example, an analogue of the α-melanocyte-stimulating hormone ([Nle^4,D-Phe^7]α-MSH) was labeled at Lys^{11} with N-succinimidyl-4-[^{18}F]fluorobenzoate (FB), which did not compromise [^{18}F]FB-α-MSH receptor binding [125]. An analogue of the vasoactive intestinal peptide (VIP-Arg^{15},Arg^{21}) was labeled with N-succinimidyl-4-(4-nitrobenzenesulfonyl)oxomethyl)benzoate, which represents the single currently known ^{18}F-labeled active ester which can be prepared in one step [66, 96]. Using the same reagent, insulin was labeled for studying insulin receptor-ligand interactions in vivo, especially in the liver and kidney [38, 113].

Octreotide is a prominent example of a selective receptor ligand for tumors expressing somatostatin receptors. This octapeptide was labeled via 4-nitrophenyl-2-[^{18}F]fluoropropionate at the N-terminal D-Phe^1 position [49] and evaluated [141] (cf. Fig. 7.4).

A major difference between ^{18}F-labeling of peptides and radiometal-labeled peptides is based on the fate of the label after metabolization or lysosomal degradation. Whereas most of the radiometals are trapped in the cells, ^{18}F and small labeled fragments leave the cell resulting in a faster decrease of target (tumor) located activity. Whereas trapping in the cell is a clear advantage for tumor imaging, reversible binding of the tracer kinetics is closer to that of the parent compound, such as found for ^{18}Foctreotide [141], is a prerequisite for studying receptor-ligand interactions and thus might become important in characterizing the tumor receptor status or for the planning and control of the therapy.

Apart from peptide receptor ligands, receptor binding steroid hormones are important, e.g., as estrogens or progesterones for mastocarcinomas or as androgen analogues for prostatic cancer. Corresponding ^{18}F-labeled radiopharmaceuticals have been worked on since 1980 [74]. 16-α-[^{18}F]fluoro-17β-

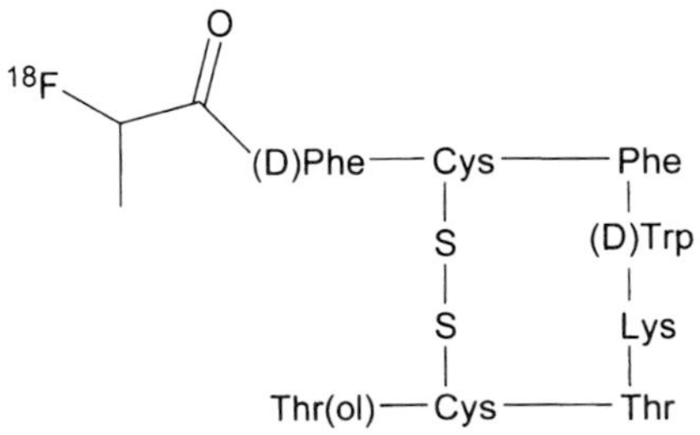

Fig. 7.4. 2-[^{18}F]fluoropropionyl-(D)phe^1-octreotide.

estradiol has been the most thoroughly researched [11, 12, 74, 91, 97, 122, 139]. In recent years, various substituted estrogen receptor ligand analogs have been synthesized (e.g., [13, 126], [^{18}F]fluorotamoxifene [60], [^{18}F]progesterone analogs such as 21-fluoro-16α,17α-furanketales and -acetales [77], 21-[^{18}F]fluoro-16α-ethyl-19-norprogesterone [32, 129], 16α-[^{18}F]fluoro-progesterone [20], 16α-[^{18}F]fluorotestosterones [30] and [^{18}F]androgen receptor ligands [13, 20, 85]). Generally, radiochemical yields of the ^{18}F-labeled ligands range from 10% to 30% following a nucleophilic synthesis. For routine oncologic applications, however, further metabolic evaluations are necessary to assess the clinical relevancy of such tracers.

7.6 Hypoxia tracers

The oxygen partial pressure (pO_2) of a tumor cell is a diagnostically as well as therapeutically relevant parameter in tumor biology [128]. Tissue hypoxia (subnormal pO_2) is the result of metabolic demand for oxygen in excess of oxygen delivery to the cell. It may result from ischemia (subnormal perfusion) at normal oxygen consumption rates or elevated metabolic demand without a compensatory increase of perfusion.

The concept of a hypoxia tracer consists of the synthesis and labeling of a molecule which can pass the membrane of both normal and tumor cells chemically intact and which – inside the cell – is sensitive to redox reactions. Under electron-rich conditions, the tracer is reduced in the cell. But in contrast to normal cells, however, the reduced tracer cannot be oxidized in hypoxic cells because of their reduced oxygen content. Thus, the tracer in its reduced state remains in the hypoxic cell, irreversibly covalently bound to intracellular proteins (cf. Fig. 7.5). The tracer accumulation would therefore be inversely related to the pO_2 value.

Molecules having 2-nitroimidazole structures display this redox behavior in cells [70, 71]. A synthetic strategy for the ^{18}F-labeling of nitroimidazoles via a [^{18}F]epifluorohydrin intermediate was developed by Grierson et al. in 1989 [45] and adapted for automated production equipment. It is now possible to obtain 2-hydroxy-3-([^{18}F]fluoropropan)-2-nitroimidazole ([^{18}F]FMISO)

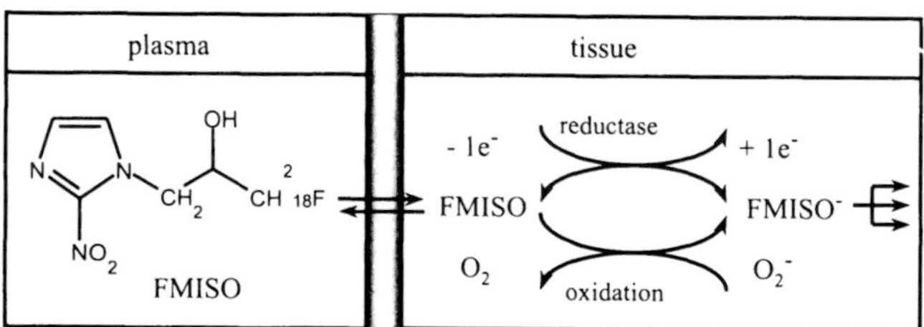

Fig. 7.5. Schematic principle of hypoxia tracers for 2-hydroxy-3-[^{18}F]fluoropropan-2-nitroimidazole ([^{18}F]FMISO).

without addition of carrier in yields of about 20% [90, 105, 118, 121]. For this tracer, studies have been carried out regarding both the visualization of hypoxic cells in tumors [77, 78, 110, 111] and hepatic hypoxia [89, 107, 109]. Comparative studies between glucose-, amino acid- and [^{18}F]FMISO images also prove an ischemia-specific accumulation of the hypoxia tracer [81].

Studies with [^{18}F]FMISO demonstrate the direct dependence of tracer accumulation on decreased O_2 concentration. Thus, the effect of low perfusion ("delayed wash-out") can clearly be excluded. Structural changes on the side chain of the molecule's basic structure result in changes of the lipophilicity and toxicity [69, 146], such as [^{18}F]fluoroethanidazole [84, 123] for example. Systematic variations of the 2-nitroimidazole moiety influence the sensitivity towards redox reactions depending on the pO_2 value [8]. An up-to-date survey can be found in [48, 87]. An interesting approach is the attachment of ribose to [^{18}F]FMISO, yielding [^{18}F]fluoroazomycinarabinoside ([^{18}F]FAZA). It is assumed to show an uptake mechanism via the thymidine transporter, while [^{18}F]FMISO clearly has to diffuse into the cell [106].

7.7 Bones

The [^{18}F]fluoride anion has not been consistently and continuously applied in the diagnosis and therapy of bone metastases or osteoporosis since its first use in the 1940s [9]. However, the reason was mainly a historical one, namely the formerly difficult production of [^{18}F]F^- by means of a reactor, and the usefulness of [^{99m}Tc]-labeled tracers for conventional nuclear medicine imaging of bone metastases. Today, the availability of ^{18}F via the (p,n)-process on highly enriched $H_2{}^{18}O$ in comparatively common particle accelerators, together with modern, high-resolution PET scanners, offers excellent conditions for a renaissance of this tracer [7, 54, 108, 112]. Detection of even small metastases and their exact localization allows the differentiation between degenerative or metastatic processes. Furthermore, quantification of metabolic bone remodeling by [^{18}F]fluoride compared to metabolic parameters determined via other tracers may result in additional information important for therapy control purposes.

7.8 Conclusions

While respecting the international acceptance of 2-[^{18}F]FDG in PET imaging of neoplasms, we are still far away from the more than 100 year old dream of Paul Ehrlich concerning a *Magic Bullet* specifically targeting a tissue, region, cell structure or physiological process of interest. However, no field in life sciences is more equipped to transfer and accumulate the advances in molecular biology, pharmaceutical research or more basic sciences. Thus, the interdisciplinarity of ^{18}F radiochemistry, radiopharmacology, and medicine will be a key and main force for future developments of biospecific tracers in oncology.

References

[1] Alauddin MM, Conti PS, Lever JR et al. (1996) Synthesis of F-18 9-[(3-fluoro-1-hydroxy-2-propoxy)-methyl]guanine (FHPG) for in vivo imaging of viral and gene therapy with PET. J Nucl Med 37:193P (abstr.)

[2] Alauddin MM, Raman RK, Kundu R et al. (1997) Evaluation of F-18 9-[(3-fluoro-1-hydroxy-2-propoxy)-methyl]guanine (F-18 FHPG) in HT-29 cells. J Nucl Med 38:176P (abstr)

[3] Alauddin MM, Conti PS (1998) Synthesis and preliminary evaluation of 9-(4-^{18}F-fluor-3-hydroxymethylbutyl)guanine (^{18}F-FHBG): a new potential imaging agent for viral infection and gene therapy using PET. Nucl Med Biol 25:175–180

[4] Bading JR, Alauddin MM, Fissekis JH et al. (1997) Pharmacokinetics of F-18 fluorohydroxypropoxymethylguanine (FHPG) in primates. J Nucl Med 38:43P (abstr)

[5] Barrio JR, Namavari N, Phelps ME, et al. (1996) Regioselective fluorination of substituted guanines with dilute F2: a facile entry of 8-fluoroguanine derivatives. J Org Chem 61:6084–6085

[6] Barrio JR, Namavari N, Satyamurthy A et al. (1996) 8-[F-18]fluoroacyclovir: an in vivo probe for gene expression with PET. J Nucl Med 37:193P (abstr.)

[7] Berding G, Burchert W, van den Hoff J et al. (1995) Evaluation of the incorporation of bone grafts used in maxillofacial surgery with [18F]fluoride ion and dynamic positron emission tomography. Eur J Nucl Med 22:1133–1140

[8] Biskupiak JE, Rasey JS, Martin GV et al. (1993) Synthesis of 4-substituted misonidazole derivatives for imaging hypoxia. J Nucl Med 34:79P (abstr.)

[9] Blau M, Nagler W, Bender MA (1962) Fluorine-18: a new isotope for bone scanning. J Nucl Med 3:332–334

[10] Bodsch W, Coenen HH, Stöcklin G et al. (1988) Biochemical and autoradiographic study of cerebral protein synthesis with F-18 and C-14-fluorophenylalanine. J Neurochem 50:979–983

[11] Bonasera TA, Pajeau TS, Dehdashti F et al. (1993) Comparison of the hepatic metabolism of 16α-[F-18]fluoroestradiol (FES) and 16β-[F-18]fluoromoxesterol (FMOX) utilizing isolated hepatocytes from different species. J Nucl Med 34:49P (abstr)

[12] Bonasera TA, Pajeau TS, Welch MJ (1994a) D3FES, a doubly labeled (F-18 and H-2) estrogen receptor ligand with reduced in vitro 17-oxidation as compared to FES. J Nucl Med 35:6P (abstr)

[13] Bonasera TA, O'Neil JP, Choe YS et al. (1994b) Imaging the prostate in baboons with fluorine-18 labeled androgen receptor ligands. J Nucl Med 35:53P (abstr)

[14] Börner AR, Mühlensiepen H, Hamacher K et al. (1998a) Uptake of cis-4-[18F]-fluoroproline in cultures of hormone sensitive and hormone resistant prostate cancer cells. Eur J Nucl Med 25:952 (abstr)

[15] Börner AR, Hamacher K, Herzog H et al. (1998b) [18F]-fluoroproline biodistribution and first results in patients with renal tumors. Eur J Nucl Med 25:952 (abstr)

[16] Börner AR, Hamacher K, Herzog H et al. (1999) cis-4-[18F]-fluoroproline PET – preliminary results in patients with urological tumors, Eur J Nucl Med 26:1016

[17] Brix G, Bellemann ME, Haberkorn U et al. (1996) Assessment of the biodistribution and metabolism of 5-fluorouracil as monitored by F-19 MRI and F-18 PET: a comparative animal study. J Nucl Med 37:249P (abstr)

[18] Brown RS, Wahl RL (1993) Overexpression of GLUT-1 glucose transporter in human breast cancer: an immunohistochemical study. Cancer 72:2979–2985

[19] Brown GD, Khan HR, Steel LJ et al. (1993) A practical synthesis of 5-[^{13}F]fluorouracil using HPLC and a study of its metabolic profile in rats. J Labelled Comp Radiopharm 32:521–522

[20] Choe YS, Lidström PJ, Bonasera TA et al. (1995) Bromo-[F-18] fluorination: a radiofluorination method applied to the synthesis of 11β-[F-18]fluoroandrogens and 6α[F-18]fluoroprogestins. J Nucl Med 36:39P (abstr)

[21] Clavo AC, Brown RS, Wahl RL (1995) Fluorodesoxyglucose uptake in human cancer cell lines is increased by hypoxia. J Nucl Med 36:1625–1632

[22] Coenen HH, Bodsch W, Takahashi K et al. (1986) Synthesis, autoradiography and biochemistry of L-[^{18}F]fluorophenylalanines for probing protein synthesis. Nuklearmedizin (Suppl) 22:600–602

[23] Coenen HH, Franken K, Metwally S et al. (1986b) Electrophilic radiofluorination of aromatic compounds with [^{18}F]F_2 and [^{18}F]CH_3CO_2F and regioselective preparation of L-p-[^{18}F]fluorophenylalanine. J Lab Compds Radiopharm 23:1179–1181

[24] Coenen HH, Franken K, Kling P, Stöcklin G (1988) Direct electrophilic fluorination of phenylalanine, tyrosine and dopa. Appl Radiat Isot 39:1243–1250

[25] Coenen HH, Kling P, Stöcklin (1989) Synthesis and cerebral metabolism of aromatic [F-18]fluoroamino acids. J Lab Compds Radiopharm 26:224–226

[26] Coenen HH, Kling P, Stöcklin G (1989) Cerebral metabolism of L-[^{18}F]fluorotyrosine, a new PET tracer of protein synthesis. J Nucl Med 30:1367–1372

[27] Coenen HH (1993) Biochemistry and evaluation of fluoroamino acids. In: Mazoyer BM, Heiss WD, Comar D (eds) PET Studies on Amino Acid Metabolism and Protein Synthesis. Kluwer Academic Publishers, Dordrecht, The Netherlands, pp 109–129

[28] Conti PS, Alauddin MM, Fissekis JD et al. (1997) Synthesis of F-18-labeled 5-fluoro-2′-deoxy-2′-fluoro-1-β-arabinofuranosyluracil ([F-18]FFAU) for PET imaging studies. J Nucl Med 38:177P (abstr)

[29] Crawford EJ, Friedekin M, Wolf AP et al. (1982) ^{18}F-5-fluorouridine, a new probe for measuring the proliferation of tissue in vivo. Adv Enzyme Regul 20:3–22

[30] Cutler PD, Dehdashti F, Siegel BA et al. (1996) Investigation of a prostate ligand 16β-[F-18]fluoro-5α-dihydrotestosterone for staging of prostate carcinoma. J Nucl Med 37:87P

[31] Davenport RJ, Visser GM, Zijlstra S et al. (1995) Facile introduction of the 4-(2-[^{18}F]fluoroethylamino) group into thymidine derivatives. A versatile approach towards labeling antisense oligodeoxynucleotides for PET. XIth Int Symp Radiopharm Chem, Proceedings, pp 332–334

[32] Dehdashti F, McGuire AH, Van Brocklin H et al. (1991) Assessment of (21-[^{18}F]-fluoro-16α-ethyl-19-norprogesterone as a positron-emitting radiopharmaceutical for the detection of progestin receptors in human breast carcinomas. J Nucl Med 32:1532–1537

[33] Dimitrakopoulou-Strauss A, Strauss LG, Krems B et al. (1996) Studies of fluorouracil (FU) pharmacokinetics using positron emission tomography (PET) and magnetic resonance spectroscopy (MRS). J Nucl Med 37:257P (abstr)

[34] Dimitrakopoulou-Strauss A, Strauss LG, Schlag P et al. (1998) Intravenous and intra-arterial oxygen-15-labeled water and fluorine-18-labeled fluorouracil in patients with liver metastases from colorectal cancer. J Nucl Med 39:465–473

[35] Dimitrakopoulou-Strauss A, Strauss LG, Schlag P et al. (1998) Fluorine-18-fluorouracil to predict therapy response in liver metastases from colorectal cancer. J Nucl Med 39:1197–1202

[36] Dollé F, Kuhnast B, Terrazino S et al. (1997) Fluorine-18 labeled oligodeoxynucleotides for in vivo PET imaging. XIIth Int Symp Radiopharm Chem, Proceedings, pp 4–6

[37] Dougan H, Hobbs JB, Lyster DM et al. (1995) Radiohalogenated DNA aptamers. XIth Int Symp Radiopharm Chem, Proceedings, pp 324–325

[38] Eastman RC, Carson RE, Jackobson KA et al. (1992) In vivo imaging of insulin receptors in monkey using 18F-labeled insulin and positron emision tomography. Diabetes 41:855–860

[39] Fowler JS, Finn RD, Lambrecht RM et al. (1973) The synthesis of 5-[^{18}F]fluorouracil. J Nucl Med 14:63–64

[40] Füchtner F, Steinbach J, Vorwieger G et al (1999) 3-O-Methyl-6-[F-18]fluoro-L-DOPA – a promising substance for tumor imaging. J Lab Compds Radiopharm 42:267–269

[41] Gambhir SS, Barrio JR, Bauer E et al. (1998) Radiolabeled penciclovir: a new reporter probe with improved imaging properties over ganciclovir for imaging herpes-simplex virus type 1 thymidine kinase reporter gene expression [abstract]. J Nucl Med 39:53P (abstr)

[42] Gambhir SS, Barrio JR, Wu L et al. (1998) Imaging of adenoviral-directed herpes-simplex virus type 1 thymidine kinase reporter gene expression in mice with radiolabeled ganciclovir. J Nucl Med 39:2003–2011

[43] Gambhir SS, Barrio JR, Herschman HR et al. (1999) Assays for noninvasive imaging of reporter gene expression. Nucl Med Biol 26:481–490

[44] Germann C, Shields AF, Grierson JR et al. (1998) 5-fluoro-1-(2′-deoxy-2′-fluoro-β-D-ribofuranosyl)uracil in Morris hepatoma cells expressing the Herpes Simplex Virus thymidine kinase gene. J Nucl Med 39:1418–1423

[45] Grierson JR, Link JM, Mathis CA et al. (1989) A radiosynthesis of fluorine-18-fluoromisonidazole. J Nucl Med 30:343–350

[46] Grierson JR, Shields AF (1995) A strategy for the labeling of [F-18]-3′-deoxy 3′-fluorothymidine: [F-18]FLT. XIth Int Symp Radiopharm Chem, Proceedings, pp 606–607

[47] Grierson JR, Shields AF, Eary JF (1997) Development of a radiosynthesis for 3′-[F-18] fluoro-3′-deoxynucleosides. XIIth Int Symp Radiopharm Chem, Proceedings, pp 60–62

[48] Grierson JR, Patt M (1999) Synthesis of PET-tracers for the detection of hypoxia. In: Machulla H-J (ed) Imaging of Hypoxia. Kluwer Academic Publishers, Dordrecht, The Netherlands, pp 75–84

[49] Guhlke S, Wester H-J, Bruns Ch et al. (1994) (2-[^{18}F]fluoropropionyl-(D)phe^{1})-octreotide, a potential radiopharmaceutical for quantitative somatostatin receptor imaging with PET: synthesis, radiolabeling, in vitro validation and biodistribution in mice. Nucl Med Biol 21:819–825

[50] Hamacher K, Coenen HH, Stöcklin G (1986) Efficient stereospecific synthesis of no-carrier-added 2-[^{18}F]fluoro-2-deoxy-D-glucose using aminopolyether supported nucleophilic substitution. J Nucl Med 27:235–238

[51] Hamacher K, Stöcklin G (1995) Synthesis of n.c.a. (2S,4R)-4-[^{18}F]fluoroproline: a potential amino acid for PET measurements of procollagen and matrix protein synthesis. XIth Int Symp Radiopharm Chem, Proceedings, pp 175–176

[52] Hamacher K, Herz M, Truckenbrodt R et al. (1996) 4-[F-18]fluoroproline: a potential tracer for collagen synthesis. Radiosynthesis and biological evaluation. J Nucl Med 37:41P (abstr)

[53] Hamacher K (1999) Synthesis of n.c.a. cis- and trans-4-[F-18]fluoroproline, radiotracers for PET investigation of disordered matrix protein synthesis. J Lab Compds Radiopharm 42:1135–1144

[54] Hawkins RA, Choi Y, Huang S-C et al. (1992) Evaluation of the skeletal kinetics of fluorine-18-fluoride ion with PET. J Nuc Med 33:633–642

[55] Hedberg E, Takechi B, Langstrøm B (1995) Oligonucleotides labeled with ^{18}F-linkers in the 5′-position. XIth Int Symp Radiopharm Chem, Proceedings, pp 335–337

[56] Heiss WD, Wienhard K, Wagner R et al. (1996) F-Dopa as an amino acid tracer to detect brain tumors. J Nucl Med 17:1180–1182

[57] Heiss P, Mayer M, Hertz M (1999) Investigation of transport mechanism and uptake kinetics of O-(2-[F-18]fluoroethyl)-L-tyrosine in vitro and in vivo. J Nucl Med 40:1368–1373

[58] Hertz M, Nguyen N, Egert S et al. (1997) 1,3,4,6-tetra-acetyl-2-[F-18]-2-deoxy-D-glucose: biochemical and kinetic studies in the isolated rat heart. XIIth Int Symp Radiopharm Chem, Proceedings, pp 707–709

[59] Higashi T, Tamaki N, Torizuka T et al. (1998) FDG uptake, GLUT-1 glucose transporter and cellularity in human pancreatic tumors. J Nucl Med 39:1727–1735

[60] Inoue T, Yang N, Oriuchi S et al. (1996) Positron emission tomography with F-18 fluorotamoxifen in patients with breast cancer. J Nucl Med 37:86P (abstr)

[61] Inoue T, Tomiyoshi K, Higuichi T et al. (1998) Biodistribution studies on L-3-[fluorine-18]fluoro-α-methyl tyrosine: a potential tumor-detecting agent. J Nucl Med 39:663–667

[62] Inoue T, Shibasaki T, Oriuchi N et al. (1999) F-18-methyl tyrosine PET studies in patients with brain tumors. J Nucl Med 40:399–405

[63] Ishiwata K, Kubota K, Murakami M et al. (1993) Re-evaluation of amino acid PET studies: can the protein synthesis rates in brain and tumor tissues be measured in vivo. J Nucl Med 34:1936–1943

[64] Ito H, Hatzazawa J, Murakami M (1995) Aging effect on neutral amino acid transport at the blood brain barrier measured with L-[2-^{18}F]fluorophenylalanine and PET. J Nucl Med 35:1232–1237

[65] Jacob R, Rösch F, Mann W (1998) ^{18}F-Fluorethyltyrosin (FET) Positronen-Emissions-Tomographie zum Nachweis von Plattenepithelkarzinomen und deren Metastasen im Kopf-Hals-Bereich. Personal communication

[66] Jagoda E, Aloj L, Seidel J et al. (1997) The biodistribution of a F-18 labeled derivative of vasoactive intestinal peptide (dVIP) in a xenograft mouse model of breast cancer. J Nucl Med 38:239P (abstr)

[67] Jeong JM, Yang DJ, Chang YS et al. (1997) Efficient radiosynthesis and biodistribution of 2′-deoxyarabino-2β-F-18-3′,5′,6′-triacetyladenine in tumor-bearing rodents: a prodrug of fluoroadenosine for PET assessment of proliferation. J Nucl Med 38:177P (abstr.)

[68] Jeong JM, Lee YJ, Kim C et al. (1997) Simple synthesis of [F-18]2′-fluoro-3′,5′-di-O-acetyl-2′-deoxyarabino-6-N-acetyladenine for detecting tumors: a prodrug of fluoroadenosine. XIIth Int Symp Radiopharm Chem, Proceedings, pp 23

[69] Jeong JM, Lee YJ, Kim C et al. (1997) PET imaging agents for hypoxic tumor: F-18 labeled nitroimidazole analogues. XIIth Int Symp Radiopharm Chem, Proceedings, pp 349–350

[70] Jerabek PA, Dischino DD, Kilbourn MR et al. (1984) Synthesis of fluorine-18 labeled 1-(2-nitro-1-imidazolyl)-3-fluoro-2-propanol: a hypoxic cell radiosensitizer. J Label Comp Radiopharm 21:1234

[71] Jerabek PA, Patrick TB, Kilbourn MR et al. (1986) Synthesis and biodistribution of ^{18}F-labeled fluoronitroimidazoles: potential in vivo markers of hypoxic tissue. Int J Appl Radiat Isot A37:599–605

[72] Jones HA, Hamacher K, Hill AA et al. (1997) PET-Messung der in vivo Aufnahme von 4-[^{18}F]Fluor-L-Prolin nach Induktion einer Lungenfibrose im Kaninchen. Nukl-Med 36:A80 (abstr)

[73] Kaufmann S (1961) The enzymatic conversion of 4-fluorophenylalanine to tyrosine. Biochim Biophys Acta 61:619–621

[74] Katzenellenbogen JA, Carlson KE, Heimann DF et al. (1980) Receptor-binding radiopharmaceuticals for imaging breast tumors: estrogen-receptor interactions and selectivity of tissue uptake of halogenated estrogen analogs. J Nucl Med 21:550–558

[75] Kim CG, Yang DJ, Tansey W et al. (1995) Assessment of tumor proliferation rate with F-18 labeled adenosine and uracil. J Nucl Med 36:148P (abstr)

[76] Kirschbaum KS, Bonasera TA, Buckman BO et al. (1995) [F-18] progestins: synthesis and tissue distribution of 21-fluoroprogestin-16α,17α-furan ketals and acetals: potential breast tumor imaging agents. J Nucl Med 36:39P (abstr)

[77] Koh W-J, Rasey JS, Evans ML et al. (1993) Imaging of hypoxia and reoxygenation in human tumors with [F-18]fluoromisonidazole. J Nucl Med 34:21P (abstr)

[78] Koh W-J, Bergman KS, Rasey JS et al. (1995) Evaluation of oxygenation status during fractionated radiotherapy in human nonsmall cell lung cancers using [F-18]fluoromisonidazole positron emission tomography. Int J Rad Onc Biol Phys 33:391–398

[79] Kubota K, Ishiwata K, Kubota R et al. (1995) F-18fluorophenylalanine, possibility for tumor imaging compared with L-methionine. J Nucl Med 36:72P (abstr)

[80] Kubota K, Ishiwata K, Kubota R et al. (1996) Feasibility of fluorine-18-fluorophenylalaine for tumor imaging compared with carbon-11-L-methionine. J Nucl Med 37:320–325

[81] Kubota K, Tada M, Yamada S et al. (1997) Intra-tumoral distribution of F-18 fluoromisonidazole, FDG and methionine. J Nucl Med 38:148P (abstr)

[82] Lemaire C (1993) Production of L-[F-18]fluoro amino acids for protein synthesis. Overview and recent developments in nucleophilic syntheses. In: Mazoyer BM, Heiss WD, Comar D (eds) PET Studies on Amino Acid Metabolism and Protein Synthesis. Kluwer Academic Publishers, dordrecht, The Netherlands, pp 89–108

[83] Lemaire C, Guillouet S, Plenevaux A et al (1999) The synthesis of 6-[F-18]fluoro-L-DOPA by chiral catalytic phase transfer alkylation. J Lab Compds Radiopharm 42:113–115
[84] Lim J-L, Berridge MS (1994) Synthesis of [F-18] fluoroetanidazole for hypoxia imaging evaluation. J Nucl Med 35:6P (abstr)
[85] Liu A, Dence CS, Welch MJ et al. (1992) Fluorine-18-labeled androgens: radiochemical synthesis and tissue distribution studies on six fluorine-substituted androgens, potential imaging agents for prostatic cancer. J Nucl Med 33:724–734
[86] Mazoyer BM, Heiss WD, Comar D (1993) PET Studies on Amino Acid Metabolism and Protein Synthesis. Kluwer Academic Publishers, Dordrecht, The Netherlands
[87] Machulla H-J (ed) (1999) Imaging of Hypoxia. Kluwer Academic Publishers, Dordrecht, The Netherlands
[88] Machulla H-J, Blocher A, Kuntzsch M et al. (2000) Simplified labeling approach for synthesizing 3′-deoxy-3′-[^{18}F]fluorothymidine. J Lab Comp Radiopharm, in press
[89] Maxwell AP, MacManus MP, Gardiner TA (1989) Misonidazole binding in murine liver tissue: a marker for cellular hypoxia in vivo. Gastroenterology 97:1300–1303
[90] McCarthy TJ, Dence CS, Welch MJ (1993) Application of microwave heating to the synthesis of [^{18}F]fluoromisonidazole. Appl Radiat Isot 44:1129–1132
[91] Mintun MA, Welch MJ, Siegel BA et al. (1988) Breast cancer: PET imaging of estrogen receptors. Radiology 169:45–52
[92] Monclus M, Luxen A, Van Naemen J et al. (1995) Development of PET radiopharmaceuticals for gene therapy: synthesis of 9-(1-[^{18}F]fluoro-3-hydroxy-2-propoxy) methylguanine. XIth Int Symp Radiopharm Chem, Proceedings, pp 193–195
[93] Monclus M, Luxen A, Cool V et al. (1997) Synthesis of (R)- and (S)-9-{(3-[^{18}F]fluoro-1-hydroxy-propoxy)methyl}guanine: radiopharmaceuticals for gene therapy. XIIth Int Symp Radiopharm Chem, Proceedings, pp 20–22
[94] Monclus M, Luxen A, Cool V et al. (1997) Development of a positron emission tomography radiopharmaceutical for imaging thymidine kinase gene expression: synthesis and in vitro evaluation of 9-{3-[^{18}F]fluoro-1-hydroxy-2-propoxy)-methyl} guanine. Bioorganic Med Chem Lett 7:1879–1882
[95] Senekowitch-Schmidtke, personal communication
[96] Moody TW, Leyton J, Unsworth E et al. (1998) (Arg(15),Arg(21))VIP: evaluation of biological activity and localization to breast cancer tumors. Peptides 19:585–592
[97] Moresco RM, Casati R, Lucignani G et al. (1994) Systemic and cerebral kinetics of 16α[F-18]fluoro-17β-estradiol. J Nucl Med 35:255P (abstr.)
[98] Murakami M, Takahashi K, Kondo Y et al. (1987) The comparative synthesis of ^{18}F-fluorophenylalanine by electrophilic substitution with ^{18}F-F$_2$ and ^{18}F-AcOF. J Lab Comp Radiopharm 25:1367–1376
[99] Murakami M, Takahashi K, Kondo Y et al. (1988) 2-F-18-phenylalanine and 3-F-18-tyrosine – synthesis and preliminary data of tracer kinetics. J Lab Compds Radiopharm 25:773–782
[100] Murakami M, Takahashi K, Kondo Y et al. (1989) The slow metabolism of L-2-F-18-fluorophenylalanine in rat. J Lab Compds Radiopharm 27:245–255
[101] Nakamichi H, Murakami M, Miura S et al. (1994) Does the anabolic metabolism of L-[2-^{18}F]fluorophenylalanine and L-[2,6-^{3}H]phenylalanine differ in the cerebrum and the cerebellum? Nucl Med Biol 21:959–962
[102] Ogawa T, Miura S, Murakami M et al. (1996) Quantitative evaluation of neutral amino acid transport in cerebral gliomas using positron emission tomography and fluorine-18 fluorophenylalanine. Eur J Nucl Med 23:889–895
[103] Pajeau TS, Welch MJ, Bonasera TA et al. (1993) The radiotoxicity of 16α[F-18]-fluorostradiol ([F-18]FES) in cell culture. J Nucl Med 34:160P (abstr)
[104] Pan D, Gambhir SS, Phelps ME et al. (1997) Synthesis of fluorinated nucleosides for antisense oligodeoxynucleotide imaging with PET. J Nucl Med 38:134P (abstr)
[105] Patt M, Knutzsch M, Machulla H-J (1999) Preparation of [^{18}F]fluoromisonidazole by nucleophilic substitution on THP-protected precursors: yield dependence on reaction parameters. J Radioanal Nucl Chem 240:925–927

[106] Patt M, Kumar P, Wiebe LI, Machulla H-J (1999) [^{18}F]fluoroazomycinarabinosid (FAZA) ein neuer Radiotracer zur Bestimmung von Gewebehypoxien. Nuklearmedizin 38:A22 (abstr.)
[107] Piert M, Machulla H-J, Dißmann PD et al. (1998) Simple SUV analysis of F-18-fluoromisonidazole uptake allows accurate measurement of regional liver hypoxia. Eur J Nucl Med 25:P981 (abstr.)
[108] Piert M, Zittel TT, Machulla H-J et al. (1998) Blood flow measurements with [15O]H_2O and [18F]fluoride ion PET in porcine vertebrae. J Bone Miner Res 13:1328–1336
[109] Piert M, Machulla H-J, Becker G et al. (1999) Introducing ^{18}F-misonidazole PET for localization and quantification of pig liver hypoxia. Eur J Nucl Med 26:95–109
[110] Rasey JS, Koh W-J, Grierson JR et al. (1989) Radiolabeled fluoromisonidazole as an imaging agent for tumor hypoxia. Int J Rad Onc Biol Phys 17:985–991
[111] Rasey JS, Koh W-J, Peterson LM et al. (1996) Evaluation of tumor hypoxic fraction using tumor : muscle ratios of [F-18]FMISO uptake. J Nucl Med 37:235P (abstr)
[112] Schiepers C, Broos P, Nuyts J, et al. (1994) Positron emission tomography using F-18 fluoride for the evaluation of femoral head osteonecrosis. Eur J Nucl Med 21:762 (abstr)
[113] Shai Y, Kirk KL, Channing MA et al. (1989) F-18-labeled insulin: a prosthetic group methodology for incorporation of a positron emitter into peptides and proteins. Biochemistry 28:4801–4806
[114] Shields AF, Grierson JR (1996) Labeled AZT and FLT for imaging cell proliferation. J Nucl Med 37:240P (abstr)
[115] Shields AF, Grierson JR (1997) F-18 FLT can be used to image cell proliferation in vivo. J Nucl Med 38:249P (abstr)
[116] Shields AF, Grierson JR, Dohmen BM et al. (1998) Imaging proliferation in vivo with [F-18]FLT and positron emission tomography (PET). Nat Med 4:1334–1336
[117] Shoup TM, Olson J, Hoffman JM et al. (1999) Synthesis and evaluation of [F-18]1-amino-3-fluorocyclobutane-1-carboxylic acid to image brain tumors. J Nucl Med 40:331–338
[118] Solbach M, Machulla H-J (1995) Yield dependence of [^{18}F]FMISO on different reaction parameters. XIth Int Symp Radiopharm Chem, Proceedings, pp 199–201
[119] Stöcklin G, Wester HJ (1998) Strategies for radioligand development. Peptides for tumor imaging. In: Gulyás B, Müller-Gärtner HW (eds) Positron Emission Tomography: A Critical Assessment of Recent Trends. Kluwer Academic Publishers, Dordrecht, Boston, London, pp. 57–90
[120] Strauss LG, Conti PS (1991) The application of PET in clinical oncology. J Nucl Med 32:623–648
[121] Tada M, Iwata R, Sugiyama H et al. (1996) A concise one-pot synthesis of [^{18}F]fluoromisonidazole from (2R)-(–)-glycidyl tosylate. J Label Comp Radiopharm 38:771–774
[122] Tewson TJ, Mankoff DA, Eary JF (1997) Metabolism and clearance of [F-18]16α-fluoroestradiol (FES) in patients. J Nucl Med 38:176P (abstr)
[123] Tewson TJ (1997) Synthesis of [F-18]fluoroethanidazole – a new nitroimidazole tracer of hypoxia. XIIth Int Symp Radiopharm Chem, Proceedings, pp 56–576
[124] Tomiyoshi K, Amed K, Muhammed S (1997) Synthesis of isomers of F-18-labelled amino acid radiopharmaceutical: position-2- and 3-L-18F-alpha-methyltyrosine using a separation and purification system. Nucl Med Commun 18:169–175
[125] Vaidyanathen G, Zalutsky MR (1997) Fluorine-18-labeled [Nle(4),D-Phe(7)]-alpha-MSH, an alpha-melanocyte stimulating hormone analogue. Nucl Med Biol 24:275–286
[126] Van Brocklin HF, Liu A, Welch MJ et al. (1994) The synthesis of 17 alpha-methyl-substituted estrogens labeled with fluorine-18: potential breast tumor imaging agents. Steroids 59:34–45
[127] Van der Ley M (1983) [F-18]Fluorine labelled amino acids. J Lab Compds Radiopharm 20:453–461
[128] Vaupel P, Kelleher DK, Günderoth M (eds) (1995) Tumor Oxygenation. Gustav Fischer Verlag, Stuttgart, Jena, New York

[129] Verhagen A, Luurtsema G, Pesser JW et al. (1991) Preclinical evaluation of a positron emitting progestin (21-^{18}F-fluor-16α-ethyl-19-norprogesterone) for imaging progesterone receptor positive tumours with positron emission tomography. Cancer Lett 59:125–132

[130] Vine EN, Young D, Vine WH et al. (1979) An improved synthesis of 5-[^{18}F]fluoruracil. Int J Appl Radiat Isot 30:401–404

[131] Vos MG, Visser GM, Pike VW et al. (1995) Synthesis of 5′-deoxy-5′-[^{18}F]-fluoro-thymidine (5′-[^{18}F]FDT). A bifunctional agent to investigate DNA synthesis rate and a useful tool as a terminal building unit in antisense ODN labelling for PET. XIth Int Symp Radiopharm Chem, Proceedings, pp 338–340

[132] Vyska K, Profant M, Schuier F et al. (1984) In vivo determination of kinetic parameters for glucose influx and efflux by means of 3-O-^{11}C-methyl-D-glucose, ^{18}F-3-deoxyfluoro-D-glucose and dynamic positron emission tomography; theory, methods and normal values. In: Knapp WH, Vyska K (eds) Current Topics in Tumor Cell Physiology and Positron Emission Tomography. Springer Verlag, Heidelberg, New York, pp 37–60

[133] Waki A, Fujibayashi Y, Magata Y et al. (1996) A new strategy for selective detection of hexokinase activity in tumor cells: lipophilic but metabolizable glucose analogue, [F-18] acetyl-FDG. J Nucl Med 37:192P (abstr)

[134] Waki A, Yonekura Y, Sadato N et al. (1997) [^{18}F]-AFDG, a 2-deoxyglucose analogue with high lipophilicity and glucose transporter-independent uptake; in vitro and in vivo characterization. XIIth Int Symp Radiopharm Chem, Proceedings, pp 671–673

[135] Waki A, Kato H, Yano R et al. (1998 a) The importance of glucose transporter activity as the rate-limiting step of 2-deoxyglucose uptake in tumor cells in vitro. Nucl Med Biol 25:593–597

[136] Waki A, Fujibayashi Y, Yokoyama A (1998 b) Recent advances in the analysis of the characteristics of tumors on FDG uptake. Nucl Med Biol 25:589–592

[137] Waki A, Fujibayashi Y, Magata Y et al. (1998 c) Glucose transporter protein-independent tumor cell accumulation of fluorine-18-AFDG, a lipophilic fluorine-18-FDG analog. J Nucl Med 39:245–250

[138] Weber W, Wester HJ, Grosu AL et al. (1999) O-(2′-[F-18]fluoroethyl)-L-tyrosine and [methyl-C-11]-L-methionine uptake in brain tumors: a comparative PET study. Eur J Nucl Med (in press)

[139] Welch MJ, Bonasera TA, Sherman EIC et al. (1995) [F-18]fluorodeoxyglucose (FDG) and 16α-[F-18]fluoroestradiol-17β (FES) uptake in estrogen-receptor (ER)-rich tissues following tamoxifen treatment: a preclinical study. J Nucl Med 36:39P (abstr.)

[140] Wester HJ, Hamacher K, Stöcklin G (1996) A comparative study of nca fluorine-18-labeling of proteins via acylation and photochemical conjugation. Nucl Med Biol 23:365–372

[141] Wester HJ, Brockmann J, Rösch F et al. (1997) PET-pharmacokinetics of ^{18}F-octreotide: a comparison with ^{68}Ga-DFO- and ^{86}Y-DTPA-octreotide. Nucl Med Biol 24:275–286

[142] Wester HJ, Hertz M, Weber W et al. (1999) Synthesis and radiopharmacology of O-(2-[^{18}F]fluoroethyl)-L-tyrosine ([^{18}F]FET) for tumor imaging. J Nucl Med 40:205–212

[143] Wester HJ, Hertz M, Senekowitsch-Schmidtke R et al. (1999) Preclinical evaluation of 4-[^{18}F]fluoroprolines: diastereomeric effects on metabolism and uptake in mice. Nucl Med Biol 26:259–265

[144] Wienhard K, Herholz K, Coenen HH et al. (1991) Increased amino acid transport into brain tumors measured by PET of L-(2-^{18}F)fluorotyrosine. J Nucl Med 32:1338–1346

[145] Yamamoto T, Seino Y, Fukumoto A et al. (1990) Overexpression of facilitated glucose transporter genes in human cancer. Biochem Biophys Res Commun 170:223–230

[146] Zheng L, Ma C, McCarthy TJ et al. (1994) Synthesis of 1-(2-nitro-1-imidazolyl-3-(2-[F-18]-fluoromethyl-1-aziridinyl)-2-propanol, a potential hypoxic radiosensitizer for PET. J Nucl Med 35:73P (abstr)

8 Cerium-doped lutetium oxyorthosilicate: a fast, efficient new scintillator

C. L. Melcher, J. S. Schweitzer

8.1 Introduction

A wide variety of applications in nuclear physics, medical imaging, high energy physics, and geophysics have spurred an interest in the development of new inorganic scintillators that would have significantly improved responses, compared with NaI(T1), for these applications [1]. A number of basic properties can be enumerated which would enhance gamma-ray detectors in all these applications: high detection efficiency, light output comparable to NaI(T1), fast scintillation decay time, rugged, non-hygroscopic and, in some cases, temperature dependence comparable to and radiation length smaller than NaI(T1).

The first significant advance was the introduction of bismuth germanate (BGO). BGO has a very high detection efficiency and short radiation length, due to its high density and high effective atomic number, is very rugged and non-hygroscopic, but has relatively low light output, is very temperature sensitive, and is even somewhat slower than NaI(T1). A number of other materials, such as barium fluoride and cadmium tungstate, show promise with regard to a number of properties, but have weaknesses that have limited their usefulness. In 1983, cerium-doped gadolinium oxyorthosilicate (GSO) was reported as having some significant advances over existing materials [2]. The scintillation properties of this rare earth oxyorthosilicate prompted an examination of other rare earth oxyorthosilicates. Yttrium oxyorthosilicate (YSO) had also been shown to have reasonably good scintillation properties [3]. Studies of these two scintillators led to the investigation of cerium-doped lutetium oxyorthosilicate (LSO). Following successful studies with phosphors, optically clear boules of cerium-doped lutetium oxyorthosilicate were successfully grown with useful properties as a gamma-ray detector.

From: 2000 IEEE. Reprinted with permission from IEEE transactions on nuclear science, vol. 39, no. 4, 1992.

Table 8.1. Physical properties.

	NaI(T1)	BGO	GSO	LSO
Density (g/cm^3)	3.67	7.13	6.7	7.4
Effective atomic no.	51	75	59	66
Radiation length (cm)	2.56	1.12	1.38	1.14
Index of refraction	1.85	2.15	1.85	1.82
Hygroscopic?	yes	no	no	no
Rugged?	no	yes	no	yes

8.2 Physical properties

The physical properties of Ce-doped lutetium oxyorthosilicate are shown in Table 8.1, together with the properties of some important existing scintillators. LSO has a good detection efficiency, with a higher density than the other materials and an effective atomic number that is only a little smaller than BGO. Its radiation length is within 2% of BGO, a significant advantage for high energy physics applications. The index of refraction of 1.82 is somewhat lower than the other scintillators, resulting in less reflection at the crystal-photomultiplier tube interface and permitting a higher fraction of the light produced by the crystal to be converted into an electrical pulse. Finally, it is not hygroscopic and is reasonably rugged, resulting in minimal difficulties for handling and packaging.

8.3 Crystal growth

The most common method for growing crystals of high-melting-point oxide materials such as LSO is the Czochralski technique in which a seed crystal is used to pull a single crystal boule from a melt. Since LSO is a new material, we did not have a seed crystal and so growth was initiated on an iridium wire instead. This technique worked surprisingly well despite a tendency for small cracks to form at the upper end of the boule during cooling, probably due to the different coefficients of thermal expansion of iridium and LSO. The cracks, however, affected only a small portion of a typical boule, and all boules had large crack-free regions. The raw materials were 99.99% pure Lu_2O_3, SiO_2, and CeO_2. After mixing and pressing the raw materials into pellets, they were melted in an iridium crucible which was inductively heated. The furnace assembly was located in a sealed chamber and crystal growth was carried out under a continuous flow of N_2+3000 ppm O_2.

We grew both undoped LSO ($Lu_2(SiO_4)O$) and Ce-doped LSO ($Lu_{2(1-x)}Ce_{2x}(SiO_4)O$). The boules were typically $\sim$20 mm in diameter and $\sim$40–60 mm long. Both the undoped and Ce-doped boules were colorless and transparent to the naked eye. The Ce-doped boules are listed in Table 8.2 along with the Ce concentration in the raw materials, i.e., the "melt". The

Table 8.2. Distribution of Ce between melts and crystals.

Crystal	Ce conc. in melt (at. % rel. to Lu)	Ce conc. in melt (ppm by weight)	Ce conc. in crystal (ppm by weight)	Dist. coeff. of Ce in LSO
# 6	0.12%	735	155	0.21
# 7	0.25%	1530	339	0.22
# 8	0.25%	1530	361	0.24
#10	0.25%	1530	353	0.23

concentration of Ce in the crystals themselves was measured by inductively-coupled-plasma mass spectrometry by X-Ray Assay Laboratories. As expected, the concentration in the crystals is much lower compared to the melt due to the fact that the Ce^{+3} ion is much larger than the Lu^{+3} ion for which it substitutes in the crystal lattice (1.034 Å vs. 0.848 Å). From these data, the crystal-to-melt distribution coefficient appears to be ~0.22.

8.4 Crystal structure

LSO is one member of the group of rare earth oxyorthosilicates reviewed by Felsche [4]. The crystal structure of these compounds is either monoclinic P or monoclinic C, depending on the radius of the trivalent rare earth ion. In the case of LSO, Lu^{+3} has a small ionic radius of 0.848 Å and so its structure is monoclinic C. The unit cell parameters reported by Felsche [5] are a = 14.254 Å, b = 10.241 Å, c = 6.641 Å, and $\gamma = 122.20°$. Figure 8.1 shows a typical X-ray diffraction pattern of a powdered sample from one of our single crystal boules. Although we have not yet calculated the unit cell parameters from these data, the pattern is representative of the monoclinic C (C2/c) structure [6].

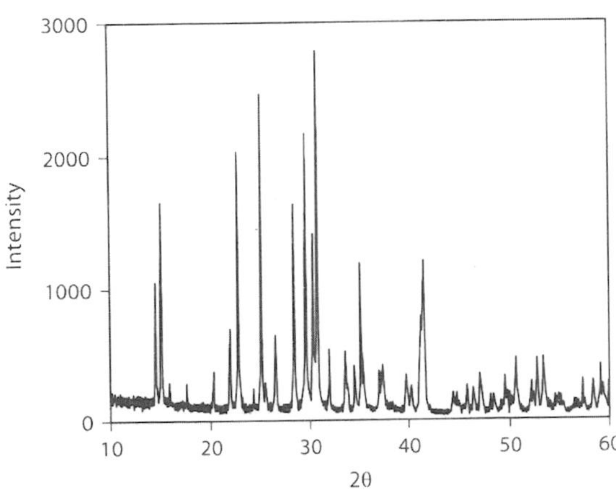

Fig. 8.1. X-ray diffraction pattern of LSO #6 displays monoclinic C (C2/c) symmetry.

The density of undoped LSO calculated from the unit cell parameters above is 7.42 g/cm^3. We measured the density of several Ce-doped crystals (0.25% Ce in the melt) with the liquid submersion technique and determined a value of 7.35 ± 0.03 g/cm^3. The small difference between the theoretical and experimental values may reflect a difference between doped and undoped crystals. The substitution of lighter Ce ions for a fraction of the heavier Lu ions as well as a possible enlargement of the unit cell due to the larger ionic radius of Ce^{+3} compared to Lu^{+3} may explain the slightly lower experimental value.

8.5 Scintillation properties

An important property of any scintillator is that it must have minimal absorbance in the wavelength region of the scintillation emission so that the emission intensity is not reduced as the light passes through the crystal itself. Figure 8.2 shows that undoped LSO has very little absorbance between 200 and 600 nm. Also shown in the figure is the absorbance spectrum of a crystal grown from a melt doped with 0.25% Ce (relative to Lu). This spectrum displays absorption bands corresponding to electronic transitions from the 4f ground state of Ce^{+3} to the split 5d levels [7].

In Fig. 8.3 we compare the emission spectrum of LSO under gamma-ray excitation (^{241}Am) to NaI(Tl), BGO, and GSO. The peak emission wavelength of LSO is ~420 nm which provides a good match to the spectral response of bialkali photomultiplier tubes. The intensity of the best crystal is about 75% of NaI(Tl) and several times greater than either BGO or GSO.

The scintillation decay was measured with the time-correlated single photon counting technique [8] and is shown in Fig. 8.4. To a good approximation, the decay can be described by a single exponential with a time

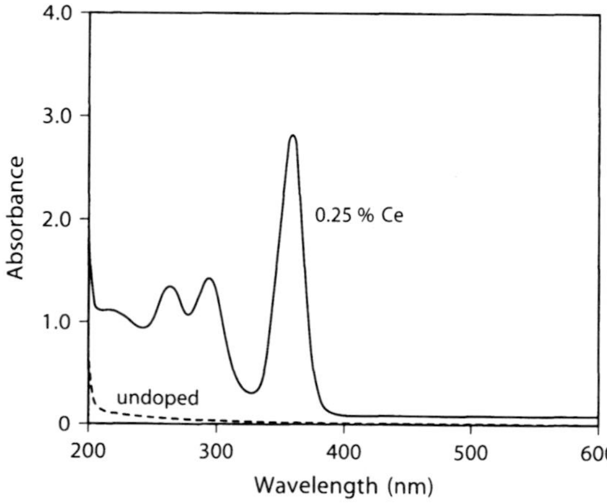

Fig. 8.2. Absorbance of undoped LSO and LSO with 0.25% Ce.

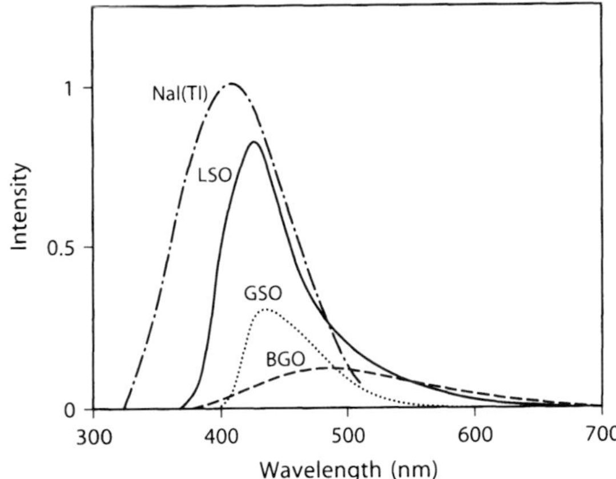

Fig. 8.3. Comparison of the emission spectrum of LSO to three well-known scintillators.

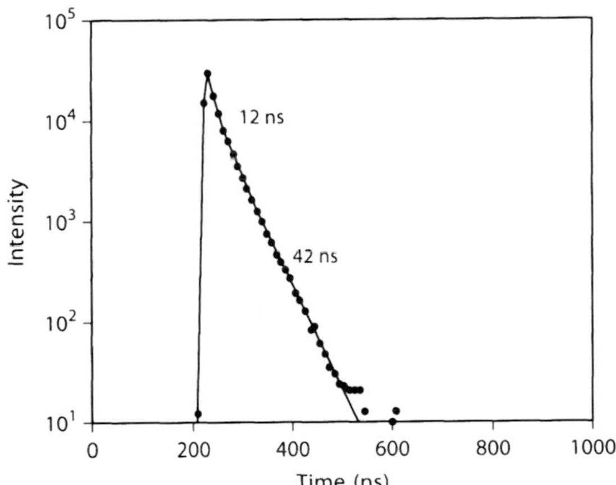

Fig. 8.4. The scintillation decay following gamma-ray excitation can be approximated by a single 40 ns component or more precisely by the sum of 12 and 42 ns components.

constant of $\sim$40 ns. However, a more careful fit to the decay data reveals two exponential components with time constants of 12 and 42 ns. The relative intensities of these components are 35 and 65% respectively for this crystal. Measurements of other crystals yielded similar results. The emission intensities and decay constants are summarized in Table 8.3.

A $10 \times 10 \times 2$ mm crystal coupled to a Hamamatsu R878 photomultiplier tube was used to measure the pulse spectrum of a 10 μCi ^{137}Cs source (Fig. 8.5). The energy resolution of the 662 keV photopeak is 10.3%. Also shown is the natural activity background spectrum which arises from the decay of ^{176}Lu which is present in the crystal with an abundance of 2.6% of natural Lu. Under the conditions of this measurement the background does not have a large effect on the spectrum. However, when the counting rate is low, proper background subtraction could become important.

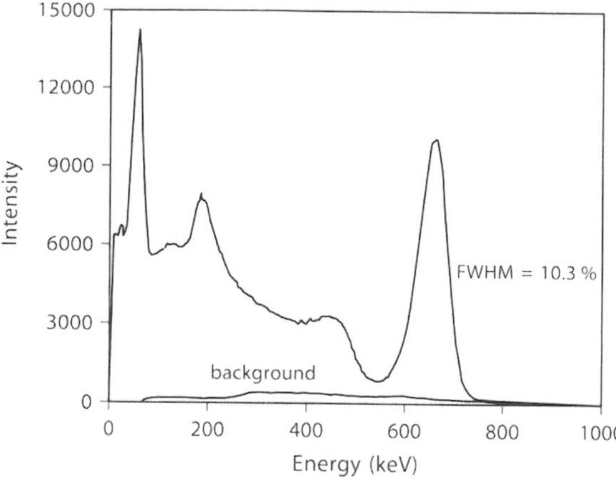

Fig. 8.5. Pulse height spectrum of a 10 μCi ^{137}Cs source measured with a 10 × 10 × 2 mm LSO crystal coupled to a Hamamatsu R878 photomultiplier tube. The background spectrum is due to the 2.6% abundant, naturally radioactive, ^{176}Lu.

Table 8.3. Scintillation properties.

Crystal	Emission intensity NaI(T1) = 400	Decay time constants (ns)
# 6	292	13 (20%) 37 (80%)
# 7	285	12 (35%) 40 (65%)
# 8	163	13 (26%) 41 (74%)
#10	135	12 (46%) 37 (54%)

8.6 Summary

The scintillation properties of Ce-doped LSO are compared to NaI(T1), BGO, and GSO in Table 8.4. In addition to desirable physical properties such as high density and high atomic number, LSO also possesses a combination of high emission intensity and fast decay which together are superior to any other known single crystal scintillator. This unique combination of physical and scintillation properties offers potential advantages in a number of applications. In medical imaging, the high density, high atomic number, and fast decay would provide high gamma-ray or x-ray detection efficiency by small detectors as well as enhanced coincidence timing to provide greater image resolution. The short radiation length and fast decay would allow smaller detectors with increased count-rate capability and timing properties for nuclear and particle physics experiments. In oil well logging or other types of geophysical exploration, the high emission intensity and favorable emission wavelength, high density, high atomic number, ruggedness, non-hygroscopic

Table 8.4. Scintillation properties of LSO compared to other scintillators. The decay constants listed for NaI(T1), BGO, and LSO are single exponential approximations. The decay times are more precisely described by the sum of multiple exponential components.

	NaI(T1)	BGO	GSO	LSO
Relative emission intensity	100	15	25	75
Peak wavelength (nm)	410	480	440	420
Decay constant (ns)	230	300	56 600	40

nature, and fast decay would provide higher gamma-ray detection efficiency, higher count-rate capability, and ease of handling compared to currently used scintillators such as NaI(T1).

References

[1] Melcher CL: Lutetium orthosilicate single crystal scintillator detector. U.S. Patent No. 4958080, (1990) and 5025151 (1991)

[2] Takagi K, Fukazawa T (1983) Cerium-activated Gd_2SiO_5 single crystal scintillator. Appl Phys Lett 42(1):43–45

[3] Brandle CD, Valentino AJ, Berkstresser GW (1986) Czochralski growth of rare-earth orthosilicates (Ln_2SiO_5). J Crystal Growth 79:308–315

[4] Felsche J (1973) The crystal chemistry of the rare-earth silicates. In: *Structure and Bonding* V13. Springer-Verlag, pp 99–197

[5] Felsche J (1971) Rare earth silicates of the type $RE_2[SiO_4]O$. Naturwissenschaften 11:565–566

[6] See, for example, JCPDS No. 36-1476 for YSO. International Centre for Diffraction Data, Swarthmore

[7] Hoshina T (1980) 5d-4f Radiative transition probabilities of Ce^{3+} and Eu^{2+} in crystals. J Phys Soc Japan 48(4):1261–1268

[8] Bollinger LM, Thomas GE (1961) Measurement of the time dependence of scintillation intensity by a delayed-coincidence method. Rev Sci Instr 32:1044–1050

9 Optimization of gamma camera coincidence systems for PET in oncology

M. Bähre

9.1 Introduction

H. Anger proposed the use of gamma camera detectors based on sodium iodide to register positron annihilation quanta as early as 1963. However, it took a relatively long time, until the year 1995, to develop tomographic imaging systems which were suited for routine applications [1]. In the few years since then, the performance of these systems has significantly risen, and their development has been predominantly aimed at improving the imaging quality of this PET variant. As a matter of fact, PET with gamma camera coincidence systems has now reached a level of performance which was hardly imaginable even a few years ago. The current imaging quality far surpasses that of the early dedicated PET scanners. This progress was made possible by advances in the design of digital gamma camera detectors as well as the availability of highly effective and fast signal processors. The performance of computers suited for complex tomographic reconstruction techniques has also risen considerably. When the first gamma camera coincidence systems for routine applications were introduced onto the market, it was apparent that the starting points of the manufacturers of such cameras were very different. Some of them focused their efforts on crystal thickness, others on signal processing or the application of transaxial septa. But these differing approaches were soon converging, optimizing tomographic resolution and providing easy system handling. Since the systems have become more alike, their imaging properties and clinical results are comparable.

However, as holds true for all imaging procedures in nuclear medicine, the clinical information provided depends to a large extent on parameters chosen by the physician. This is particularly relevant in this field of complex multiparametric scintigraphic techniques. The following factors, which have relevant effects on the image quality and diagnostic benefits of gamma camera coincidence systems in oncology and which can be controlled by the physician, are discussed from the point of view of a clinician.

9.2 Hardware-based optimization

Transaxially orientated septa simulating 2D-acquisition of dedicated PET systems have been introduced by several companies. The function of these septa, sometimes incorrectly referred to as "filters", is to efficiently absorb quanta incident at an angle of more than 12–15 degrees to the transversal plane. The septa represent one basis for high quality tomographic imaging, because they prevent non-coincident quanta from patient regions inside and outside the field of view from being detected. This has two positive effects: First, the percentage of random coincidences within the field of view is decreased. Thus, the proportion of quanta with incorrect positioning information deteriorating the resulting tomograms is reduced. Second, signal processing by the detector is less affected by dead time effects caused by the detection of quanta irrelevant for imaging. Consequently, higher activities can be administered to the patients – an essential fact in view of the lower system sensitivity of gamma camera-based systems when compared to dedicated PET scanners (see below).

The central role of the *crystal thickness* with regard to the sensitivity and also the imaging properties of gamma camera coincidence systems was soon well understood. Doubling of the crystal thickness increases the gain of coincident quanta by a factor of 4, since the chance of detecting both annihilation quanta is doubled resulting in a quadratic increase of the rate of true coincidences. This reversed the tendency towards thin detector crystals optimized for high-resolution detection of low energy single photons. In 1997 most new systems were already equipped with 15 to 19 mm crystals. The resolution of the scintigrams when detecting low-energy quanta was slightly lower, but this effect was found to be negligible for routine applications [5]. Since the system resolution depends both on collimator and intrinsic resolution, it can be deduced that a LEUHR collimator can compensate for the discrete loss of the detector resolution. In the meantime, it was proved under routine conditions that the choice of collimators does indeed influence imaging quality to a comparable or even larger extent than crystal thickness. At present, the use of sodium iodide for scintillation crystals of 15 or preferably of 19 mm thickness is strongly recommendable for hybrid gamma camera systems. New *scintillation materials*, which in principle offer the chance to improve the system sensitivity and to reduce the system dead time, are not yet routinely available. Up to now, these approaches seem to play an important role merely in marketing strategies.

Another important feature, the *wiring of photomultipliers in groups*, has been implemented by several manufacturers. This modification of detector circuitry is aimed at further reducing dead time effects: after the detection of one annihilation quantum not the complete detector, but only a subgroup of multipliers is temporarily blocked for subsequent incidents. This is another strategy to detect more than one quantum within different sections of the detector and to raise the quanta yield at a given activity. Furthermore, this option makes it possible to increase the applied tracer activities to usual levels when using dedicated PET scanners.

9.3 Software-based optimization

Because of the lower sensitivity of gamma camera coincidence systems, the choice of an appropriate *tomographic reconstruction technique* is more critical than it is in conventional PET. The comparably low quanta yield from the volume under investigation results in a considerable amount of radial artifacts when using filtered backprojection (FBP) for tomographic reconstruction. As was proved in SPET applications, well-suited iterative reconstruction techniques significantly decrease the number of artifacts of this type [4]. Without doubt this is of special importance when tomograms are to be quantified. It is sometimes argued that only iteratively reconstructed tomograms provide sufficient precision and allow any quantitative evaluation of PET studies. In addition, recognizability of small lesions with increased tracer uptake is diminished by a high rate of artifacts. This results in a loss of sensitivity in detecting tumors at a very early stage, which is unacceptable in view of the strategic role of PET in oncology.

For these reasons filtered backprojection should generally not be used for tomographic reconstruction in gamma camera-based systems. *Iterative techniques* should be used instead. Different algorithms are available, such as EM-ML or OSEM. Reconstruction based on a multiplicative iterative reconstruction technique developed by Luig et al. primarily for tomographic reconstruction in SPET applications was also reported to be very efficient [2, 3, 6].

It is still under discussion whether or not *attenuation correction* is necessary in PET with dedicated systems. In principle, two different techniques of attenuation correction have to be distinguished: the less complex variant is based on calculating attenuation during tomographic reconstruction by applying a fixed attenuation coefficient. This requires a valid criterion for the determination of the body outline. The alternative technique includes the use of an external radiation source to measure regional attenuation coefficients in the individual patient. It is yet unclear which of these techniques provide superior information and should thus be used. Imaging results of organs with very low attenuation as well as low tracer activity are generally less correct and not convincing ("hot" display of the lungs) when simply calculating the attenuation based on a constant coefficient. Consequently, a correction based on direct measurement of absorption appears to be superior. On the other hand, calculated attenuation compensation using the reconstruction technique developed by Luig et al. has produced satisfactory clinical results [2, 6]. At present, in gamma camera coincidence PET it appears to be necessary to perform one of these types of attenuation correction to close the gap to high-end PET imaging with dedicated systems. The best-suited variant will have to be determined in the near future.

During rebinning, no photo-compton or compton-compton coincidences should be accepted. Restriction to *photo-photo coincidences* minimizes weak or incorrect information entering the tomographic reconstruction process. Since a considerable number of random coincidences from inside the field-of-view are always present, the admitting of invalid quanta would unnecessarily decrease the imaging quality of the obtained tomograms even further.

9.4 Actual performance of gamma camera-based PET systems

With respect to some of the factors which reflect the tomographic imaging power in PET, gamma camera-based systems have already reached the standards of dedicated systems. This is especially true for *system resolution*, which in the meantime has been reaching the values of low or midrange dedicated systems in transaxial as well as in axial orientation (Table 9.1).

The most important disadvantage of gamma camera-based PET systems is the still *limited system sensitivity*, which currently stands at about 1:7 when compared with standard systems. Modified detector technology and triple head systems as mentioned above might contribute towards reducing the gap to dedicated PET cameras to a factor of 2–3. Therefore, in order to ensure a high diagnostic benefit of this PET variant in clinical oncology and to approach the information provided by dedicated systems, all factors influencing the imaging properties have to be carefully optimized to compensate for the restrictions. The measures have to aim at minimizing signal-to-noise ratios of all steps of imaging and at achieving a maximum quanta yield during the limited time of data acquisition.

9.5 Patient preparation

The preparation of the patients is as important as it is in standard PET investigation protocols. An appropriate *fasting period* of more than 5 hours leading to a blood glucose level of less than 120 mg/dl is standard for adequate imaging of tumor manifestations. Patients with diabetes often need individual preparation to fulfill this criterion and to avoid poor diagnostic output. As is usual, muscle activity has to be kept at a low level to exclude high and eventually misleading tracer uptake. Hydrating patients to reduce bladder activity is the same as it is in conventional PET investigations.

When gamma camera-based systems are used, the *activity applied* is more critical than is the case with standard PET scanners. Obviously, some early systems on the market could be used only at comparably low tracer activities. This was probably due to the non-availability of transversal septa.

Table 9.1. System resolution and sensitivity of a gamma camera coincidence system (Prism 2000 XP PCD, Picker) compared with dedicated PET scanners (modified after Kunze et al. and Schwaiger & Ziegler [5, 7]).

	Resolution (x, y, z) [mm]	Sensitivity [kcps/μCi/ml]
GE Advance 2D	4.4 × 4.0 × 4.2	128
Siemens ECAT EXACT HR+	4.5 × 4.5 × 4.1	158
Siemens ECAT EXACT 47 2D	5.8 × 5.8 × 5.0	216
GE Quest 3D	5.8 × 5.8 × 6.4	400
Prism 2000 XP PCD	5.5 × 6.5 × 8	30

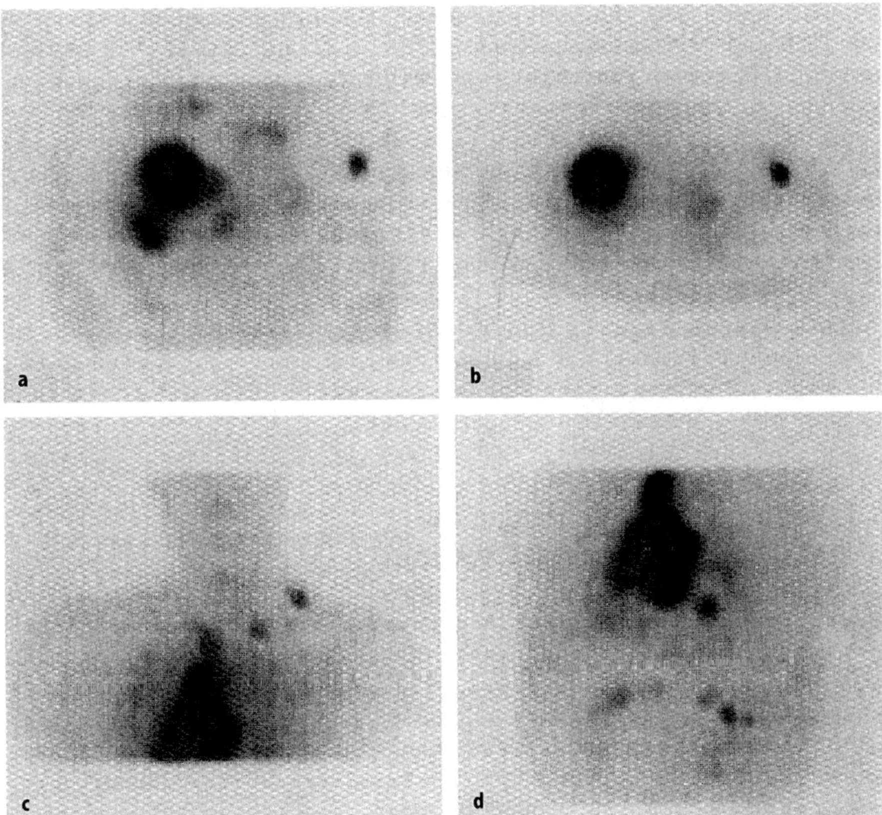

Fig. 9.1. Results of gamma camera-based PET (Prism 2000 XP PCD, Picker) using transversal septa and the multiplicative iterative reconstruction technique with implemented attenuation correction (Luig et al.). All tomograms exhibit a high degree of constancy of the image amplitudes, a correct delineation of superficial body sections (no superelevation of amplitudes near the body contour) and absence of radial artifacts within and outside the body contour. Pat. M. P. with breast cancer (on the left) and four liver metastases, including one with a large central necrosis in coronal (**a**) and transverse slices (**b**); Pat. M. S. with multiple metastases of a NSCLC, coronal slices of the upper (**c**) and the lower thorax and upper abdomen (**d**).

Recommended activities amounted to 200 MBq [^{18}F]FDG when using detectors without septa. However, the use of transversal septa allows to enhance activities up to 300 or 350 MBq in tall or obese patients even in coincidence systems of the first generation [3].

9.6 Clinical results of gamma camera coincidence systems

Published original articles covering extensive clinical studies about the clinical information provided by this PET variant are not available yet. At present, its benefits in clinically routine applications can only be estimated from known physical data and from preliminary studies published as abstracts of the 1998 and 1999 annual meetings of the SNM and EANM. The physical properties of current gamma camera coincidence systems point to limitations when recognizing small lesions of approx. 8–12 mm in diameter. This was confirmed by a number of studies [3, 8, 9]. On the other hand, informative and clinical value provided in cases with cancer of the head and neck, in patients with lymphoma, breast cancer and melanoma were found to be relatively high [2, 4, 8, 9]. Interestingly it was proved that the accuracy of gamma camera-based PET exceeded that of X-ray mammography even at this early stage of the development of these systems [3]. The results match the author's experience in more than 900 PET investigations performed with the new technique. Based on the published information, it can be assumed that the results of optimized gamma camera coincidence PET systems come close to those of low and midrange standard systems.

9.7 Perspectives of the routine use of gamma camera-based systems

Already at the present stage of their development, gamma camera coincidence systems have been found to be very useful in oncological diagnostics [8, 9]. Especially in cases with suspected or present colorectal cancer, in lymphoma, in differentiating solitary pulmonary nodules or in cases with malignant melanoma, the method is very valuable. Thus, this PET variant can contribute to a breakthrough in diagnostics based on [^{18}F]FDG imaging in oncology as well as in a non-oncological context.

Using gamma camera-based systems for PET can considerably reduce the high costs of this kind of diagnosis – a potential key for the widespread use of PET in medicine. Two factors contribute to cost reduction: moderate prices for cameras, on the one hand, and the possible use of the systems for conventional nuclear medicine procedures when they are not needed for PET applications. These factors can help increase the clinical relevance of nuclear medicine and enhance its role in imaging diagnostics in medicine.

Without doubt there is a large potential for further advances in gamma camera-based systems, since the next steps (triple head cameras, "measured" attenuation correction) are emerging. As was the case with conventional PET, corrections for random coincidences, scattered quanta and dead time effects can be awaited. It is expected that the diagnostic efficiency of gamma-based systems will reach that of conventional PET, because gamma camera coincidence systems have just started to evolve and will probably improve very quickly, as was the case with conventional PET cameras some years ago.

References

[1] Anger H (1963) Gamma-ray and positron scintillation camera. Nucleonics 21:1056
[2] Bähre M, Meller B, Lauer I, Luig H, Richter E (1998) PET with a gamma camera coincidence system: phantom studies and first clinical results. J Nucl Med 39:108P (abstr)
[3] Bähre M, Dormeier A, Meller B, Lauer I, Haase A, Richter E (1999) Diagnostic efficacy of gamma camera coincidence PET in breast cancer. J Nucl Med 40:134P (abstr)
[4] Delbeke D, Sandler MP, Al-Sugair A, Martin WH, Coleman RE (1998) Comparison of dedicated and camera-based PET imaging of FDG in patients with focal pulmonary lesions. J Nucl Med 39:108P (abstr)
[5] Kunze WD, Baehre M, Richter E (2000) PET with a dual-head coincidence camera: spatial resolution, scatter fraction and sensitivity. J Nucl Med 41 (in press)
[6] Luig H, Eschner W, Bähre M, Voth E, Nolte G (1988) An iterative strategy for determination of the source distribution in Single-Photon Emission Tomography with a rotating gamma camera. Nucl Med 27:140-146
[7] Schwaiger M, Ziegler S (1997) PET mit Koinzidenzkamera versus Ringtomograph, Fortschritt oder Rückschritt? Nuklearmedizin 36:3–5
[8] Segall GM, Carlisle M, Bocher M (1999) Prospective comparison of coincidence imaging versus dedicated PET in patients with cancer. J Nucl Med 40:135P (abstr)
[9] Shreve P, Steventon RS, Deters E, Gross MD, Wahl RL (1998) Lesion detection in oncologic diagnosis: comparison of dual head coincidence with dedicated PET FDG imaging. J Nucl Med 39:109P (abstr)

10 Combined PET/CT imaging using a single, dual-modality tomograph: a promising approach to clinical oncology of the future

T. Beyer, D.W. Townsend, R. Nutt, M. Charron, P.E. Kinahan, C. Meltzer

10.1 Diagnostic imaging in clinical oncology

Computed tomography (CT) is a widely-used anatomical imaging modality that was introduced in the early 1970s [1] and appeared in clinical practice a few years later [18, 32]. CT offers good spatial resolution and low levels of statistical noise, resulting in morphological images of high quality. In general, radiological imaging techniques reveal anatomical changes, such as tumor development, associated with the underlying functional abnormality.

The development and progression of malignant disease is a consequence of underlying functional or metabolic changes that will, in general, precede any associated anatomical change. Metabolic abnormalities are best visualized by a functional imaging approach such as positron emission tomography (PET) [11, 47]. The sensitivity of PET to identify malignant disease is based on metabolic changes associated with tumors, such as increased rates of glucose transport, protein synthesis [52], and DNA production. The magnitude of the metabolic changes may thus be indicative of the aggressiveness of the disease process [22, 47].

Currently, CT is the most widely-used imaging modality for cancer. However, since CT detects only anatomical changes associated with the disease, functional imaging approaches are increasingly being adopted in an attempt to image the underlying metabolic modifications before significant anatomical change occurs. For example, whole-body PET imaging with 2-[^{18}F]fluoro-2-deoxy-D-glucose (FDG), a radioactively-labeled glucose analog, is used to image the increased glucose transport and decreased hexokinase enzymatic activity associated with tumor growth [47, 52]. While FDG is not a tracer specific to cancer, FDG-PET is nevertheless an effective imaging procedure for diagnosis and staging of malignancy, and the localization of disseminated metastatic disease in almost any region of the body [22, 40, 42]. Regions of abnormally increased FDG uptake are considered suspicious for malignancy, and whole-body PET scanning is thus becoming a widely used procedure for imaging cancer [4, 12].

FDG-PET is also proving to be a useful technique for monitoring the effects of both radiation and chemotherapy, and in distinguishing the effect of surgical intervention from tumor recurrence. The role of FDG-PET is complementary to the anatomical imaging techniques widely used to monitor treatment effects. The functional change resulting from treatment is at least as significant as the anatomical, or size, change, and in many circumstances a functional change will occur earlier than a size change.

10.2 Retrospective image alignment: challenges in diagnostic oncology

A major and widely recognized difficulty with FDG-PET imaging is the absence of recognizable anatomical features that would allow accurate localization of focal lesions to specific structures. In theory, CT and PET images acquired for a patient on different scanners can be aligned using computer algorithms developed for the brain [35, 53]. In brain studies, image alignment is based on algorithms such as in reference [54] that minimize the differences between the functional and anatomical images acquired on different scanners, thus, bringing the two image sets into registration. This approach works well for fixed organs such as the brain, where a linear transformation with six degrees of freedom can generally be found to map the anatomical image into the functional space. The procedure is also aided by the presence of some low-resolution anatomy in the FDG image. However, such an approach is far less successful for the rest of the body where a suitable coordinate transformation may be difficult, or even impossible, to determine due to internal organ motion, patient positioning errors, physical differences between scanners, and an absence of even low resolution anatomical landmarks in the functional image. Some image registration has been successful in the thorax [43] and the abdomen [49], although the application of these algorithms outside the brain often requires manual intervention, or the use of 3D elastic transformations. Nevertheless, the importance of having fused anatomy and function has now been recognized for all parts of the body, not only to enable more accurate localization of functional abnormalities but also for correlation of functional and anatomical changes in monitoring response to therapy.

To overcome the problems of the software approach for fused image tomography outside the brain, the concept of physically combining a PET scanner with a CT scanner has been explored. Such an approach represents a synergy between the two complementary imaging modalities: PET providing functional information and CT providing anatomical information. The design to be presented here incorporates separate clinical PET and clinical CT scanners, without compromising the performance of either modality. The advantages of such a dual-modality approach include 1) accurate co-registration of anatomical and functional images for any region of the body, 2) precise patient positioning using CT, 3) the possibility to perform low-noise PET attenuation correction based on uncontaminated, post-injection CT transmission scans acquired with very short scan times, 4) the potential to employ the available CT transmission information in a scatter correction algorithm, and 5) guiding a statistical image reconstruction algorithm based on the anatomical information from the CT.

10.3 Design concept of a combined PET/CT tomograph

10.3.1 Prototype design

To address the above issues, a prototype dual-modality PET/CT tomograph has been designed and built as a joint effort between the University of Pittsburgh Medical Center and CTI PET Systems. The PET/CT tomograph is based on combining a commercial low-cost CT scanner with the PET components from a rotating partial ring tomograph inside a single, compact gantry. The CT tomograph is a third generation, helical tomograph (Somatom AR.SP) manufactured by Siemens Erlangen, Germany. The PET components are identical to the ECAT ART, a commercial rotating partial ring tomograph [3, 46]. Since the packing density of the CT components precluded the possibility to mount the PET detectors on the same side of the rotating support as the CT, the closest integration of the two scanners was to mount the CT and PET components back-to-back on a common rotating support. The CT components are installed in the front of the combined gantry (Fig. 10.1 a), while the PET components are mounted on a common support and attached to the rear of the combined gantry (Fig. 10.1 b). The combined detector assembly rotates at 30 rpm and is housed within a single gantry with dimensions of 168 cm in height and 170 cm in width. The patient entry port is 60 cm in di-

(a) 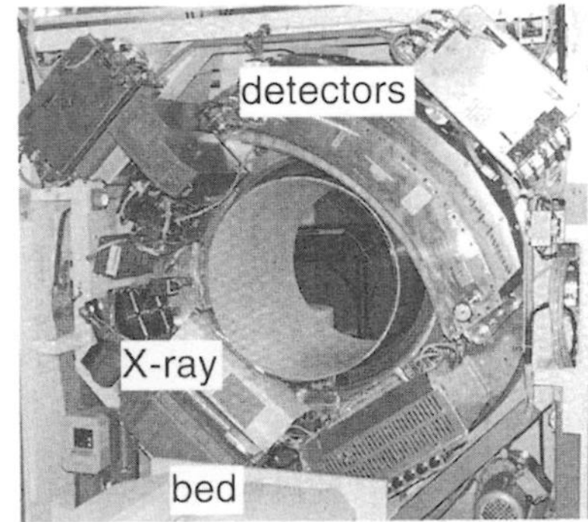

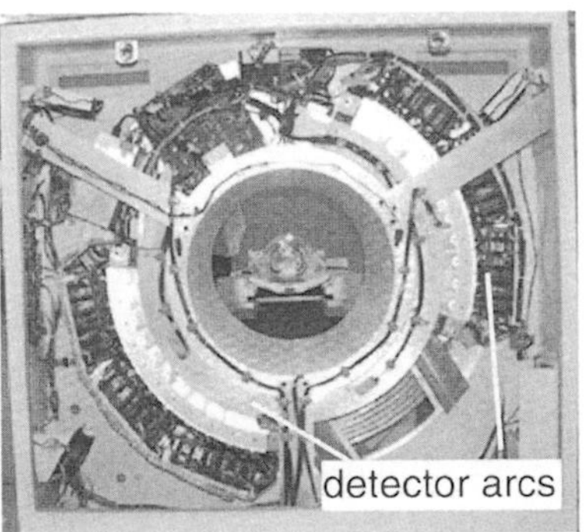 (b)

Fig. 10.1. Front (**a**) and rear (**b**) view of the combined PET/CT tomograph.

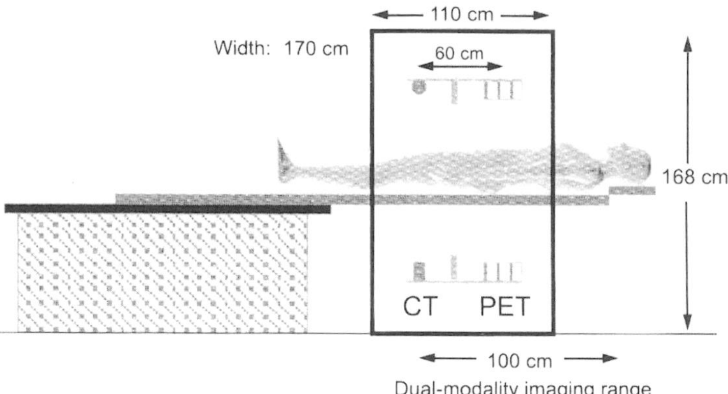

Fig. 10.2. Schematic of the design of the prototype PET/CT scanner. The combined dual-modality imaging range with this scanner is 100 cm.

Table 10.1. System parameters for the CT components of the combined PET/CT tomograph (identical to system parameters of Somatom AR.SP).

Tube voltage [kV_p]	110, 130
Tube current [mA]	63, 83, 105
Scan time per slice [s]	1.3, 1.9
Slice thickness [mm]	1, 2, 3, 5, 10
Focus to isocenter [mm]	890
Fan beam opening [°]	52.2
Transaxial FOV [mm]	450

Table 10.2. System parameters for the PET components of the combined PET/CT tomograph (identical to system parameters of an ECAT ART).

Detector block size [mm^3]	$54 \times 54 \times 20$
Crystal size [mm^3]	$6.75 \times 6.75 \times 20$
Crystal rings	24
Plane spacing [mm]	3.375
Axial field-of-view [mm]	162
Ring diameter [mm]	824
Transaxial FOV [mm]	600

ameter and the depth of the tunnel is 110 cm (Fig. 10.2). The centers of the two tomographs are axially offset by 60 cm.

A common patient handling system is installed at the front of the combined gantry, and enables positioning of the patient anywhere along the 180 cm longitudinal travel range with sub-millimeter accuracy once the patient table is raised to a vertical height between 74.5 cm and 78.0 cm above ground level. Owing to the axial displacement of the two imaging modalities (Fig. 10.2), dual-modality PET and CT images can only be acquired for a longitudinal travel range of 100 cm, which is, however, sufficient to cover the range for most patients from chin to lower thigh. Additional design parameters of the CT and PET components of the dual-modality tomograph are similar to the parameters of either tomograph alone (Tables 10.1 and 10.2) [5].

10.3.2 Operation of the combined PET/CT tomograph

The PET and CT components can be operated in the combined mode as a PET/CT scanner, or separately in the CT or PET mode. Since all major hardware characteristics of the Somatom AR.SP and the ECAT ART were left unchanged in the combined design, the individual performance of both modalities is comparable to that of a commercial AR.SP (Table 10.3) and commercial ART (Table 10.4) tomograph. However, for any combination of the two tomographs in a dual-modality device cross-talk between the two imaging modalities may affect the PET and CT performance of the combined system and must be evaluated. The effect of heat dissipation from operating the X-ray tube, and cross-contamination of the CT transmission and PET emission data thereby deserve particular attention [5].

During the operation of the combined dual-modality PET/CT scanner, the occupational dose limits to the medical personal on site must not be exceeded. While the medical personal is not anticipated to access the patient during CT operation, the total occupational dose is determined by the scattered X-rays [41] during CT operation. The occupational dose can be estimated from

Table 10.3. Performance of the CT components (Somatom AR.SP) of the combined PET/CT tomograph.

Transaxial resolution [mm]	0.45 (at 1.9 s scan time)
CT value of air [HU]	-1000 ± 10
CT value of water [HU]	0 ± 4
Cross-field uniformity	± 2.5
Contrast scale	$(1.90 \pm 0.03) \cdot 10^{-4}$
Contrast resolution	2.5 mm/5 HU/1.9 s

Table 10.4. Performance parameters of the PET components (ECAT ART) of the combined PET/CT tomograph and a standard ECAT ART.

Performance	PET/CT	ECAT ART
Transaxial spatial resolution [mm]		
– at center	6.4 ± 0.1	6.2 ± 0.3
– 10 cm off-center	6.4 ± 0.1	6.5 ± 0.1
Axial spatial resolution [mm]		
– center	n.a.	6.0
Sensitivity [cps/Bq/mL]	8.2	8.4
Scatter fraction	0.34 ± 0.01	0.36 ± 0.02
Maximum NEC [kcps]	36.4 (at 15 kBq/ml)	39.5 (at 18 kBq/ml)

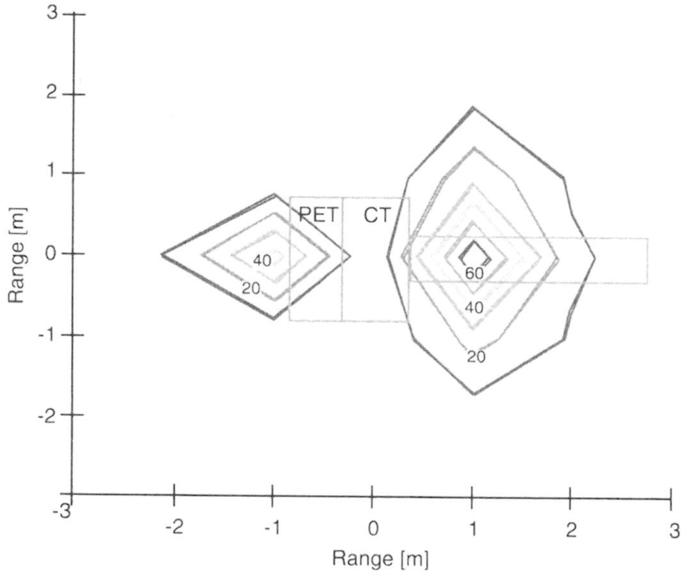

Fig. 10.3. Isodose curves [μGy] measured in the vicinity of the PET/CT scanner with the CT operated at 1000 mAs (equal to five scans of 100 mA with a 2 s scan time).

the isodose curves measured around the tomograph with the X-ray tube in operation. As shown in Fig. 10.3 the isodose curves are skewed to the rear of the combined PET/CT scanner and spread out to the front, most likely as a consequence of the asymmetric distribution of scattering media in the combined gantry [20]. The total occupational dose from the combined PET/CT scanner is, however, similar to the dose from the operation of a Somatom AR.SP.

If installed in a nuclear medicine department, additional lead shielding [2] is warranted primarily for the side of the scanner room facing the control area, due to the limited occupancy of medical personal around the PET/CT suite. The walls and the door facing the control area can be lined with 1 mm thick lead foils. The remaining walls, if made of concrete, can be left intact. Lead glass windows with an attenuation thickness of 1 mm lead-equivalent must be installed in the scanner suite if the patients are to be monitored during PET/CT scans.

10.4 Combined PET/CT scanning protocols using a single tomograph

10.4.1 Scan range and total scan time

For patient studies with the dual-modality prototype tomograph, PET and CT data are acquired consecutively because of the 60 cm axial displacement of the two imaging modalities (Fig. 10.2). CT scans are usually acquired first, before the patient bed is repositioned axially to acquire the corresponding PET scan. Unlike standard clinical CT procedures, patients are not required to hold their breath during the CT acquisition of a combined PET/CT study. An axial range of 40 cm, for example, sufficient to cover the entire thorax, can then be scanned in little more than a minute using a slice width of 5 mm and pitch 1.6.

The axial examination range naturally depends on the clinical indication for the PET/CT scan, and may involve scanning several contiguous PET bed positions when scanning patients with cancers of unknown primary. If indicated, a single bed position over a specific region of interest can be acquired for a longer scan duration in addition to a whole-body scan. Most patient studies with the prototype PET/CT tomograph are performed over three bed positions while a few may extend over as many as six bed positions when imaging patients with disseminated, metastatic disease.

Scan times per bed position are typically between 5 min and 20 min for clinical oncology scans. Of all PET/CT scans to date, 63% were performed in less than 50 min including the time for the corresponding CT examination. While this total scan time is comparable to other scan times reported for whole-body PET scans, combined PET/CT exams also provide reconstructed PET emission data of exceptional quality with low-noise attenuation and scatter correction on routine basis.

10.4.2 Acquisition protocols

Although PET/CT imaging is not restricted to a particular tracer, all oncology studies to date with the prototype tomograph were performed with FDG as a tracer of glucose metabolism. Most patients are injected with 260–270 MBq of FDG and positioned on the examination table after a 60 min uptake period (range from 30 min to 2 h). Prior to the scan procedure the subjects are asked to void and remove any metal objects, such as necklaces, bracelets, and belts before being positioned on the examination table. The patients are preferentially positioned head first supine (Fig. 10.2). Owing to the long scan time of the combined PET/CT procedure compared to a standard CT protocol, the subjects must keep the arms in a comfortable position close to their body. While the presence of the arms inside the transaxial field-of-view may lead to beam hardening [14, 16] or truncation artifacts in the CT images [31], most patients are in a clinical condition that does not allow them to keep their arms over their head outside the imaged area for the duration of the PET scan.

Prior to the start of the PET/CT scan, the examination table is advanced vertically to the center of the field-of-view of the CT. A laser positioning system is used to define the first scan position. A CT topogram is performed to determine the axial range of the helical CT scan. The maximum axial extent of a single helical CT scan depends on the defined slice width and pitch. The total axial length to be scanned is subdivided into contiguous, 15 cm long, segments. The helical scan of each segment takes about 40 s, and X-ray cooling may sometimes be required between segments. Patients are generally required to hold their breath during the scan. For patients who cannot hold their breath, either short axial segments are selected or the patients are instructed to breathe shallowly. The time for the complete helical CT scan ranges typically from 5 min to 10 min in total.

Once the helical scans covering the required axial examination range are completed, the patient is moved to the start position of the multi-bed PET acquisition, and the PET scan is initiated. An emission scan time of 6–10 min per bed position is selected depending on the number of bed positions, resulting in a total PET examination time of 45–60 min. Typically, an axial overlap of 4 cm is used between bed positions for the PET emission scan [3, 46]. The ranges scanned for CT and PET are matched to ensure the CT-based attenuation correction factors are available for all PET sections, and to avoid unnecessary X-ray exposure of the patient in regions where PET emission data are not acquired.

10.4.3 CT-based quantitative corrections

In addition to the complementary and accurately aligned metabolic and morphological information of the PET and CT, the available CT images may theoretically be used for quantitative corrections of the PET emission data. Since the CT images contain low-noise transmission information of the patient, low-noise attenuation correction factors for the PET emission data may be calculated, and noise amplification during CT-based attenuation correction is limited. The challenge of CT-based attenuation correction, however, is to account for the difference in energy at which the CT transmission data are acquired (continuously between 40 keV and 140 keV), and the emission energy of the PET data (mono-energetic at 511 keV). Nevertheless, the use of transmission data acquired at energies different from those of an emission data set for the purpose of attenuation correction is not new [28, 29]. It was originally proposed for a hybrid emission-transmission computed tomography acquisition system [29], and applied in simulations [28] and practice [44, 45] to estimate CT-based attenuation maps for single photon emission tomography (SPECT) data.

For CT-based attenuation correction of the PET emission data from the prototype PET/CT tomograph, the CT transmission images are scaled from an effective CT energy (70 keV) to 511 keV using the hybrid segmentation and scaling method described in [27]. This attenuation correction method is applied routinely to all studies from the prototype PET/CT scanner. Figure 10.4 shows transverse sections through the upper thorax of a patient referred for recurrence of esophageal cancer: (a) the original CT scan, (b) the

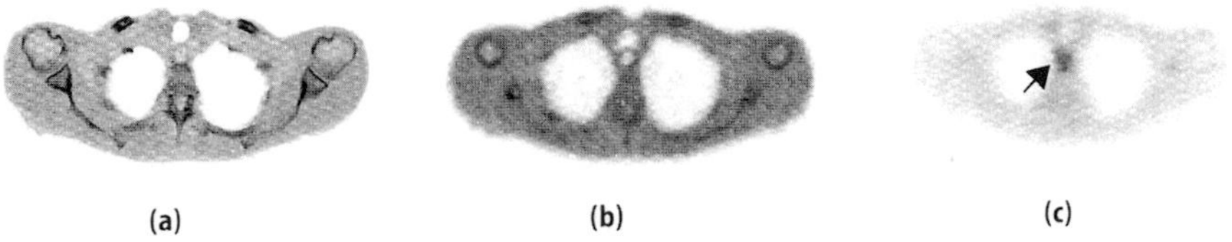

(a) (b) (c)

Fig. 10.4. CT-based attenuation correction [33]. **a** original CT image of the upper thorax, **b** attenuation map at 511 keV derived from the CT image in **a**, and **c** corresponding CT-based attenuation-corrected PET emission image. A region of focal FDG accumulation can be seen in **c** consistent with esophageal cancer.

Table 10.5. Measured CT attenuation values [HU] for three NEMA inserts (materials) and water-filled background without (pre-injection) and with (post-injection) emission activity in the phantom.

Material	Pre-injection	Post-injection
Air	-997.5 ± 0.8	-998.4 ± 0.8
Water	0.2 ± 0.3	$0.8 \pm \pm 0.4$
Spongiosa	319.9 ± 0.6	319.0 ± 1.0
Cortical	1389 ± 3	1389 ± 3

smoothed CT scan transformed to a photon energy of 511 keV, and (c) the PET emission scan corrected for attenuation using the image in (b).

For clinical, attenuation-corrected, whole-body PET imaging with FDG, it is important to acquire the transmission data post-injection to avoid having the patient occupying the scanner for the full uptake period of FDG. While standard PET transmission scans are sensitive to the presence of emission activity and thus require additional scans to correct for the emission contamination [36], the accuracy of post-injection CT transmission scans is not affected by emission activities inside the field-of-view of the tomograph. This is illustrated in Table 10.5, which lists the mean attenuation values of three NEMA phantom [25] inserts and the water-filled background. The phantom was scanned twice with the same CT scan parameters, with (post-injection) and without (pre-injection) emission activity in the phantom. Pre-injection corresponds to no emission activity inside the phantom, and post-injection corresponds to emission activity present in the phantom. Prior to the post-injection study ^{18}F was added to the water-filled NEMA phantom to yield an activity concentration of 3.7 kBq/ml, a concentration that is slightly higher than the concentrations typically encountered in whole-body imaging situations with about 260 MBq FDG injected into the patient. The insensitivity of the CT attenuation measurements to the presence of relatively high emission activity concentrations in the scan field of the CT can be explained by the high source strength of the X-ray tube. According to [6] the non-attenuated X-ray photon flux during the operation of the Somatom AR.SP can be estimated as 4×10^{15} photons/s, which corresponds to an equivalent non-attenuated activity of 2×10^{9} MBq (seven orders of magnitude more than the activity injected into patients for whole-body scans).

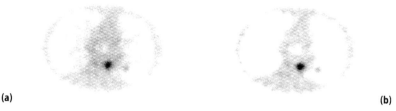

Fig. 10.5. Transaxial PET emission images of a thoracic phantom after CT-based attenuation correction, **a** with and **b** without CT-based scatter correction was applied. Note the increased contrast of the cold lesion in the center of the image (mediastinum) after CT-based scatter correction (**b**).

The scaled CT transmission information can also be used to provide the geometrical distribution of the scattering media, from which the scattered contribution to any point in an emission projection view can be calculated [51]. Figure 10.5 shows the results of CT-based scatter correction for a thorax phantom study with active (hot) and non-active (cold) simulated lesions in a background filled with a uniform activity of ^{18}F in water (3.7 kBq/ml). CT-based scatter correction significantly reduces the scatter contribution and improves contrast for the cold, spherical lesion between the lungs.

10.4.4 Image reconstruction and dual-modality image display

After CT-based scatter and attenuation correction, the 3D PET emission data are rebinned into 2D sinograms using the Fourier rebinning algorithm (FORE) [13] and reconstructed using the OSEM algorithm [24]. FORE + OSEM reconstruction has been shown to improve image quality in count-limited situations, such as in whole-body PET scans, compared to standard filtered-backprojection [26]. Alternatively the emission data may be reconstructed using a penalized weighted least-squares (PWLS) algorithm [17], which is well suited for reconstructing FORE rebinned data with an appropriate statistical model [9]. The idea is to constrain the reconstruction of the emission activity distribution by introducing penalty weights that are derived from anatomical information that is available from the CT (e.g., [30, 55]). The penalty weights encourage smoothness inside, but not across, the anatomical regions, and are typically generated from the binary use of voxel labels [10]. Figure 10.6 shows the potential advantage of using CT-derived anatomical prior information in statistical image reconstruction of PET emission data. For example, the contrast of a small lesion in the upper mediastinal region of a thoracic phantom similar to the phantom, shown in Fig. 10.5, is significantly improved with the use of CT-based anatomical priors (Fig. 10.6b). As in all imaging situations involuntary patient motion is un-

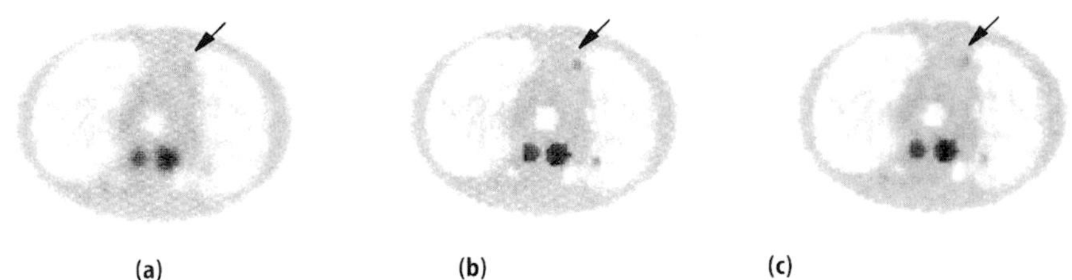

Fig. 10.6. A transverse section through the reconstructed image (FORE+PWLS) of a torso phantom with four hot spheres and three cold spheres of different sizes: **a** no anatomical prior information, **b** with anatomical prior information (voxel labels), and **c** with blurred labels. Note the improved lesion contrast in the upper mediastinal lesion (arrow) compared to the lesion in the image reconstructed without anatomical prior (**a**). Figure curtesy of Claude Comtat and Paul Kinahan.

avoidable. Anatomically constrained image reconstruction can account for mismatches between anatomical and functional data due to respiratory [39] and cardiovascular motion [38] by 'blurring' the voxel labels. Although the use of blurred voxel labels reduces apparent lesion contrast (Fig. 10.6 c) compared to the aligned images with non-blurred labels (Fig. 10.6 b), image quality is better than the quality of the images reconstructed without anatomical priors (Fig. 10.6 a).

The diagnostic power of fused PET/CT image display has been recognized in diagnostic oncology, and is sometimes referred to as *anato-metabolic imaging*, a term introduced by Wahl et al. [49]. Ideally, complementary functional and anatomical images should be displayed side by side or combined as a fused image in a single display tool. Therefore a viewing tool has been developed with the prototype tomograph to display transverse, coronal and sagittal sections of the PET and CT image volumes either adjacently with linked cross-hairs, or in fused mode with the PET images superimposed on the CT images. All images are viewed at the pixel resolution (512×512) of the original CT images. Fused PET/CT images use an interlaced pixel display with a grayscale and a hot metal scale assigned by default to CT and PET images, respectively. This fusion method corresponds to the alternating pixel method of Rehm et al. [37]. The maximum intensity of each image in both separate and fused mode can be scaled independently. As this image fusion method may obscure low-contrast objects [37], the CT display panel can be toggled between CT only and fused PET/CT mode. The display scale of each image in both separate and fused mode can be adjusted independently. Zooming and regions-of-interest capabilities are useful for diagnostic purposes and are also provided with this display tool.

10.5 Clinical applications of dual-modality PET/CT imaging

10.5.1 Introduction

Since the installation of the prototype PET/CT tomograph at the University of Pittsburgh Medical Center in May 1998, almost 70 combined PET/CT studies of clinical patients (31 males, 39 females, average age: 57 years) were performed through July 1999. Most patients (52%) presented with malignancies involving the lungs, head and neck, and pancreas, in addition to metastatic melanomas and lymphomas. A few patients with colon cancer, renal cell carcinomas and cholangiocarcinomas were also imaged on the prototype tomograph. A cross-section of clinical patient studies performed on the PET/CT is presented in the following sections to demonstrate the applicability of dual-modality imaging using a single PET/CT tomograph in clinical oncology [8]. Unless stated otherwise, the patient was injected with 260 MBq of FDG, and an uptake period of 60 min allowed prior to commencing the PET/CT scan described in section 10.4.2.

10.5.2 Abdominal imaging

PET imaging of the abdomen is generally difficult owing to the low-count statistics due to the high tissue absorption of the annihilation photons. Increased fraction of scatter and random coincidences arising from activity concentrations outside the field-of-view, such as the bladder and the myocardium may further degrade overall image quality. The discrimination of physiologic accumulation of FDG in the abdomen is therefore a particularly challenging task as illustrated in the following case study of a patient with pancreatic cancer.

A 38-year-old female was diagnosed in February 1998 with non-resectable pancreatic carcinoma. A stent was placed and during surgery liver metastasis were noted. Separate CT scanning (10 mm slices) revealed a non-specific hypodense lesion in the lower abdomen and a minimal decrease in pancreatic mass compared to the previous follow-up scan. Coronal whole-body PET images (70 min uptake period) demonstrated increased FDG accumulation in the upper mid-abdomen (Fig. 10.7a). It was not clear if this uptake was located in the transverse colon or in the pancreas because of the close proximity of structures. Fused PET/CT images (Fig. 10.7b) localized the increased FDG accumulation (SUV $\sim$ 5.3) to the pancreas, and not to the transverse colon. Transverse sections through the PET volumes further revealed the presence of two metastases that were localized by means of PET/CT image fusion to the right posterior chest wall (Fig. 10.7c) and the left aorto-pulmonary window region of the mediastinum (Fig. 10.7d).

This case study illustrates two advantages of combined PET/CT imaging over single-modality imaging. First, non-specific FDG uptake can be accu-

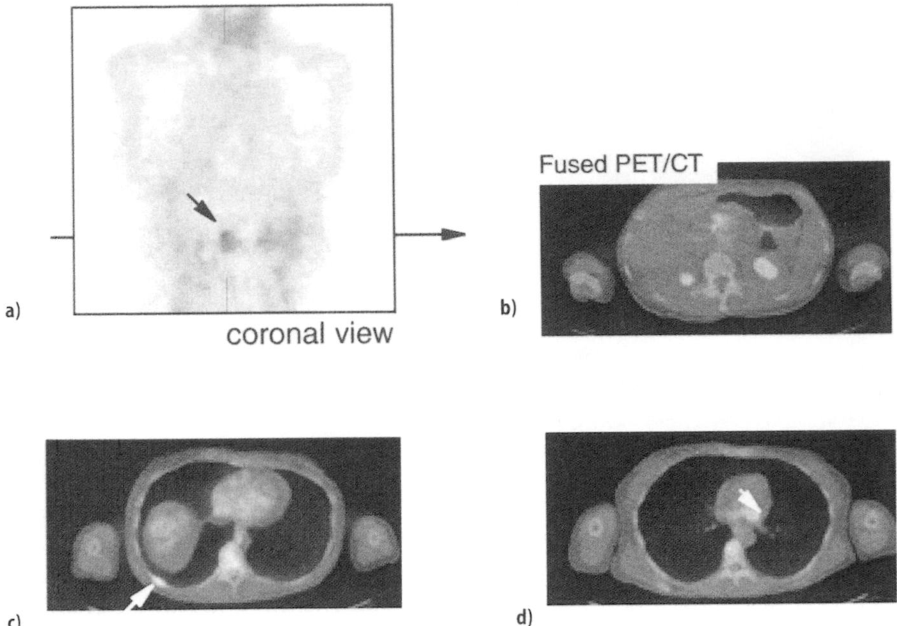

Fig. 10.7. PET/CT study of patient with pancreatic cancer. Coronal view of whole-body FDG-PET image showed primary tumor (**a**, arrow) in mid-abdomen. Image fusion of transaxial CT and PET images localized FDG accumulation to pancreas near the stent (**b**). Fused PET/CT images showed additional foci of FDG uptake in right posterior chest wall (**c**), and in mediastinum (**d**), suspicious of metastatic disease.

rately localized with respect to the anatomy of the patient, which is a challenge if only PET images were available. Second, estimates of the SUV of FDG are provided by the low-noise CT-based attenuation correction, and may be used to differentiate malignant from benign disease. Furthermore, standardized uptake values can help estimate the prognostic value for patients suffering from pancreatic adenocarcinoma [34].

Separate CT and PET imaging already have a rather high sensitivity and accuracy (about 90%) for the detection of pancreatic masses [15, 34]. The combined interpretation of independently acquired PET and CT data, however, can help to detect pancreatic malignancies with a sensitivity of 100% and an accuracy above 90% as shown recently by Diederichs et al. [15].

Another example of abdominal cancer for which the availability of accurately aligned functional and anatomical information is particularly beneficial is renal cell carcinoma. Since accurate pre-operative knowledge of vascular involvement by renal cancer is more important to the surgeon than the presence of extracapsular spread [32], CT is used almost exclusively in the evaluation of solid renal masses due to its superior anatomic resolution. Combined PET/CT imaging has been shown to anecdotally assist surgical treatment planning for this type of cancer. A 49-year-old male suffering from

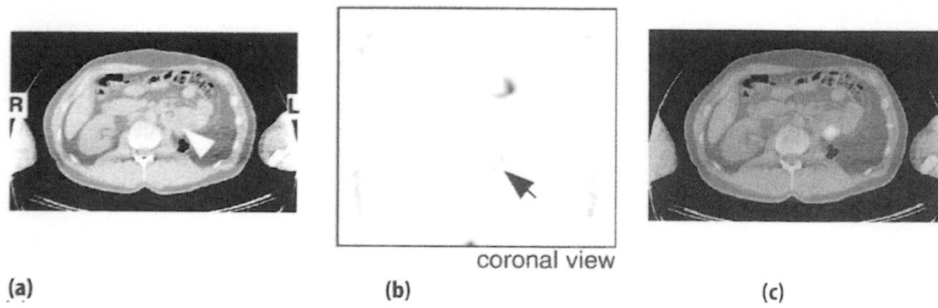

Fig. 10.8. Patient with renal cell carcinoma after resection of the left kidney and post-therapy with interleukin-2 and interferon. CT scan showed large uniform mass in the surgical bed (**a**, arrow). Whole-body PET scan showed high accumulation of FDG in the same area (**b**). Fused PET/CT imaging localized the FDG uptake to the anterior portion of the lesion (**c**) whereby the larger lateral part did not take up FDG, consistent with necrosis.

metastatic renal cell carcinoma of the left kidney presented for a PET/CT scan in January 1999. The patient had undergone a left nephrectomy in October 1998 and post-surgical treatment with interleukin-2 and interferon. The follow-up CT scan showed no progression of the disease (Fig. 10.8 a). Multiple spots in the abdomen were inconsistent with malignancy, and the CT exam was negative for disease. The PET images (Fig. 10.8 b) demonstrated a focal area of elevated FDG uptake (SUV 3.6±0.6) corresponding to the lobulated, uniform soft tissue mass in the left renal surgical bed (Fig. 10.8 a). The lateral larger portion of the lesion (a) did not take up FDG and was centrally hypodense, consistent with necrosis (c).

10.5.3 Thoracic imaging

The advantages of using complementary PET and CT information in tumor imaging of lung cancer was emphasized by Wahl and colleagues in 1993 [49]. The authors state that image fusion '...provides unique information about the primary lung lesion that in some cases cannot be obtained with PET alone and may allow development of algorithms that increase the accuracy of PET and CT. ...' [50]. This statement can be supported by the following case study. A CT scan of a 78-year-old man with a history of T2, N2 squamous cell carcinoma of the right lung demonstrated a large right upper lobe mass without lymphadenopathy (Fig. 10.9a). Metastatic workup was negative preoperatively. The patient was referred for a PET/CT scan that was performed over the region of the thorax. The PET scan duration was 8 min per bed position. The large isodense mass in the upper lobe of the right lung appears on the fused PET/CT image as a highly metabolic rim surrounding a necrotic center (Fig. 10.9 c). In addition a lymph node with increased FDG uptake was seen in the hilum.

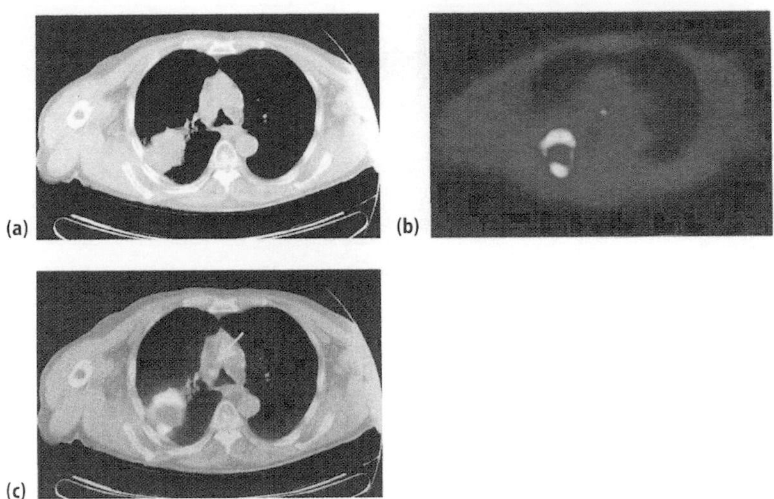

Fig. 10.9. A 78-year-old male with squamous cell carcinoma of the lung. The large isodense mass seen on CT (**a**) appears on the PET scan (**b**) as a hypermetabolic rim of increased FDG uptake, with a necrotic center (**c**). A lymph node in the hilum (arrow) also demonstrated increased FDG uptake.

Although the combined prototype tomograph achieves the best possible co-registration overall between PET and CT images, a variety of periodic and aperiodic physiologic motions during CT and PET scanning may result in some intrinsic misalignment of the complementary images. Most misalignments arise from the fact that different scan times are needed for the PET and CT scans. Helical CT allows one to scan the entire patient thorax in a single breathold and thus limits respiratory motion artifacts in contrast, PET scans image tracer distributions over several respiratory cycles. In contrast to CT acquisitions, the patient breathes normally during the PET scan, and the resulting PET image is an integration over many respiratory and cardiac cycles. Therefore, misalignment of the PET tracer distribution and the corresponding morphology seen on CT images is observed occasionally.

Figure 10.10 illustrates the misalignment of two thoracic lesions seen on CT and PET in a patient with emphysema who was scanned on the PET/CT for two contiguous bed positions covering the entire thorax. Two lesions, suspicious for malignancy, were found in the PET images. Although two nodules were also seen in the CT volume, these lesions were not brought into alignment by simple fusion of the PET and CT images. While the anterior nodule on CT corresponded to the focal FDG uptake in the PET image (Fig. 10.10 a), the lesion close to the chest wall was offset from the corresponding focal FDG accumulation by about 8 mm in the horizontal and 13 mm in the vertical direction (Fig. 10.10 b).

Misalignment of thoracic structures in CT and PET images due to respiratory motion may further affect the quality of the reconstructed PET images if CT-based attenuation correction is used. Figure 10.11 shows the transaxial

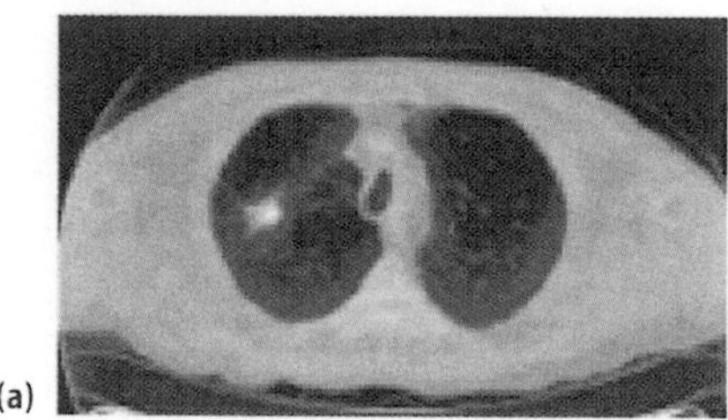
(a)

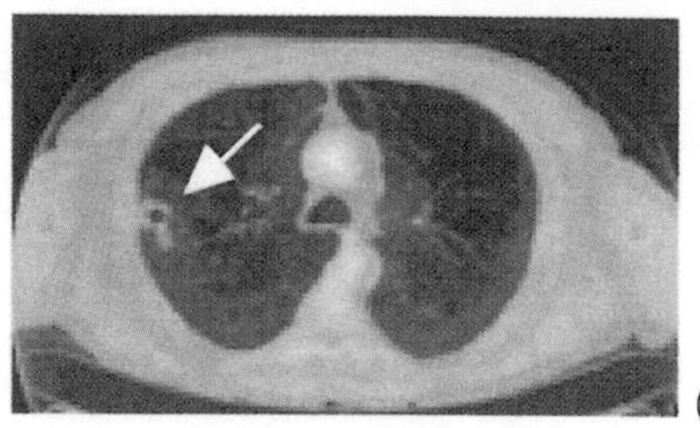
(b)

Fig. 10.10. Misalignment of lung nodule in the mid-thorax. An anterior lesion (**a**) and a lesion close to the chest wall (**b**) were uniquely identified on PET and CT images, but only one lesion (**a**) was accurately aligned after PET/CT image fusion.

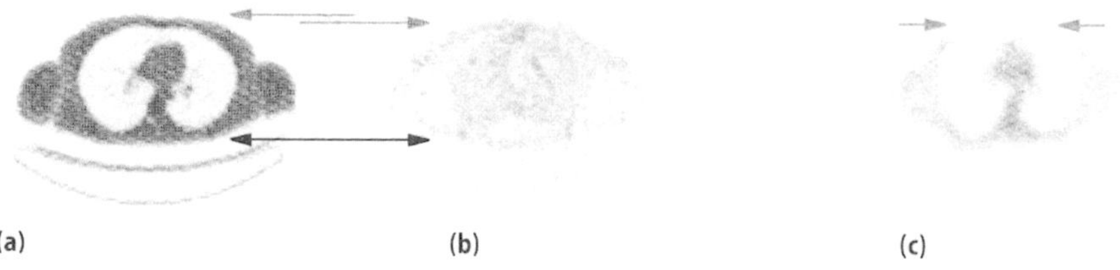

Fig. 10.11. Transaxial section through (**a**) the CT and (**b**) the PET volume of the thorax of a patient undergoing a combined PET/CT scan. The CT scan was acquired during breath-hold with the lungs inflated. The anterior chest wall seen on CT (**a**) was displaced from its average position during respiration (**b**). The use of the CT transmission data (**a**) for CT-based attenuation correction of the available emission data (**b**) introduced a bias into the corrected emission image, seen as a disappearing anterior chest wall (**c**).

cross-sections through the CT and non-gated PET volume of the thorax of a PET/CT patient. The CT scan was acquired during breath-hold with the lungs inflated, while the PET scan was acquired during respiration over a period of 10 min. The misalignment of the anterior chest wall in both scans is clearly seen (Fig. 10.11 a, b). When using the CT transmission images for attenuation correction [27], this misalignment led to an underestimation of the attenuation along lines-of-responses passing through that portion of the chest wall, with subsequent underestimation of true tracer concentration in this region. As a result the anterior chest wall 'disappeared' in the corrected emission images (Fig. 10.11 c). One may compensate for the misalignment of the chest wall by non-stationary blurring of the CT image to smooth the most anterior portion of chest wall in the posterior direction, and to match the blurring in the PET data that occurs due to the emission data being acquired over many respiratory cycles. Alternatively the patients may be allowed to breathe shallowly during the CT exam to avoid situations of misalignment of portions of the anterior chest wall in respiration-CT and PET images.

While the misalignment artifacts described above are observed on a random basis, dual-modality PET/CT imaging can, in our experience, be suc-

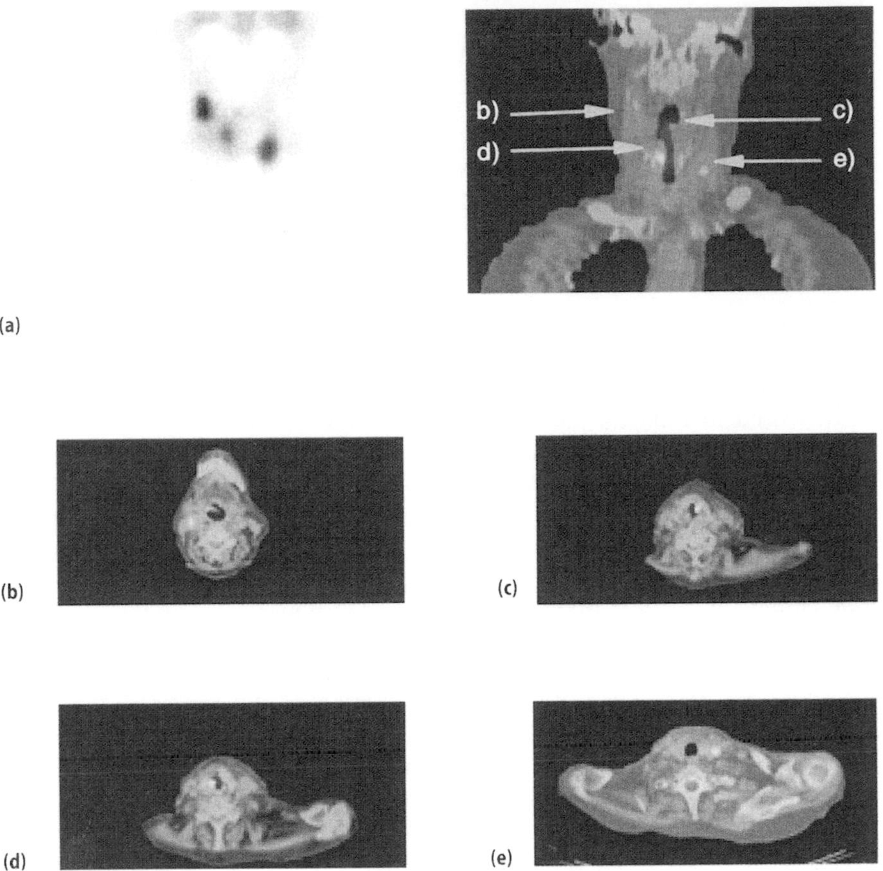

Fig. 10.12. PET/CT study of patient with persistent laryngeal carcinoma. Coronal section (**a**) through PET before attenuation correction (left) and fused PET/CT (right) demonstrated four focal areas of increased FDG uptake in the neck. Transaxial fused PET/CT images (**b–e**) are shown through the center of each of the four foci seen in (**a**).

cessfully applied to diagnose and stage thoracic disease. A 71-year-old female with a known recurrence of head and neck carcinoma after resection and chemotherapy presented for a PET/CT scan in May 1999 (Fig. 10.12). PET/CT images demonstrated a focal area of markedly elevated FDG uptake (SUV 28.6±7.7) corresponding to the laryngeal soft tissue mass (Fig. 10.12 c, d). There were also focal areas of similarly elevated FDG uptake in a soft tissue mass (Fig. 10.12 b) in the right neck at the same level and in the left neck (Fig. 10.12 e) adjacent to the jugular vein at the level of the cricoid cartilage of SUVs 21.4±5.6 and 47.8±4.2, respectively. These findings were consistent with malignant laryngeal tumor and bilateral malignant adenopathy. Also noted was a small focal area of low level FDG uptake in the left upper lung (not shown) corresponding to a possible, ill-defined opacity on the CT. This finding was somewhat suspicious for malignancy and further evaluation was recommended.

While follow-up imaging in head and neck cancers is often required due to the high incidence of recurrent disease, proof of recurrence is difficult because of post-operative scar tissue and displacement of vessels, lymph nodes and other anatomical landmarks after surgical intervention. Therefore, combined PET/CT imaging can be effective in diagnosing and staging head and neck cancer.

10.5.4 Metastatic disease

PET is used in imaging metastatic disease and was shown to be very accurate in determining extra-lymphatic, metastatic spread, such as lymphoma [21, 33] and melanoma [19, 23]. PET was also shown to provide reliable early staging in patients with untreated malignant lymphoma [40] and melanoma [48]. In contrast to functional imaging with FDG-PET, staging and grading with CT is based on size criteria of the lymph nodes. However, small nodes may contain metastatic disease, while enlarged nodes may be the result of a benign process. In one study, disease was present in up to 70% of normally sized lymph nodes [33]. It is interesting to note that accurate anatomical localization of all lesions in extensive disseminated disease may not be required. Combined PET/CT imaging could, however, be used to monitor therapy response, as illustrated in the following example. While PET alone plays an important role in the evaluation of residual mass in CT after therapy [7], only limited data exist regarding the role of PET after lymphoma therapy [48], and to our knowledge no study has yet been performed on the use of combined PET and CT imaging for therapy follow-up in metastatic disease.

A 49-year-old male with metastatic melanoma was scanned on the PET/CT before and after chemotherapy in November and December 1998. The patient underwent abdominal ultrasound where a large retroperitoneal adenopathy was seen. Subsequent CT showed extensive lymphadenopathy in the hilar and periaortic region. The PET study before treatment demonstrated many areas of focally abnormal FDG uptake that were highly suspicious of malignancy (Fig. 10.13 a, b). A second PET study, one month post-chemotherapy showed partial response to therapy (Fig. 10.13 a, c), which was estimated more carefully on the basis of the lesion size in the reconstructed emission images corrected for attenuation and scatter using the available CT transmission images. The lesion in the mediastinum, for example, measured 8.5 cm by 7.2 cm and 6.4 cm by 3.2 cm before and after therapy, respectively. The smaller of the peripancreatic nodes disappeared after therapy, while the larger was stable at around 1.4 cm. High uptake was noted in the pancreatic head prior to therapy. After therapy, uptake was mild, and lesion diameter decreased from 1.8 to 1.2 cm. A periaortic node seen on the pre-treatment images measured 1 cm and appeared three times larger on the post-treat-

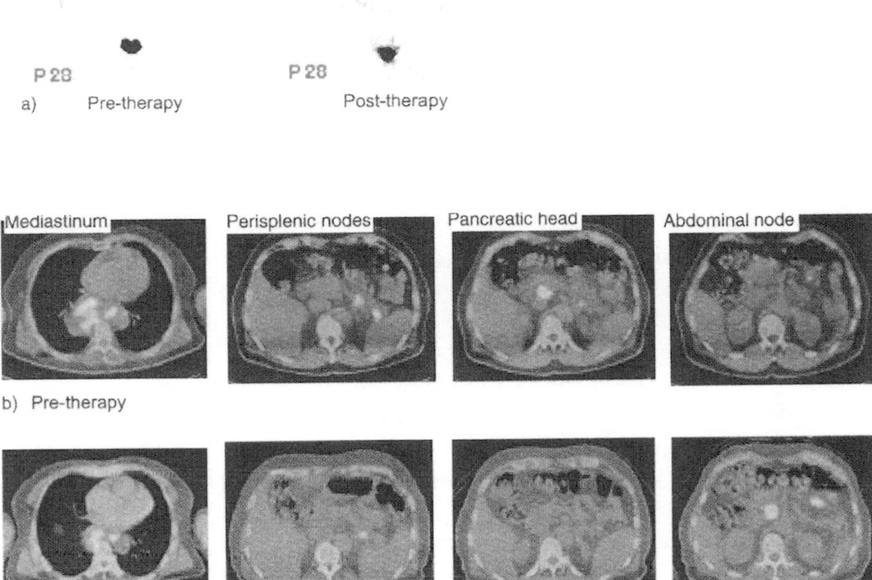

Fig. 10.13. Patient with metastatic melanoma. Whole-body PET study before chemotherapy (**a**, left) revealed multiple areas of abnormal FDG accumulation in the chest and abdomen. A PET study performed one month after chemotherapy showed partial clinical response (right). Independent PET/CT studies before (**c**) and after (**d**) chemotherapy helped to evaluate treatment response.

ment images, suggestive of further advanced malignancy in that area. A second node was seen with intense FDG uptake, and measured 2.7 cm by 3.9 cm. This case study demonstrates the utility of combined PET/CT imaging for staging and therapy follow-up that is facilitated by providing accurately aligned CT and PET images, which are also fully quantitative owing to the low-noise CT-based attenuation correction [27] applied to the PET emission data prior to reconstruction.

10.6. Future directions

The existence of technology to image both function and anatomy with a single device will begin to blur the previously well-established boundaries between radiology and nuclear medicine. The interpretation of fused PET/CT images will necessitate input not only from conventional imaging disciplines, such as radiologists and nuclear medicine specialists, but also from the referring physicians such as surgeons and medical oncologists. Compared to standard PET imaging, the studies presented here clearly demonstrate improved localization of functional abnormalities that can help significantly in the preoperative assessment of primary and metastatic lesions, in the differentiation of normal physiologic uptake from pathology, and in the separation of postoperative surgical scar tissue from tumor recurrence. Furthermore, the evaluation of response to therapy, both radiation and chemotherapy, is an application in which co-registered functional images can significantly enhance the efficacy of current procedures based on anatomical images only.

The use of CT transmission images to provide noiseless attenuation correction factors for PET enables high quality, fully quantitative PET images to be obtained in a time significantly shorter than currently possible with standard PET transmission sources. However, issues still remain to be addressed, including effects due to the arms of the patient being in the field-of-view (increased beam hardening and truncated CT images), and CT images acquired with a contrast medium that may affect the segmentation procedure. Considerably more problematic may be the effects of respiration and cardiac motion, and movement of the patient during the combined imaging procedure, which may limit the image alignment accuracy that can ultimately be achieved.

It is anticipated that the commercial availability of combined PET/CT scanners will further extend the areas of application of this approach. Of particular interest will be the availability of functional information in radiotherapy treatment planning, currently based exclusively on CT images. The use of functional images to more clearly define regions of malignancy within a tumor, and distinguish active tumor from necrosis, may avoid unnecessary radiation. A further possibility is the potential of fused PET/CT images to reduce the sampling error in fine needle biopsies by guiding the needle into regions of active tumor seen on the PET scan. Finally, with the anticipated development of increasingly tumor-specific PET tracers, the provision of co-registered anatomical images will be even more important owing to the absence of recognizable landmarks such as brain, heart, kidneys and bladder seen on standard FDG scans.

The combination of clinical CT with clinical PET within a single device as described here is an integrating force that can bring nuclear medicine and radiology closer together. However, as with any new approach that could potentially change clinical practice, while general acceptance may be slow, it is hoped that it will not be unduly delayed by unnecessary conflicts between different medical specialties.

Acknowledgments. We thank Werner Ertel and Frank Schimmel, from Siemens Erlangen (Germany) for their assistance. We also thank Marsha Dachille, James Ruszkiewicz, and Donna Milko from the University of Pittsburgh Medical Center (USA). We are grateful to Keith Vaigneur, Thomas Bruckbauer, Charles Watson, Ken Baker, Doug Adams, Tony Brun,

Jef Jerin, and Matthias Schmand from CTI PET Systems, Knoxville (USA), and Lary Byars (Byars Consulting) for their help and advice during the design and assembly of the PET/CT scanner at CTI. This project was initially funded by the National Cancer Institute (CA 65856) and has benefited from recent support by Siemens Medical, Hoffman Estate (USA).

References

[1] Ambrose J (1973) Computerized transverse axial scanning (tomography): Part 2. Clinical application. British Journal of Radiology 46:1023–1047

[2] Archer BR, Thorby JI, Bushong SC (1983) Diagnostic X-ray shielding design based on an empirical model of photon attenuation. Health Physics 44(5):507–517

[3] Bailey DL, Young H, Bloomfield PM, Meikle SR, Glass D, Myers MJ, Spinks TJ, Watson CC, Luk P, Peters AM, Jones T (1997) ECAT ART – a continuously rotating PET camera: performance characteristics, initial clinical studies and installation considerations in a nuclear medicine department. European Journal of Nuclear Medicine 24:6–25

[4] Baum RP, Weidmann E, Adams S, Hertel A, Knupp B, Elsner E, Mitrou PS, Hoelzer D, Hör G (1996) Serial whole-body FDG-PET compared to conventional diagnostic imaging in patients with malignant lymphomas: results of a prospective study. European Journal of Nuclear Medicine 23:1208

[5] Beyer T, Townsend DW, Brun T, Kinahan PE, Charron M, Roddy R, Jerin J, Young J, Nutt R, Byars LG (2000) A combined PET/CT tomograph for clinical oncology. Journal of Nuclear Medicine 41:8

[6] Birch B, Marshall M (1979) Catalogue of spectral data for diagnostic X-rays. Hospital Physicists Association, London

[7] Bumann D, Wit MD, Beyer W, Beese M, Lübeck M, Bücheler E, Clausen M (1998) Computertomographie und F-18-FDG-Positronen-Emissions-Tomographie im Staging maligner Lymphome: ein Vergleich. Fortschr Röntgenstr 165(5):457–465

[8] Charron M, Beyer T, Kinahan PE, Meltzer CC, Dachille MA, Townsend DW (1999) Whole-body FDG PET and CT imaging of malignancies using a combined PET/CT scanner. The Journal of Nuclear Medicine 40(5):256P

[9] Comtat C, Kinahan PE, Fessler JA, Beyer T, Townsend DW, Defrise M, Michel C (1998) Reconstruction of 3D whole-body PET data using blurred anatomical labels. IEEE Medical Imaging Conference, Toronto

[10] Comtat C, Kinahan PE, Fessler JA, Beyer T, Townsend DW, Defrise M, Michel C (2000) Reconstruction of 3D whole-body PET data using blurred anatomical labels. IEEE Transactions on Medical Imaging (submitted)

[11] Conti PS, Lilien DL, Hawley K, Keppler J, Grafton ST, Bading JR (1996) PET and [18F]-FDG in oncology: a clinical update. Nuclear Medicine and Biology 23:717–735

[12] Dahlbom M, Hoffman EJ, Hoh CK, Schiepers C, Rosenqvist G, Hawkins RA, Phelps, ME (1992) Whole-body positron emission tomography: Part I Methods and performance characteristics. Journal of Nuclear Medicine 33:1191–1199

[13] Defrise M, Kinahan PE, Townsend DW (1997) Exact and approximate rebinning algorithms for 3D PET data. IEEE Transactions on Medical Imaging 16:145–158

[14] deMan B, Nuyts J, Dupont P, Marchal G, Suetens P (1999) Metal streak artifacts in X-ray computed tomography: a simulation study. IEEE Transactions on Nuclear Science 46(3): 691–696

[15] Diederichs CG, Sokiranski R, Pauls S, Schwarz M, Staib L, Guhlmann CA, Glatting G, Moller P, Berger HG, Brambs H-J, Reske SN (1998) Prospective comparison of FDG-PET of pancreatic tumors with high end spiral CT and MRI. The Journal of Nuclear Medicine 39(5):81P

[16] Duerinckx AJ, Macovski A (1978) Polychromatic streak artifacts in computed tomography images. Journal of Computer Assisted Tomography 2(4):481–487

[17] Fessler JA (1994) Penalized weighted least-squares image reconstruction for positron emission Ttomography. IEEE Transactions on Medical Imaging 13(2):290–300
[18] Fishman EK, Kuhlman JE, Schuchter LM, Miller JA, Magid D (1990) CT of malignant melanoma in the chest, abdomen, and musculoskeletal system. RadioGraphics 10(4): 603–620
[19] Gritters LS, Francis IR, Zasadny KR, Wahl RL (1993) Initial assessment of Positron Emission Tomography using 2-fluorine-18-fluoro-2-deoxy-D-glucose in the imaging of malignant melanoma. The Journal of Nuclear Medicine 34(9):1420–1427
[20] Harpen MD (1998) An analysis of the assumptions and their significance in the determination of required shielding of CT installations. Medical Physics 25(2):194–196
[21] Hoh CK, Glaspy JA, Hawkins RA, Yao WJ, Harris GC, Flores JA, Jacob PK, Maddahi J, Phelps ME (1994) Utility of FDG whole-body PET in the staging of Hodgkin's disease and lymphoma. Journal of Nuclear Medicine 35(5):221P
[22] Hoh CK, Hawkins RA, Glaspy JA, Dahlbom M, Tse NY, Hoffman EJ, Schiepers C, Choi Y, Rege S, Nitzsche E, Maddahi J, Phelps ME (1993) Cancer detection with whole-body PET using 2-[18F]fluoro-2-deoxy-D-glucose. Journal of Computer Assisted Tomography 17(4):582–589
[23] Holder WD, White RL, Zuger JH, Easton EJ, Greene FL (1998) Effectiveness of positron emission tomography for the detection of melanoma metastases. Annals of Surgery 227(5):764–769
[24] Hudson HM, Larkin RS (1994) Accelerated image reconstruction using ordered subsets of projection data. IEEE Transactions on Medical Imaging 13:601–609
[25] Karp JS, Daube-Witherspoon ME, Hoffman EJ, Lewellen TK, Links JM, Womg W-H, Hichwa RD, Casey ME, Colsher JG, Hitchens RE, Muehllehner G, Stoub EW (1991) Performance standards in positron emission tomography. Journal of Nuclear Medicine 12(32):2342–2350
[26] Kinahan PE, Michel C, Defrise M, Townsend DW, Sibomana M, Lonneux M, Comtat C, Luketich JD (1997) Accelerated statistical reconstruction methods for PET and coincidence-SPECT whole-body oncology imaging. The Journal of Nuclear Medicine 38(5):102
[27] Kinahan PE, Townsend DW, Beyer T, Sashin D (1998) Attenuation correction for a combined 3D PET/CT scanner. Medical Physics 25(10):2046–2053
[28] LaCroix KJ, Tsui BMW, Hasegawa BH, Brown JK (1994) Investigation of the use of X-ray CT images for attenuation correction in SPECT. IEEE Transactions on Nuclear Science 41:2793–2799
[29] Lang TF, Hasegawa BH, Liew SC, Brown JK, Blankespoor SC, Reilly SM (1992) Description of a prototype emission-transmission computed tomography imaging system. Journal of Nuclear Medicine 33:1881–1887
[30] Leahy R, Yan X (1991) Incorporation of anatomical MR data for improved functional imaging with PET. XIIth IPMI International Conference, Wye, UK
[31] Lehr JL (1983) Truncated-view artifacts: clinical importance on CT. American Journal of Roentgenology 141(1):183–191
[32] Miles KA, London NJ, Lavalle JM, Messios N, Smart JG (1991) CT staging of renal carcinoma: a prospective comparison of three dynamic computed tomography techniques. European Journal of Radiology 13(1):37–42
[33] Moog F, Bangerter M, Dietrichs CG, Guhlmann A, Kotzerke JR, Merkle E, Kolokythas O, Herrmann F, Reske SN (1997) Lymphoma: role of whole-body 2-deoxy-2-[F-18] fluoro-D-glucose (FDG) PET in nodal staging. Radiology 203:795–800
[34] Nakata B, Chung Y-S, Nishimura S, Nishihara T, Sajurai Y, Sawada T, Okamura T, Kawabe J, Ochi H, Sowa M (1997) [18F]-fluorodeoxyglucose positron emission tomography and the prognosis of patients with pancreatic adenocarcinoma. Cancer 15:695–699
[35] Pelizzari CA, Chen GTY, Spelbring DR, Weichselbaum RR, Chen C-T (1989) Accurate three-dimensional registration of CT, PET, and/or MRI images of the brain. Journal of Computer Assisted Tomography 13(1):20–26

[36] Ranger NT, Thompson CJ, Evans AC (1989) The application of a masked orbiting transmission source for attenuation correction in PET. Journal of Nuclear Medicine 30:1056–1068
[37] Rehm K, Strother SC, Anderson JR, Schaper KA, Rottenberg DA (1994) Display of merged multimodality brain images using interleaved pixels with independent color scales. Journal of Nuclear Medicine 35(11):1815–1821
[38] Ritchie CJ, Godwin JD, Crawford CR, Stanford W, Anno H, Kim Y (1992) Minimum scan speeds for suppression of motion artifacts in CT. Radiology 185(1):37–42
[39] Ritchie CJ, Hsieh J, Gard MF, Godwin JD, Kim Y, Crawford CR (1994) Predictive respiratory gating: a new method to reduce motion artifacts on CT scans. Radiology 190 (3):847–852
[40] Schönberger JA, Stollfuß JC, Kocher F, Tobuschat J, Bangerter M, Frickhofen N, Heimpel H, Reske SN (1994) Whole-body 18-FDG-PET for staging of malignant lymphomas. European Journal of Nuclear Medicine 21:727
[41] Simpkin DJ (1990) Transmission of scatter radiation from computed tomography (CT) scanners determined by a Monte Carlo calculation. Health Physics 58(3):363–367
[42] Steinert HC, Schulthess GK v, Weder W (1998) Effectiveness of whole-body FDG PET imaging in staging of non-small-cell lung cancer (NSCLC). The Journal of Nuclear Medicine 39(5):80P
[43] Tai YC, Lin KP, Hoh CK, Huang H, Hoffman EJ (1997) Utilization of 3-D elastic transformation in the registration of chest X-ray CT and whole body PET. IEEE Transactions on Nuclear Science 44(4):1606–1612
[44] Tang HR, Blankespoor SC, Brown JK, Hasegawa BH (1996) Effect of iodine contrast media in quantitative SPECT with emission-transmission imaging systems. Journal of Nuclear Medicine 37(5):218P
[45] Tang HR, Brown JK, Silva AJD, Matthay KK, Price D, Huberty JP, Hawkins RA, Hasegawa BH (1999) Implementation of a combined X-ray CT scintillation camera imaging system for localizing and measuring radionuclide uptake: experiments in phantoms and patients. IEEE Transactions on Nuclear Science 46:551–557
[46] Townsend DW, Beyer T, Jerin J, Watson CC, Young J, Nutt R (1999) The ECAT ART scanner for positron emission tomography: 1. Improvements in performance characteristics. Clinical Positron Imaging 2(5):5–15
[47] Wahl RL (1997) Clinical oncology update: the emerging role of positron emission tomography: Part I PRO updates. Principles and Practice of Oncology 11(1):1–18
[48] Wahl RL (1997) Clinical oncology update: The emerging role of positron emission tomography: Part II PRO updates. Principles and Practice of Oncology 11(2):1–24
[49] Wahl RL, Quint LE, Cieslak RD, Aisen AM, Koeppe RA, Meyer CR (1993) "Anatometabolic" tumor imaging: Fusion of FDG-PET with CT or MRI to localize foci of increased activity. Journal of Nuclear Medicine 34:1190–1197
[50] Wahl RL, Quint LE, Greenough RL, Meyer CR, White RI, Orringer MB (1994) Staging of mediastinal non-small cell lung cancer with FDG-PET, CT and fusion images: preliminary prospective evaluation. Radiology 191:371–377
[51] Watson CC, Newport D, Casey ME (1996) A single scatter simulation technique for scatter correction in 3D PET. In: Grangeat P, Amans J-L (eds) Three-dimensional Image Reconstruction in Radiology and Nuclear Medicien. Kluwer Academic, Dordrecht, pp 255–268
[52] Weber G (1977) Enzymology of cancer cells. The New England Journal of Medicine 296(10):541–551
[53] Woods RP, Cherry SR, Mazziotta JC (1992) Rapid automated algorithm for aligning and reslicing PET images. Journal of Computer Assisted Tomography 16(4):620–633
[54] Woods RP, Mazziotta JC, Cherry SR (1993) MRI-PET registration with automated algorithm. Journal of Computer Assisted Tomography 17(4):536–546
[55] Yan X, Leahy R, Wu Z, Cherry S (1993) MAP estimation of PET images using prior anatomical information from MR scans. IEEE Medical Imaging Conference, San Francisco

11 Brain tumors

T. Kuwert, D. Delbeke

11.1 Epidemiology and classification

Brain tumors are relatively rare: in post-mortem statistics, their incidence is approximately 6.7% in Eastern Germany and between 2.2 and 15.8% in other countries (for a review, see [68]). Only between 1 and 4% of all malignancies in adults are brain tumors. In children, the percentage is higher, ranging between 20 and 25%.

Various histopathological types of tumors can affect the brain. Nearly 50% of all neoplasms arising in the brain are derived from glial cells, the so-called gliomas. The remaining 50% include various other tumors, among which metastases and meningiomas are the most common. Glioma is the only brain tumor that has been extensively evaluated by PET. Therefore, this chapter will discuss predominantly the role of PET in the management of patients with gliomas.

11.2 Differentiation between a malignant brain tumor and nonneoplastic cerebral lesion

Magnetic resonance imaging (MRI) and X-ray computerized tomography (CT) are the two imaging modalities used conventionally for the detection and differential diagnosis of cerebral lesions. However, in some cases, morphological imaging techniques may not reliably distinguish between neoplastic and nonneoplastic processes. The administration of an intravenous contrasting agent allows evaluation of the integrity of the blood-brain barrier. Alteration of the blood brain-barrier (enhancement after intravenous contrast) is characteristic of certain types of lesion. For non-enhancing lesions on CT and MRI, the differentiation between low-grade glioma and chronic inflammation may occasionally be difficult; for enhancing lesions, MRI and CT can not differentiate high-grade brain tumors and benign processes such as toxoplasmosis or hemorrhagic infarction.

Functional imaging with radiolabeled amino acids may be helpful in that regard. Amino acids can be labeled with positron emitters (^{11}C or ^{18}F) or single photon emitters (^{123}I). Some studies suggest that [^{11}C]methionine or

[^{11}C]tyrosine [31, 45] as well as [^{123}I]α-methyltyrosine [43] may concentrate in non-enhancing low-grade gliomas, but not in chronic inflammatory processes. A variety of ^{18}F-labeled amino acids such as [^{18}F]α-methyl tyrosine and [^{18}F]ethyl-tyrosine are currently being validated for clinical usefulness and may in the future be available on a larger scale [30, 35, 36, 86]. To differentiate benign processes from low-grade gliomas, the accuracy of emission tomography with radiolabeled amino acids is approximately 75% [31, 43]. PET using [^{18}F]fluorodeoxyglucose (FDG) as radiopharmaceutical is not suitable for this purpose since low-grade gliomas do not concentrate FDG.

Most high-grade gliomas exhibit higher FDG uptake than contralateral cortex (Fig. 11.1); therefore, FDG-PET can be used to distinguish between high-grade gliomas and nonneoplastic enhancing processes. For example, it has been shown that FDG-PET can differentiate accurately between hemorrhagic infarctions and malignant astrocytomas. However, acute inflammatory processes such as brain abscesses may also accumulate FDG (Fig. 11.2); therefore, FDG-PET is less useful for differentiating between high-grade astrocytomas and acute inflammatory processes [61, 76]. In patients with acquired immune deficiency syndrome (AIDS), FDG-PET allows the distinction between toxoplasmosis and lymphoma with an accuracy ranging from 80 to 95% [32, 70, 85]. Accuracy in the same range has been reported for SPECT imaging with thallium [51, 52, 75].

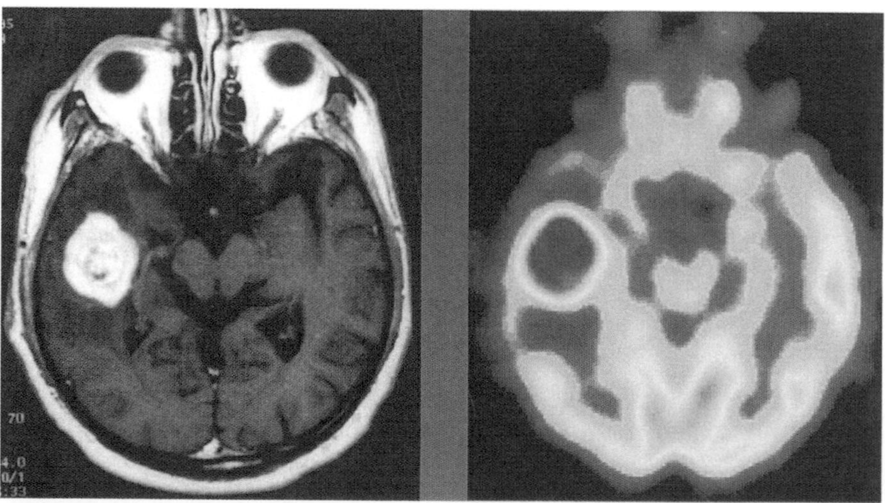

Fig. 11.1. FDG-PET (right) and T1-weighted post-gadolinium MR (left) in a 63-year-old patient with a right-temporal astrocytoma III. The FDG uptake in the tumor is markedly increased when compared to that of contralateral cortex. The PET image is calibrated to its own maximum; in this and the following images red indicates the highest values, followed by yellow, green, and blue.

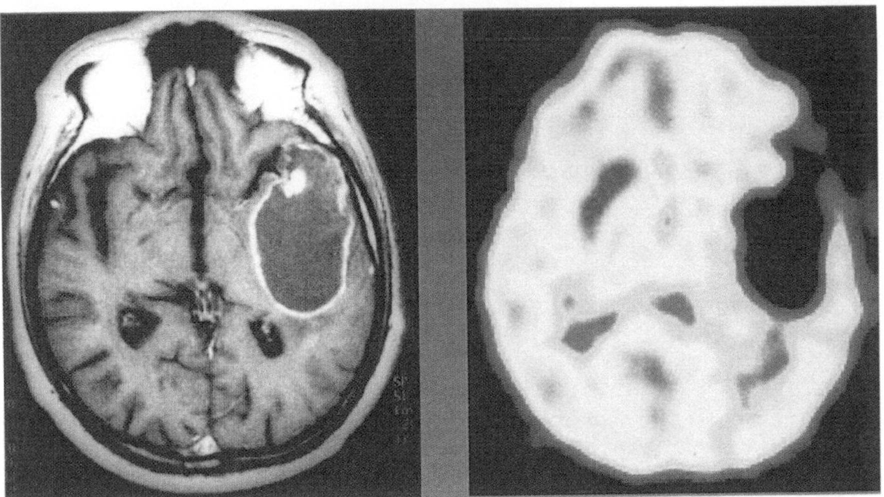

Fig. 11.2. FDG-PET (right) and T1-weighted post-gadolinium MR (left) in a 71-year-old patient with a brain abscess right-temporal astrocytoma III. Due to partial volume artifacts, FDG uptake in the rim of the lesion is underestimated. The FDG uptake in the anterior nodular structure which measures 1 cm in diameter is lower than that of contralateral cortex, in agreement with the nonneoplastic nature of the lesion.

11.3 Grading brain tumors

The main CT- or MR-criterion for differentiating high-grade from low-grade gliomas is contrast enhancement of the lesion. The specificity of contrast enhancement is in the range of 80% because some low-grade gliomas may enhance after administration of intravenous contrast medium (for a review, see [9]). The degree of FDG accumulation in gliomas correlates with the degree of malignancy (Figs. 11.1 and 11.3; Table 11.1). FDG-PET imaging can differentiate high-grade from low-grade gliomas with an accuracy ranging between 75 and 96% in different studies [16]. The degree of FDG uptake in cerebral lesions can be quantified with semiquantitative indices using uptake in different regions of the brain as reference, including white matter and cortex. White matter has two to four times less uptake than cortex. As gliomas arise from white matter, the level of FDG uptake of low-grade gliomas is close to that of white matter. The level of uptake in high-grade gliomas can vary from two times the level of uptake in the white matter to above the level of uptake in cortex. MRI and FDG-PET are complementary, and in some cases correlation of FDG-PET images with gadolinium-enhanced MR images is critical to differentiate uptake in high-grade tumor from uptake in normal cortex. False positive FDG-PET images can occur in patients with pilocystic astrocytoma (glioma grade 1), characterized by a relatively high uptake of FDG, and some low-grade oligodendrogliomas [39].

Other types of central nervous system tumors, such as meningiomas [20], and schwannomas [7] have been evaluated with FDG-PET. The glucose meta-

Table 11.1. FDG-PET in gliomas: accuracy for assessing malignancy grade.

Author	n	Percentage of low-grade tumors [%]	Sensitivity [%]	Specificity [%]	Accuracy [%]	Analysis	Gold standard	Remarks
Di Chiro et al. 1986	100	40	100	90	96	Visual	Clinical course and histology	No information on pretreatment
Kim et al. 1991	20	20	85	75	75	Visual	Histology	Majority pretreated
Delbeke et al. 1995	58	45	94	77	86	Quantitative	Histology	Before therapy; 20 non-gliomas
Olivero et al. 1995	32	28	87	100	91	Visual	Clinical course and histology	Majority pretreated
Woesler et al. 1997	23	39	93	89	91	Quantitative	Histology	7/23 pretreated
Kaschten et al. 1998	45	53	NA	NA	82	Quantitative	Predominantly histology	All before treatment

NA Not available; *Visual* Visual evaluation conforming to Kim et al. 1991; *Quantitative* Quantification as ratios between tumor and unaffected reference tissue

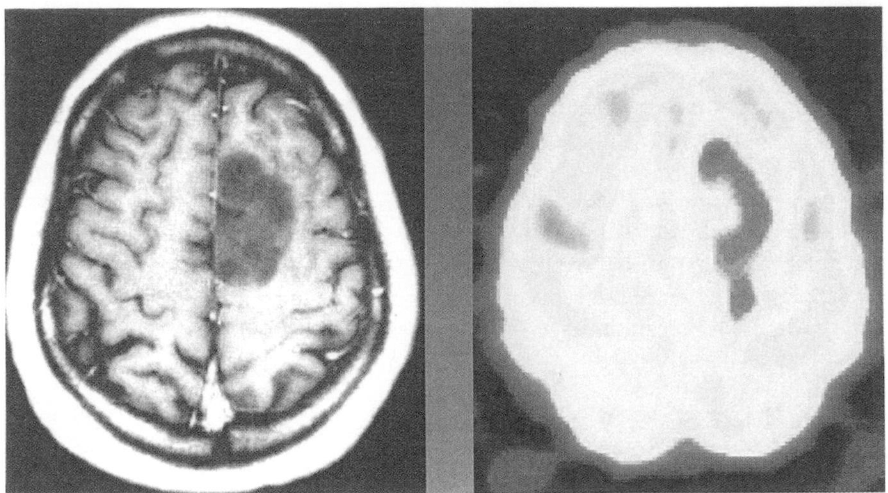

Fig. 11.3. FDG-PET (right) and T1-weighted post-gadolinium MR (left) in a 44-year-old patient with an astrocytoma II. The FDG uptake in the lesion is lower than that of cortex.

bolic rate in these tumors appears to be a good predictor of their biological behavior and aggressiveness. Metastases from primaries outside the central nervous system seem to exhibit more variable uptake [27]. Pituitary adenomas are benign tumors but usually have marked uptake [14]. Data about non-gliomatous tumors have been reported only in small series of patients. Therefore, evaluation of non-gliomatous brain tumors is only a relative indication for FDG-PET imaging (classification 1b).

Approximately 50% of low-grade gliomas dedifferentiate within the first seven years after diagnosis. This is accompanied by a marked worsening of prognosis [50, 55]. The dedifferentiation can be reliably demonstrated with FDG-PET imaging [15, 23]. This has therapeutic consequences as these patients can then be subjected to more aggressive treatment such as surgery, external radiation or chemotherapy (classification 1 a).

The degree of uptake of radiolabeled amino acids as well as that of ^{201}Tl also correlates with the degree of malignancy of gliomas [17, 43, 66, 79]. Data in the literature comparing the relative merit of these radiopharmaceuticals and FDG for grading brain tumors is scarce, and do not clearly prove the superiority of FDG-PET [87].

11.4 Guidance for the site of biopsy

The most important prognostic factor in brain tumors is proliferative activity since distant metastases are rare. The gold standard for determining the degree of malignancy is the histopathological examination of biopsies or surgical specimens.

High-grade gliomas are heterogeneous: some regions can be relatively well differentiated and be adjacent to anaplastic or necrotic tissue [69]. The prognosis is related to the most undifferentiated region of the tumor.

Stereotactic biopsy is usually performed with reference to MR- or CT-images. This procedure is associated with a sampling error of approximately 10% [8, 11, 68]. Several studies have shown that the regional uptake of FDG correlates with the degree of malignancy in gliomas [25, 26, 29]. FDG-PET may help provide guidance during biopsy at the site of maximum activity which is the most undifferentiated region [68]. Performing biopsies using FDG-PET images as a reference increases the diagnostic accuracy to nearly 100% [48, 53]. Therefore, FDG-PET is clearly indicated for guiding biopsy (classification 1 a) [42].

11.5 Delineation of the extension of brain tumors

At diagnosis, high-grade gliomas have usually infiltrated adjacent brain tissue. This does not necessarily lead to changes in cerebral macrostructure [59]. Furthermore, well-differentiated regions of gliomas do not exhibit contrast enhancement so that their extent may not be reliably determined using CT or MRI. The extension of tumor regions with high uptake of amino acids is significantly larger than that of regions exhibiting increased contrast enhancement or FDG accumulation [4, 22, 31, 39, 60, 64, 81]. Therefore, PET with radiolabeled amino acids is better suited for delineating gliomas than the other two mentioned modalities. This assumption has been confirmed with reference to neuropathology [56]; therefore, delineation of the extent of gliomas is accepted as a relative indication for PET using radiolabeled amino acids (classification 1 b).

11.6 Monitoring of therapy

For high-grade gliomas, surgical resection followed by external radiation therapy is the standard care. The usefulness of other conservative therapeutic modalities, and in particular that of chemotherapy, is a debated issue. Therefore, methods allowing the evaluation of the success of these therapeutic modalities on an individual basis would be useful.

Changes in FDG uptake in gliomas following radiation therapy have been demonstrated in small series of patients. Several hours after radiation therapy, FDG uptake has been shown to increase, followed by a decrease approximately three days thereafter to the original level; this phenomenon can be interpreted as a stress reaction of damaged tumor cells [72]. Early effects of chemotherapy have also been demonstrated [34, 46, 74]. The prognostic value of these early metabolic effects of radiation therapy or chemotherapy is, however, still unclear. Some months after radiation therapy or chemotherapy

Table 11.2. FDG-PET in gliomas: accuracy for diagnosing recurrence.

Author	n	Percentage of radionecroses [%]	Sensitivity [%]	Specificity [%]	Accuracy [%]	Analysis	Gold standard	Remarks
Doyle et al. 1987	9	22	100	100	100	Visual	Histology and clinical course	
Di Chiro et al. 1988	95	11	100	100	100	Visual	Histology	
Valk et al. 1988	38	55	88	81	84	Visual	Clinical course	Additional brachytherapy
Glantz et al. 1991	32	41	100	83	97	Visual	Histology and clinical course	PET < 3 months after initial therapy: (early recurrences) 3 non-gliomas
Ogawa et al. 1991	15	33	80	100	90	Visual	Histology	4 Non-gliomas
Janus et al. 1993	20	40	77	71	75	Visual	Histology	In 10 patients intensified radiation therapy[1)]
Black et al. 1994	35	0	91	NA	NA	Visual	Histology	
Kahn et al. 1995	21	24	81	40	71	Visual	Clinical course	2 Non-gliomas

NA not available; *Visual* Diagnosis of a recurrence when the lesion in question had a visually higher FDG uptake than contralateral tissue;
[1)] Intensified radiation therapy: hyperfractionation, additional brachytherapy or stereotactic irradiation

the decrease of FDG accumulation correlates with therapeutic success [58]. Currently, the data are insufficient to recommend FDG-PET imaging for this indication. Preliminary studies suggest that radiolabeled amino acids may be more useful for this purpose, but this need further confirmation [78, 88].

11.7 Diagnosis of recurrence

Usually, the therapy of high-grade gliomas consists of tumor resection followed by radiation therapy. Six to 12 months following radiation therapy, CT and MRI frequently demonstrate contrast-enhancing areas at the original site of the tumor, changes that may be secondary either to radionecrosis or tumor recurrence. On CT and MRI, radionecrosis and tumor recurrence can not be reliably differentiated [9, 47]. The distinction between these two conditions may have therapeutic consequences at least in those patients that may still benefit from surgery since resection of recurrent tumor has been shown to improve survival and quality of life [84].

Recurrent high-grade tumor has higher FDG uptake than radionecrosis; furthermore, there is a significant inverse correlation between the degree of FDG uptake in contrast-enhancing posttherapeutic lesions and the survival rate [2, 3, 67]. The accuracy of FDG-PET for distinguishing between radionecrosis and high-grade tumor recurrence ranges between 71 and 100% (Table 11.2). Therefore, differentiation of radionecrosis from recurrent high-grade tumor is an approved indication for FDG-PET imaging (classification 1a; Fig. 11.4). However, the reliability of FDG-PET for this indication decreases

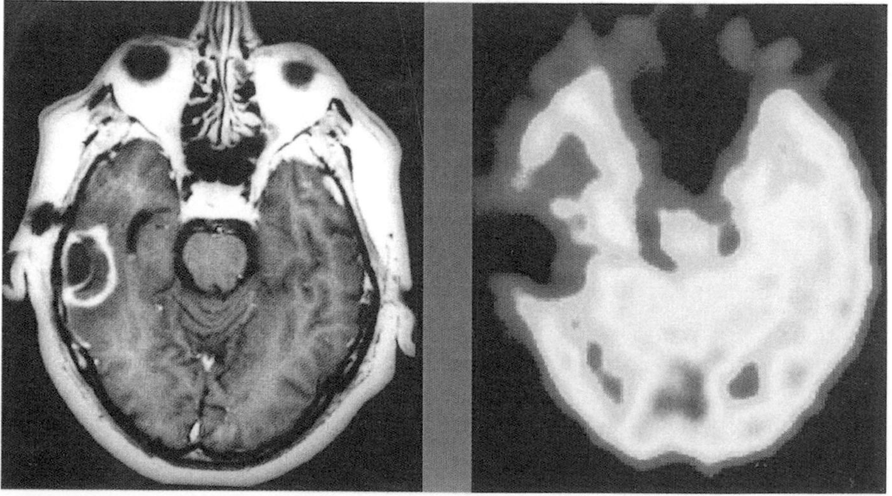

Fig. 11.4. FDG-PET (right) and T1-weighted post-gadolinium MR (left) in a 63-year-old patient with a radionecrosis. The contrast-enhancing lesion is hypometabolic.

with more aggressive radiation therapy regimens because they produce more aggressive necroses which may accumulate FDG to a higher degree [37].

Radiolabeled amino acids can also be used for differentiating tumor recurrence and radionecrosis [31, 49, 62] and have the advantage over FDG to demonstrate well-differentiated, low-grade, tumor recurrences. Since low-grade gliomas do not accumulate FDG, and do not enhance on post-contrast CT and MRI, functional imaging with radiolabeled amino acids is the only modality that can demonstrate low-grade tumor recurrence. Therefore, evaluation of low-grade tumor recurrence is an approved indication for imaging with radiolabeled amino acids (classification 1a).

A third possibility to differentiate tumor recurrence from benign posttherapeutic lesions includes SPECT with ^{201}Tl or ^{99m}Tc-MIBI [10, 54]. Published comparative studies do not prove the superiority of FDG-PET over SPECT imaging with single photon emitters, but suffer from methodological problems, in particular, the limited number of subjects studied [6, 38].

11.8 Future directions

PET with FDG and radiolabeled amino acids definitely has a role in managing patients with brain tumors and in particular with gliomas. Functional imaging with PET does not replace CT or MRI but provides additional, complementary information which can not be obtained by CT or MRI. Functional imaging, however, does not have the resolution and the anatomic landmarks provided by morphological imaging. One of the major issues is to integrate functional and morphological data for precise localization of lesions that have increased metabolism. Image fusion is a potentially powerful diagnostic tool to improve the planning and performance of surgical resection and radiation therapy in brain tumors [60]. New developments in hardware and software are currently being investigated to improve registration of both sets of images to provide optimal fusion images.

SPECT imaging with single photon emitters, such as ^{201}Tl, is still more widely available than PET and may be a diagnostic alternative to PET for specific indications. Large prospective studies should be performed to confirm preliminary data obtained on small numbers of patients.

One of the major problems of functional imaging of tumors with the currently available radiopharmaceuticals, including FDG, is the nonspecific uptake by inflammatory cells. Evaluation of new radiopharmaceuticals, for example imaging DNA metabolism, may circumvent this problem [77, 80, 83]. Another possibility would be evaluating radioligands, for example against peripheral benzodiazepine receptors [57].

New approaches for therapy of brain tumors are also under current investigation, in particular gene therapy and radioimmunotherapy [41, 71].

References

[1] Alavi JB, Alavi A, Goldberg HI, Dann R, Hickey W, Reivich M (1987) Sequential CT and PET studies in a patient with malignant glioma. Nucl Med Commun 8:457–468
[2] Alavi JB, Alavi A, Chawluk J, Kushner M, Powe J, Hickey W, Reivich M (1988) Positron emission tomography in patients with glioma – a predictor of prognosis. Cancer 62:1074–1078
[3] Barker FG, Chang SM, Valk PE, Pounds TR, Prados MD (1997) 18 Fluorodeoxyglucose uptake and survival of patients with suspected recurrent malignant glioma. Cancer 79:115–126
[4] Bergström M, Collins VP, Ehrin E, Ericson K, Eriksson L, Greitz T, Halldin C, von Holst H, Langström B, Lilja A, Lundqvist H, Nagren K (1983) Discrepancies in brain tumor extent as shown by computed tomography and positron emission tomography using [^{68}GA] EDTA, [^{11}C] glucose and [^{11}C] methionine. J Comput Assist Tomogr 7:1062–1066
[5] Black KL, Hawkins RA, Kim KT, Becker DP, Lerner C, Marciano D (1989) Use of thallium-201 SPECT to quantitate malignancy grade of gliomas. J Neurosurg 71:342–346
[6] Black KL, Emerick T, Hoh C, Hawkins RA, Mazziotta J, Becker DP (1994) Thallium-201 SPECT and positron emission tomography equal predictors of glioma grade and recurrence. Neurol Res 16:93–96
[7] Borbely K, Fulham MJ, Brooks RA, Di Chiro G (1992) PET-fluorodeoxyglucose of cranial and spinal neuromas. J Nucl Med 33:1931–1934
[8] Brucher JM (1993) Neuropathological diagnosis with stereotactic biopsies. Possibilities, difficulties and requirements. Acta Neurochir 124:37–39
[9] Byrne TN (1994) Imaging of gliomas. Semin Oncol 21:162–171
[10] Carvalho PA, Schwartz RB, Eben A et al. (1992) Detection of recurrent gliomas with quantitative thallium-201/technetium-99m HMPAO single-photon emission computerized tomography. J Neurosurg 77:565–570
[11] Chandrasoma PT, Smith MM, Appuzzo MLJ (1989) Stereotactic biopsy in the diagnosis of brain masses: comparison of results of biopsy and resected surgical specimen. Neurosurgery 24:160–165
[12] Chang LT (1978) A method for attenuation correction in radionuclide computed tomography. IEEE Trans Nucl Sci NS-26/2:2780–2789
[13] Cremerius U, Striepecke E, Henn W, Weis J, Mull M, Lippitz B, Gilsbach J, Schröder JM, Zang KD, Böcking A, Büll U (1994) ^{18}FDG-PET in intracranial meningeomas versus grading, proliferation index, cellular density, and cytogenetic analysis. Nuklearmedizin 33:144–149
[14] De Souza B, Brunetti A, Fulham MJ, Brooks RA, DeMichele D, Cook P, Nieman L, Doppman JL, Oldfield EH, Di Chiro G (1990) Pituitary microadenomas: a PET study. Radiology 177:39–44
[15] De Witte O, Levivier M, Violon P, Salmon S, Damhaut P, Wikler D, Hildebrand J, Brotchi J, Goldman S (1996) Prognostic value of positron emission tomography with [18] fluorodeoxyglucose in the low-grade glioma. Neurosurgery 39:470–477
[16] Delbeke D, Meyerowitz C, Lapidus RL, Maciunas RJ, Jennings MT, Moots PL, Kessler RM (1995) Optimal cutoff levels of F-18 fluorodeoxyglucose uptake in the differentiation of low-grade from high-grade brain tumors with PET. Radiology 195:47–52
[17] Derlon JM, Bourdet C, Bustany P et al. (1989) [11C] L-Methionine uptake in gliomas. Neurosurgery 30:225–232
[18] Di Chiro G, Oldfield E, Wright DC, De Michele D, Katz DA, Patronas NJ, Doppman JL, Larson SM, Ito M, Kufta CV (1988) Cerebral necrosis after radiotherapy and/or intraarterial chemotherapy for brain tumors: PET and neuropathological studies. AJR 150:189–197
[19] Di Chiro G (1986) Positron emission tomography using [^{18}F] fluorodeoxyglucose in brain tumors: a powerful diagnostic and prognostic tool. Invest Radiol 22:360–371

[20] Di Chiro G, Hatazawa J, Katz DA, Rizzoli HV, De Michele DJ (1987) Glucose utilization by intracranial meningeomas as an index of tumor aggressivity and probability of recurrence: a PET study. Radiology 164:521–526

[21] Doyle WK, Budinger TF, Valk PE, Levin VA, Gutin PH (1987) Differentiation of cerebral radiation necrosis from tumor recurrence by [^{18}F] FDG and ^{82}Rb positron emission tomography. J Comput Assist Tomogr 11:563–570

[22] Ericson K, Lilja A, Bergström M, Collins VP, Eriksson L, Ehrin E, von Holst H, Lundqvist H, Langström B, Mosskin M (1985) Positron emission tomography with ([^{11}C] methyl)-L-methionine, [^{11}C] D-glucose, and [^{68}GA] EDTA in supratentorial brain tumors. J Comput Assist Tomogr 9:683–689

[23] Francavilla TL, Miletich RS, Di Chiro G, Patronas NJ, Rizzoli HV, Wright DC (1989) Positron emission tomography in the detection of malignant degeneration of low-grade gliomas. Neurosurgery 24:1–5

[24] Glantz MJ, Hoffman JM, Coleman RE, Friedman AH, Hanson MW, Burger PC, Herndon JE II, Meisler WJ, Schold SC (1991) Identification of early recurrence of primary central nervous system tumors by [^{18}F] fluorodeoxyglucose positron emission tomography. Ann Neurol 29:347–355

[25] Goldman S, Levivier M, Pirotte B, Brucher J-M, Wikler D, Damhaut P, Stanus E, Brotchi J, Hildebrand J (1996) Regional glucose metabolism and histopathology of gliomas. Cancer 78:1098–1106

[26] Goldman S, Levivier M, Pirotte B, Brucher J-M, Wikler D, Damhaut P, Dethy S, Brotchi J, Hildebrand J (1997) Regional methionine and glucose uptake in high-grade gliomas: a comparative study on PET-guided stereotactic biopsy. J Nucl Med 38:1459–1462

[27] Griffeth LK, Rich KM, Dehdashti F, Simpson JR, Fusselman MJ, McGuire AH, Siegel BA (1993) Brain metastases from non-central nervous system tumors: evaluation with PET [see comments]. Radiology 186:37–44

[28] Guth-Tougelides B, Müller St, Mehdorn MM, Knust EJ, Dutschka K, Reiners C (1995) Anreicherung von DL-3-^{123}I-Jod-Methyltyrosin in Hirntumorrezidiven. Nuklearmedizin 34:71–75

[29] Herholz K, Pietrzyk U, Voges J, Schröder R, Halber M, Treuer H, Sturm V, Heiss W-D (1993) Correlation of glucose consumption and tumor cell density in astrocytomas. A stereotactic PET study. J Neurosurg 79:853–858

[30] Heiss P, Mayer S, Herz M, Wester HJ, Schwaiger M, Senekowitsch-Schmidtke R (1999) Investigation of transport mechanism and uptake kinetics of O-(2-[18F]fluoroethyl)-L-tyrosine in vitro and in vivo. J Nucl Med 40:1367–173

[31] Herholz K, Hölzer T, Bauer B, Schröder R, Voges J, Ernestus RI, Mendoza G, Weber-Luxenburger G, Löttgen J, Thiel A, Wienhard K, Heiss W-D (1998) C-11-Methionine PET for differential diagnosis of low-grade gliomas. Neurology 50:1316–1322

[32] Hoffman JM, Waskin HA, Schifter T, Widemann B, Schröder R, Neubauer I, Heiss WD (1993) FDG-PET in differentiating lymphoma from nonmalignant central nervous system lesions in patients with AIDS. J Nucl Med 34:567–575

[33] Holthoff VA, Herholz K, Berthold F, Widemann B, Schröder R, Neubauer I, Heiss WD (1993) In vivo metabolism of childhood posterior fossa tumors and primitive neuroectodermal tumors before and after treatment. Cancer 72:1394–1403

[34] Holzer T, Herholz K, Jeske J, Heiss WD (1993) FDG-PET as a prognostic indicator in radiochemotherapy of glioblastoma. J Comput Assist Tomogr 17:681–687

[35] Inoue T, Shibasaki T, Oriuchi N, Aoyagi K, Tomiyoshi K, Amano S, Mikuni M, Ida I, Aoki J, Endo K (1999) 18F alpha-methyl tyrosine PET studies in patients with brain tumors. J Nucl Med 40:399–405

[36] Inoue T, Tomiyoshi K, Higuichi T, Ahmed K, Sarwar M, Aoyagi K, Amano S, Alyafei S, Zhang H, Endo K (1998) Biodistribution studies on L-3-[fluorine-18]fluoro-alpha-methyl tyrosine: a potential tumor-detecting agent

[37] Janus TJ, Kim E, Tilbury R, Bruner JM, Yung WKA (1993) Use of [^{18}F] fluorodeoxyglucose positron emission tomography in patients with primary malignant brain tumors. Ann Neurol 33:540–548

[38] Kahn D, Follett KA, Bushnell DL, Nathan MA, Piper JG, Madsen M, Kirchner PT (1994) Diagnosis of recurrent brain tumor: Value of ^{201}Tl SPECT vs ^{18}F-fluorodeoxy-glucose PET. AJR 163:1450–1465

[39] Kaschten B, Stevenaert A, Sadzot B, Deprez M, Degueldre C, Del Fiore G, Luxen A, Reznik M (1998) Pre-operative evaluation of 54 gliomas by PET with fluorine-18-fluorodeoxyglucose and/or carbon-11-methionine. J Nucl Med 39:778–785

[40] Kim CK, Alavi JB, Alavi A, Reivich M (1991) New grading system of cerebral gliomas using positron emission tomography with F-18 fluorodeoxyglucose. J Neuro-Oncol 10:85–91

[41] Kramm CM, Sena-Esteves M, Barnett FH, Rainov NG, Schuback DE, Yu JS, Pechan PA, Paulus W, Chiocca EA, Breakefield XO (1995) Gene therapy for brain tumors. Brain Pathology 5:345–381

[42] Kuwert T, Morgenroth C, Woesler B, Matheja P, Palkovic S, Vollet B, Samnick S, Maasjosthusmann U, Lerch H, Gildehaus F-J, Wassmann H, Schober O (1996) Uptake of iodine-123-methyl tyrosine by gliomas and non-neoplastic brain lesions. Eur J Nucl Med 23:1345–1353

[43] Kuwert T, Bartenstein P, Grünwald F, Herholz K, Larisch R, Sabri O, Biersack H-J, Moser E, Müller-Gärtner H-W, Schober O, Schwaiger M, Büll U, Heiss W-D (1998) Klinische Wertigkeit der Positronen-Emissions-Tomographie in der Neuromedizin. Nervenarzt 69:1045–1060

[44] Kuwert T, Woesler B, Morgenroth C, Lerch H, Schäfers M, Palkovic P, Matheja P, Brandau W, Wassmann H, Schober O (1998) Diagnosis of recurrent glioma with SPECT and iodine-123-methyl tyrosine. J Nucl Med 39:23–27

[45] Kole AC, Pruim J, Nieweg OE, van Ginkel RJ, Hoekstra HJ, Schraffordt Koops H, Vaalburg W (1997) PET with L-[1-carbon-11]-tyrosine to visualize tumors and measure protein synthesis rates. J Nucl Med 38:191–195

[46] Langen K-J, Roosen N, Kuwert T, Herzog H, Kiwit JC, Rota Kops E, Muzik O, Bock WJ, Feinendegen LE (1989) Early effects of intra-arterial chemotherapy in patients with brain tumours studied with PET: preliminary results. Nucl Med Commun 10:779–790

[47] Leeds NE, Jackson EF (1994) Current imaging techniques for the evaluation of brain neoplasms. Curr Opin Oncol 6:254–261

[48] Levivier M, Goldman S, Pirotte B, Brucher JM, Balériaux D, Luxen A, Hildebrand J, Brotchi J (1995) Diagnostic yield of stereotactic brain biopsy guided by positron emission tomography with [^{18}F] fluorodeoxy-glucose. J Neurosurg 82:445–452

[49] Lilja A, Lundqvist H, Olsson Y, Spännare B, Gullberg P, Langström B (1989) Positron emission tomography and computed tomography in differential diagnosis between recurrent or residual glioma and treatment-induced brain lesions. Acta Radiol 30:121–128

[50] Loiseau H, Bousquet P, Rivel J, Vital C, Kantor G, Rougier A, Dartigues JF, Cohadon F (1995) Astrocytomes de bas grade sustentoriels de l'adulte: Facteurs prognostics et indications thérapeutiques – á propos d'une série de 141 patients. Neurochirurgie 41:38–51

[51] Lorberboym M, Estok L, Machac J, German I, Sacher M, Feldman R, Wallach F, Dorfman D (1996) Rapid differential diagnosis of cerebral toxoplasmosis and primary central nervous system lymphoma by thallium-201 SPECT. J Nucl Med 37:1150–1154

[52] Lorberboym M, Wallach F, Estok L, Mosesson RE, Sacher M, Kim CK, Machac J (1998) Thallium-201 retention in focal intracranial lesions for differential diagnosis of primary lymphoma and nonmalignant lesions in AIDS patients. J Nucl Med 39:1366–1369

[53] Maciunas RJ, Kessler RM, Maurer C, Mandava V, Watt G, Smith G (1992) Positron emission tomography imaging directed stereotactic neurosurgery. Stereotact Funct Neurosurg 58:134–140

[54] Maffioli L, Gasparini M, Chiti A, Gramaglia A, Mongioj V, Pozzi A, Bombardieri E (1996) Clinical role of technetium-99m sestamibi single-photon emission tomography in evaluating pretreated patients with brain tumors. Eur J Nucl Med 23:308–311

[55] McCormack BM, Miller DC, Budzilovich GN, Vorhees GJ, Ransohoff J (1992) Treatment and survival of low-grade astrocytoma in adults: 1977–1988. Neurosurgery 31:636–642

[56] Mosskin M, Ericson K, Hindmarsh T, von Holst H, Collins VP, Bergström M, Eriksson L, Johnström P (1989) Positron emission tomography compared with magnetic resonance imaging and computed tomography in supratentorial gliomas using multiple stereotactic biopsies as reference. Acta Radiol 30:225–232

[57] Miettinen H, Kononen J, Haapasalo H, Helen P, Sallinen P, Harjuntausta T, Helin H, Alho H (1995) Expression of peripheral-type benzodiazepine receptor and diazepam binding inhibitor in human astrocytomas: relationship to cell proliferation. Cancer Res 55:2691–2695

[58] Mineura K, Yasuda T, Kowada M, Ogawa T, Shishido F, Uemura K (1987) Positron emission tomography evaluation of radiochemotherapeutic effect on regional cerebral hemocirculation and metabolism in patients with gliomas. J Neuro-Oncol 5:277–285

[59] Nagano N, Sasaki H, Aoyagi M, Hirakawa K (1993) Invasion of experimental brain tumor: early morphological changes following microinjection of C6 glioma cells. Acta Neuropathol 86:117–125

[60] Nariai T, Senda M, Ishii K, Maehara T, Wakabayashi S, Toyama H, Ishiwata K, Hirakawa K (1997) Three-dimensional imaging of cortical structure, function and glioma for tumor resection. J Nucl Med 38:1563–1568

[61] Newsholme P, Newsholme EA (1989) Rates of utilization of glucose, glutamine, and oleate and formation of end-products by mouse peritoneal macrophages in culture. Biochem J 261:211–218

[62] Ogawa T, Kanno I, Shishido F, Inugami A, Higano S, Fujita H, Murakami M, Uemura K, Yasui N, Mineura K, Kowada M (1991) Clinical value of PET with ^{18}fluoro-deoxyglucose and L-methyl-11C-methionine for diagnosis of recurrent brain tumor and radiation injury. Acta Radiol 32:197–202

[63] Ogawa T, Shishido F, Kanno I et al. (1993) Cerebral glioma: evaluation with methionine PET. Radiology 186:45–53

[64] Ogawa T, Shishido F, Kanno I et al. (1996) Clinical positron emission tomography for brain tumors: comparison of fluorodeoxyglucose ^{18}F and L-methyl-^{11}C-methionine. AJNR 17:345–353

[65] Olivero WC, Dulebohn SC, Lister JR (1995) The use of PET in evaluating patients with primary brain tumors: is it useful? J Neurol Neurosurg Psychiatr 58:250–252

[66] Oriuchi N, Tomiyoshi K, Inoue T et al. (1996) Independent thallium-201 accumulation and fluorine-18-fluorodeoxyglucose metabolism in glioma. J Nucl Med 37:457–462

[67] Patronas NJ, Di Chiro G, Kufta C, Bairamian D, Kornblith PL, Simon R, Larson SM (1985) Prediction of survival in glioma patients by means of positron emission tomography. J Neurosurg 62:816–822

[68] Paulus W (1995) Tumoren des Nervensystems. In: Peiffer J, Schröder JM (eds) Neuropathologie. Morphologische Diagnostik der Krankheiten des Nervensystems, der Skelettmuskulatur und der Sinnesorgane. Springer, Berlin, pp 217–262

[69] Paulus W, Peiffer J (1989) Intratumoral histologic heterogeneity of gliomas. Cancer 64:442–447

[70] Pierce MA, Johnson MD, Maciunas RJ, Murray MJ, Allen GS, Harbison MA, Creasy JL, Kessler RM (1995) Evaluating contrast-enhancing brain lesions in patients with AIDS using positron emission tomography. Ann Intern Med 123:594–598

[71] Riva P, Arista A, Franceschi G, Frattarelli M, Sturiale C, Riva N, Casi M, Rossitti R (1995) Local treatment of malignant gliomas by direct infusion of specific monoclonal antibodies labeled with 131I: comparison of the results obtained in recurrent and newly diagnosed brain tumors. Cancer Res 55 (23 Suppl): 5952S–5956S

[72] Rozental JM, Levine RL, Nickles RJ (1991) Changes in glucose uptake by malignant gliomas: preliminary study of prognostic significance. J Neuro-Oncol 10:75–83

[73] Rozental JM, Levine RL, Mehta MP, Kinsella TJ, Levin AB, Algan O, Mendoza M, Hanson JM, Schrader DA, Nickles RJ (1991) Early changes in brain tumor metabolism after treatment: the effects of stereotactic radiotherapy. Int J Radiat Oncol Biol Phys 20:1053–1060

[74] Rozental JM, Cohen JD, Mehta MP, Levine RL, Hanson JM, Nickles RJ (1993) Acute changes in glucose uptake after treatment: the effects of carmustine (BCNU) on human glioblastoma multiforme. J Neuro-Oncol 15:57–66
[75] Ruiz A, Ganz WI, Post MJ, Camp A, Landy H, Mallin W, Sfakianakis GN (1994) Use of thallium-201 brain SPECT to differentiate cerebral lymphoma from toxoplasma encephalitis in AIDS patients. AJNR 15:1885–1894
[76] Sasaki M, Ichija Y, Kuwabara Y, Otsuka M et al. (1990) Ringlike uptake of [^{18}F]FDG in brain abscess: a PET study. J Comput Assist Tomogr 14:660–661
[77] Shields AF, Grierson JR (1997) F-18-FLT can be used to image cell proliferation in vivo. J Nucl Med 38 (Suppl):249P
[78] Schmidt D, Wunderlich G, Langen KJ et al. (1996) I-123-Methyl tyrosine (IMT) SPECT for evaluation of chemotherapy in cerebral gliomas. J Nucl Med 37 (Suppl): 354
[79] Schober O, Meyer G-J, Duden C et al. (1987) Die Aufnahme von Aminosäuren in Hirntumoren mit der Positronenemissionstomographie als Indikator für die Beurteilung von Stoffwechselaktivität und Malignität. Fortschr Röntgenstr 147:503–509
[80] Tjuvjajev J, Macapinlac H, Daghighian F, Scott A, Ginos J, Finn R, Kothari P, Desai R, Zhang J, Beattie B, Graham M, Larson St, Blasberg R (1994) Imaging of brain tumor proliferative activity with Iodine-131-iododeoxyuridine. J Nucl Med 35:1407–1417
[81] Tovi M, Lilja A, Bergström M, Ericsson A, Bergström K, Hartman M (1990) Delineation of gliomas with magnetic resonance imaging using Gd-DTPA in comparison with computed tomography and positron emission tomography. Acta Radiol 31:417–429
[82] Valk PE, Budinger TF, Levin VA, Silver P, Gutin PH, Doyle WK (1988) PET of malignant cerebral tumors after interstitial brachytherapy. J Neurosurg 69:830–838
[83] Van der Borght T, Pauwels S, Lambotte L, Labar D, de Maeght S, Stroobandt G, Laterre C (1994) Brain tumor imaging with PET and 2-[carbon-11] thymidine. J Nucl Med 35:974–982
[84] Vick NA, Ciric IS, Eller TW, Cozzens JW, Walsh A (1989) Reoperation for malignant astrocytoma. Neurology 39:430–432
[85] Villringer K, Jager H. Dichgans M, Ziegler S, Poppinger J, Herz M, Kruschke C, Minoshima S, Pfister HW, Schwaiger M (1995) Differential diagnosis of CNS lesions in AIDS patients by FDG-PET. J Comput Assist Tomogr 19:532–536
[86] Wester HJ, Herz M, Weber W, Heiss P, Senekowitsch-Schmidtke R, Schwaiger M, Stöcklin G (1999) Synthesis and radiopharmacology of O-(2-[F18]fluoroethyl)-L-tyrosine for tumor imaging. J Nucl Med 40:205–212
[87] Woesler B, Kuwert T, Morgenroth C, Matheja P, Palkovic S, Schäfers M, Vollet B, Schäfers K, Lerch H, Brandau W, Samnick S, Wassmann H, Schober O (1997) Non-invasive grading of primary brain tumors: results of a comparative study between SPECT with ^{123}I-methyl tyrosine and PET with ^{18}F-deoxyglucose. Eur J Nucl Med 24:428–434
[88] Würker M, Herholz K, Voges J, Pietrzyk U, Treuer H, Bauer B, Sturm V, Heiss WD (1996) Glucose consumption and methionine uptake in low-grade gliomas after iodine-125 brachytherapy. Eur J Nucl Med 23:583–586

12 The role of FDG-PET in the management of oral squamous cell carcinoma (ICD-0-DA M-8070/3)

M. Kunkel

12.1 Incidence, etiology and epidemiology of oral cancer

Worldwide, oral and pharyngeal squamous cell carcinoma account for an estimated incidence of about 575000 tumors and 366000 tumor deaths every year and, therefore, represent the majority of all head and neck neoplasms [55]. Regarding the entirety of tumor death in the United States, the proportion of oral and pharyngeal cancer approximates 3.8% for males and 1.3% for females, while in the western parts of Germany rates are 6.7% for males and 1.1% for females [13, 47]. The cancer registry of the "DÖSAK" (Deutsch Österreichisch Schweizerischer Arbeitskreis für Tumoren im Kiefer-Gesichtsbereich) recognized an average-relative 5-year survival rate of 49% on the basis of about 10000 documented cases [16]. For decades, smoking and alcohol abuse have been identified as substantial risk factors [8, 14, 56], approximately two-thirds of oropharyngeal cancer manifestations are related to smoking in the western world. By contrast, in India and Sri Lanka this kind of cancer reaches a proportion of about 40% of all neoplasm and is associated with the long-term consumption of betel. In these countries, the majority of oral cancer patients are females [37].

12.2 Therapeutic aspects of oral cancer

Extensive local infiltration as well as early regional nodal spread are the dominating clinical features of oropharyngeal cancer. Thus, curative surgery includes both radical resection of the primary tumor preserving a 10 mm margin of safety and regional lymph node dissection. While the evidence of nodal spread is consistently accepted as an indication for a complete neck dissection, there is an ongoing clinical controversy with respect to the necessity and extent of surgical lymph node therapy in the N_0 neck [10]. Regarding the estimated ratio of occult lymph node metastases of about 15% to 45% [9, 50], elective surgical neck treatment is often recommended as the standard therapeutic procedure [22, 45, 57, 58]. By contrast, other research groups suggest a more conservative watch and wait policy, based on thorough clinical and ultrasound observation in combination with ultrasound-guided fine needle aspiration [52], on CT examination [50], or on a therapeutic decision with respect to tumor depth [12] or a score of several histologic parameters of the primaries [15].

Within the clinical study groups associated with the DÖSAK cancer registry, however, at least a partial consensus has been achieved on this issue, based on the criteria tumor localization and histological evaluation of frozen sections obtained from intraoperative lymph node biopsy [4]. According to these recommendations, the N_0 neck is treated by an anterolateral supraomohyoidal neck dissection when the primarius is located in the anterior or lateral oral cavity. When intraoperative biopsy of the jugulodigastric or other suspicious lymph nodes reveal metastases, complete neck dissection is performed. This protocol suggests complete prophylactic lymph node dissection for posterior (retromolar) localization of the primary tumor. The patients reported in this chapter have been treated according to these recommendations.

There is convincing evidence that combined therapy including surgery, high-dose irradiation and/or chemotherapy result in an improved survival rate in advanced tumor stages of oral cancer. Thus, a great variety of adjuvant and neo-adjuvant treatment protocols coexist to date [29, 36, 44, 53]. The approach of our group to T3 and T4 tumors includes preoperative radiation therapy (36 Gy), preoperative chemotherapy (5×20 mg cisplatin/m^2) and subsequent radical surgery within the pretherapeutic borders of the tumor and a safety margin of 10 mm ("Essen" scheme [35]).

12.3 Data acquisition and interpretation

Through 1996 we used a GEMS 4096 plus® (General Electrics Medical Systems) scanner; since 1997, PET scans were performed using a Siemens ECAT Exact® whole-body camera. Emission measurements were obtained 30 min after administration of FDG, lasting 11 minutes per bed position. Three to four bed positions were scanned for imaging the viscerocranium, the neck, the thorax and the epigastric region. Transmission scanning was performed with a ^{68}germanium ring source for attenuation correction after the emission scanning. The patients fasted a minimum of 6 h before the PET study. During and after administration of FDG, patients were advised to remain at rest, to avoid speaking and to minimize swallowing for reduction of local unspecific FDG uptake due to muscular activation.

Visual interpretation considered focally increased or asymmetric FDG uptake to be suspicious for tumor manifestations. For semiquantitative evaluation, Standardized Uptake Values (SUV) were calculated for Regions Of Interest (ROIs), which included the suspected pathologic lesions, an intraoral reference region (contralateral identical anatomical site) and an extraoral reference region (dorsal neck without apparent lymph nodes). For previously untreated head and neck tissues, an SUV > 2.0 was considered as pathologic

[48]. Our experience is now based on about 175 PET studies applied for staging, monitoring radiation therapy and surveillance for recurrence.

Today, CT and MR imaging represent the gold standard for staging of head and neck neoplasms and, therefore, served as diagnostic reference. In our group, for CT evaluation, axial images were obtained in sections of 3 mm for the suspected site the tumor and the viscerocranium and of 4 mm for the neck before and after administration of contrast material (Ultravist 300®). MR imaging was performed biplanar (axial and coronary) in 4 mm sections before and after administration of gadolinium (Magnevist®).

Focal tissue masses or asymmetry, contrast material enhancement, destruction of tissue planes and focal necrosis were considered signs of neoplasm. Lymph nodes were evaluated according to the criteria contrast material enhancement, minimal axial diameter, central necrosis (rim enhancement) and multiplicity of lymph nodes [11, 50, 51].

12.4 The special diagnostic aspects of oral cancer

12.4.1 Staging of the primaries

12.4.1.1 Clinical problems and aims of PET for staging the primary tumor

In general, clinical investigation and morphological imaging (CT, MRI, ultrasound) allow for adequate assessment of oral cancer with respect to size, extent of invasion and topographic relation to surrounding anatomic structures. Thus, concurrently, FDG-PET is not regularly included in the initial T-staging for oral cancer, except for the identification of unknown primary locations when conventional imaging modalities failed to depict the origin of cervical lymph node metastasis [1, 6]. The impact of FDG-PET for solving this CUP (Carcinoma of Unknown Primary) problem is addressed in chapter 14 of this book.

Due to the long-term toxic effects of alcohol and tobacco abuse, oral cancer patients suffer significant co-morbidity of cardiovascular, pulmonic, hepatorenal and psychiatric diseases which are all substantial risk factors for anesthesiologic and perioperative management especially when extended ablative surgery requires complex and time consuming reconstruction procedures. When patients suffering advanced tumor stages are treated according to combined protocols, objective and early assessment of treatment response to radiation and/or chemotherapy is helpful for a rational decision on further therapeutic options. Non-responders require radical salvage surgery even despite substantial perioperative risks when curative treatment objectives are held, while complete or subtotal response may give reasons for continuing the conservative radiation treatment.

12.4.1.2 Results of PET for staging the primary tumor

Although like in several other FDG-PET studies [20, 33, 41, 43], where all previously untreated malignant primary lesions within the fields of view were detectable with SUVs ranging from 2.1 to 14.9, FDG-PET could not provide additional relevant information like tumor size or tumor invasion and did not allow for an exact topographic orientation with respect to surgical treatment. In a multivariate analysis by Minn et al. [34], the uptake index SUV could not be confirmed as an independent prognostic factor for survival. Therefore, reviewing the literature and considering our own experience we could not see a substantial impact of FDG-PET staging the primarius on therapeutic management of oral squamous cell carcinoma.

To date, FDG-PET diagnosis of the primaries focus on monitoring treatment response to radio- and chemotherapy. In 30 patients treated according to our aforementioned protocol (preoperative radiotherapy, simultaneous preoperative chemotherapy, subsequent radical surgery uncompromised by tumor response) for advanced stages of oral cancer, we compared the post-radiotherapeutic FDG uptake, measured by PET, with the histologic degree of tumor response. In complete responders, when histology of the resection specimen confirmed complete devitalization of the tumor without residual viable malignant cells (R_0), an average SUV of 2.3 ($\pm$0.4) was determined. The mean SUV for patients whose specimen showed microscopic residual tumor cells (R_1) was 2.9 ($\pm$1.4), whereas in cases of poor treatment response with pathohistologically proven, macroscopically visible residual tumors (R_2) SUV measured 3.8 ($\pm$1.9) on average. For all these patients, a complete radical resection of the primaries was performed, and Spearman's rank correlation coefficient confirmed a significant correlation between FDG uptake and histologic degree of tumor response ($p=0.045$). In this study, low to moderate uptake (≈ 2) was seen in both responders and non-responders, while increased glucose metabolism almost always indicated viable tumor. The Reciever-Operating Characteristic (ROC) of these data suggested SUV > 2.75 as a clinically practicable threshold value for the confirmation of suspected non-responders resulting in a specifity of 88% and a positive predictive value of 94%.

These histological data of a series of complete resection specimen (certainty level IV) confirm earlier clinical observations of other groups who recognized reduced FDG uptake in clinical responders and progressive FDG uptake in clinical non-responders to radiotherapy [33, 38]. Reisser et al. [41] reported similar results for squamous cell carcinomas of the head and neck treated by cisplatin and 5-fluorouracil. Keyes et al. [25] pointed out that persistent FDG uptake within one month after radiotherapy strongly indicates residual tumor. Thus, persistent FDG uptake can be claimed to be a rather specific, early marker for non-responders and we believe that monitoring of tumor response in oral squamous cell carcinoma by PET may be beneficial for patients with very extended tumors implying substantial operative risks for resection or whose co-morbidity poses general limits to operative therapy. In these "borderline" cases of operability, a specific method for the detection of residual malignancy may be the rationale to run an operative risk.

12.4.2 Staging of lymph nodes

12.4.2.1 Clinical problems and aims of PET for staging lymph nodes

There is worldwide consensus on the outstanding relevance of regional nodal spread for the therapeutic management of oral cancer. The absence or presence of cervical lymph node metastases has been confirmed as one of the most important prognostic factors for survival after radical resection of oral neoplasms [18, 45]. As cervical lymph node dissection implies significant therapeutic morbidity [42, 46], precise preoperative lymph node assessment is mandatory for the correct decision on the individual extent of lymph node surgery. Clinical problems arise, on the one hand, in the management of the N_0 neck due to the occurrence of occult metastases and, on the other hand, due to the high proportion of false positive lymph nodes in conventional imaging techniques. Understaging cervical lymph node status may result in the loss of local tumor control, while overstaging the neck may cause unnecessary therapeutic morbidity. The 8th report of the DÖSAK cancer registry [24] may accentuate the dimension of this clinical problem. About 23% of 1564 histologically proven metastases measured less than 10 mm in diameter and would thus be addressed as not typically suspicious for metastases according to established morphologic criteria in conventional imaging techniques. By contrast, although lymph node metastases were suspected initially in 62%, nodal spread could only be confirmed histologically in 36% of the lymph node specimen leaving 26% false positive neck sides. These figures underline the need for improved staging procedures to achieve more accurate pretherapeutic assessment of cervical lymph node status.

12.4.2.2 Results of PET for staging lymph nodes

Based on the hypothesis that, due to the nature of the method, PET has the potential to identify lymph node involvement even before structural signs of malignancy (diameter, rim enhancement, etc.) exceed threshold values of morphological imaging, FDG-PET has been applied to cervical lymph node staging at several institutions. The data given in Table 12.1 show the range of sensitivity and specifity typically found in studies that addressed this issue.

At our institution we surveyed 44 patients with advanced stages of oral cancer undergoing FDG-PET for initial staging of cervical lymph nodes; all of them had either complete histologic lymph node dissection specimens or selective neck dissection and follow-up of more than 12 months which allow

Table 12.1. Staging for lymph nodes in squamous cell carcinomas of the head and neck.

–	Patients	Sensitivity [%]	Specificity [%]	Reference	Comment
Braams et al. 1995 [5]	11	91	88	Histology (15 neck sides)	Any visually positive hot spot was regarded as a metastatic lymph node
McGuirth et al. (1995) [31]	49	83	82	Histology (45 neck sides), CT	>50% laryngopharyngeal primary tumors
Laubenbacher et al. (1995) [28]	22	89	100	Histology (34 neck sides)	Lymph node involvement: SUV > 2
Rege et al. (1994) [38]	19	82	88	Histology (9 neck sides)	
Present results	44	72	90	Histology (60 neck sides), follow up for >12 months	Oral cancer

for a definite statement on factual lymph node status in 88 neck sides. Seventy-five out of eighty-eight neck sides were correctly staged as N_+ or N_0, six neck sides were staged false positive, and seven neck sides were judged false negative, resulting in a sensitivity of 72% and a specificity of 90%. However, compared to the conventional morphological imaging, additional regions of involved lymph nodes were identified in only 3 out of 88 neck sides. Only in a single patient was the concept of lymph node therapy modified due to the PET result. Although PET was able to depict some metastases down to 5 mm, we could not rely on safe detection of small and "micro"-metastases. Several groups reported either similar [31] or superior accuracy [28, 38] of FDG-PET compared to CT or MRI findings. Braams et al. [5] even identified a metastasis of 4 mm by its FDG uptake. Although sensitivity of FDG-PET might surpass the limits of conventional imaging techniques and sometimes allow for spectacular results in revealing surprisingly small lymph nodes bearing tumor, the clinical problem of occult metastases remains unsolved. Moreover, PET cannot replace CT or MRI because it lacks the detailed anatomic information that is mandatory for planning the individual operative procedure. Thus, considering the high additional costs, the moderate gain of clinically relevant information and the rather poor impact on factual therapeutic management, we do not expect FDG-PET to be instrumental for a significant improvement of lymph node staging in oral cancer.

12.4.3 Staging for distant metastasis and synchronous tumors

12.4.3.1 Clinical problems and aims of PET for staging distant metastasis and synchronous tumors

Operability is the most important prognostic factor for survival in advanced oral cancer. Regarding tumor stage, operability is limited either by extensive local invasion or by the occurrence of distant metastasis. While initial staging depicts only rare cases of distant metastasis [24], autopsy findings reveal general spread in approximately 50% in the late course of the disease [26]. Among these, the high proportion ($\approx 1/3$) of mediastinal nodal involvement may support the assumption of early spread beyond the continuity of the cervical lymphatic system. Thus, in advanced stages of oral cancer, requiring extensive ablative surgery implying consecutive functional defects, thorough examination for the exclusion of early tumor generalization is indispensable to avoid unnecessary iatrogenic morbidity in cases of infaust prognosis. Moreover, the significant incidence of multiple primary tumors due to the causative toxic agents [23, 54] may limit a patient's prognosis and has to be ruled out prior to radical surgery.

12.4.3.2 Results of PET for staging distant metastasis and synchronous tumors

The initial FDG-PET staging of 64 patients presenting with advanced oral cancer revealed five simultaneous primary tumors located in hypopharynx, esophagus, lung and thyroid gland. In three patients, PET identified distant metastasis (lung, liver, mediastinal lymph nodes). In two out of these eight tumor sites, conventional imaging could not detect a morphological correlative at the time of initial staging. These tumor manifestations had significant clinical relevance for therapeutic management and, except for one carcinoma of the thyroid gland, proved to be the decisive factor for patient prognosis. One intraepithelial carcinoma of the esophagus was missed by PET.

Although one can argue that the majority (3/4) of distant metastasis and simultaneous primary tumors could be visualized by morphological investigation techniques, the economic superiority of multi-step conventional whole-body staging (chest CT, abdomen CT, bone scan, bronchoscopy, esophagoscopy, pharyngeal endoscopy) has to be questioned when real costs and logistic effort are weighted against diagnostic gain. At least, data on whole-body staging for Hodgkin's disease and lymphoma [19] suggest lower costs for a staging algorithm based on FDG-PET and selective morphological imaging.

12.4.4 Screening and re-staging for recurrent disease

12.4.4.1 Clinical problems and aims of PET in the detection of recurrent oral cancer

In spite of radical tumor and lymph node resection in combination with high dose radiation, oral squamous cell carcinoma mortality is predominantly determined by local tumor recurrence, regional lymph node metastases and metachronous secondary carcinomas [7, 49]. Therefore, surveillance of local tumor control is of utmost importance in the diagnostic follow-up of patients treated for oral cancer. However, after ablative radical tumor surgery and radiation therapy, posttreatment altered tissue texture and changes of regional anatomy, like edema, extensive scarring, loss of tissue planes, radiation fibrosis, bone plates and complex bulky reconstruction flaps, interfere with early clinical detection of local recurrent and secondary disease. Delimitating fatty tissues between anatomic structures, otherwise a morphologic sign of structural integrity, are often obliterated due to soft tissue and lymph node dissection. For these reasons, even the findings of modern imaging techniques based on morphologic criteria for tumor detection are often equivocal, advocating either clinical and radiological follow-up or surgical biopsy. While in the case of recurrence, each day of follow-up delays initiation of salvage therapy, unnecessary surgical intervention may contribute to considerable needless morbidity in non-recurrence cases. Moreover, a negative biopsy does not always exclude the presence of recurrent disease.

Early detection of regional recurrent oral squamous cell carcinoma remains the major diagnostic challenge in oncologic surveillance, because it may improve the treatment results of salvage therapy which are currently poor [39, 49], as 2-year survival rates seldom exceed 20%. Consequently there is a continuing need for improved re-staging procedures to exclude or verify tumor recurrence in stages that allow for successful therapy.

12.4.4.2 Results of PET in the detection of recurrent oral cancer

At our institution, 50 FDG-PET investigations were performed in 44 patients for surveillance of oral squamous cell carcinoma. All patients had R_0 resections during initial radical surgical therapy; 32 patients had adjuvant radiation therapy. Twenty-three PET studies aimed at re-staging for local or regional recurrence, suspected by clinical investigation and/or anatomic imaging. The remaining patients were screened without clinical suspicion either because they were considered to belong to a "high-risk" group for recurrent disease or because of impaired access for clinical investigation. In case of focal FDG uptake, biopsies were taken at the corresponding anatomic sites. If either FDG-PET did not show any suspicious uptake or biopsies did not reveal tumor recurrence, patients were followed for a minimum of 6 months ($\varnothing = 17$ months) to confirm true status of the suspected site.

Histologic findings and follow-up revealed 16 sites of local recurrence or metachronous secondary tumor, 10 lymph node metastases and 10 distant metastases in 22 patients. A total of 32 out of 36 locations were identified by FDG-PET imaging, resulting in an excellent overall sensitivity of 88%. Only three cervical lymph node metastases and one pulmonary metastasis were missed by PET. These lymph nodes could neither be verified by clinical investigation nor by CT or MRI and were detected during surgical exploration or within the histologic workout of the resection specimen. In six patients, sites of FDG accumulation interpreted as recurrence or metastasis could not be verified by clinical investigation, morphological imaging or surgical exploration. However, in the follow-up these patients exhibited tumor manifestation within 2 to 6 months exactly where the PET study suggested the pathologic lesion.

At the time of the PET investigation (Fig. 12.1), MRI only depicted local recurrence as the morphologic correlative of the left-sided focal uptake zone. Even surgical exploration could not identify the lesion of the right side that, however, 10 weeks later proved to be a lymph node metastasis. In the case shown in Fig. 12.2, FDG-PET identified a secondary lymph node metastasis that could not be detected by CT scanning. Moreover PET revealed a suspicious pulmonary lesion in the right hilus region. In this specific case, definitive morphologic correlation to a pulmonary metastasis was not confirmed until 5 months later.

Sixteen areas of FDG accumulation suggesting tumor recurrence proved false positive by biopsy and follow-up, the majority (thirteen sites) were located in the region of the primary tumor. Although we initially expected radiation therapy to be responsible for an increased rate of false positive sites of FDG accumulation, until now statistical evaluation could not confirm that previous radiation, completed more than 4 months before the time of investigation, interferes with the specificity of FDG-PET.

Recently, FDG-PET has been successfully introduced in the surveillance of various cancers. Jerusalem et al. [21] reported superior accuracy of FDG-PET

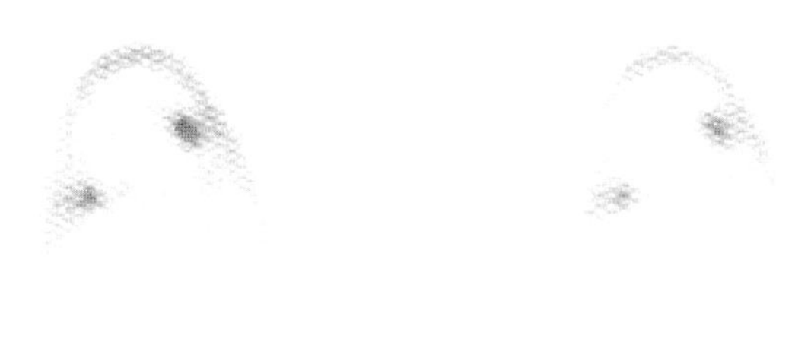

Fig. 12.1. Local recurrence (left) and contralateral lymph node metastasis as depicted by FDG-PET. Neither MR imaging nor surgical exploration could identify a morphological correlative of the right-sided uptake zone at the time of the PET investigation. A lymph node metastasis was confirmed 10 weeks later.

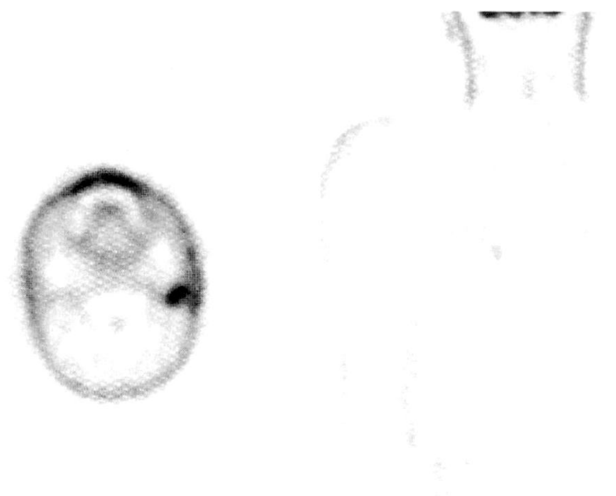

Fig. 12.2. FDG-PET showed a craniocervical secondary lymph node metastasis missed by CT (primary tumor: squamous cell carcinoma of the soft palate). In addition, FDG-PET suggested a simultaneous suspicious pulmonary lesion in the right hilus region. Morphologically, this lesion was not confirmed until 5 months later.

in re-staging lymphoma compared to CT, MRI and gallium scintigraphy which concurrently represented the gold standard of diagnostics. Similar results have been achieved for breast cancer [17] and other types of tumors so that FDG-PET is meanwhile advocated for surveillance of high-grade glioma, differentiated thyroid cancer, colorectal cancer and bronchial carcinoma (non-oat cell carcinoma) by the consensus paper of the German society of nuclear medicine [40].

Regarding head and neck cancer, the results of case series by Anzai et al. [2] and Lapela et al. [27] who identified 6 out of 7 and 15 out of 16 tumor sites have meanwhile been confirmed by larger studies of Fischbein et al. [13] and Keyes et al. [25] supporting that sensitivity of FDG-PET for detecting recurrent oral and pharyngeal squamous cell carcinoma may approximate 90% in a regular clinical setting. These data suggest FDG-PET to be superior to all alternative methods of determining tumor recurrence in the area.

As radiation-induced depression of FDG uptake may outlast the duration of radiotherapy, a clinical question arises with respect to an adequate timing of PET after radiotherapy. This issue has been addressed by the group of McGuirt et al. [32] who recommended an interval of 4 months after cessation of radiotherapy. At this time, lack of pathologic FDG uptake strongly predicts local tumor control [30]. Most of the cited data has been obtained in patients treated by radiotherapy alone; however, the results of our studies indicate that similar results can be achieved in a population treated according to a combined protocol including chemotherapy, radiotherapy and surgical resection.

We therefore recommend two clinical indications of FDG-PET in the post-therapeutic follow-up of oral cancer patients:

- Screening for recurrence 4 months after completion of combined therapy in patients who either face an increased risk for recurrence (advanced stages of the primaries, former recurrence) or allow only limited access for clinical investigation (retromolar localization, bulky reconstruction flaps, extensive scarring or fibrosis).
- Confirmation and staging for recurrence when clinical investigation or morphological imaging suggests tumor manifestation.

12.5 Conclusions

In recent years, FDG-PET has evolved as a major perspective in the diagnosis of oral cancer as it complements conventional morphological imaging techniques. However, due to the limited availability and the considerable costs that preclude the wide-spread routine application in the near future, indications that provide an optimal benefit for the patient have to be worked out. In our opinion, applying FDG-PET to pretherapeutic staging of oral squamous cell carcinoma will seldom influence therapeutic management except for advanced stages with borderline operability that exhibit a high proportion of atypical nodal spread or distant metastases. In spite of initially promising results of lymph node staging, suggesting impressive sensitivity and specifity, the factual impact of FDG-PET findings on clinical management appears rather poor, as the problem of occult metastasis in the supposed N_0 neck could not be resolved. Reviewing the literature and our own data, we could not identify sufficient evidence to discard the concept of prophylactic (diagnostic!) lymph node dissection on the basis of a PET study suggesting N_0 status.

At our institution, PET has proved helpful for an objective evaluation of treatment response in cases of borderline operability as it can indicate residual tumor after radiation therapy within an interval that allows for successful salvage surgery. Due to the high positive predictive value of the PET, pathologic uptake in the early postradiotherapeutic stage confirms the therapeutic indication of surgery even inspite of increased operative risks.

However, we expect the primary clinical value in the post-therapeutic surveillance of oral cancer patients for recurrent disease. In this application, FDG-PET apparently provides superior diagnostic accuracy and allows for sensitive and early detection of local recurrence, regional secondary metastasis, secondary primaries and late distant metastasis in a single step diagnostic procedure. Thus for the first time, we face the perspective of a true secondary prophylaxis in the oncologic aftercare of oral squamous cell carcinoma.

12.6 Recommendations for patient selection and practical clinical application

- Selection of patients/ diagnostic indications
  - initial staging in advanced stages of oral cancer
  - staging for recurrence
  - screening for recurrence (4–6 months after completion of radiotherapy and surgery)
- Instructions for the patient
  - fasting for a minimum of 6 hours
  - avoid speaking and minimize swallowing after administration of FDG
  - bedding has to be compatible to morphologic imaging, the anatomic Frankfurt plane should parallel the Gantry
- Attenuation correction:
  - transmission scanning after emission scanning, ^{68}germanium ring source
- Reconstruction:
  - filtered back projection, Hanning filter (cut-off frequency: 6.75 mm)
- Image interpretation/ pitfalls:
  - preferably combined interpretation of CT/MRI and PET
  - practicable threshold value for early monitoring of radiotherapy: SUV > 2.75
  - missing of lymph nodes sited in close contact with the primarius
  - misinterpretation of physiologic FDG uptake (Waldeyer's tonsillar ring, constrictor pharyngis muscle) as local recurrence
  - short-term follow-up in case of suspected false positive FDG uptake as tracer accumulation may precede morphologic detection for > 3 months.

Acknowledgment. The "oral cancer" PET-study group: Department of oral and maxillofacial surgery: M. Kunkel, U. Wahlmann, HD Kuffner, W. Wagner; Department of nuclear medicine: G. Foerster, P. Bartenstein; Department of neuroradiology: F. Müller-Forell, P. Stoeter; PET at the University of Mainz: P. Benz, J. Spitz.

References

[1] Aassar SO, Fischbein NJ, Caputo GR, Kaplan MJ, Price DC, Singer MI, Dillon WP, Hawkins RA (1999) Metastatic head and neck cancer: role and usefulness of FDG-PET in locating occult primary tumors. Radiology 210:177–181

[2] Anzai Y, Carroll WR, Quint DJ, Bradford CR, Minoshima S, Wolf GT, Wahl RL (1996) Recurrence of head and neck cancer after surgery or irradiation: prospective comparison of 2-deoxy-2-[F-18]-fluoro-D-glucose PET and MR imaging diagnoses. Radiology 200:135–141

[3] Becker N, Wahrendorf J (eds) (1997) Atlas of Cancer Mortality in the Federal Republic of Germany. 3. edn. Springer, Berlin Heidelberg New York, p 70

[4] Bier J (1982) Definitionen zum radikalchirurgischen Vorgehen bei Plattenepithelkarzinomen der Mundhöhle. Dtsch Z Mund Kiefer GesichtsChir 6:369–372

[5] Braams JW, Pruim J, Freling NJN, Nikkels PGJ, Roodenburg JLN, Boering G, Vaalburg W, Vermey A (1995) Detection of lymph node metastases of squamous-cell cancer of the head and neck with FDG-PET and MRI. J Nucl Med 36:211–216

[6] Braams JW, Pruim J, Kohle AC, Nikkels PGJ, Vaalburg W, Vermey A, Roodenburg JLN (1997) Detection of unknown primary head and neck tumors by positron emission tomography. Int J Oral Maxillofac Surg 26:112–115

[7] Brennan CT, Sessions DG, Spitznagel EL, Harvey JE (1991) Surgical pathology of cancer of the oral cavity and oropharynx. Laryngoscope 101:1175–1197

[8] Brugere J, Guenel P, Leclerc A, Rodriguez J (1985) Differential effects of tobacco and alcohol in cancer of the larynx, pharynx and mouth. Cancer 57:391–395

[9] Byers RM, Weber RS, Andrews T, McGill D, Kare R, Wolf P (1997) Frequency and therapeutic implications of "skip metastases" in the neck from squamous carcinoma of the oral tongue. Head Neck 19:14–19

[10] Clayman GL, Frank DF (1998) Selective neck dissection of anatomically appropriate levels is as efficacious as modified radical neck dissection for elective treatment of the clinically negative neck in patients with squamous cell carcinoma of the upper respiratory and digestive tracts. Arch Otolaryngol Head Neck Surg 124:348–352

[11] Engelbrecht V, Pisar E, Fürst G, Mödder U (1995) Verlaufskontrolle und Rezidivdiagnostik maligner Kopf- und Halstumoren nach Radiochemotherapie. Fortschr Röntgenstr 162:304–310

[12] Fakih AR, Rao RS, Borges AM, Patel AR (1989) Elective versus therapeutic neck dissection in early carcinoma of the oral tongue. Am J Surg 158:309–313

[13] Fischbein NJ, Aassar OS, Caputo GR, Kaplan MJ, Singer MI, Price DC, Dillon WP, Hawkins RA (1998) Clinical utility of positron emission tomography with ^{18}F-fluordeoxyglucose in detecting residual/recurrent squamous cell carcinoma of the head and neck. Am J Neuroradiol 19:1187–1196

[14] Graham S, Daygal H, Rohrer T, Swanson M, Sultz H, Shedd D, Fischman S (1977) Dentition, diet, tobacco and alcohol in the epidemiology of oral cancer. J Natl Cancer Inst 59:1611–1616

[15] Giacomarra V, Tirelli G, Papanikolla L, Bussani R (1999) Predictive factors of nodal metastases in oral cavity and oropharynx carcinomas. Laryngoscope 109:795–799

[16] Hassek S, Reicherts M, Kainz M, Howaldt H-P (1999) Zentralregister des Deutsch-Österreichisch-Schweizerischen Arbeitskreises für Tumoren im Kiefer- und Gesichtsbereich (DÖSAK): 9. Projektbericht

[17] Hathaway PB, Mankoff DA, Maravilla KR, Austin Seymour MM, Ellis GK, Gralow JR, Cortese AA, Hayes CE, Moe RE (1999) Value of combined FDG PET and MR imaging in the evaluation of suspected recurrent local-regional breast cancer: preliminary experience. Radiology 210:807–814

[18] Howaldt HP, Kainz M, Vorast H, Cappel I (1998) Prognostische Überlegungen zum Mundhöhlenkarzinom auf der Grundlage des DÖSAK-Tumorregisters. In: Esser E (ed) Disputation anläßlich des 48. Kongresses der Deutschen Gesellschaft für Mund-, Kiefer- und Gesichtschirurgie 03.06. 1998, Osnabrück, S 9–61

[19] Hoh CK, Glaspy J, Rosen PF, Dahlbom M, Lee SJ, Kunkel L, Hawkin RA, Maddhi J, Phelps ME (1997) Whole-body FDG-PET imaging for staging of Hodgkin's disease and lymphoma. J Nucl Med 38:343–348

[20] Ichiya Y, Kuwabara Y, Otsuka M, Tahara T, Yoshikai T, Fukumura T, Jingu K, Masuda K (1991) Assessment of treatment response to cancer therapy using fluorine-18-fluorodeoxyglucose and positron emission tomography. J Nucl Med 32:1655–1660

[21] Jerusalem G, Beguin Y, Fasotte MF, Najjar F, Rigo P, Fillet G (1999) Whole-body positron emission tomography using ^{18}F-fluordeoxyglucose for posttreatment evaluation in Hodgkin's disease and non-Hodgkin's lymphoma has higher diagnostic and prognostic value than classical computed tomography scan imaging. Blood 94:429–433

[22] Johnson JT (1998) Selective neck dissection in patients with squamous cell carcinoma of the upper respiratory and digestive tracts (comment). Arch Otolaryngol Head Neck Surg 124:353

[23] Jones AS, Morar P, Philips DE, Field JK, Husband D, Helliwell TR (1995) Second primary tumors in patients with head and neck squamous cell carcinoma. Cancer 75:1343–1353

[24] Kainz M, Howaldt HP (1997) 8. Projektbericht des Zentralen Tumorregisters des DÖSAK. Klinikum der Justus-Liebig Universität, Gießen

[25] Keyes JW, Watson NE, Williams DW, Greven KM, McGuirth WF (1997) FDG-PET in head and neck cancer. Am J Radiol 169:1663–1669

[26] Kotwall C, Sako K, Razack MS, Rao U, Bakamjian V, Shedd DP (1987) Metastatic patterns in squamous cell cancer of the head and neck. Am J Surg 154:439–442

[27] Lapela M, Grénman R, Kurki T, Joensuu H, Leskinen S, Lindholm P, Haaparanta M, Ruotsalainen U, Minn H (1995) Head and neck cancer: detection of recurrence with PET and 2-[F-18]-fluoro-2-deoxy-D-glucose. Radiology 197:205–211

[28] Laubenbacher C, Saumweber D, Wagner-Manslau C, Kau RJ, Herz M, Avril N, Ziegler S, Kruschke C, Arnold W, Schwaiger M (1995) Comparison of fluorine-18-fluorodeoxyglucose, PET, MRI and endoscopy for staging head and neck squamous cell carcinomas. J Nucl Med 26:1747–1757

[29] Loré JM, Diaz-Ordaz E, Spaulding M, Chary K, Kaufman S, Lawrence W, Hong F, Gerold T, Sundquist N, Barrali RA (1995) Improved survival with preoperative chemotherapy followed by resection uncompromised by tumor response for advanced squamous cell carcinoma of the head and neck. Am J Surg 170:506–511

[30] Mancuso AA, Drane WE, Mukherji SK (1994) The promise FDG in diagnosis and surveillance of head and neck cancer. Cancer 74:1193–1195

[31] Mc Guirth WF, Williams DW, Keyes JW, Greven KM, Watson NE, Geisinger KR, Capellari JO (1995) A comparative diagnostic study of head and neck nodal netastases using positron emission tomography. Laryngoscope 105:373–375

[32] McGuirth WF, Greven K, Williams D, Keyes JW, Watson N, Capellari JO, Geisinger KR (1998) PET scanning in head and neck oncology: a review. Head and Neck 20:208–215

[33] Minn H, Paul R, Ahonen A (1988) Evaluation of treatment response to radiotherapy in head and neck cancer with fluorine-18 fluorodeoxyglucose. J Nucl Med 29:1521–1525

[34] Minn H, Lapela M, Klemi PJ, Grénman R, Leskinen S, Lindholm P, Bergman J (1997) Prediction of survival with fluorine-18-fluorodeoxyglucose and PET in head and neck cancer. J Nucl Med 38:1907–1911

[35] Mohr C, Bohndorf W, Gremmel H, Härle F, Hausamen JE, Hirche H, Molls M, Renner KH, Reuther J, Sach H, Schettler D, Scheunemann H, Thelen M (1992) Präoperative Radio-Chemotherapie und radikale Operation fortgeschrittener Mundhöhlenkarzinome – Abschlußergebnisse einer prospektiven Therapiestudie des DÖSAK. Fortschr Kiefer Gesichtschir 37:13–17

[36] Mohr C (1998) Der heutige Stellenwert adjuvanter Verfahren im Behandlungskonzept des Plattenepithelkarzinoms der Mundhöhle und/oder des Oropharynx. In: Esser E (ed) Disputation anläßlich des 48. Kongresses der Deutschen Gesellschaft für Mund-, Kiefer- und Gesichtschirurgie 03. 06. 1998, Osnabrück, S 106–134

[37] Nandakumar A, Thimmasetty KT, Sreeramareddy NM, Venugopal Rajanna TC, Vinutha Srivinas AT, Bhargava MK (1990) A population-based case-control investigation on cancers of the oral cavity in Bangalore, India. Br J Cancer 62:847–851

[38] Rege S, Maass A, Chaiken L, Hoh CK, Choi Y, Lufkin R, Anzai Y, Juillard G, Maddahi J, Phelps ME (1994) Use of positron emission tomography with fluordeoxyglucose in patients with extracranial head and neck cancers. Cancer 73:3047–3058

[39] Reich RH, Wegener G, Hausamen JE, Knobbe H (1990) 10-Jahres Studie zum Überleben nach ablativer Chirurgie von nicht vorbehandelten Mundhöhlenkarzinomen. Fortschr Kiefer Gesichtschir 37:30–33

[40] Reske SN (1997) Konsensus-Onko-PET. Nuklearmedizin 36:45–46

[41] Reisser Ch, Haberkorn U, Dimitrakopoulou-Strauss A, Seifert E, Strauss LG (1995) Chemotherapeutic management of head and neck malignancies with positron emission tomography. Arch Otolaryngol Head and Neck Surg 121:272–276

[42] Remmler D, Byers R, Scheetz J, Shell B, White G, Zimmermann S, Goepfert H (1986) A prospective study of shoulder disability resulting from radical and modified neck dissections. Head Neck Surg 8:280–286

[43] Sakamoto H, Nakai Y, Ohashi Y, Okamura T (1997) Positron emission tomographic imaging in head and neck lesions. Eur Arch Otorhinolaryngol 254:123–126

[44] Schuller DE, Grecula JC, Gabauer RA, Bauer C, Au JLS, Smith RE, Haller JR, Mountain RE, Young DC, Nag S (1997) Intensified regimen for advanced head and neck squamous cell carcinomas. Arch Otolaryngol Head Neck Surg 123:139–144

[45] Shah JP, Candela FC, Poddar AK (1990) The patterns of cervical lymph node metastases from squamous carcinoma of the oral cavity. Cancer 66:109–113

[46] Shone GR, Yardley MP (1991) An audit into the incidence of handicap after unilateral radical neck dissection. J Laryngol Otol 105:760–762

[47] Statistisches Bundesamt, Wiesbaden (1997) Gesundheitswesen: Reihe 4, Todesursachen in Deutschland 1996. Metzler Poeschel, Stuttgart

[48] Strauss LG, Conti PS (1991) The application of PET in clinical oncology. J Nucl Med 32:623–648

[49] Sun LM, Leung SW, Su CY, Wang CJ (1997) The relapse patterns and outcome of postoperative recurrent tongue cancer. J Oral Maxillofac Surg 55:827–831

[50] Umeda M, Nishimatsu N, Teranobu O, Shimada K (1998) Criteria for diagnosing lymph node metastasis from squamous cell carcinoma on the oral cavity: a study of the relationship between computed tomographic and histologic findings and outcome. J Oral Maxillofac Surg 65:585–593

[51] Van den Brekel MWM, Stel HV, Castelijns JA, Nauta JJP, van der Waal I, Valk J, Meyer CJLM, Snow GB (1990) Cervical lymph node metastasis: assessment of radiologic criteria. Radiology 177:379–384

[52] Van den Brekel MWM, Castelijns JA, Reitsma LC, van der Waal I, Snow GB (1999) Outcome of observing the N0 neck using ultrasonographic-guided cytology for follow up. Arch Otolaryngol Head Neck Surg 125:153–156

[53] Wanebo HJ, Glicksman AS, Landman Ch, Slotman G, Doolittle Ch, Clak J, Koness RJ (1995) Preoperative cisplatin and accelerated hyperfractionated radiation induces high tumor response and control rates in patients with advanced head and neck cancer. Am J Surg 170:512–516

[54] Wangerin K, Schow J (1992) Multiple primäre maligne Tumoren in Kiefer-Gesichtsbereich und oberem Aerodigestivtrakt. Fortschr Kiefer Gesichtschir 37:65–68

[55] World Cancer Research Fund/American Institute for Cancer Research (1997) Food, nutrition and the prevention of cancer: a global perspective. BANTA Book Group, Menasha

[56] Wynder EL, Bross IJ, Feldman RM (1957) A study of the etiological factors in cancer of the mouth. Cancer 10:1300–1323

[57] Yii NW, Patel SG, Rhys-Evans PH, Breach NM (1999) Management of the N0 neck in early cancer of the tongue. Clin Otolaryngol 24:75–79

[58] Zupi A, Califano L, Mangone GM, Longo F, Piombiono P (1998) Surgical management of the neck in squamous carcinoma of the floor of the mouth. Oral Oncol 34:472–475

13 PET in head and neck tumors

H. Bender, H. J. Straehler-Pohl

13.1 Introduction

Tumors of the head and neck region comprise a heterogeneous group of neoplastic processes. Due to the complicated anatomical situation, head and neck tumors exhibit characteristic epidemiological, pathological and therapeutic features. Despite these differences, there are certain common properties concerning the anatomy of the regional drainage of lymph nodes and lymph vessels of the head and neck, the pathology, staging and screening, as well as pertaining therapeutic approaches. As a result, the head and neck have been subdivided into the following regions: nasal cavity, paranasal sinus, nasopharynx, oral cavity, oropharynx, hypopharynx and larynx.

13.2 Incidence, etiology, epidemiology

Head and neck tumors represent around 3–5% of all malignant tumors and occur predominantly in men (male : female = 6 : 1). In recent decades, the incidence has significantly risen in females, probably due to nicotine abuse. Overall, the incidence worldwide is around 20 in 100 000 males. Thus, 15 000 new cases are diagnosed annually in Germany and 63 000 in the United States [11]. In 1994, the mortality rate was 6.3 per 100 000 males and 1.1 per 100 000 females. Interestingly, there are major regional differences, (e.g., Hungary: 14 per 100 000; France: 13 per 100 000), with roughly 1/3 of the patients dying due to the tumor. An increasing incidence has been mainly observed in females and certain ethnic groups. The age peak is around the 5th and 6th decade, with a shift to younger age groups.

Major risk factors are tobacco (smoking and chewing) and alcohol abuse [24, 44]. There is a good correlation of exposure quantity and duration [24]. In addition, inadequate mouth hygiene as well as chronic mechanical irritations are discussed. In tumors originating in paranasal sinus, nasopharynx, tongue, and larynx, chronic exposure to nickel, chromium, and dust (wood, leather, synthetics, etc.) are known risk factors. There is also some evidence that the Epstein-Barr virus might play a role in the induction of nasopharynx cancer [13, 33].

Lately, the importance of genetic factors has been emphasized, e.g., differences in the metabolism of carcinogens or aberrant metabolic pathways of nitrosamines originating from smoke. Predominantly, females and African-Americans seem to be much more sensitive to assumed risk factors [39]. Furthermore, an elevated incidence has been observed in chronic vitamin deficiency, Plummer-Vinson syndrome and other various genetically transmitted diseases (Xeroderma pigmentosa, Fanconi anemia, etc.) [14, 40].

13.3 Histopathology

Most tumor lesions are histopathologically squamous cell carcinoma, which are graded depending on the degree of hornification: Grade 1: well differentiated with a hornification >75%; Grade 2: medium differentiated with a hornification 25–75% and Grade 3: dedifferentiated with a hornification <25%. Other variants of squamous cell carcinoma are verrucous ca., sarcomatous ca., and lymphoepihelial ca. In addition, adenocarcinoma, lymphoma, sarcoma and metastases (kidney, thyroid, breast, lung, prostate) can be found [39].

13.4 Role of FDG-PET

13.4.1 Background of clinical application

The diagnosis of a head and neck tumor (HNT) is predominantly based on the physical examination, which is complemented by sonography, computed tomography (CT), magnetic resonance imaging (MRI), and biopsy. Overall, physical palpation exerts a higher specificity as compared to morphological imaging, also providing information concerning structure and consistency. The use of morphological imaging methods allows better estimation of size, structure, relation to neighboring tissues and the extent of the disease. Introduction of CT and MRI has significantly improved the sensitivity of the overall tumor staging, associated with objective documentation. The major limitations which are (a) small lesions without characteristic morphological changes, e.g., micrometastases, or small metastases in normal-sized lymph nodes, (b) enlarged lymph nodes lacking typical signs of malignancy, and (c) distorted anatomy due to surgery and/or radiation therapy, complicate differentiation between scar and tumor tissue. Application of functional imaging methods has been suggested to improve the evaluation of tissue grading and probably provide hints concerning histology (e.g., due to expression of typical antigens). This is of major concern, since tumors exert rather typical functional changes already in early stages, often a long time before morphological changes can be detected. Various tumors, including squamous cell carcinoma, adenocarcinoma, etc., exert a highly enhanced glucose utilization, which provides the basis for FDG-PET. Fluoro-18-deoxyglucose (FDG) is a derivative of D-glucose, which is taken up by cells via specific glucose transporters and phosphorylated intracellularly to FDG-6-phosphate (FDG-6P) by hexokinase. Hydrophilic FDG-6P lacks further metabolization and is unable to penetrate the cell membrane; thus, it is trapped. The combination of a significantly enhanced rate of glucose utilization ($>$ 10-times) in malignant tumors compared to normal tissues with a high-resolution PET scanner also allows the detection of small lesions ($<$ 1 cm).

13.4.2 Technique

13.4.2.1 Patient preparation

Patients should be fasted ($>$ 4 h, better over night) but well hydrated. Blood sugar values should be 120 mg%, at time of injection. Between 185–740 MBq FDG are intravenously injected and patients should be kept lying in a separate room with dimmed light. In order to improve clearance from the urinary system, patients should drink 0.7–1 liter water, within 30 min after FDG injection.

13.4.2.2 Acquisition

Performance of a cold transmission scan (minimum from base of the skull to the lower edge of the liver) 7–10 min per bed position, depending on the age of the source (e.g., rotating ^{68}Ge/^{68}Ga line sources) in supine position. If the patient is moved, the exact position has to be marked (e.g., 3-point marks).

Emission scans (10 min per bed position) are started at least 45 min after injection covering the above mentioned regions. In order to exclude distant metastases, short emission scans (3–5 min per bed position) of the abdomen and pelvis should be included. In the case of cancer of unknown primary (CUP), a complete body-trunk investigation (base of the skull to pelvis) employing transmission and emission scans is recommended.

13.4.2.3 Image reconstruction and evaluation

Images are reconstructed either by filtered back-projection (Hanning filter; cutoff frequency 0.4/cycle; decay correction, x-y-z smoothing) or iterative reconstruction. In order to allow quantitative assessment (standard uptake value, SUV), images can be normalized for body weight (kg) or surface (sqm) and injected dose (MBq). Images are qualitatively evaluated ("hot-spot imaging") and coronal, sagittal and transversal slices are documented as black-and-white or color hardcopy. For the assessment of pathological lesions the use of a qualitative 4-point scoring system has been proven to be useful, employing individual normal organs as references: (1) uptake comparable cerebellum activity = malignancy; (2) uptake comparable between liver and cerebellum activity = malignancy suspicious; (3) uptake comparable liver activity = unspecific; (4) uptake comparable background activity (e.g., in morphologically documented lesions) = normal/no evidence of disease.

Malignant lesions typically show high contrast compared to surrounding tissue and present with a rather round shape. Streak-artifacts, e.g., due to improper reposition, movements (head, arms, legs) might mimic focal uptake, which are not reproducible on all three orthogonal projections. In order to minimize interpretation mistakes, use of fixed upper and lower thresholds are helpful and cerebellum should be used as the reference for maximum activity. In addition, while FDG is a rather unspecific substance, proper preselection of patients, e.g., exclusion of inflammatory processes, significantly enhances specificity (malignant versus benign). Detailed clinical information (surgery, radiation therapy, etc.) as well as inclusion of results of morphological diagnostics (CT, MRI) are prerequisites for final image assessment

13.4.3 Physiological FDG distribution in the head and neck region

With the exception of brain (cortex, basal ganglia and cerebellum) and myocardium (postprandial), most normal tissues show minimal or moderate FDG accumulation. In our experience tracer uptake in cerebellum, mediastine and liver is comparably constant, and thus can be used as reference organs. The eyes usually present as round activity defects with V-shaped tracer uptake in the eye muscles. No uptake is observed in the eye balls und maxillary sinus. Maxilla and mandible show a U-shaped activity defect in the region of the dental lamina. The mucosa of the nasal and oral cavity can be delineated by a moderate and homogeneous tracer accumulation and is best seen in the sagittal views. The palatine and pharyngeal tonsils often show moderate to intense uptake and present as two symmetrical (hot) spots dorsal to the maxilla/mandible. Along the neck, in the region of the larynx, a V-shaped uptake can be irregularly observed, which has been suggested to be the vocal muscles as a result of speaking after tracer injection. In tense patients, cervical muscles mainly sternocleidomastoid muscle show moderate to intense uptake which limits interpretation of lymph node involvement. FDG uptake in the mediastine is moderate and rather homogeneous, with irregular presentation of the hilum of the lungs. Depending on the fasting status, the myocardium shows intense tracer uptake after a meal as well as often after chemotherapy, and background activity after a prolonged fasting period (> 4 h). The lung presents with minimal tracer accumulation and can be well differentiated from the thorax wall, mediastine and abdomen (liver, stomach, spleen).

13.4.4 Primary tumors

The diagnosis of head-and neck tumors is predominantly the result of the physical examination and the histology after biopsy. Further assessment of the local tumor (size, infiltration into surrounding tissue, etc.) is the domain of ultrasound, CT and rarely MRI. Functional imaging methods, including FDG-PET usually play no role in this phase of the diagnostic evaluation.

In order to assess the potential value of FDG-PET in head and neck tumors, different groups have studied tumor patients before and after surgery as well as after chemo- and radiation therapy [3, 18, 19, 36]. The results demonstrated intense FDG uptake in histologically confirmed malignant tumors, with rather uniform distribution, also in large vital tumor masses (Fig. 13.1). No uptake was observed in necrotic tissues and cysts. Overall, high sensitivities (95–100%) and specificities and an excellent grade of differentiation between malignant and benign processes have been documented. False-negative results were mainly due to micrometastases (< 7 mm) and false-positive findings observed in pleomorphic adenoma, Warthin's tumor and benign adenopathy due to toxoplasmosis [17, 20].

Our own results in 50 prospectively studied patients, with palpable tumors (pT = 2), support these results (sensitivity 100%). Intense FDG uptake was seen in vital tumor tissue (Fig. 13.1) in contrast to necrotic areas, cysts and scar tissue. All false-positive findings (n = 4) were histologically pleomorphic adenoma [4, 46].

13.4.5 Lymph node staging

Accurate lymph node (LN) staging in HNT has a significant impact, since LN involvement has to be expected to be high at the time of primary diagnosis (Table 13.1) and, in addition, it is the most important prognostic factor

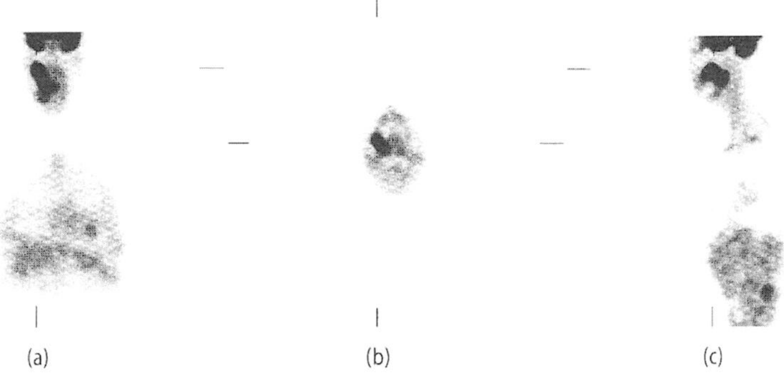

Fig. 13.1. Typical example of a large palpable tumor in the right neck showing intense FDG uptake. Uptake is comparable to that of cerebellum and thus graded as "malignancy likelyl". Histology: Squamous cell carcinoma. Right: coronal image; Middle: transaxial image; Left: sagittal image.

Table 13.1. Incidence, gender distribution, rate of cervical metastases und prognosis of head and neck tumors as a function their localization.

Localization	Incidence/ 100 000	M:F	Metastases (cervical)	5-year Survival
Nose/Sinus	0.75	2:1	20% (clinical) 15% bilateral	I: 70% IV: 15%
Lips			< 20% (late)	I: > 90%
Nasopharynx	1.0	2–3:1	60–80% 53% (bilateral)	I: 60% IV: 15%
Oral cavity	13	3:1		I: 30-60% IV: < 20%
– Floor of the mouth	0.6	3:1	T1: 12%; T4: 50%	I: > 85% IV: < 30%
– Tongue	3	3:1		I: > 75% IV: 30%
Oropharynx	2	3–5:1	70%–85%	I-II: 40-60% III–IV: 13–30%
– Tonsils			T1–2: 38% T3 > 70%	I: > 90% IV: < 20%
Larynx	6	2:1		
– Glottis			< 10% 70%	I: > 90%
– Supraglottis			T1: > 60% 20% bilateral	35–50%
– Subglottis			20-30%	I: > 80% IV: 20–80%
Hypopharynx	2		70–80%	I: 35–60% IV: < 20%
Salivary glands	0.5–1	1:1	35–40%	25-80%

[39]. While 60% of the patients present with LN involvement according to the clinical assessment (palpation), only 40% can histologically be confirmed.

LN metastases exert intense FDG uptake and can be delineated with high contrast from normal surrounding tissue (Fig. 13.2). The lower detection limit are in the range of 5–7 mm. Comparison of the diagnostic value of FDG-PET based on histological confirmation following neck dissection shows a sensitivity of 71–84% [3, 25]. The accuracy was comparable to CT (PET vs. CT: 82% vs. 84%), but significantly improved compared to the clinical investigation (71%) [15]. Similar results have also been reported by Jabour et al. [19] and Rege et al. [34]. It is worthy to note that, while radiological methods are often limited in clear differentiation of malignant versus benign LN involvement (either normal sized or borderline enlarged), functional information (FDG-PET) significantly improves the safety and accuracy of the final interpretation. Our own experiences indicate that this benefit is mostly valued in presurgical patients. Recently, Adams et al. [1] published the results of a study evaluating 1284 lymph nodes with 114 LN metastases. FDG-PET presented with a sensitivity and spec-

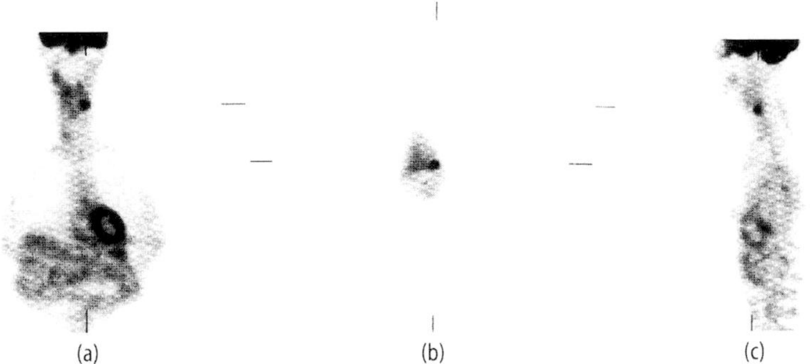

Fig. 13.2. Typical example of a small solitary cervical lymph node metastasis easily deliniated by the normal tissue due to intense FDG uptake. Uptake is comparable to that of cerebellum and thus graded as "malignancy likely". Histology: Squamous cell carcinoma. Right: coronal image; Middle: transaxial image; Left: sagittal image.

ificity of 90% and 94%, respectively. Sensitivity and specificity by CT was 82% and 85%, respectively, and by MRI 80% and 79%, respectively. Similar results have also been reported by others [8, 22, 26].

We have prospectively studied presurgically more than 150 patients with large tumors (pT=2), palpable tumors or suspected LN metastases under routine clinical conditions, with comparable results. Our data demonstrate that FDG-PET identified 19 of 141 lesions (13%) as metastases which were not graded as malignant by CT scan. On the other hand, 17 lesions (12%) were suspicious in CT, but true negative in FDG-PET, as confirmed by histology. Thus, in around 25% of all patients, FDG-PET had an influence on the final diagnosis, resulting in an improvement of the accuracy by 10%. In addition, in 19 patients (14%) lymph node metastases within the mediastine were detected first by FDG-PET and could be confirmed by CT and/or clinical follow-up. In 13 patients (9%) scheduled for surgery, FDG-PET indicated distant metastases (lung, liver and/or bone) in the whole-body scan. In conclusion, our experience underscores the benefit of FDG-PET in the presurgical assessment of lymph node status in presumedly resectable primaries as well as the exclusion of distant metastases. First, FDG-PET allows better assessment of the dignity (malignant versus benign) of palpably or morphologically inconclusive findings; second, FDG-PET is able to detect small LN metastases (0.5–1.2 cm), which are considered normal by CT criteria, and third, is able to exclude tumor involvement in morphologically enlarged or borderline lymph nodes with a high degree of accuracy.

13.4.6 Local recurrence/secondary tumors

Follow-up studies in HNT after surgery and/or radiation therapy employing physical examinations and morphological imaging modalities are crucial.

Changes of the normal anatomy following surgery and fibrotic and sclerotic processes after radiation therapy limit their primary diagnostic value. Often only follow-up studies with signs of volume enlargement are conclusive. Under these circumstances, the use of functional methods seems to be ideal [23, 35]. FDG accumulation in morphologically suspicious lesions are indicative of vital tumor tissue [16], if acute inflammatory processes have been excluded. In contrast, absence of FDG uptake usually contradicts tumor remnants or recurrence [5, 6, 32]. Direct comparison of conventional clinical investigations and FDG-PET underscores the advantage of functional imaging in the accurate detection of tumor recurrence in malignant HNT.

In our own experience [4, 6] prospectively evaluating 34 patients with suspected tumor recurrence, based on clinical examinations and CT scans, FDG-PET was able to confirm the presence of tumor tissue in 20 of 22 (91%) histologically proven cases, as compared to CT (19/22, 86%). Interestingly, 3/22 (13%) were missed by CT, but detected by FDG-PET and 2/22 (11%) were missed by FDG-PET. These two false-negative findings were due to thin submucosal growth (2 mm). Overall, both methods showed sensitivities and specificities of > 85%. It should be emphasized that the additional functional information "malignancy-typical glucose utilization" significantly improved the decisiveness of the final interpretation of the acting surgeous preoperatively reviewing the collected results. Thus, the decision to proceed with further therapeutic measurements or to recommend a "wait-and-watch policy", was heavily based on the functional imaging results. Morphological imaging, at least in our experience, often lacked an unambiguous conclusion, but rather recommended a follow-up study in a few months. This is not only associated with significant psychological distress of the patient, but might have also impact on tumor progression and development of metastases. Thus, FDG-PET allows early-on collection of the missing and critical information. Interestingly, in 23 of 34 patients (67%) FDG-PET detected both lymph node and/or distant metastases, with 6 metastatic sites (26%), primarily visualized by FDG-PET. These data underscore the potential improvements concerning the restaging, if FDG-PET is used as a part of the current diagnostic algorithm, resulting in a better and probably more cost-effective therapy management.

13.4.7 Cancer of unknown primary (CUP syndrome)

The detection of the primary tumor site in patients diagnosed with cervical lymph node metastases is assumed to improve prognosis and overall survival. This effect is probably due to possible complete tumor resection and adapted chemo- and/or radiation therapy. The published experience concerning the use of FDG-PET in patients with CUP syndrome demonstrates considerably higher sensitivity, with detection rates between 20 and 50% in patients where conventional imaging results were negative [2, 5, 9, 21, 28, 31, 34, 41].

Our own results in 25 patients with CUP syndrome allowed the detection of the primary tumor in 6 cases (24%) by FDG-PET, which was negative in the preceding studies. Noteworthy, in 8 of these 25 patients (32%) distant metastases were already observed due to the routinely applied whole-body scanning [4, 6, 45, 46].

13.4.8 Therapy monitoring

HNT are often diagnosed at a rather late tumor stage. Nevertheless, large tumor volumes of the primary with or without locoregional LN involvement are also primarily treated with a curative intension. Effective tumor therapy requires a combination of surgery, radiation and/or chemotherapy. While this concept is often less effective than anticipated, methods allowing early evaluation of the response are needed. Major concerns are (a) early proof of therapeutic effectiveness, (b) evidence or exclusion of vital tumor remnants and (c) early detection of recurrence. Observations that uptake of FDG correlates not only with the cell number but mainly with the proliferation rate [17, 29, 38] provide the basis to employ FDG-PET for therapy monitoring. Previous follow-up studies indicated that diminishing glucose utilization after chemotherapy and/or radiation therapy was associated with therapy response, while unchanged glucose utilization was indicative of therapy resistance [7, 10, 16, 18, 35, 37, 38, 42]. Notable, Haberkorn et al. [17, 18] reported that therapy effectiveness is heterogeneous in the same patient concerning responses and resistance of various tumor sites. There was good correlation of therapy outcome and the effects on FDG uptake (glucose utilization) in the various lesions.

While this diagnostic option is intriguing, the currently high costs of FDG-PET are the major limiting factor. Additionally, several parameters are not yet fully established: (a) minimum or best interval between therapy and FDG scan; (b) optimal method of quantification (absolute or relative values); (c) establishment of threshold values which allow accurate differentiation between positive and negative therapy response.

13.5 Summary and future aspects

FDG-PET is a topofunctional imaging modality with increasing impact on the oncological diagnostics. While FDG is a rather unspecific substance, multiple tumor-associated alterations allow a comparably specific (malignant versus benign) diagnosis. Active trapping of FDG, predominantly in highly malignant tissues, grants images with high contrast and outstanding resolution, including small lesions. Faint to moderate uptake of FDG in normal tissues provides the basis for excellent anatomical landmarking. Nevertheless, morphological resolution of FDG-PET is limited and visual correlation of functional and morphological (CT/MRI) data is needed, mainly in small lesions.

Currently, the major benefit of FDG-PET has been established in LN staging and differentiation of scar versus tumor relapse, which is limited in morphological methods. Further assessment of various factors of the employed study techniques (head fixation, scan times, detector resolution, etc.) might enhance the detection rate of small metastases or even micrometastases. In addition, automatic or semiautomatic image fusion techniques, e.g., a combination of CT and PET, should allow one to obtain attenuation corrected images, based on the CT scan combined with a rather perfect image overlay. Thus, images with higher resolution, improved contrast, and reduced artifacts could be expected.

Generation of more data concerning therapy monitoring [7] should provide the basis to move this technique from preclinical to clinical application. At the same time, development and availability of new tracers, e.g., amino acids, RNA/DNA precursors, might open up new options in tumor diagnosis as well as the cancer management.

13.6 Hints for the practical use and interpretation of FDG-PET results in head and neck tumors

- Patient preparation: Fasting >4 h (better overnight)
  water ad libitum
  blood sugar <120 mg%
- Data acquisition: Whole-body mode with overlapping bed positions (10 min per bed position)
  45–60 min after injection of 185–370 MBq FDG;
  0.7–1 l water to clear kidneys and urinary bladder
- Attenuation correction: Due to activity overestimation in the surface regions, attenuation correction based on measured transmission is recommended (7–10 min per bed position; $^{68}Ge/^{68}Ga$ line source)
- Reconstruction: e.g., filtered backprojection, Hanning filter (cut off frequency 0.4/cycle), decay correction, x-y-z-smoothing
- Image evaluation: Comparison with recent CT/MRI scans; if possible image fusion

1. Visual/qualitative:
   comparison of FDG uptake in tumor (Tmax) with contralateral side and cerebellum.
   Scoring system:
   - intense uptake: equal to cerebellum = malignancy likely;
   - moderate uptake: lower than cerebellum but higher than liver/mediastine = malignancy suspicious;
   - minimal uptake: equal to liver: non-malignant/unspecific;

- no enhanced uptake (background), e.g. in morphologically documented lesions: no evidence of disease
2. Semiquantitative/ROI analyses: threshold values not yet established
3. Quantitative analyses (standard uptake values): threshold values not yet established

References

[1] Adams S, Baum RP, Stuckensen T, et al. (1998) Prospective comparison of 18F-FDG PET with conventional imaging modalities (CT, MRI, US) in lymph node staging of head and neck cancer. Eur J Nucl Med 25:1255–1260
[2] Assar OS, Fischbein NJ, Caputo GR, et al. (1999) Metastastatic head and neck cancer: role and usefullness of FDG-PET in locating occult primary tumors. Radiology 210:177–181
[3] Bailet JW, Abemayor E, Jabour BA, et al. (1992) Positron emission tomography: a new, precise imaging modality for detection of primary head and neck tumors and assessment of cervical adenopathy. Laryngoscope. 102: 281–288
[4] Bender H, Straehler-Pohl HJ, Schomburg A, et al. (1997) Value of F-18-DG-PET in the assessment of head and neck tumors. J Nucl Med 38:153 (abstr)
[5] Bender H, Straehler-Pohl HJ, Frohmann JP et al. (1998) FDG-PET as a clinical routine tool for the staging of selected tumors: results and implications In: Limouris GS, Bender H, Biersack HJ (eds) Radionuclides for therapy. Mediterra Publishers Athens
[6] Bender H, Straehler-Pohl HJ, Linke D, et al. (1998) Klinische Bedeutung von 18FDG-PET in der Diagnostik von Kopf-Hals-Tumoren. Nuklearmedizin 37:30 (abstr)
[7] Bender H, Metten N, Bangard N, et al. (1999) Possible role of FDG-PET in the early prediction of therapy outcome in liver metastases of colorectal carcinoma. Hybridoma 18: 87–91
[8] Braams JW, Pruim J, Freling NJ, et al. (1995) Detection of lymph node metastases of squamous-cell cancer of the head and neck with FDG-PET and MRI. J Nucl Med 36: 211–216
[9] Braams JW, Pruim J, Kole AC, et al. (1997) Detection of unknown primary head and neck tumors by positron emission tomography. Int J Oral Maxillofac Surg 26:112–115
[10] Berlangieri SU, Brizel DM, Scher RL, et al. (1994) Pilot study of positron emission tomography in patients with advanced head and neck cancer receiving radiotherapy and chemotherapy. Head Neck 16:340–346
[11] Cancer Statistics (1994) Cancer journal for clinicians. American Cancer Society 44:9–26
[12] Donald PJ (1986) Marijuana smoking: possible cause of head and neck carcinoma in young patients. Otolaryngol Head Neck Surg 94:517–519
[13] Fahraeus R, Fu HL, Ernberg I, et al. (1988) Expression of Epstein-Barr virus-encoded proteins in nasopharyngeal carcinoma. Int J Cancer 42:329–331
[14] German J (1983) Chromosome Mutation and Neoplasia. Alan R Liss, New York
[15] Greven KM, McGuirt WF, Watson X, et al. (1995) PET in the evaluation of laryngeal carcinoma. Ann Otol Rhinol Laryngol 104:274–278
[16] Greven KM, Williams DW 3rd, Keyes JW Jr et al. (1994) Positron emission tomography of patients with head and neck carcinoma before and after high dose irradiation. Cancer 74:1355–1359
[17] Haberkorn U, Strauss LG, Dimitrakopoulou A, et al. (1993) Fluorodeoxyglucose imaging of advanced head and neck cancer after chemotherapy. J Nucl Med 34:12–17
[18] Haberkorn U, Strauss LG, Reisser C, van Kaick G, et al. (1992) Positron emission tomography (PET) in the evaluation of tumor proliferation and follow-up of therapy in ear, nose and throat tumors. Radiologe 32:296–301

[19] Jabour BA, Choi Y, Hoh CK, et al. (1993) Extracranial head and neck: PET imaging with 2-[F-18]fluoro-2-deoxy-D-glucose and MR imaging correlation. Radiology 186:27–35
[20] Keyes JW, Harkness BA, Greven KM, et al. (1994) Salivary gland tumors: pretherapy evaluation with PET. Radiology 1992:99–102
[21] Kole AC, Nieweg OE, Pruim J, et al. (1998) Detection of unknown occult primary tumors using positron emission tomography. Cancer 82:1160–1166
[22] Laubenbacher C, Saumweber D, Wagner Manslau C et al. (1995) Comparison of fluorine-18-fluorodeoxyglucose PET, MRI and endoscopy for staging head and neck squamous-cell carcinomas. J Nucl Med 36:1747–1757
[23] Mancuso AA, Drane WE, Mukherji SK (1994) The promise FDG in diagnosis and surveillance of head and neck cancer. Cancer 74:1193–1195
[24] Mashberg A, Garfinkel L, Harris S (1981) Alcohol as a primry factor in oral squamous carcinoma. CA Cancer J Clin 31:146–148
[25] McGuirt WF, Greven KM, Keyes JW et al. (1995) Positron emission tomography in the evaluation of laryngeal carcinoma. Ann Otol Rhinol Laryngol 104:274–278
[26] McGuirt WF, Keyes JW, Greven KM et al. (1995) Preoperative identification of benign versus malignant parotid masses: a comparative study including positron emission tomography. Laryngoscope 105:579–584
[27] McGuirt WF, Williams DW 3rd, Keyes JW Jr, et al. (1995) A comparative diagnostic study of head and neck nodal metastases using positron emission tomography. Laryngoscope 105:373–375
[28] Mendenhall WM, Manusco AA, Parsons JT, et al. (1998) Diagnostic evaluation of squamous cell carcinoma metastatic to cervical lymph nodes from an unknown head and neck primary site. Head-Neck 20:739–744
[29] Minn H, Clavo AC, Grenman R, Wahl RL (1995) In vitro comparison of cell proliferation kinetics and uptake of tritiated fluorodeoxyglucose and L-methionine in squamous cell carcinoma of the head and neck. J Nucl Med 36:252–258
[30] Moser E, Krause T (1997) Konsensus – Onko-PET: Arbeitsausschuß Positronen-Emissions-Tomographie der DGN, Vorsitz Reske SN, 2. Konsensuskonferenz in Ulm. Nuclearmedizin 36:45–46
[31] Mukherji SK, Drane WE, Mancuso AA, et al. (1996) Occult primary tumors of the head and neck: detection with 2-[F-18] fluoro-2-deoxy-D-glucose SPECT. Radiology 199:761–766
[32] Mukherji SK, Drane WE, Tart RP, et al. (1994) Comparison of thallium-201 and F-18 FDG SPECT uptake in squamous cell carcinoma of the head and neck. Am J Neuroradiol 15: 1837–1842
[33] Old LJ, Boyse EA, Oettgen, et al. (1966) Precipitating antibody in human serum to an antigen present in cultured Burkitt's lymphoma cells. Proc Natl Acad Sci USA 56:1699–1701
[34] Rege S, Maass A, Chaiken L, et al. (1994) Use of positron emission tomography with fluorodeoxyglucose in patients with extracranial head and neck cancers. Cancer 73: 3047–3058
[35] Rege SD, Chaiken L, Hoh CK, et al. (1993) Change induced by radiation therapy in FDG uptake in normal and malignant structures of the head and neck: quantitation with PET. Radiology 189:807–812
[36] Reisser C, Haberkorn U, Strauss LG (1991) PET scan in tumor diagnosis in the head and neck. Laryngorhinootologie 70:214–217
[37] Reisser C, Haberkorn U, Strauss LG (1992) Diagnosis of energy metabolism in ENT tumors – a PET study. HNO 40:225–231
[38] Reisser C, Haberkorn U, Strauss LG (1993) The relevance of positron emission tomography for the diagnosis and treatment of head and neck tumors. J Otolaryngol 22: 231–238
[39] Schantz SP, Harrison LB, Forastiere AA (1997) Tumors of the nasal cavity and paranasal sinuses, nasopharynx, oral cavity and orophrarunx. In: DeVita VT, Hellman S,

Rosenberg SA (eds) Cancer, Principles and Practice of Oncology. Lippincott-Raven Publ New York, pp 741–801

[40] Schantz SP, Hsu TC (1989) Head and neck cancer patients express increased clastogen-induced chromosome fragility. Head Neck 11:337–339

[41] Schipper JH, Schrader M, Arweiler D, et al. (1996) Positron emission tomography for primary tumor detection in lymph node metastases with unknown primary tumor. HNO 44:254–257

[42] Seifert E, Schadel A, Haberkorn U, Strauss LG (1992) Evaluating the effectiveness of chemotherapy in patients with head-neck tumors using positron emission tomography (PET scan). HNO 40:90–93

[43] Shemen LJ, Klotz J, Shottenfeld D, Strong EW (1984) Increase of tongue cancer in young men. JAMA 252:1857–1859

[44] Spitz MR, Fuegger JJ, Goeffert H, et al. (1988) Squamous cell carcinoma of the upper aerodigestive tract: a case comparison analysis. Cancer 61:203–209

[45] Straehler-Pohl HJ, Bender H, Linke D, et al. (1998) Value of F-18-DG-PET in the assessment of head and neck tumors: clinical experience in 152 patients. J Cancer Res Clin Oncol 124:R10

[46] Straehler-Pohl HJ, Bender H, Linke D, et al. (1998) Value of F-18-DG-PET in the staging of head and neck tumors under clinical routine conditions. Eur J Nucl Med 25:1032 (abstr)

14 Carcinoma of unknown primary

K. Scheidhauer, N. Avril, V. M. Bonkowsky

14.1 Incidence, aetiology and epidemiology

The management of metastases of unknown primary origin presents considerable challenges to the treating physician, because therapy decisions are often determined by the nature of the primary tumor. Metastases originating from an unknown source are known as "CUP tumors" (carcinoma of unknown primary). Incidence of CUP tumors ranges from 0.5 to 10% of all newly diagnosed tumors [2, 8, 11, 15, 19, 26]; they are more prevalent in males and the mean age of diagnosis is about 60 years. Frequent first sittings for the metastatic lesions are lymph nodes (37%); of these, 31% are located in the head and neck region, which is the most common site for metastases of unknown origin [14].

14.2 Histopathological classification and prognostic factors

Treatment decisions in carcinoma are frequently based on the histology and localization of the primary tumor. Where the tumor source is unknown, such decisions are complicated and the prognosis is more uncertain. Systemic metastases may become evident before the manifestation of the primary tumor and in such instances the metastatic signs and symptoms may not be typical of those of the primary tumor. Reasons for this dissimilarity include the facts that

- primary tumors normally metastasize into regional lymph nodes (lymphogen) or distant capillary beds (hematogen), although a first location may be skipped [22],
- tumor cells from metastases have a greater tendency for dissemination than tumor cells from primary tumors [27], and
- growth rates of primary tumors can decrease under loco-regional immunological influences resulting in tumor involution during disease progression [7].

Five year survival rates for patients with CUP syndrome vary enormously between 6% and 70% [3, 25] and are largely determined by histology and location of the metastases. Patients with undifferentiated tumors and adenocarcinomas have a poorer prognosis than those with squamous cell carcinomas. Cervical metastases offer a better prognosis than metastases in the lung or liver [17]. Overall, however, the general prognosis for CUP tumor patients is poor. Identification of the primary tumor enables a rational approach to treatment; although paradoxically upon identification of the primary tumor, the metastases can no longer be defined as CUP tumors.

It is clear, therefore, that it is becoming increasingly necessary to use new diagnostic tools and concepts to uncover occult primary tumors even if these do not yet play a role in routine diagnostic work. Technical developments in conventional imaging techniques, such as sonography, computed tomography and magnetic resonance imaging, lead to improved sensitivity and specificity in the diagnosis of malignancies in general. To date, there exists comparatively little published work discussing the merits of employing conventional imaging techniques in the management of CUP syndrome. However due to the relatively good prognosis of patients with a CUP syndrome located in the head and neck and the expected favorable cost effectiveness, most research examining the use of FDG-PET in CUP syndrome has been published. The use of FDG-PET in CUP syndrome is, however, still limited due to availability and relatively high costs as well as its yet not fully established, proven clinical benefit in this area.

14.3 General diagnostic investigations

As the median survival of patients with CUP syndrome is short, the remainder of the patients' lives should not be passed in an endless round of fruitless diagnostic studies causing discomfort and frustration. Basic investigations for patients with CUP syndrome and cervical lymph node metastases include history taking, physical examination (with inspection and palpation of the oropharynx), endoscopy of the nasopharynx and hypopharynx, laryngoscopy, sonography of the neck (including salivary glands), thyroid and abdomen and serology (Table 1) [15, 29, 30]. If fine needle aspiration cytology is insufficient for diagnostic certainty, an excisional biopsy is recommended for histological diagnosis of cervical lymph node metastasis.

Table 14.1. Diagnostic procedures performed on patients with CUP syndrome presenting with cervical lymph node metastases.

- Sonography of neck and abdomen
- Panendoscopy (oropharynx, larynx, nasopharynx, hypopharynx)
- Fine needle biopsy of suspicious lymph nodes/regions
- CT and/or MRI of head, neck and thorax
- Bone scintigraphy
- Serum analysis (ESR, electrolytes, blood counts, GOT, GPT, CHE, amylase and phosphatase)
- Tumor markers evaluation (Ca 19-9, CEA, EBV-AVC)

Immunohistochemistry is often valuable in locating tumor characteristics such as thyroglobulin, cytokeratines, the S-100 antigen, prostate specific antigen and estrogen receptors, which in turn may lead to histological tumor identification [9, 13]. Tumor masses such as differentiated thyroid cancer and non-Hodgkin's lymphoma are, therefore, rarely causes of CUP syndrome simply because the primary tumor is identifiable. Undifferentiated tumors, such as squamous cell carcinoma, adenocarcinoma and neuroectodermal tumors often feature in CUP syndrome because the primary tumor is not identifiable. As additional information is gathered, additional diagnostic tests might be indicated which in turn influence therapy decisions and prognosis.

14.4 Standard diagnostic tests

X-ray of the thorax and, if non-diagnostic, a CT of the thorax are essential. In the case of adenocarcinoma, a CT/MRI of the abdomen is highly recommended. Endoscopy of the upper aerodigestive tract (including esophagoscopy and bronchoscopy), together with systematic biopsies, should be performed for all patients with CUP of the cervical lymph nodes. A tonsillectomy may also be indicated but gastroscopy is only recommended for adenocarcinomas [14–16]. Additional diagnostic procedures of asymptomatic organs, such as contrast enemas of the bowel or urogenital tract, mammography, thyroid scintigraphy or endoscopy of other tracts, are of little diagnostic value. Most serum markers are non-specific for tumor localization [20]. However, the Epstein-Barr virus is associated with an increased incidence of lymphoepithelial tumors of the nasopharynx, as are high IgA antibody values against viral Capsid-antigen [31].

14.5 Nuclear medicine imaging and FDG-PET

Selective tumor imaging using radioactive tracers is the domain of diagnostic nuclear medicine. Immunoscintigraphy with specific monoclonal antibodies, against for example CEA, melanoma associated antigens or squamous cell carcinoma, was clinically evaluated but failed to fulfill the high expectations for tumor imaging [24]. However, PET imaging of increased glucose metabolism, using FDG, has been found to be of value despite the rather unspecific metabolic processes involved. As most malignant tumors have a high glucose metabolism compared to normal tissue, a high tumor-to-background contrast can be achieved which is, in turn, frequently of benefit when "screening" for unknown primary tumors.

14.5.1 FDG-PET imaging

A dose of 350–400 MBq (~10 mCi) of [^{18}F]FDG is most often recommended in oncological acquisitions. Likewise, it is also useful in patients with CUP syndrome as small lesions need high counts for good image quality. Additional activities to promote clearer imaging include flushing with saline after tracer injection and abducting and elevating the arm after injection to improve venous flow. Patient preparation is as for other oncological studies, namely fasting for at least six hours (preferably from the evening before), calmly waiting in a quiet room prior to scanning and lying completely still once scanning has commenced in a position that is as comfortable as possible. Scanning is usually performed in the supine position with the arms at the side. Acquisition time is dependent on the amount of activity injected, scanner characteristics, size of the field of view, and the number of required bed positions for the particular acquisition. The latter is, in turn, dependent on the locality and histology of known metastases. Longer than generally recommended acquisitions may be desirable in some locations to assist in the identification of the primary tumor, which is likely to be small, not having been identified earlier by other diagnostic procedures. Recommended acquisition times are 10 to 15 minutes per bed position for emission scans and 5 to 10 minutes for transmission scans, the latter depending mainly on the activity of the transmission sources. Dynamic acquisitions are generally unnecessary, and quantification (SUV) may be omitted [6, 10]. A measured attenuation correction (transmission scan) is widely recommended as the tumors sought are often small and difficult to locate. In the head and neck region, attenuation correction improves orientation and fewer artifacts appear. In whole-body studies, transmission scans may be omitted if time is an issue. Emission and transmission scans should be done consecutively to minimize the impact of potential patient movement. Movement, resulting in a difference in positioning, can lead to artifacts in attenuation corrected images and subsequently to misinterpretations.

14.5.2 Image interpretation

For routine clinical purposes, visual and qualitative image interpretation is often sufficient. Such interpretation should be performed on all orthogonal slices (transaxial, coronal, sagittal), particularly those of the head. Unusual focal FDG uptake should be considered indicative of malignancy and investigated further. Artifacts attributable to patient movement or poor transmission scans should be ignored. False-positive findings may occur if biopsies and other invasive procedures are performed shortly before the PET study; likewise inflammation or muscle tension increases glucose metabolism thereby raising the probability of false-positive results being obtained. Anatomical orientation from transmission images or on-screen magnification of the suspected area (Fig. 14.1) may be of benefit in determining the correct results.

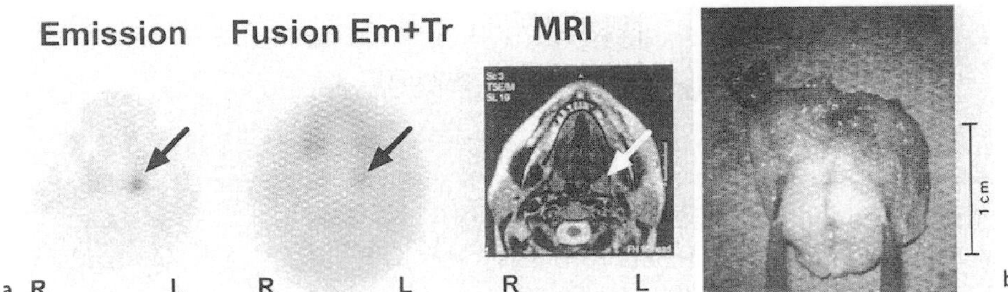

Fig. 14.1. FDG-PET, MRI and surgical specimen (tonsil) of a 46-year old woman suffering from lymph node metastases (squamous cell carcinoma) of the left submandibular region and unknown primary tumor. **a** Transverse imaging slices of the head in identical positions: Left: FDG-PET attenuation-corrected emission scan with focal FDG accumulation (arrow) on the left side dorsal from the teeth (='cold' areas). Middle: fusion of attenuation-corrected emission scan and transmission scan in order to enhance the localization of the FDG focus (arrow) on the left side dorsal from the teeth (='dark' areas). Right: MRI at the same level and of comparable size, showing both tonsils of the same size (arrow). **b** Surgical specimen (cut) of the visually unsuspicious left tonsil: 7 mm (max. diameter) white tumor. Histology: undifferenciated squamous cell carcinoma.

When evaluating whole-body studies, FDG imaging presents with some difficulties:

- in the brain, due to high physiological glucose metabolism,
- in the kidneys, due to renal excretion of FDG, and
- in the lymphatic system of the head and neck region (nasopharynx, tonsils) due to physiological uptake [28].

14.6 Clinical use and results

Several, mainly anecdotal, reports have described the detection of unknown primary tumors in patients with cervical lymph node metastases with FDG-PET [21]. In a recently published study, 29 patients with metastases from unknown primaries were examined with FDG-PET following unsuccessful, conventional diagnostic imaging procedures [12]; FDG-PET detected a primary tumor in 24% of these patients with no false-positive findings. Another study of 17 patients with CUP syndrome found an even higher sensitivity for detection of a primary tumor (53%) although there were 3 false-positive findings [1].

At a university outpatient ENT unit (Cologne, Germany) 16 out of 477 patients with malignant disease (3.3%) were diagnosed with a CUP syndrome. Malignant lymphadenopathy was the main reason for referral to the hospital. Fine needle aspiration cytology or excisional biopsy confirmed provisional diagnosis. All patients with proven malignancy underwent the conventional diagnostic procedures listed in Table 14.1. In all patients included in the study, lymph node metastases were found in the head and neck region. No primary tumor was located elsewhere despite clinical study, routine diagnostic imaging and tumor staging procedures, all completed within four weeks of the first out-patient attendance.

Histological diagnosis of lymph node metastases was made following unilateral or bilateral, functional or radical neck dissection. Additionally, bronchoscopy was performed on four patients and gastroscopy on three; no primary tumors were located. FDG-PET imaging was completed in 1 to 4 overlapping positions, corresponding to an axial field extension of 16–60 cm. Primary tumors were detected (and histologically confirmed) in 7 of the 16 patients examined by FDG-PET: three bronchial carcinomas, two nasopharygeal and one adenocarcinoma of the parotid gland. As a result of FDG-PET imaging, a potentially curative therapy was identified for five patients and in four other patients additional, previously unidentified, lymph node metastases were found (although these had no impact on patient management). In nine patients of the study group of 16, a primary tumor could not be located. There were no false-positive findings. Figure 14.1 shows a tonsillary carcinoma, having a maximum diameter of 7 mm, which was missed during clinical investigations as well as by magnetic resonance imaging. Only a very limited number of studies [12, 18, 23] and just one case report [4] have been published dealing with CUP syndrome and metastases in the cervical region. Consequently comparison of the merits of various imaging techniques, including FDG-PET, is not possible at this time.

14.7 Conclusions

CUP syndrome is often overdiagnosed as a result of conventional, morphological imaging techniques. Intensive investigations for unknown primary tumors are only valid if there is benefit for the patient upon location (therapeutic or palliative) [2, 12–14, 22]. Prognosis increases considerably for patients with CUP syndrome and curable TNM staging, if the primary tumor is found before the start of therapy [22].

FDG-PET is potentially an important diagnostic tool in the search for unknown primary tumors in manifest malignant disease. It offers high sensitivity and represents a whole-body imaging technique, recommending it for early use. In the line-up of the various diagnostic procedures available in the search for unknown primary tumors, FDG-PET should be placed closely behind the conventional primary staging techniques (clinical examination, sonography) and probably even before panendoscopy for use, particularly, if cervical lymph node metastases are present. It should be considered for use before routinely performed morphological imaging techniques, such as CT and MRI of the head, neck, thorax and abdomen.

14.8 Recommendations for FDG-PET imaging in CUP tumors

Patient preparation:
- fasted for >6 hours
- hydration (glucose-free, e.g., NaCl infusion)

	– + furosemide Lasix® (abdominal field-of-view)
	– history: biopsies, inflammation, therapies?
	– relaxation, no talking after FDG application
Scanning:	– Patient in supine position, arms at the side (fixed)
	– head & neck (incl. attenuation corr., trunk)
Field-of-view:	– cervical lymph nodes: head/neck/thorax;
	– in the case of adeno-carcinomas, also abdomen
Data acquisition:	– starting 45–60 minutes after tracer injection
	– 2D mode; 10–15 minutes emission per bed position, transmission 5-10 minutes per bed position
Image reconstruction:	– filtered back projection (Hanning 0.4–0.5 cycles per bin)
	– or iterative reconstruction (e.g., OSEM, 4 subsets, 8 iterations)
Quantification	– calculate SUV of suspicious lesions
Image interpretation:	– visual image analysis (non-physiological, focally increased FDG uptake is suspicious)

Acknowledgment. We gratefully acknowledge the editorial help of Leishia Tyndall-Heynes in preparing the manuscript.

References

[1] Aassar OS, Fischbein NJ, Caputo GR, Kaplan MJ, Price DC, Singer MI, Dillon WP, Hawkins RA (1999) Radiology 210:177–181

[2] Abbruzzese JL, Abbruzzese MC, Hess KR, Raber MN, Lenzi R, Frost P (1994) Unknown primary carcinoma: natural history and prognostic factors in 657 consecutive patients. J Clin Oncol 12:1272–1280

[3] Altmann E, Cadmann E (1986) An analysis of 1539 patients with cancer of unknown primary site. Cancer 57:120–124

[4] Bailet JW, Abemayor E, Jabour BA, Hawkins RA (1992) HoC; Ward PH:Positron emission tomography: a new, precise imaging modality for detection of primary head and neck tumors and assessment of cervical adenopathy. Laryngoscope 102:281–288

[5] Brewin T (1981) The cancer patient – too many scans and X-rays? Lancet 1:1098–1099

[6] DiChiro G, Brooks RA (1988) PET quantitation: blessing and curse. J Nucl Med 29:1603–1604

[7] Frost P (1991) Unknown primary tumors: an example of accelerated (type 2) tumor progression. In: Sudilovski O (Ed) Boundaries between Promotion and Progression during carcinogenesis. New York: Plenum Press, pp 233–241

[8] Gitten R, Horton MB (1990) Issues in the management of patients with carcinoma of unknown primary site. Curr Concepts Oncol 9:7–15

[9] Hainsworth JD, Wright EP, Johnson DH, Davis BW, Greco FA (1991) Poorly differentiated carcinoma of unknown primary site: clinical usefulness of immunoperoxidase staining. J Clin Oncol 9:1931–1938

[10] Keyes JW (1995) SUV: standard uptake or silly useless value? J Nucl Med 36:1836–1839

[11] Kirsten F, Chi CH, Leeary JA, Ng AB, Hedley DW, Tattersall MH (1987) Metastatic adeno- or undifferentiated carcinoma from an unknown primary site – Natural history and guidelines for identification of treatable subsets. Q J Med 62:143–161

[12] Kole A, Nieweg O, Pruim J, et al (1998) Detection of unknown occult primary tumors using positron emission tomography. Cancer 82:1160-1166
[13] Kruger R, de Leon F, Maihoff J (1992) Der Wert der Immunhistochemie in der histologischen Routinediagnostik von Metastasen unbekannter Primartumoren Pathologe 13:65–72
[14] Lefebvre JL, Coche-Dequeant B, Ton Van J, Buisset E, Adenis A (1990) Cervical lymph nodes from an unknown primary tumor in 190 patients. Am J Surg 160:443–446
[15] Leonard RJ, Nystrom JS (1993) Diagnostic evaluation of patients with carcinoma of unknwown primary tumor site. Sem Oncol 20(3)244–250
[16] Lote K (1989) Metastatic cancer from unknown primary site. In: Veronesi U, Arnesjo B, Burn I, Denis L, Mazzeo F (ed) Surgical Oncology. A European Handbook. Springer, Berlin Heidelberg New York, pp 976–983
[17] Mohit-Tabatabai MA, Dasmahapatra KS, Rush BF, Ohanian M (1986) Management of squamous cell carcinoma of unknown origin in cervical lymph nodes. Am J Surg 52:152–154
[18] Mukherji S, Drane W, Mancuso A, Parsons J, Mendenhall W, Stringer S (1996) Occult primary tumors of the head and neck: detection with 2-(F-18) fluoro-2-deoxy-D-glucose SPECT. Radiology 199:761–766
[19] Nystrom SJ, Weiner JM, Wolf RM, Bateman JR, Viola MV (1979) Identifying the primary site in metastatic cancer of unknown origin. Inadequacy of roentgenographic procedures. JAMA 241:381–383
[20] Panza N, Lombardi G, Rosa M, Pacilio G, Lapenta L, Salvatore M (1987) High serum thyroglobulin levels, diagnostic indicators in patients from unknown primary sites. Cancer 60:2233–2236
[21] Rege S, Maass A, Chaiken L, et al (1994) Use positron emission tomography with fluorodeoxyglucose in patients with extracranial head and neck cancers. Cancer 73:3047–3058
[22] Scanlon EF (1985) The process of metastasis. Cancer 55:1163–1166
[23] Schipper JH, Schrader M, Arweiler D, Müller S, Sciuk J (1996) Positron emission tomography to locate primary tumor in patients with cervical lymph node metastases from an occult tumor. HNO 44:254–257
[24] Schomburg A, Hotze A, Walther E, Alberty J, Bender H, Herberhold C, Biersack HJ (1993) Radioimmunoimaging of head and neck cancer. Onkologie 16:465–469
[25] Smith PE, Krementz ET, Chapman W (1967) Metastatic cancer without a detectable primary site. Am J Surg 113:633–637
[26] Stewart JF, Tattersall MNH, Woods RL, Fox RM (1979) Unknown primary adenocarcinoma: incidence of overinvestigation and natural history. Br Med J 1:1530–1533
[27] Talmadge JE, Fidler IJ (1982) Enhanced metastatic potential of tumor cells harvested from spontaneous metastases of heterogeneous murine tumors. JNCI 69:975–980
[28] Uematsu H, Sadato N, Yonekura Y, Tsuchida T, Nakamura S, Sugimoto K, Waki A, Yamamoto K, Hayashi N, Ishii Y (1998) Coregistration of FDG PET and MRI of the head and neck using normal distribution of FDG. J Nucl Med 39:2121–2127
[29] Van den Brekel MPM, Castelijns JA, Steel H, Golden RP, Meyer, Snow G (1993) Modern imaging techniques and ultrasound – guided aspiration cytology for the assessment of neck node metastasis. A prospective comoparative study. Eur Arch Otorhinolaryngol 250:11–17
[30] Wang RC, Goepfert H, Barber AE, Wolf P (1990) Unknown primary squamous cell carcinoma metastatic to the neck. Arch Otolaryngol Head Neck Surg 116:1388–1393
[31] zur Hausen H, Schulte-Holthausen H, Klein G, et al (1970) EBV DNA in biopsies of Burkitt tumors and anaplastic carcinomas of the nasopharynx. Nature 228:1056–1058

15 Thyroid carcinomas

K. Tatsch

15.1 Fundamentals

15.1.1 Incidence, etiology and epidemiology

About 95% of primary tumors of the thyroid gland are carcinomas. In comparison, non-epithelial tumors of the thyroid, such as lymphomas, sarcomas, teratomas or hemangioendotheliomas, are relatively rare and are not included in this discussion.

The yearly incidence of thyroid carcinomas stands at about three to five new cases per 100 000 persons. The associated mortality is 0.5 deaths per 100 000 persons, which is rather low, compared with other malignancies. Thyroid carcinoma represents the eleventh most common cause of cancer deaths. Women are affected about two to three times more frequently than males. Both incidence and prevalence increase with age in both sexes [28].

Broken down into its subtypes, thyroid carcinomas are papillary carcinomas in about 50–80% of cases, followed by follicular carcinoma in 20–40%, medullary carcinoma in 5–8% and anaplastic carcinoma in about 2%. While the overall prognosis in thyroid carcinoma is generally rather good, carcinoma type and stage are decisive in each individual case. Papillary microcarcinomas have the best prognosis, represented by a 10-year survival rate exceeding 99%. In general, the 10-year survival rate for papillary carcinomas stands at 80–90%, while those for follicular and medullary carcinomas are given at 60–70% and 50–70%, respectively. Conversely, the undifferentiated anaplastic carcinoma has an extremely poor prognosis, with a 10-year survival rate of practically zero [28, 29].

One unequivocal etiologic risk factor for the development of thyroid carcinoma is the external exposure of the neck region to ionizing radiation, particularly when this occurs in childhood or adolescence. These include both therapeutic measures (e.g., local radiation of the neck region in the management of Hodgkin's disease) [23, 38] and radiation accidents, such as the Ukrainian reactor catastrophe in Chernobyl in 1986 [24, 30]. Further factors including the amount of iodine intake, pre-existing thyroid autonomy or autoimmune thyroiditis remain controversial. There does not seem to be any pathogenetic connection between hyperthyroidism, radioiodine therapy or endemic goiter and thyroid carcinoma. While studies of tumor genetics, including oncogenes and tumor suppressor genes, have identified corresponding specific changes in only 3–30% of patients with differentiated thyroid carcinomas [10], the genetic basis is much better understood in medullary thyroid carcinomas and, in the case of the hereditary autosomal dominant form, has led to the development of a routinely applied genetic screening method [10, 15].

15.1.2 Histopathological classification

According to the WHO classification (1986), malignant epithelial tumors of the thyroid gland are divided into five groups (Table 15.1). This classification, however, is based more on prognostic features than histological subtypes. Following these criteria, follicular carcinomas are divided into minimally invasive, encapsulated and widely invasive forms. Metastasis is predominantly hematogenous, affecting the lung and skeletal structures. The oxyphilic cell type or Hürthle cell carcinomas are considered to be variations of follicular carcinomas when criteria indicative of papillary carcinomas are not fulfilled. Assigned to the class of papillary carcinomas are microcarcinomas, encapsulated, diffuse sclerosing and oxyphilic cell type variants. If a follicular carcinoma includes papillary elements, this mixed type is considered as belonging to the papillary carcinomas. Papillary carcinomas metastasize predominantly through the lymphatic system, affecting the cervical lymph nodes, while invasively spreading carcinomas may in some cases be associated with lung metastases. Medullary carcinomas are split into sporadic (approx. 75%) and hereditary (approx. 10–20%) forms. The latter may occur as an isolated disease or as part of type II multiple endocrine neoplasia (MEN II). Metastases are both lymphogenous and hematogenous. Patients' prognoses depend to a great extent on the degree of lymph node involve-

Table 15.1. Classification of malignant epithelial tumors of the thyroid (according to WHO: Histological typing of thyroid tumors, 1986).

1. Follicular carcinoma
Minimally invasive (encapsulated)
Widely invasive
Oxyphilic cell type (Hürthle cell carcinoma)
Clear cell variant
2. Papillary carcinoma
Papillary microcarcinoma
Encapsulated variant
Follicular variant
Diffuse sclerosing variant
Oxyphilic cell type
3. Medullary thyroid carcinoma
4. Undifferentiated (anaplastic) carcinomas
5. Others

ment. Anaplastic carcinomas are undifferentiated tumors which infiltrate rapidly into perithyroid tissues and, as noted above, are associated with an extremely poor prognosis [29].

15.1.3 Diagnosis of thyroid carcinoma

In this discussion, we will differentiate between primary tumor diagnosis and the work-up for recurrent and metastatic disease.

Primary tumor diagnosis includes the following obligatory measures, such as a detailed history, documentation of patient's complete physical examination findings and laboratory evaluation of thyroid parameters. Diagnostic imaging in these cases consists of ultrasound and radionuclide imaging with [^{99m}Tc]pertechnetate. Scintigraphically cold areas and suspicious areas or nodular structures visualized at ultrasound should be evaluated further by fine needle puncture. The latter method is associated with a sensitivity of about 80% and a specificity of about 90%. In the case of inadequate cytology findings, or if nodules increase in size, repeated punctures may be necessary. Since normal findings at cytology do not definitively exclude carcinoma of the thyroid, patients in whom carcinoma is suspected should be referred for surgical exploration.

Other diagnostic procedures which may help clarify equivocal findings include computed tomography (CT), magnetic resonance imaging (MRI) and, in some cases, excision of cervical lymph nodes. The role of color-coded duplex ultrasound has not yet been sufficiently explored. Positron emission tomography (PET) using [^{18}F]fluorodeoxyglucose (FDG) has not yet gained any significance in the primary work-up of thyroid carcinoma.

The diagnosis of recurrent and metastatic disease is based on a variety of methods and parameters. In patients with differentiated papillary and follicular thyroid carcinomas and their subtypes who have undergone thyroidectomy and successful ablation of residual thyroid tissue, follow-up includes regular laboratory monitoring of the thyreoglobulin level and, at certain intervals, ^{131}I studies following obligatory interruption of thyroid hormone substitution. If the findings of these studies show increasing thyreoglobulin levels and ^{131}I uptake at sites of recurrent or metastatic disease, patients may undergo therapeutic administration of ^{131}I. In patients in whom radioiodine diagnostics are negative despite increasing levels of the tumor marker thyreoglobulin, the general practise in the past included the use of various morphologic methods (ultrasound, CT, MRI) as well as the diagnostic administration of unspecific oncotropic radiopharmaceuticals (e.g., [^{201}Tl]chloride, [^{99m}Tc]sestamibi, [^{99m}Tc]tetrofosmine), whose uptake in tumor cells depends on a different mechanism than for iodine uptake, which is a function of the sodium iodide symporter. In recent years, there has been increased interest in the role of FDG-PET in the diagnosis of recurrent or metastatic thyroid carcinoma. Based on preliminary findings, a superiority of this method over the above-mentioned non-specific tumor detection methods has been postulated. In medullary carcinoma of the thyroid, follow-up is based primarily on monitoring of the calcitonin level supplemented by morphologic imaging of the neck region and other possible affected locations elsewhere in the body. Additional nuclear medicine methods include the use of pentavalent [^{99m}Tc] DMSA, [^{99m}Tc]sestamibi, [^{123}I]MIBG or [^{111}In]octreotide. Preliminary findings are also available for the usefulness of FDG-PET in the evaluation of this disease entity.

15.2 Positron emission tomography (PET)

15.2.1 Radiopharmaceuticals

To date, studies of PET's capabilities in the diagnosis of primary, recurrent and metastatic thyroid carcinoma have almost exclusively used [^{18}F]FDG as a tracer. Since FDG uptake in thyroid carcinomas basically depends on the same mechanisms as in other tumors, the reader is referred for details to previous chapters in this book ('FDG,' 'current development of PET tracers in tumor diagnostics'). One peculiarity of FDG uptake in thyroid carcinoma does, however, deserve mention at this point, namely, that there is a certain degree of correlation between glucose uptake and the TSH level. Filetti et al. [13] have studied the relationship between glucose transport and the TSH level in vitro on rat thyroid cell cultures and have identified a significant correspondence. These in vitro findings have been supported by casuistic in vivo observations by Sisson et al. [41]. The latter authors conducted FDG-PET examinations for detection of metastases in a patient with papillary thyroid carcinoma both under TSH stimulation and TSH suppression. They found that both visually and using quantitative parameters (SUV values, FDG influx rate, tumor/lung ratios) the accumulation of FDG in a lung metastasis was significantly higher during TSH stimulation than under suppression of the thyroid feedback system. We will discuss the potential consequences of observations that FDG-PET may yield more sensitive results under TSH stimulation in section 15.2.5.

15.2.2 Method and interpretation of FDG-PET studies

The use of positron emission tomography (PET) in the diagnosis of thyroid carcinoma depends on the same principles governing its use in other malignancies. The basic technologies involved in PET data acquisition and processing have already been discussed in detail in previous chapters of this book ('Fundamentals, physics, quality control', 'Image reconstruction, quantification, SUV'). Briefly, PET studies can consist of whole-body examinations or focus on specific regions and may or may not include transmission correction. Quantitative data derived from dynamic acquisition sequences (e.g., thyroid region) appear to be most useful as part of primary diagnostics. Acquisition (e.g., acquisition in 2D or 3D mode, transmission correction with measured or calculated transmission) and evaluation (reconstruction methods, quantification, etc.) protocols, however, remain to be standardized and are characterized by the capabilities of the individual PET system utilized for a given examination.

15.2.3 Primary diagnosis

To date, few data have been published to delineate FDG-PET's role in the primary diagnosis of carcinomas of the thyroid gland. This is possibly due to the fact that the first publication addressing this issue by Joensuu et al. [22] took a relatively critical view of FDG-PET's usefulness. At present, published data regarding pre-operative FDG uptake patterns in cases with thyroid carcinoma later verified by histology are probably not available for much more than 20 patients in the world literature.

As noted above, Joensuu et al. [22] published in 1988 their initial findings on the use of FDG-PET in the preoperative work-up of patients with suspected thyroid carcinoma. In that study, a total of 14 patients were examined, including eight cases with benign changes (follicular adenomas, nodular goiter) and six cases with histologically confirmed carcinomas (papillary, three cases; Hürthle cell and anaplastic, one case each) or lymphoma of the thyroid. While the papillary carcinomas either showed no or only slightly increased FDG uptake, both the Hürthle cell and anaplastic carcinomas, as well as the thyroid lymphoma, were characterized by a moderately increased FDG accumulation. Since three of the eight benign entities also showed a moderate to pronounced FDG accumulation, the authors concluded from their data that FDG-PET would play no more than a subordinate role in the preoperative diagnosis of thyroid carcinomas. Critical review of Joensuu's study reveals that scans were conducted using a conventional Anger camera with a special 511 keV collimator, and not a dedicated PET scanner. This should be kept in mind when considering their data.

In 1993, Bloom et al. [3] reported on FDG-PET examinations conducted in a group of 19 patients, four of whom were found at post-operative histology to have thyroid carcinomas (papillary, three cases; follicular, one case), while the remaining 15 exhibited benign changes (follicular adenomas, eight cases; nodular goiter, seven cases). In this study, all carcinoma forms (including the papillary carcinoma) showed higher uptake values than did benign changes. There was no recognizable overlap between the groups. Adler et al. [1], part of the same research group, reported at the same time on a somewhat smaller collective of nine patients. They reported similar results, though it was apparent that they had been based on the same patient group.

Later, in 1995, Uchida et al. [43] reported on results of FDG-PET examinations of 17 patients, of whom a total of eleven (carcinomas, four cases; benign disorders, seven cases) patients were examined pre-operatively. The carcinomas were not broken down with regard to the histological diagnosis. Although the primarily malignant changes had a significantly higher SUV value than did benign changes, there was a partial overlap between the groups.

In a case report published in 1995, Scott et al. [39] stated that the FDG uptake is not only increased in a primary thyroid carcinoma but that FDG uptake in lymph node metastases can be detected pre-operatively.

A larger collective of 22 patients with thyroid carcinoma undergoing FDG-PET was studied by Sasaki and co-workers [34] in 1997. Only two of these patients, however, had been examined pre-operatively with newly diagnosed thyroid carcinoma. These two patients both suffered from papillary thyroid carcinoma whose SUV values were significantly higher than that of normal controls and patients with follicular ademonas.

The most current study, published recently by Uematsu et al. [44], also supports the observations of the previous investigations. The authors pre-operatively examined 11 patients with nodular changes in the thyroid. In these patients, not only were the SUV values documented, but, in addition, a dynamic SPECT scan was performed up to 60 min after infusion in order to obtain time-activity curves to evaluate the kinetics of FDG accumulation. In this study collective, all four patients with papillar carcinoma had significantly increased SUV values, while five other patients with follicular adenoma showed significantly lower FDG accumulation as did a patient with nodular goiter. A false-positive result was obtained in one patient with chronic thyreoiditis, who exhibited a relatively high SUV value.

There is also a paucity of data regarding the capabilities of FDG-PET in the primary diagnosis of patients with medullary thyroid carcinoma. In 1997, Gasparoni et al. [16] reported on the preoperative work-up in a series of five patients, three of whom were found to suffer from medullary carcinoma. In all three cases, the primary tumor was visualized at FDG-PET, which also detected lymph node metastases in two of these cases, as well as a lung metastasis in one case.

Table 15.2 summarizes the most important quantitative findings derived from the literature. The available data permit us to make the following conclusions: a) the original negative evaluation of FDG-PET's role in the primary work-up of thyroid carcinoma [22] was not supported in all respects by later studies; b) all histological subtypes of thyroid carcinoma (papillary, follicular, Hürthle cell, medullary, anaplastic) appear to exhibit increased FDG uptake, although the extent to which this depends on the individual tumor's degree of differentiation has not yet been satisfactorily studied; c) benign conditions (nodular goiter, follicular adenomas) may also show increased FDG uptake, although adequate differentiation between benign and malignant changes seems possible [3, 34, 44].

Although current review articles dealing with the role of PET in oncology [6, 33, 35] and consensus conferences (e.g., by the German Society for Nuclear Medicine [31, 32]) do not consider FDG-PET to be a useful method in

Table 15.2. Results of quantitative FDG-PET investigations in the preoperative work-up of patients with suspected thyroid carcinomas.

Reference	Diagnosis	N	SUV	Comment
[3]	Nodular goiter	7	3.00 ± 2.00	
	Follicular adenoma	8	4.30 ± 2.00	
	Carcinoma (3 × pap., 1 × foll.)	4	10.8 ± 3.20	No overlap
[43]	Benign lesions	7	2.00 ± 0.80	
	Carcinoma	4	4.10 ± 2.10	Partial overlap
[34]	Controls	5	0.98 ± 0.22	
	Follicular adenoma	3	2.12 ± 0.32	
	Papillary carcinoma	2	6.70 ± 5.09	No overlap
[44]	Nodular goiter	1	4.34	
	Chronic thyreoiditis	1	6.30	
	Follicular adenoma	5	1.89 ± 0.72	
	Papillary carcinoma	4	9.07 ± 5.25	No overlap

the primary diagnosis of thyroid carcinomas, a final decision, in my opinion, cannot be made on the basis of the currently available data. The fact that more recent studies do not share the negative opinion characterizing earlier investigations suggests that it would be useful to explore this issue prospectively in a larger number of patients with more sophisticated methodology (dynamic PET scans, valid SUV determinations).

15.2.4 Diagnosis of recurrent and metastatic disease

A much larger body of data is available in the literature to underscore the efficacy of FDG-PET as a diagnostic tool for detecting recurrent and metastatic carcinomas of the thyroid gland than for its role in the work-up of primary disease.

As early as 1987, Joensuu et al. [21] published a case report about three patients with metastatic thyroid carcinomas (papillary, one case; follicular, two cases) who had undergone FDG-PET and radioiodine scans. Their fundamental observation that metastases may show increased uptake either of FDG or of radioiodine alone or of both substances – whereby this type of metabolic heterogeneity may affect different metastases in the same individual – was thereafter confirmed by a series of later studies based on larger patient collectives. In 1994, Schmidt et al. [37] noted in a publication based on four patients that FDG-PET can be used for differentiation of suspected metastases in patients not showing radioiodine uptake. With the availability of whole-body PET scanners, both Conti et al. [7] and Lawson et al. [25] have reported on the advantages of this technique in comparison to conventional procedures using ^{131}I or ^{201}Tl.

The results of the first systematic investigations based on larger numbers of cases were presented by Feine et al. in 1995 [11] and 1996 [12]. These authors identified five possible patterns of FDG and radioiodine uptake. Because of the larger number of patients involved (24 vs. 41 patients), we will examine the latter study in more depth. In 34 of 41 patients studied, elevated thyreoglobulin levels at the time of the examination suggested the presence of recurrent or metastatic disease. In the remaining seven patients, laboratory findings for this tumor marker were negative; patients had been referred for further work-up on the basis of suspicious findings at palpation or ultrasound. In 32 of 34 patients with increased thyreoglobulin levels, pathologic findings were returned either by PET alone (FDG positive, radioiodine negative; 17 cases), with radioiodine alone (radioiodine positive, FDG negative; six cases) or by both methods (both FDG positive and radioiodine negative, and FDG negative and radioiodine positive foci [mixed type, five cases] or both FDG and radioiodine positive [four cases]). This represents a sensitivity of about 94%. FDG-PET returned pathologic findings in 28 of 34 patients, whereas positive radioiodine findings alone were rather infrequent being observed in only six of 34 patients. The various combinations of findings were observed in both differentiated papillary and follicular carcinomas. In Hürthle cell carcinomas (four cases), the only pattern observed was FDG positive/radioiodine negative.

These observations lead to the following conclusions: a) recurrent or metastatic disease can be detected in a majority of patients with increasing thyreoglobulin levels but negative radioiodine scans using FDG-PET; b) the observed constellations of findings allow for hypothetical correlations with the degree of differentiation in the recurrent or metastatic lesions. FDG uptake in the absence of radioiodine uptake is associated with moderate to poorly differentiated malignant tissue, while, conversely, positive radioiodine uptake in the absence of FDG uptake suggests a high degree of differentiation. It has also been a matter for discussion whether statements regarding patients' prognoses can be made on the basis of the observed uptake constellations.

Grünwald and co-workers reported similar findings in 1996 [19] and again in 1997 [17] on a larger collective of 54 patients. Furthermore, these authors have also shown that certain correlations may be drawn between the pattern of FDG uptake and the primary tumor stage and tumor grading. Their findings also suggest that FDG-PET may be of significant importance in the work-up of those patients showing elevated thyreoglobulin levels but no evidence of radioiodine uptake. Although morphologic imaging methods such as ultrasound, CT and MRI may point to the presence of malignant tissue, the low specificity associated with these methods and other limitations may restrict their usefulness in thyroid carcinomas. In these studies, one subcollective of patients participated in a comparison between FDG-PET and scans using [^{99m}Tc]sestamibi as a tracer. Results showed that the findings returned by these two methods correlate better with one another than with the findings of radioiodine scans; these differences were explained on the basis of the specific uptake mechanisms of the respective radiopharmaceuticals. As a whole, the direct FDG/[^{99m}Tc]sestamibi comparison demonstrated a slight advantage for PET technology. Similar findings were reported by Fridrich et al. [14], although this group found a slightly higher sensitivity for [^{99m}Tc] sestamibi than for FDG.

Dietlein et al. [8, 9] employed FDG-PET, [^{99m}Tc]sestamibi and radioiodine in the follow-up of patients with differentiated thyroid carcinoma with the goal of developing a useful diagnostic algorithm for the detection of recurrent and metastatic disease. Based on their data, they calculated a sensitivity for FDG-PET alone of 50%, for radioiodine scans of 61% and up to 86% for a combination of the two methods. Restricting the use of FDG-PET only to patients with increasing thyreoglobulin levels with concomitant negative radioiodine findings, increased the sensitivity to 82%. The diagnostic value of FDG-PET and [^{99m}Tc]sestamibi were considered about equal. On the other hand, critical examination of the data showed that neither method proved capable of identifying patients with lung metastases smaller than 1 cm in diameter. Because these lesions were visualized at spiral CT imaging, the authors' recommendation was to combine FDG-PET (or [^{99m}Tc]sestamibi) with spiral CT in patients with the constellation of rising thyreoglobulin levels and negative radioiodine studies for exclusion of small lung metastases. Tatsch et al. [42] restricted the use of FDG-PET to those patients with rising thyreoglobulin levels and with negative findings at both radioiodine and [^{99m}Tc]sestamibi examinations. In this highly selected collective, FDG-PET identified locally recurrent or metastatic disease in 10 of 14 patients (3/4 with papillary, 5/8 with follicular and 2/2 with Hürthle cell carcinoma). Brandt-Mainz et al. [4] investigated whether [^{99m}Tc]furifosmine may play an analogous role to [^{99m}Tc]sestamibi in the follow-up of differentiated thyroid carcinoma. The authors reported significantly poorer results, however, in comparison with FDG-PET. In another recent publication Altenvoerde et al. [2] reported on positive PET findings in 6 of 12 patients with differentiated thyroid carcinoma, elevated thyreoglobulin levels and otherwise negative "conventional" diagnostic procedures including ^{131}I scans, cervical and abdominal ultrasound, and X-ray of the chest. Interestingly the PET-positive group presented with higher thyreoglobulin levels (23–277 ng/ml) than the PET-negative one (1.5–17 ng/ml).

Wang et al. [45] concluded from their study of 37 patients with differentiated thyroid cancer that FDG-PET is helpful particularly in a subgroup of patients (17/37) with negative diagnostic ^{131}I scans and elevated thyreoglobulin levels. PET localized occult disease in 12 of 17 of those cases (71%), was false positive in one, and false negative in 5 patients, the majority of whom had minimal cervical adenopathy. Furthermore the authors stated that, all in all, FDG-PET results changed the clinical management in 19 of their 37 patients. Schlueter et al. [36] also pointed out that PET is a useful diagnostic tool to guide early surgical therapy in patients with suspected recurrent or metastatic disease. They retrospectively analyzed the data of 13 patients operated on after positive PET findings. Thirteen of 16 operations in these 13 patients confirmed the suspected involvement of thyroid cancer. The false

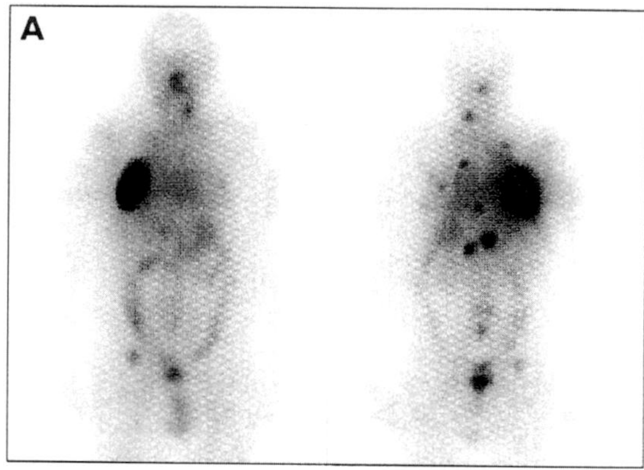

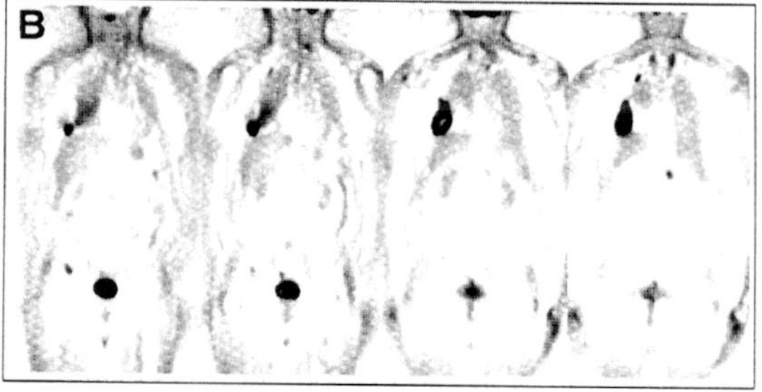

Fig. 15.1. Comparison of radioiodine and FDG-PET findings in a 79 yr old male with follicular thyroid carcinoma who underwent a total of ten courses of radioiodine therapy within the last 9 years with a cumulative dose of 72 GBq ^{131}I. The scan performed after the last ^{131}I therapy scan shows several ^{131}I positive metastases in the chest, lungs, vertebra, and pelvis (**A**). In the FDG-PET scan corresponding to the radioiodine scan, several foci with increased glucose metabolism were seen; however, many of the radioiodine-positive metastases were negative in the FDG-PET scan (**B**).

positive findings were caused by inflamed lymph nodes in two cases and benign thymus tissue in one case. In another study recently published by Chang et al. [5] it was also concluded that FDP-PET is helpful in determining the surgical management of patients with cervical and mediastinal lymph node metastasis. The authors focused their study on patients with papillary carcinoma and negative ^{131}I whole-body scans and showed in particular that FDG-PET is helpful to detect metastasis even in normal sized lymph nodes.

The role of FDG-PET in the diagnosis of recurrent and metastatic medullary thyroid carcinoma has been much less extensively investigated. In a group of three patients with medullary carcinoma (MEN II) and pathologically elevated calcitonin levels, Feine et al. [12] found no lesions with increased FDG uptake. Simon et al. [40] reported on one patient with medullary thyroid carcinoma and increasing calcitonin levels but negative pentavalent [^{99m}Tc]DMSA and [^{131}I]MIBG scans, in whom PET identified sites of increased FDG uptake suggestive of recurrent disease or lymph node metastases. The correct diagnosis based of FDG-PET findings was confirmed by

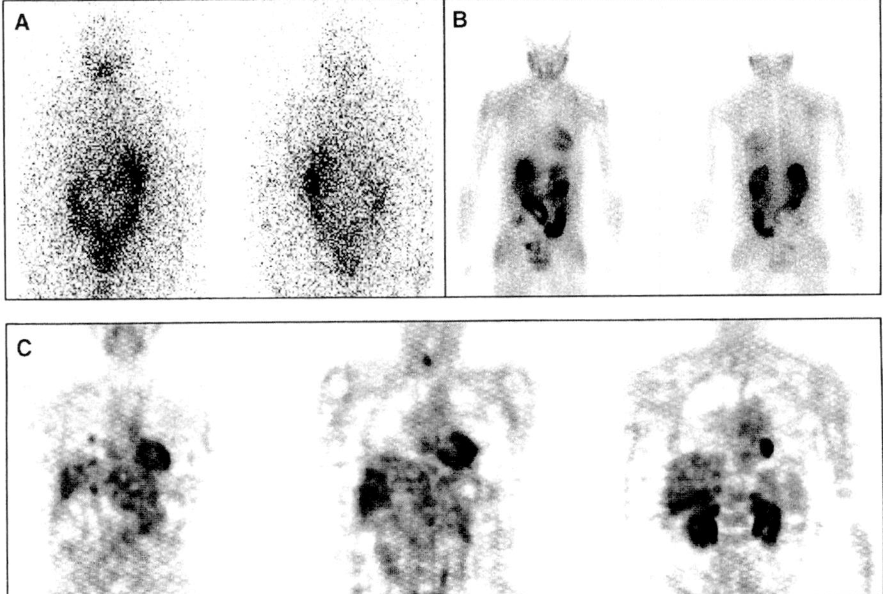

Fig. 15.2. Diagnosis of local recurrency and metastases of differentiated thyroid carcinoma with FDG PET. In a 50 yr old patient with Hürthle cell carcinoma, recurrent or metastatic disease was suspected due to increasing thyreoglobulin levels (107 ng/ml). A diagnostic radioiodine scan (**A**) performed under TSH stimulation was negative, also a [^{99m}Tc]sestamibi scan (**B**). The FDG PET study clearly shows local recurrency as well as two lung metastases (**C**).

postoperative histological examination. Gasparoni et al. [16] reported on five patients, although only two of these were suspicious for recurrent disease. In one of these two cases, only FDG-PET detected the mediastinal recurrence. In the second case, a patient with medullary thyroid carcinoma with concomitant MEN II, neither FDG-PET nor other diagnostic imaging methods proved capable of detecting laparoscopically verified micrometastases (diameters: 2–5 mm) of the liver. Musholt et al. [27] compared FDG-PET with CT and MRI findings in 10 patients with medullary thyroid carcinoma. Of 31 sites of increased FDG uptake, only 11 were detected with morphologic imaging methods. The number of false negative findings were twice as high with CT and MRI than with PET. Since the various morphologic (ultrasound, CT, MRI) and functional (^{201}Tl, pentavalent [^{99m}Tc]DMSA, [^{131}I]MIBG, [^{111}In]octreotide, etc.) imaging techniques are capable of detecting recurrent and metastatic lesions with a sensitivity of only 60%, the use of PET may easily be justified even though the currently available data do not (yet) show a clear advantage for this method.

15.3 Perspectives

Of fundamental interest in the immediate future is the question whether and to what degree the uptake of FDG in thyroid carcinomas and their metastases is influenced by the patient's TSH level. Confirmation that FDG-PET returns significantly better findings in subjects under TSH stimulation than in those receiving TSH-suppressive thyroid hormone preparations would force us to discard one presumed advantage of PET investigations, namely, that use of the method does not require interruption of hormone substitution therapy with all the associated adverse effects (Fig. 15.3). Indeed Moog et al. [26] most recently reported on an intraindividual comparison of FDG-PET findings in patients studied under TSH suppression and TSH stimulation. This group studied 10 patients with 17 lesions. In 15 of 17 lesions with positive FDG uptake, TSH stimulation was associated with an increase of the tumor to background ratio as compared to the study performed under TSH suppression. Furthermore, in 3 of 10 patients, TSH stimulation resulted either in detection of new lesions or in classifying FDG uptake patterns as typical for malignancy. These findings do not only suggest that FDG uptake in recurrent and metastatic thyroid cancer depends on the TSH level but also to preferably perform PET examinations under TSH stimulation. This would,

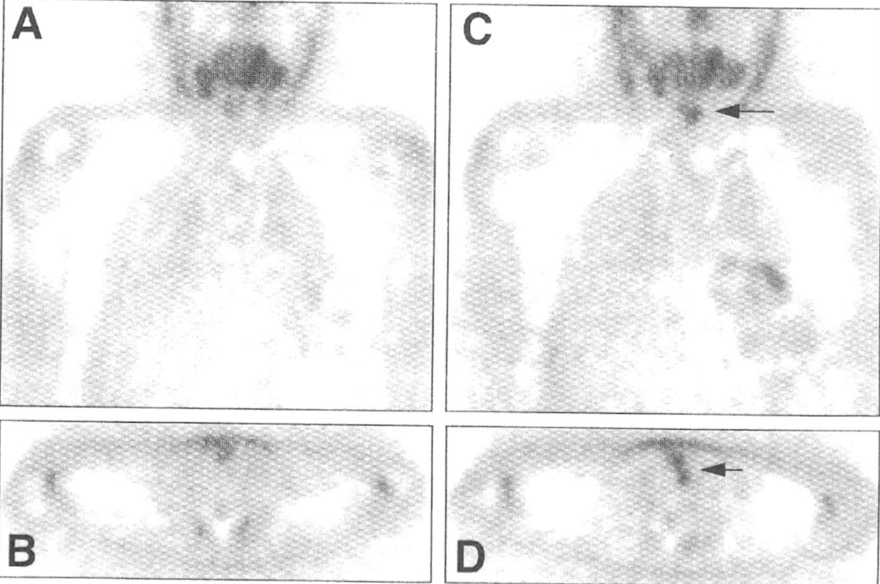

Fig. 15.3. Influence of the TSH level on FDG uptake in recurrent and metastatic differentiated thyroid carcinoma. FDG-PET in an 82 yr old female with follicular carcinoma presenting with a negative ^{131}I scan and increasing thyreoglobulin level shows unsuspicious findings under TSH suppressive therapy with thyroxin (**A**, B). One month later, under conditions of hypothyroidism, findings suspicious for malignancy are seen in the left paralaryngeal area (arrows) (**C**, **D**). Local recurrent disease was histologically verified 4 weeks later.

as in the case of radioiodine studies, simply have to be accepted in order to optimize the quality of the FDG-PET examination. It may be possible in the near future to achieve a satisfactory increase in FDG uptake by the use of recombinant human TSH [20], thus sparing patients the unpleasant phase of pre-PET hypothyroidism.

The diagnostic role of FDG-PET in patients with differentiated thyroid carcinomas, which have lost the capacity for radioiodine uptake, who are undergoing an attempt at redifferentiation therapy with retinoic acid, must also remain open at present. Preliminary studies [18] have yet to yield conclusive findings. Based on the assumption that FDG uptake depends on the degree of differentiation of the given patient's malignancy and that decreasing differentiation correlates with increased FDG accumulation, it would be expected that patients with successful redifferentiation would show decreased FDG uptake at sites of recurrent or metastatic disease. Whether such considerations or observations will warrant FDG-PET's use in monitoring the success of this type of therapy must be answered by future studies.

Most PET studies to date in patients with carcinomas of the thyroid gland are based on determinations of glucose utilization, i.e., they involve the use of [^{18}F]FDG. Whether other radiopharmaceuticals, whose accumulation in malignant cells is controlled by other physiological mechanisms (e.g., [^{11}C]methionine or [^{18}F]tyrosine as markers for the amino acid metabolism or [^{11}C]thymidine or [^{18}F]deoxyuridine as markers of cell proliferation), may prove superior to FDG must be answered in future investigations.

References

[1] Adler LP, Bloom AD (1993) Positron emission tomography of thyroid masses. Thyroid 3:195–200

[2] Altenvoerde G, Lerch H, Kuwert T, Matheja P, Schäfers M, Schober O (1998) Positron emission tomography with F-18-deoxyglucose in patients with differentiated thyroid carcinoma, elevated thyroglobulin levels, and negative iodine scans. Langenbeck's Arch Surg 383:160–163

[3] Bloom AD, Adler LP, Shuck JM (1993) Determination of malignancy of thyroid nodules with positron emission tomography. Surgery 114:728–735

[4] Brandt-Mainz K, Müller SP, Sonnenschein W, Bockisch A (1998) Technetium-99m-furifosmin in the follow-up of differentiated thyroid carcinoma. J Nucl Med 39:1536–1541

[5] Chung JK, So Y, Lee JS, et al. (1999) Value of FDG PET in papillary thyroid carcinoma with negative ^{131}I whole-body scan. J Nucl Med 40:986–992

[6] Conti PS, Lilien DL, Hawley K, et al. (1996) PET and [^{18}F]-FDG in oncology: a clinical update. Nucl Med Biol 23:717–735

[7] Conti PS, Wdowczyk J, Grafton ST, Bacqui F, Singer PA, Nickoloff JT (1994) Improved detection of locally recurrent and metastatic thyroid cancer in patients with persistently elevated thyroglobulin using FDG PET scanning. Eur J Nucl Med 21:S10 (abstr)

[8] Dietlein M, Scheidhauer K, Voth E, Theissen P, Schicha H (1997) Fluorine-18 fluorodeoxyglucose positron emission tomography and iodine-131 whole-body scintigraphy in the follow-up of differentiated thyroid cancer. Eur J Nucl Med 24:1342–1348

[9] Dietlein M, Scheidhauer K, Voth E, Theissen P, Schicha H (1998) Follow-up of differentiated thyroid cancer: what is the value of FDG and sestamibi in the diagnostic algorithm? Nuklearmedizin 37:6–11

[10] Duh QY, Grossman RF (1995) Thyroid growth factors, signal transduction pathways, and oncogenes. Surg Clin North Am 75:421–437
[11] Feine U, Lietzenmayer R, Hanke J-P, Wöhrle H, Müller-Schauenburg W (1995) ^{18}FDG-Ganzkörper-PET bei differenzierten Schilddrüsenkarzinomen. Flipflop im Speichermuster von ^{18}FDG und ^{131}I. Nuklearmedizin 34:127–134
[12] Feine U, Lietzenmayer R, Hanke J-P, Held J, Wöhrle H, Müller-Schauenburg W (1996) Fluorine-18-FDG and iodine-131-iodide uptake in thyroid cancer. J Nucl Med 37:1468–1472
[13] Filetti S, Damante G, Foti D (1987) Thyrotropin stimulates glucose transport in cultured rat thyroid cells. Endocrinology 120:2576–2581
[14] Fridrich L, Messa C, Landoni C et al. (1997) Whole-body scintigraphy with ^{99m}Tc-MIBI, ^{18}F-FDG and ^{131}I in patients with metastatic thyroid carcinoma. Nucl Med Commun 18:3–9
[15] Goretzki PE, Schulte K-M (1998) Bedeutung von Onkogenen in Entstehung und Prognose von differenzierten Schilddrüsenkarzinomen. Internist 39:584–587
[16] Gasparoni P, Rubello D, Ferlin G (1997) Potential role of fluorine-18-deoxyglucose (FDG) positron emission tomography (PET) in the staging of primitive and recurrent medullary thyroid carcinoma. J Endocrinol Invest 20:527–530
[17] Grünwald F, Menzel C, Bender H, et al. (1997) Comparison of ^{18}FDG-PET with ^{131}iodine and ^{99m}Tc-sestamibi scintigraphy in differentiated thyroid cancer. Thyroid 7:327–335
[18] Grünwald F, Pakos E, Bender H et al. (1998) Redifferentiation therapy with retinoic acid in follicular thyroid cancer. J Nucl Med 39:1555-1558
[19] Grünwald F, Schomburg A, Bender H, et al. (1996) Fluorine-18-fluorodeoxyglucose positron emission tomography in the follow-up of differentiated thyroid cancer. Eur J Nucl Med 23:312–319
[20] Hörmann R (1998) Rekombinantes TSH und TSH-Analoga. Therapeutische Implikationen. Internist 39:607–609
[21] Joensuu H, Ahonen A (1987) Imaging of metastases of thyroid carcinoma with fluorine-18-fluorodeoxyglucose. J Nucl Med 28:910–914
[22] Joensuu H, Ahonen A, Klemi PJ (1988) ^{18}F-fluorodeoxyglucose imaging in preoperative diagnosis of thyroid malignancy. Eur J Nucl Med 13:502–506
[23] Kaplan MM, Garnick MB, Gelber R, et al. (1983) Risk factors for thyroid abnormalities after neck irradiation for childhood cancer. Am J Med 74:272–280
[24] Kazakov VS, Demidchik EP, Astakhova LN (1992) Thyroid cancer after Chernobyl. Nature 359:21–22
[25] Lawson M, Duick D, Bandy D, Chen K, Koleske S, Palant A (1995) Comparison of F-18 and Tl-201 for detection of recurrent metastatic differentiated thyroid cancer. J Nucl Med 36:203P (abstr)
[26] Moog F, Linke R, Tiling R, Manthey N, Knesewitsch P, Tatsch K, Hahn K (2000) Influence of TSH levels on the uptake of fluorodeoxyglucose in recurrent and metastatic differentiated thyroid carcinoma. J Nucl Med 41, in press
[27] Musholt TJ, Musholt PB, Dehdashti F, Moley JF (1997) Evaluation of fluorodeoxyglucose-positron emission tomographic scanning and its association with glucose transporter expression in medullary thyroid carcinoma and pheochromocytoma: a clinical and molecular study. Surgery 122:1049–1061
[28] Oberwittler H, Nawroth PP, Ziegler R, Seibel MJ (1998) Klinik des Schilddrüsenkarzinoms. Tumordiagn Ther 19:52–55
[29] Pfannenstiel P, Hotze LA, Saller B (1997) Maligne Tumoren der Schilddrüse. In: Henning Berlin (eds) Schilddrüsenkrankheiten: Diagnose und Therapie. Berliner Med Verl-Anst, Berlin, pp 262–289
[30] Reiners C (1994) Prophylaxe strahleninduzierter Schilddrüsenkarzinome bei Kindern nach der Reaktorkatastrophe von Tschernobyl. Nuklearmedizin 33:229–234
[31] Reske SN (1998) Positronen-Emissionstomographie in der Onkologie. Dtsch Ärzteblatt 95:C1370–1372

[32] Reske SN, Bares R, Büll U, et al. (1996) Klinische Wertigkeit der Positronen-Emissions-Tomographie (PET) bei onkologischen Fragestellungen: Ergebnisse einer interdisziplinären Konsensuskonferenz. Nuklearmedizin 35:42–52
[33] Rigo P, Paulus P, Kaschten BJ, et al. (1996) Oncological applications of positron emission tomography with fluorine-18 fluorodeoxyglucose. Eur J Nucl Med 23:1641–1674
[34] Sasaki M, Ichiya Y, Kuwabara Y, et al. (1997) An evaluation of FDG-PET in the detection and differentiation of thyroid tumors. Nucl Med Commun 18:957–963
[35] Schiepers C, Hoh CK (1998) Positron emission tomography as a diagnostic tool in oncology. Eur Radiol 8:1481–1494
[36] Schlüter B, Grimm-Riepe C, Beyer W, Lübeck M, Schirren-Bumann K, Clausen M (1998) Histological verification of positive fluorine-18 fluorodeoxyglucose findings in patients with differentiated thyroid cancer. Langenbeck's Arch Surg 383:187–189
[37] Schmidt D, Herzog H, Langen K-J, Müller-Gärtner H-W (1994) Glucose metabolism in thyroid cancer metastases. A pilot study using 18 fluoro-2-deoxy-D-glucose and positron emission tomography. Exp Clin Endocrinol 102 (Suppl 3):51–54
[38] Schneider AB (1990) Radiation induced thyroid tumors. Endocrinol Metab North Am 19:495–509
[39] Scott GC, Meier DA, Dickinson CZ (1995) Cervical lymph node metastasis of thyroid papillary carcinoma imaged with fluorine-18-FDG, technetium-99m-pertechnetate and iodine-131-sodium iodide. J Nucl Med 36:1843–1845
[40] Simon GH, Nitzsche EU, Laubenberger JJ, Einert A, Moser E (1996) PET imaging of recurrent medullary thyroid cancer. Nuklearmedizin 35:102–104
[41] Sisson JC, Ackermann RJ, Meyer MA, Wahl RL (1993) Uptake of 18-fluoro-2-deoxy-D-glucose by thyroid cancer: implications for diagnosis and therapy. J Clin Endocrinol Metab 77:1090–1094
[42] Tatsch K, Weber W, Roßmüller B, et al. (1996) F-18 FDG-PET in der Nachsorge von Schilddrüsencarcinom-Patienten mit hTG-Anstieg aber fehlender Iod- und Sestamibi-Speicherung. Nuklearmedizin 35:A34 (abstr)
[43] Uchida Y, Matsuno N, Minoshima S, Imazeki K, Uno K, Kitahara H (1995) Diagnostic value of ^{18}F-FDG PET in primary and metastatic thyroid cancer. J Nucl Med 36:196P (abstr)
[44] Uematsu H, Sadato N, Ohtsubo T, et al. (1998) Fluorine-18-fluorodeoxyglucose PET versus thallium-201 scintigraphy evaluation of thyroid tumors. J Nucl Med 39:453–459
[45] Wang W, Macapinlac H, Larson SM, et al. (1999) [^{18}F]-2-Fluoro-2-deoxy-D-glucose positron emission tomography localizes residual thyroid cancer in patients with negative diagnostic ^{131}I whole body scans and elevated serum thyroglobulin levels. J Clin Endocrinol Metab 84:2291–2302

16 Lung cancer

B. Klemenz, K. M. Taaleb

16.1 Epidemiology and etiology

Lung cancer is one of the most prevalent cancers in the world and a leading cause of cancer death both in men and women. Thus, it is a major health problem with 180000 new cases in the United States in 1996. Men are five times more affected than women due to the different smoking habits [29, 42]. In men 90% and in women 30–60% of all lung cancers are attributed to cigarette smoking. The proportion of smoking women is continuously increasing; thus, in the United States lung cancer has surpassed breast carcinoma as the leading cause of cancer death in women in the late 1980s [29]. Small cell lung cancer (SCLC) is the most rapidly increasing cell type in women [42]. Occupational exposure to carcinogens also has a role although smaller in carcinoma induction. There is no significant correlation between lung cancer and residential radon nor air pollution exposure [29, 42].

Lung cancer has a very poor prognosis (5 year survival rate less than 9% in men and 17% in women). Resection at an early stage of non-small cell lung cancer (NSCLC; primary tumor <3 cm, Table 16.1) resulted in an increase of the survival rate at 5 years up to 50–80% [64, 101].

Despite the curative intention to treat the limited disease, 5–7% of patients (pts) have unresectable disease at surgery, and 14% die within the first year after "curative" surgery [56]. These results increased the need to improve the diagnostic strategy in bronchogenic carcinoma. Patients should be spared as much as possible the increased risk of morbidity and mortality of invasive diagnostic procedures [12, 14, 36, 66].

Positron emission tomography (PET) imaging can exploit the biochemical processes in malignant tumors contrary to the detection of morphological changes by conventional imaging methods, e.g., computed tomography (CT) or magnetic resonance imaging (MRI) [66]. In clinical oncology 2-[^{18}F] fluoro-2-deoxy-D-glucose (FDG) is the most commonly used radiopharmaceutical. As mentioned above (see chapter 6), the increased intratumoral FDG-uptake is the result of the high activity of transmembranous glucose transporters, hexokinase, and the low activity of glucose-6-phosphatase [21, 22, 80]. The high tumor-to-background contrast in lung parenchyma is due to the relatively low FDG extraction rate by parenchyma [26, 71]. Thus FDG-PET is particularly suitable in the diagnostic work-up of thoracic lesions [2, 10, 11].

Because of its long half-life (109.8 min) ^{18}F-labeled FDG is used in a so-called satellite system (regional distribution of FDG for institutions with a PET scanner without a cyclotron). In this chapter we will concentrate on FDG-PET in staging and restaging of lung tumors. Its value in patients with solitary pulmonary nodules (SPN), the acquiring of semiquantitative parameters and the importance of a standardized protocol will be discussed.

16.2 Histopathological classification

The histopathological differentiation between non-small cell lung cancer (NSCLC) and small cell lung cancer (SCLC) is essential for the therapeutic regimen and the prognosis of the patient.

16.2.1 Small cell lung cancer: SCLC

Small cell lung cancer comprises about 20% of all primary lung cancers [42]. The prognosis of SCLC is very poor with a survival rate of less than 1% at 5 years. SCLC is classified as "limited disease" (tumor is limited to the hemithorax and regional as well as contralateral mediastinal lymph nodes) and "extended disease" ("limited disease" plus other manifestations); the latter diagnosed in 70% of all patients at the first presentation [42, 67]. There is a limited number of PET studies with FDG concerning this tumor type [49, 50].

16.2.2 Non-small cell lung cancer: NSCLC

Non-small cell lung cancer is often limited to the thorax at the initial staging. Thus surgical procedures and radiotherapy are possible with a curative intent [67]. The most frequent histological subtypes of NSCLC are squamous cell carcinoma, adenocarcinoma, large-cell carcinoma, and bronchioloalveolar carcinoma.

Table 16.1. TNM classification of non-small cell lung cancer (NSCLC) (UICC 1997) [20].

TX	Positive cytology
T1	≤ 3 cm
T2	> 3 cm, main bronchus > 2 cm apart of the carina, invasion of visceral pleura, partial atelectasis
T3	Chest wall, diaphragm,pericardium, mediastinal pleura, main bronchus < 2 cm apart of the carina, total atelectasis
T4	Mediastinum, heart, great vessels, carina, trachea, esophagus, separate lesions foci in the same lobe, malignant effusion
N1	Ipsilateral peribronchial/hilar lymph nodes
N2	Ipsilateral mediastinal/subcarinal lymph nodes
N3	Contralateral mediastinal, hilar, ipsi- or contralateral scalene or supraclavicular lymph nodes
M1	Distant metastases, separate lesions in the other lobe

Table 16.2. Clinical stages of bronchogenic carcinoma (UICC 1997) [21].

Stage	TNM classification		
Occult carcinoma	TX	N0	M0
0	T cis [a]	N0	M0
IA	T1	N0	M0
IB	T2	N0	M0
IIA	T1	N1	M0
IIB	T2	N1	M0
	T3	N0	M0
IIIA	T1	N2	M0
	T2	N2	M0
	T3	N1, N2	M0
IIIB	T4	any N	M0
	any T	N3	M0
IV	any T	any N	M1

The clinical staging of NSCLC is based upon the recommendations of the Union Internationale Contre le Cancer (UICC) [100]. Table 16.1 shows an overview of the actual TNM classification. There are significant differences in the 5-year survival rates concerning the stage of NSCLC: stage I, 60–70%; stage II, 30–50%; stage III, 5–30%, while stage IV is less than 2% [42] (Table 16.2). The histopathological grading system is scaled from G1 (well differentiated) up to G4 (poorly differentiated).

Rare intrapulmonary tumors are carcinoid tumors, adenoidcystic carcinomas (cylindroma) und mesotheliomas [29, 67].

16.3 Radiopharmaceuticals

The greatest clinical experience has been achieved with [^{11}C]methionine ([^{11}C]MET). The pathophysiological basis is the increased transmethylation rate in malignant tumors. Thus [^{11}C]MET uptake is correlated to the protein biosynthesis [54]. Early [^{11}C]MET studies by Kubota et al. did not show significant differences in comparison to FDG-PET in patients with NSCLC [52, 53]. This observation was also confirmed by others [70, 98]. [^{11}C]MET uptake in the inflammatory lesions, esophagus and bronchi deteriorates the specificity of the visual assessment of intrapulmonary lesions though there is faster blood clearance [98]. Because of the short half-life of ^{11}C (only 20 min) it is not routinely used.

16.4 Indications

Since 1998 Medicare has paid for FDG-PET scans for patients with indeterminant solitary pulmonary nodules and the initial staging of lung cancer in

Table 16.3. Indications for FDG-PET in lung cancer (reimbursement by Medicare) [16].

Initial staging of lung cancer in patients with pathologically diagnosed NSCLC
Evaluation of indeterminant solitary pulmonary nodules (SPN)

Table 16.4. Recommendations for FDG-PET in patients with lung cancer from the German Consensus Conference 1997 [28].

Ia	– Peripheral solitary nodule in high risk patients – Local recurrence – Lymph node staging
Ib	–
IIa	– Therapy control
IIb	– Distant metastases
III	–

[a] *Ia* adequate, *Ib* acceptable, *IIa* helpful, *IIb* unreliable as yet, *III* not useful

those patients, who have histologically confirmed NSCLC [16] (Table 16.3). The FDG-based strategy in the diagnostic process of bronchogenic carcinoma is cost effective, as has been shown by Gambhir et al. The major cost savings result from avoiding unnecessary surgical procedures in patients with unresectable disease [27].

Germany is the European country with the most installed PET scanners. A consensus conference has made recommendations for the use of FDG-PET in lung cancer [78]. The clinical usefulness is classified as follows: Ia adequate, Ib acceptable, IIa helpful, IIb unreliable as yet, III not useful (Table 16.4).

16.5 Staging

16.5.1 Clinical situation and conventional diagnostic methods

Screening for lung cancer is not recommended, because there is no significant improvement of mortality rates by such measures [23, 29].

An intrapulmonary lesion is often an accidental finding detected by ordinary chest X-ray. Radiological criteria of a benign process are central, concentric calcification and growth-stability over 2 years [13, 33, 45, 76, 97]. Malignancy is suspected in nodules with irregular margins, absence of calcification, and a diameter of more than 3 cm [13, 45, 101]. Despite advances in computed tomography of the chest, 20–40% of all resected tumors are benign in nature. These patients are liable to unnecessarily increased peri- and postoperative risk of morbidity and mortality associated with surgery [66, 80, 101].

Clinical findings at the initial stage of bronchogenic carcinoma are often inconspicuous and nonspecific [29]. Unequivocal symptoms and signs appear in advanced disease: hemoptysis, weight loss, Horner's syndrome. In these cases a curative therapeutic regimen is generally not feasible any more.

Sputum cytology is of no great value in early stages of disease because of its low sensitivity in peripheral lesions (up to 60%) [45, 97, 101]. The histological classification is based upon invasive procedures with their coherent risk of morbidity and mortality. Even these methods have a limited sensitivity and specificity. Bronchoscopy has a relatively low complication rate and is indicated in endobronchial lesions [97]. However in pulmonary nodules of less than 2 cm diameter a definite diagnosis is made only in less than 40% of cases [13, 101]. Transthoracal needle biopsy (TTNB) in peripheral solitary pulmonary nodules (SPN) is effective in the diagnosis of 80–90% of malignant tumors [3, 45, 56]. Drawbacks of TTNB are its limited value in benign lesions [101] as well as its complications, e.g., pneumothorax in 15–46% [12–14, 44, 93, 101] and hemoptyses [13]. Thoracotomy has a variable risk of mortality depending on the extent of the surgical procedure: 1.4% in wedge resection, 3% in lobectomy, and 6% in pneumonectomy [101].

After the diagnosis of malignancy, tumor spread has to be examined with different measures, e.g., CT of the chest and upper abdomen. Mediastinal invasion by the tumor, lymph node involvement, and distant metastases have direct consequences on the therapeutic regimen and prognosis [93]. Up to stage IIb, surgical resection is the therapy of choice with a curative intent. At present from stage IIIa onward adjuvant and neoadjuvant chemotherapy and radiotherapy is discussed. There is no indication for surgery when the tumor has spread to contralateral lymph nodes (stage IIIb) [29, 62].

Rationale for the FDG-PET is the non-invasive differentiation between benign and malignant lesions without the increased risk of morbidity and mortality [58].

16.5.2 Tumor stage

Concerning the differentiation of intrapulmonary lesions FDG-PET is more accurate than conventional imaging techniques such as CT [15]. It also has a higher specificity in the diagnosis of benign tumors in comparison to invasive procedures, e.g., TTNB [18]. Lowe et al. reported a sensitivity of 97% and a specificity of 89% in 60 patients with malignant SPNs (reference value: mediastinal FDG uptake [59]). In most studies the sensitivity of FDG-PET was higher than 90% with visual assessment as well as with the assessment of the semiquantitative standardized uptake values (SUV). The specificity was in the range of 70–100% (Table 16.5, Fig. 16.1). Comparing morphologic images, e.g., CT, with FDG-PET is recommended, whereas image fusion is not always necessary [93, 94, 96]. Differentiation between NSCLC and SCLC is not possible with FDG-PET. In previous studies of Nolop et al. and Gupta

Table 16.5. FDG-PET in the staging of intrapulmonary lesions.

Author	Year	Patients [a]	Prevalence [b]	Sensitivity	Specifity	SUV [c]
Lowe [58]	1998	89	60/89 (67%)	55/60 (92%)	26/29 (90%)	+
Nettelbladt [70]	1998	19	15/19 (79%)	14/15 (93%)	3/4 (75%)	+
Dewan [15]	1997	52	37/52 (71%)	35/37 (95%)	13/15 (87%)	–
Gupta [34]	1996	61	42/61 (69%)	39/42 (93%)	17/19 (89%)	+
Sazon [82]	1996	107	82/107 (77%)	82/82 (100%)	12/25 (48%)	–
Duhaylongsod [18]	1995	87	59/87 (68%)	57/59 (97%)	23/28 (82%)	+
Dewan [14]	1995	35	26/35 (74%)	26/26 (100%)	7/9 (78%)	–
Hübner [40]	1995	23	17/23 (74%)	17/17 (100%)	4/6 (67%)	+
Lowe [59]	1994	88	61/88 (69%)	59/61 (97%)	24/27 (89%)	+
Scott [84]	1994	62	47/62 (76%)	44/47 (94%)	12/15 (80%)	+
Wahl [96]	1994	23	19/23 (83%)	19/19 (100%)	4/4 (100%)	+
Patz [75]	1993	51	33/51 (65%)	29/33 (88%)	18/18 (100%)	+
Slosman [86]	1993	31	26/31 (84%)	29/31 (93%)	3/5 (60%)	–
Dewan [45]	1993	30	20/30 (67%)	19/20 (95%)	8/10 (80%)	+

[a] number of patients; [b] based on the number of patients; [c] +/–: SUV determined/not determined

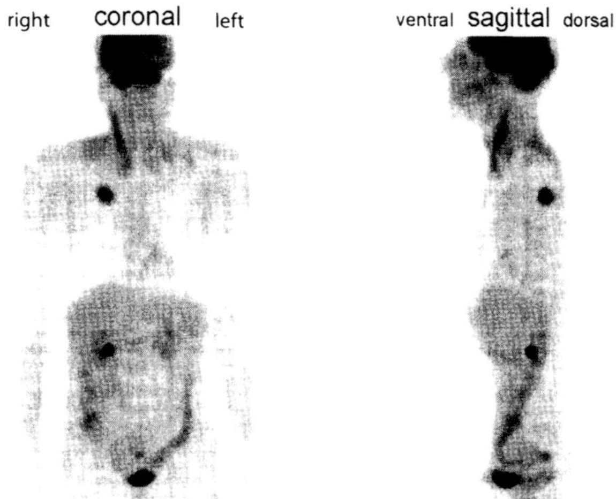

Fig. 16.1. Squamous cell carcinoma of the right upper lobe (posterior segment) (SUV_{max}: 6.2; male, 59 years). Neck dissection on the right and radiotherapy 6 months ago because of palatinal carcinoma (SUV_{max}: 3.4). Physiological FDG uptake in the renal pelvis on the right, the urinary bladder, descending colon, and sigmoid (maximum intensity projections; Siemens/CTI ECAT EXACT).

et al., it was shown that intratumoral FDG uptake is heterogeneous even in the same tumor subtype [33, 71].

There is a great challenge for FDG-PET with regard to the solitary pulmonary nodules (SPN), in which only 30–50% are malignant in nature [45, 58]. Lesion detection in PET depends on its size, resolution of the scanner, tissue concentration of the radiotracer and other factors (e.g., motion artifacts of intrathoracical organs due to breathing). Partial volume effects of currently used PET scanners must be considered in small lesions (<2–3 cm). In these

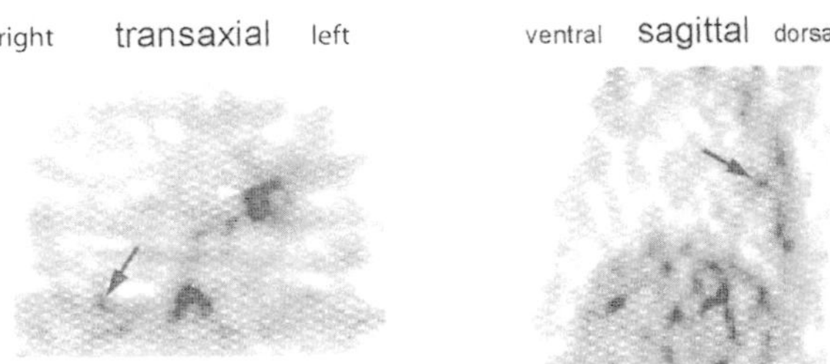

Fig. 16.2. Solitary pulmonary nodule of 1.2 cm diameter, right lower lobe (superior segment; black arrow; male, 45 years). SUV_{max}: 2.2 (uncorrected for partial volume effect); SUV_{max}: 5.5 (corrected for partial volume effect, recovery coefficient 0.4). Tubulopapillary adenocarcinoma. White arrow: myocardium (attenuation-corrected images; Siemens/CTI ECAT EXACT).

foci an underestimation of the activity concentration can result in missed malignant tumors, consequently leading to a decrease in sensitivity of PET [39]. Attenuation correction is recommended to detect small intrapulmonary foci with increased FDG uptake [13, 80]. High FDG uptake in small lesions localized in the posterior basal parts of the lungs might be missed due to a higher background of normal lung tissue and to scatter from myocardium and liver [68]. The accuracy of PET in SPNs can be improved by the determination of recovery coefficients and correction of semiquantitative parameters [39, 68] (Fig. 16.2) (see chapter 4). FDG-PET in combination with CT is cost effective in patients with SPNs [28].

The acquisition of transmission data is essential to determine the semiquantitative parameters, e.g., SUV, that are important for follow-up and therapy control. Several studies have confirmed that the accuracy of attenuation-corrected FDG-PET data is in the same order as invasive procedures [6] (Table 16.5).

SUV represents the intratumoral activity concentration in relation to the activity in the whole body of the patient (chapter 3). There are different reference values: most PET studies used the body weight, a few the lean body mass [102], body mass index, or body surface area [46]. A cut-off level of 2.5 is reported for the differentiation of benign and malignant tumors [20, 59, 74, 83]. Rationale of SUVs is the higher reproducibility compared to the visual assessment of FDG-PET emission data [66]. A standardized data acquisition and reconstruction protocol is obligatory (see below): a fixed time of the emission scan, and a standardized size of the region of interest (ROI). The maximum SUV (SUV_{max}) as well as the mean SUV (SUV_{mean}) should be determined in small ROI of 1 cm^2 [4, 13, 33, 34, 46, 66, 98, 102].

False-positive results. High FDG uptake is found in granulomatous infections, e.g., sarcoidosis, tuberculosis, aspergillosis, and plasma cell granuloma [13, 48, 59, 75, 86, 87]. Likewise pneumonic infiltrates show increased FDG uptake [70, 71].

False-negative results. A relatively low FDG uptake is consistently reported in bronchioloalveolar carcinoma [47, 74, 84]. Higashi et al. reported false-negative FDG-PET results in 4 of 7 cases with bronchioloalveolar carcinoma [38]. Because of few viable cancer cells in the fibrous tissue, FDG uptake in scar carcinoma is also low [13, 84, 86].

As a rule FDG-PET is negative in carcinoid tumors. In the majority of patients the differentiated, slow growing subtype is found (in 90% of all cases) [20, 77].

FDG-PET is useful for the differentiation of pleural lesions, e.g., a suspected pleural effusion or mesothelioma [37, 60, 89]. In a recent review Rigo et al. reported that FDG-PET can reduce the number of both open pleural biopsies and thoracotomies for benign pleural disease. An intense FDG uptake can be used for biopsy guidance [80].

16.5.3 Staging of lymphogenic metastases

Lymphogenic metastases of NSCLC usually appear before the distant hematogenous spread occurs [29]. T1–T3 tumors and ipsilateral hilar and mediastinal lymph nodes (N1–N2) are operated upon with a curative intent, whereas only palliative treatment is applied in T4 tumors or in case of contralateral nodal involvement (N3) [29].

The main criterion of conventional imaging methods in the assessment of lymph nodes is nodal size. A node with a short axis diameter of more than 1 cm is suspected to be malignant [30, 76]. The sensitivity of this parameter is relatively low, because malignant cells can occur in normal-sized nodes [32, 57, 76, 93]. On the other hand, benign hyperplastic lymph nodes due to inflammatory disease are often enlarged and cause false-positive CT results [62, 63, 76]. McLoud et al. found benign lesions in 37% of mediastinal lymph nodes with a diameter of 2–4 cm [62]. Other studies have confirmed the low sensitivity and specificity of CT [59, 62, 81, 88, 93, 95].

FDG-PET is the non-invasive method of choice in the nodal staging of NSCLC (Table 16.6). Nodal involvement in normal-sized lymph nodes is reliably detected. In case of a low FDG uptake in enlarged lymph nodes, metastases can be excluded with high accuracy. Recently Vansteenkiste et al. found that the very high negative predictive value of mediastinal PET could substantially reduce the need for mediastinal invasive surgical staging in NSCLC [95]. Valk et al. reported that FDG-PET accurately differentiates 14 of 29 false-positive CT results [93]. Patz et al. postulated that a negative PET result makes preoperative mediastinoscopy unnecessary, whereas a positive PET result determines the surgical approach [73]. Although the detection of hilar and lobar lymph nodes (N1) is improved by FDG-PET in comparison to chest CT, the sensitivity and specificity are lower than in mediastinal lymph nodes (N2) [73] (Table 16.6). The differentiation of peribronchial hilar from adjacent mediastinal lymph nodes is difficult (N1 versus N2) [80, 84, 96]. An analysis by Malenka et al. indicated that a noninvasive method for mediastinal staging would have the same life-expectancy outcome as strategies in-

Table 16.6. FDG-PET in lung cancer: lymph node staging.

Author	Year	Pts (n)	Prevalence[b]	Sensitivity a. hilar/lobar (N1) b. mediastinal (N2)	Specifity a. hilar/lobar (N1) b. mediastinal (N2)
Vansteenkiste [95]	1998	690[a]	47/690 (89%)	a.+b. 42/47 (89%) CT: 22/47 (47%)	a.+b. 636/643 (99%) CT: 616/643 (96%)
Steinert [88]	1997	112[a]	28/112 (47%)	a.+b. 25/28 (89%) CT: 16/28 (57%)	a.+b. 83/84 (99%) CT: 79/84 (94%)
Sazon [82]	1996	32	16/32 (50%)	a.+b. 16/16 (100%) CT: 13/16 (81%)	a.+b. 16/16 (100%) CT: 9/16 (56%)
Sasaki [81]	1996	71[a]	17/71 (24%)	a.+b. 13/17 (76%) CT: 11/17 (65%)	a.+b. 53/54 (98%) CT: 47/54 (87%)
Gupta [34]	1996	12	7/12 (58%)	a.+b. 7/7 (100%)	a.+b. 5/5 (100%)
Chin [9]	1995	30	9/30 (30%)	a.+b. 7/9 (78%) CT: 5/9 (56%)	a.+b. 17/21 (81%) CT: 18/21 (86%)
Valk [93]	1995	76[a]	31/76 (41%)	a. 4/7 (57%) CT: 1/7 (14%) b. 20/24 (83%) CT: 15/24 (63%)	b. 49/52 (94%) CT: 38/52 (73%)
Patz [73]	1995	62[a]	23/62 (37%)	a. 8/11 (73%) CT: 3/11 (27%) b. 11/12 (92%) CT: 7/12 (58%)	a. 22/29 (76%) CT: 25/29 (86%) b. 10/10 (100%) CT: 8/10 (80%)
Scott [84]	1994	25	3/25 (12%)	a.+b. 2/3 (67%)	a.+b. 19/22 (86%)
Wahl [96]	1994	27[a]	11/27 (41%)	a.+b. 9/11 (82%) CT: 7/11 (64%)	a.+b. 13/16 (81%) CT: 7/16 (44%)

[a] lymph node regions; [b] based on the number of patients or lymph nodes

volving surgical staging if the specificity of the noninvasive diagnostic method is 90% or higher [61] (Table 16.6).

If the patient has not fasted for more than 4 hours, the assessment of mediastinal lymph nodes is restricted by high myocardial FDG uptake. Scatter is reduced by attenuation correction. The mediastinal blood pool activity is used as a reference parameter (SUV: 2.0–2.5) [96].

A standardized lymph node mapping scheme was introduced in 1997 by the American Joint Committee on Cancer (AJCC) and the Union Internationale Contre le Cancer (UICC), thus, providing a basis for unequivocal nomenclature by radiologists, nuclear medicine physicians, surgeons, and pathologists [69].

False-positive results. As in primary lung tumors, granulomatous lesions and nodular hyperplasia can intensely concentrate FDG [5, 84, 93, 96].

False-negative results. Detection of involved subcarinal lymph nodes can be difficult because of the relatively high background activity in the lower lung fields. Likewise microscopic metastases are sometimes missed with FDG-PET [93].

16.5.4 Staging of hematogenous metastases

The main manifestations of hematogenous metastases in lung cancer are the liver, brain, skeleton, bone marrow, and adrenal cortex, but all other organ systems may also be affected. In autopsy studies metastases are detectable in about 50% of squamous cell lung cancer, in 80% of adenocarcinoma and large cell carcinoma, and in more than 95% of SCLC [10, 29].

Several publications have confirmed the value of whole-body FDG-PET in the staging of distant metastases in NSCLC [4, 7, 8, 56, 77, 93, 99]. With a whole-body PET scan all potential sites of metastases are examined in about one hour. Bury et al. reported an up- or down-staging of nodal disease after FDG-PET in 21% and in distant metastases in 10% of their patients [8]. The investigators concluded that whole-body FDG-PET provides more accurate thoracic and extrathoracic staging of NSCLC than conventional imaging methods (CT of the chest and abdomen, bone scintigraphy). The same study group reported that FDG-PET could accurately confirm the absence of osseous involvement in 87 out of 89 patients (bone scintigraphy: 54 of 89 patients) [7].

Indeterminant morphological findings by CT and MRI are better clarified with functional PET imaging that serves as a complementary diagnostic method [46, 76, 81, 88]. Boland et al. reported that FDG-PET correctly identified all malignant adrenal lesions (14 of 24 adrenal masses) that occur usually in about one third of all enlarged adrenal glands in cancer patients [4, 19].

The higher sensitivity of FDG-PET versus CT is confirmed by Valk et al., who reported metastases in 11 of 99 patients with a normal CT scan. In addition a correct diagnosis of a benign lesion in FDG-PET was achieved in 18 of

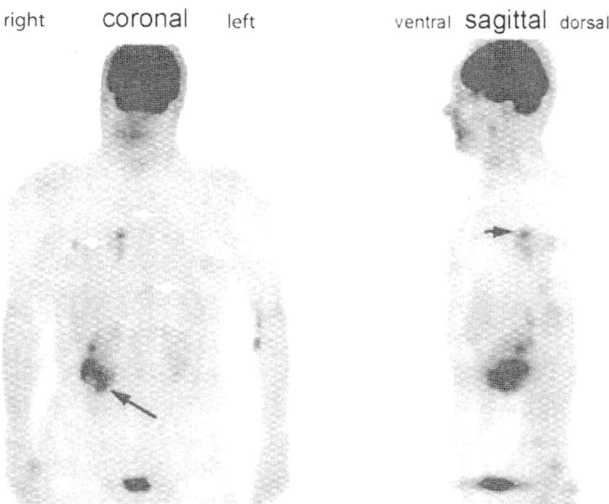

Fig. 16.3. Restaging of an undifferentiated adenocarcinoma (female, 53 years). Renal metastasis on the right (long black arrow), skeletal metastases (white arrows), local recurrence (short black arrow) (maximum intensity projections; Siemens/CTI ECAT EXACT).

19 patients, in whom CT results were suspicious for malignancy. The investigators conclude that an improved accuracy of nonsurgical staging in lung cancer patients can be achieved by replacing abdominal and pelvic CT with whole-body PET. Chest CT is needed for an accurate determination of tumor stage and the evaluation of thoracic anatomy [93].

16.6 Restaging

After therapy, follow-up of the primary site of lung cancer is indicated to detect local tumor recurrence in an early stage and prevent the metastatic spread by the effective retreatment [24]. Thus, the prognosis will be improved if an asymptomatic local recurrence of cancer is detected early, and it will respond more favorably to retreatment due to its small tumor burden [24]. Drawbacks of conventional imaging methods are the distorted or the absent anatomical structures after surgery [77]. In addition the differentiation of postradiation fibrosis from tumor recurrence is difficult with conventional imaging methods [31, 84].

Several studies reported a high sensitivity of FDG-PET in the restaging of lung cancer (95–100%) [24, 43, 74]. Specificity in most studies ranged from 89% [24] - 100% [18, 74]. Inoue et al. correctly detected local recurrence in all 26 patients with FDG-PET, but specificity was only 61% (8/13 pts) [43].

Variable inflammatory tissue reactions with potential high FDG uptake can occur after radiotherapy of lung cancer: edematous and chronic inflammatory or fibrotic lesions, radiation pneumonitis, and peritumoral inflammatory reactions [24] (Fig. 16.1). Therefore, a time interval of at least six months for a PET scan is recommended after tumor radiotherapy [24].

16.7 Therapy monitoring

Only few data have been published concerning the diagnostic value of FDG-PET in monitoring therapy of patients with lung cancer [41, 85, 90]. FDG-PET after radiotherapy or chemotherapy in patients with SCLC was more accurate in response evaluation and differentiation of responders/non-responders in comparison to CT [89]. False-positive results are due to postirradiation pneumonitis [43]. Important points to consider are time interval after therapy, standardized data acquisition, a standard protocol for image reconstruction and interpretation [65, 66].

16.8 Grading

Grading of lung cancer as a prognostic parameter is of no great importance as in other tumor entities, e.g., carcinoma of the bladder, prostatic carcinoma, non-Hodgkin lymphoma [16]. To correlate the intratumoral FDG uptake and the histological tumor differentiation, the calculation of semiquantitative parameters is necessary, e.g., standardized uptake values (SUV).

Although Duhaylongsod et al. have reported a direct correlation between tumor growth and FDG uptake [17], in other studies the extent of FDG uptake was not related to the histopathological differentiation of bronchogenic carcinoma, nor could it differentiate NSCLC from SCLC [14, 33, 35, 43, 55, 71, 79, 89]. These divergent results might be contributed in particular to heterogeneous tumor tissues and the variable extent of inflammatory peritumoral reactions [14].

In bronchioloalveolar carcinoma which often grow slowly, FDG uptake was not increased in most studies [38, 58, 84]. Fujiwara et al. found higher uptake of [^{11}C]methionine in large cell carcinomas compared to squamous cell carcinomas [25]. Higashi et al. reported the correlation of FDG uptake with grading of adenocarcinomas [38]. In addition, in a recent retrospective study FDG uptake correlated with survival in patients with bronchogenic carcinoma [1].

16.9 Outlook

PET scanning offers additional information of the biochemical processes in intrathoracic lesions. This is complementary to conventional imaging methods and might influence the therapeutic regimen of the oncologist, as well as improve the very poor prognosis of lung cancer.

The introduction of FDG-PET as a new diagnostic method is associated with high costs, but the studies have confirmed its cost effectiveness in patients with lung cancer. Thus, reimbursement of FDG-PET by Medicare has increased the number of patients with lung cancer undergoing this examination [11].

Radiolabeled chemotherapeutic drugs for the pretherapeutic evaluation of tumor sensitivity have been recently studied for other tumor entities [89]. ^{18}F-labeled tracers are of great promise to evaluate different functional aspects of malignant tumors: amino acid transport using [^{18}F]tyrosine, [^{18}F] methyltyrosine [72], DNA synthesis (fluorodeoxyuridine, [^{18}F]uridine, fluorouracil, ^{18}F-labeled chemotherapeutic drugs ([^{18}F]fluorouracil)), differentiation of hypoxic tumor tissue (Cu-62-ATSM) [51, 91, reviews: 92].

A reduction of the injected dose and acquisition time might be achieved as the technique of data acquisition improves, e.g., gated scanning to minimize respiratory based motion artifacts, with the introduction of 3D-acquisition, and iterative reconstruction algorithms [80, 81, review: 6]. All these factors will contribute to establishing FDG-PET in clinical oncology as a routine examination in the diagnostic work-up of patients with lung cancer.

16.10 Recommendations of performing and interpreting FDG-PET in lung cancer patients

- **Preparation of patients:**
  - Fasting state (NPO) for 12 h.
  - Blood glucose level < 100 mg/dl.
- **Data acquisition:**
  - "Cold" transmission of the chest (10 min for each bed position).
  - Intravenous application of 370 MBq [^{18}F]FDG.
  - Whole-body emission scan 60 min after application (10 min/bed position, caudocranial direction; start from the proximal third of the thigh up to the base of the skull). Imaging of the chest 90–110 min after application.
  - If "cold" transmission is not feasible, "hot" transmission is recommended.
- **Reconstruction:**
  - Filtered backprojection (Hanning, filter factor 0.3).
  - Iterative reconstruction, if available.
- **Interpretation:**
  - Visual: Emission images (reference: mediastinal FDG uptake)
Attenuation-corrected images
  - SUV: SUV_{max} (cutoff level 2.5)
SUV_{mean} ROI area 1 cm^2
(reference: body weight).

References

[1] Ahuja V, Coleman RE, Herndon J, Patz EF (1998) The prognostic significance of fluorodeoxyglucose positron emission tomography imaging for patients with non-small cell lung carcinoma. Cancer 83:918–924

[2] Al-Sugair A, Coleman RE (1998) Applications of PET in lung cancer. Sem Nucl Med 28:303–319

[3] Austin JHM, Cohen MB (1993) Value of having a cytopathologist present during percutaneous fine-needle biopsy of lung: report of 55 cancer patients and metaanalysis of the literature. Chest 160:175–177

[4] Boland GW, Goldberg MA, Lee MJ, Mayo-Smith WW, Dixon J, McNicholas MM, Mueller PR (1995) Indeterminate adrenal mass in patients with cancer: evaluation at PET with 2-[F-18]-fluoro-2-deoxy-D-glucose. Radiology 194:131–134

[5] Brudin LH, Valind SO, Rhodes CG, Pantin CF, Sweatman M, Jones T, Hughes JMB (1994) Fluorine-18 deoxyglucose uptake in sarcoidosis measured with positron emission tomography. Eur J Nucl Med 21:297–305

[6] Budinger T (1998) PET instrumentation: what are the limits? Sem Nucl Med 28:247–267

[7] Bury T, Barreto A, Daenen F, Barthelemy N, Ghaye B, Rigo P (1998) Fluorine-18 deoxyglucose positron emission tomography for the detection of bone metastases in patients with non-small cell lung cancer. Eur J Nucl Med 25:1244–1247

[8] Bury T, Dowlati A, Paulus P, Hustinx R, Radermecker M, Rigo P (1996) Staging of non-small-cell lung cancer by whole-body fluorine-18 deoxyglucose positron emission tomography. Eur J Nucl Med 23:204–206
[9] Chin R, Ward R, Keyes JW, Choplin RH, Reed JC, Wallenhaupt S, Hudspeth AS, Haponik EF (1995) Mediastinal staging of non-small-cell lung cancer with positron emission tomography. Am J Respir Crit Care Med 152:2090–2096
[10] Chiti A, Schreiner FAG, Crippa F, Pauwels EKJ, Bombardieri E (1999) Nuclear medicine procedures in lung cancer. Eur J Nucl Med 26:533–555
[11] Coleman RE (1999) PET in lung cancer. J Nucl Med 40:814–820
[12] Conces DJ, Tarver RD, Gray WC, Pearcy EA (1988) Treatment of pneumothoraces utilizing small caliber chest tubes. Chest 94:55–57
[13] Dewan NA, Gupta NC, Redepenning LS, Phalen JJ, Frick MP (1993) Diagnostic efficacy of FDG-PET imaging in solitary pulmonary nodules. Chest 104:997–1002
[14] Dewan NA, Reeb SD, Gupta NC, Gobar LS, Scott WJ (1995) PET-FDG imaging and transthoracic needle lung aspiration biopsy in evaluation of pulmonary lesions. Chest 108:441–446
[15] Dewan NA, Shehan CJ, Reeb SD, Gobar LS, Scott WJ, Ryschon K (1997) Likelihood of malignancy in a solitary pulmonary nodule. Comparison of Bayesian analysis and results of FDG-PET scan. Chest 112:416–422
[16] Donhuijsen K (1998) Histologisches Malignitätsgrading. Dt Ärztebl 95:2391–2395
[17] Duhaylongsod FG, Lowe VJ, Patz EF, Vaughn AL, Coleman RE, Wolfe WG (1995) Lung tumor growth correlates with glucose metabolism measured by fluoride-18 fluorodeoxyglucose positron emission tomography. Ann Thorac Surg 60:1348–1350
[18] Duhaylongsod FG, Lowe VJ, Patz EF, Vaughn AL, Coleman RE, Wolfe WG (1995) Detection of primary and recurrent lung cancer by means of F-18 fluorodeoxyglucose positron emission tomography (FDG PET). J Thorac Cardiovasc Surg 110:130–140
[19] Dunninck NR (1990) Adrenal imaging: current status. AJR 154:927–936
[20] Erasmus JJ, McAdams HP, Patz EF, Coleman RE, Ahuja V, Goodman PC (1998) Evaluation of primary pulmonary carcinoid tumors using FDG PET. AJR 170:1369–1373
[21] Fischman AJ, Alpert NM (1993) FDG-PET in oncology: there's more to it than looking at pictures. J Nucl Med 34:6–10
[22] Flier JS, Mueckler M, Usher P, Lodish HF (1987) Elevated levels of glucose transport and transporter messenger RNA are induced by ras or src oncogenes. Science 235:1492–1495
[23] Fontana RS, Sanderson DR, Woolner LW, Taylor WT, Miller WE, Muhm JR, Bernatz PE, Payne WS, Pairolero PC, Bergstralh EJ (1991) Screening for lung cancer – a critique of the Mayo lung project. Cancer 67:1155–1164
[24] Frank A, Lefkowitz D, Jaeger S, Gobar L, Sunderland J, Gupta N, Scott W, Mailliard J, Lynch H, Bishop J, Thorpe P, Dewan N (1995) Decision logic for the treatment of asymptomatic lung cancer recurrence based on positron emission tomography findings. Int J Radiation Oncology Biol Phys 32:1495–1512
[25] Fujiwara T, Matsuzawa T, Kubota K, Abe Y, Itoh M, Fukuda H, Hatazawa J, Yoshioka S, Yamaguchi K, Ito K, Watanuki S, Takahasi T, Ishiwata K, Iwata R, Ido T (1989) Relationship between histologic type of primary lung cancer and carbon-11-L-methionine uptake with positron emission tomography. J Nucl Med 30:33–37
[26] Gallagher BM, Fowler JS, Gutterson NI, MacGregor RR, Wan CN, Wolf AP (1978) Metabolic trapping as aprinciple of radiopharmaceutical design: some factors responsible for the biodistribution of [^{18}F] 2-deoxy-2-fluoro-D-glucose. J Nucl Med 19:1154–1161
[27] Gambhir SS, Hoh CK, Phelps ME, Madar I, Maddahi J (1996) Decision tree sensitivity analysis for cost-effectiveness of FDG-PET in the staging and management of non-small-cell lung carcinoma. J Nucl Med 37:1428–1436
[28] Gambhir SS, Shepherd JE, Shah BD, Hart CK, Valk PE, Emi T, Phelps ME (1998) Analytical decision model for the cost-effectiveness management of solitary pulmonary nodules. J Clin Oncol 16:2113–2125

[29] Ginsberg RJ, Vokes EE, Raben A (1997) Non-small cell lung cancer. In: DeVita VT, Hellman S, Rosenberg SA (eds) Cancer: Principles and Practice of Oncology. Lippincott-Raven, Philadelphia, pp 858–911

[30] Glazer GM, Gross BH, Quint LE, Francis IR, Bookstein FL, Orringer MB (1985) Normal mediastinal lymph nodes: number and size according to American Thoracic Society mapping. AJR 144:261–265

[31] Glazer HS, Lee JKT, Levitt RG, Heiken JP, Ling D, Totty WG, Balfe DM, Emani B, Wasserman TH, Murphy WA (1985) Radiation fibrosis: differentiation from recurrent tumor by MR - work in progress. Radiology 156:721–726

[32] Gross BH, Glazer GM, Orringer MB, Spizarny DL, Flint A (1988) Bronchogenic carcinoma metastatic to normal-sized lymph nodes: frequency and significance. Radiology 166:71–74

[33] Gupta NC, Frank AR, Dewan NA, Redepenning LS, Rothberg ML, Mailliard JA, Phalen JJ, Sunderland JJ, Frick MP (1992) Solitary pulmonary nodules: detection of malignancy with PET with 2-[F-18]-fluoro-2-deoxy-D-glucose. Radiology 184:441–444

[34] Gupta NC, Maloof J, Gunel E (1996) Probability of malignancy in solitary pulmonary nodules using fluorine-18-FDG and PET. J Nucl Med 37:943–948

[35] Hamberg LM, Hunter GJ, Alpert NM, Choi NC, Babich JW, Fischman AJ (1994) The Dose Uptake Ratio as an index of glucose metabolism: useful parameter or oversimplification? J Nucl Med 35:1308–1312

[36] Haramati LB, Austin JHM (1991) Complications after CT-guided needle biopsy through aerated versus nonaerated lung. Radiology 181:778

[37] Hellwig A, Hellwig D, Ukena D, Sybrecht GW, Kirsch CM (1998) FDG-PET zur Differenzierung zwischen benignen und malignen Pleuraergüssen. Nuklearmedizin 37:A70 (abstr)

[38] Higashi K, Ueda Y, Seki H, Yuasa K, Oguchi M, Noguchi T, Taniguchi M, Tonami H, Okimura T, Yamamoto I (1998) Fluorine-18-FDG PET imaging is negative in bronchioloalveolar lung carcinoma. J Nucl Med 39:1016–1020

[39] Hoffman EJ, Huang SC, Phelps ME (1979) Quantitation in positron emission computed tomography: 1. Effect of object size. J Comput Assist Tomogr 3:299–308

[40] Hübner KF, Buonocore E, Singh SK, Gould HR, Cotten DW (1995) Characterization of chest masses by FDG positron emission tomography. Clin Nucl Med 20:293–298

[41] Ichiya Y, Kuwabara Y, Sasaki M, Yoshida T, Omagari J, Akashi Y, Kawashima A, Fukumura T, Masuda K (1996) A clinical evaluation of FDG-PET to assess the response in radiation therapy for bronchogenic carcinoma. Ann Nucl Med 10:193–200

[42] Ihde DC, Pass HI, Glatstein E (1997) Small cell lung cancer. In: DeVita VT, Hellman S, Rosenberg SA (eds) Cancer: Principles and Practice of Oncology. Lippincott-Raven, Philadelphia, pp 911–949

[43] Inoue T, Kim EE, Komaki R, Wong FCL, Bassa P, Wong WH, Yang DJ, Endo K, Podoloff DA (1995) Detecting recurrent or residual lung cancer with FDG-PET. J Nucl Med 36:788–793

[44] Kazerooni EA, Lim FT, Mikhail A, Martinez FJ (1996) Risk of pneumothorax in CT-guided transthoracic needle aspiration biopsy of the lung. Radiology 198:371–375

[45] Khouri NF, Meziane MA, Zerhouni EA, Fishman EK, Siegelman SS (1987) The solitary pulmonary nodule - assessment, diagnosis, and management. Chest 91:128–133

[46] Kim CK, Gupta NC, Chandramouli B, Alavi A (1994) Standardized uptake value of FDG: body surface area correction is preferable to body weight correction. J Nucl Med 35:164–167

[47] Kim BT, Kim Y, Lee KS, Yoon SB, Cheon EM, Kwon OJ, Rhee JH, Han J, Shin MH (1998) Localized form of bronchioloalveolar carcinoma: FDG PET findings. AJR 170:935–939

[48] Knopp MV, Bischoff HG (1994) Beurteilung von pulmonalen Herden mit der Positronenemissionstomographie. Radiologe 34:588–591

[49] Knopp MV, Bischoff H, Rimac A, Doll J, Oberdorfer F, Lorenz WJ, van Kaick G (1994) Clinical utility of positron emission tomography with FDG for chemotherapy response monitoring - a correlative study of patients with small cell lung cancer. J Nucl Med 35:75P (abstr)

[50] Knopp MV,Strauss LG, Haberkorn U et al. (1990) Positron emission tomography (PET) with ^{18}F-deoxyglucose in the imaging and staging of bronchogenic carcinoma. Eur J Nucl Med 16:560

[51] Koh WJ, Bergman KS, Rasey JS, Peterson LM, Evans ML, Graham MM, Grierson JR, Lindsley KL, Lewellen TK, Krohn KA, Griffin TW (1995) Evaluation of oxygenation status during fractionated radiotherapy in human nonsmall cell lung cancers using [F-18]fluoromisonidazole positron emission tomography. Int J Radiat Oncol Biol Phys 33:391–398

[52] Kubota K, Matsuwaza T, Fujiwara T, Ito M, Hatazawa J, Ishiwata K, Iwata R, Ido T (1990) Differential diagnosis of lung tumor with positron emission tomography: a prospective study. J Nucl Med 31:1927–1933

[53] Kubota K, Matsuzawa T, Masatoshi I, Ito K, Fujiwara T, Abe Y, Yoshioka S, Fukuda H, Hatazawa J, Iwata R, Watanuki S, Ido T (1985) Lung tumor imaging by positron emission tomography using C-11-Methionine. J Nucl Med 26:37–42

[54] Kubota K, Yamada S, Ishiwata K, Ito M, Ido T (1992) Positron emission tomography for treatment evaluation and recurrence detection compared with CT in long-term follow-up cases of lung cancer. Clin Nucl Med 17:877–881

[55] Langen KJ, Braun U, Rota-Kops E, Herzog H, Kuwert T, Nebeling B, Feinendegen LE (1993) The influence of plasma glucose levels on fluorine-18-fluorodeoxyglucose uptake in bronchial carcinomas. J Nucl Med 34:355–359

[56] Lewis P, Griffin S, Marsden P, Gee T, Nunan T, Malsey M, Dussek J (1994) Whole-body ^{18}F-fluorodeoxyglucose positron emission tomography in preoperative evaluation of lung cancer. Lancet 344:1265–1266

[57] Libshitz HI, McKenna RJ, Haynie TP, McMurtrey MJ, Mountain CT (1984) Mediastinal evaluation in lung cancer. Radiology 151:295–299

[58] Lowe VJ, Fletcher JW, Gobar L, Lawson M, Kirchner P, Valk P, Karis J, Hubner K, Delbeke D, Heiberg EV, Patz EF, Coleman RE (1998) Prospective investigation of positron emission tomography in lung nodules. J Clin Oncol 16:1075–1084

[59] Lowe VJ, Hoffman JM, DeLong DM, Patz EF, Coleman RE (1994) Semiquantitative and visual analysis of FDG-PET images in pulmonary abnormalities. J Nucl Med 35:1771–1776

[60] Lowe VJ, Patz E, Harris L, Hoffman JM, Hanson M, Goodman P, Coleman RE (1997) FDG-PET of pleural abnormalities. J Nucl Med 37(Suppl):228P (abstr)

[61] Malenka DJ, Colice GL, Beck JR (1991) Does the mediastinum of patients with non-small cell lung cancer require histologic staging? Future standards for computed tomography. Am Rev Respir Dis 144:1134–1139

[62] McLoud TC, Bourgouin PM, Greenberg RW, Kosiuk JP, Templeton PA, Shepard JO, Moore EH, Wain JC, Mathisen DJ, Grillo HC (1992) Bronchogenic carcinoma: analysis of staging in the mediastinum with CT by correlative lymph node mapping and sampling. Radiology 182:319–323

[63] Medina Gallardo JF, Borderas Naranjo F, Torres Cansino M, Rodriguez-Panadero F (1992) Validity of enlarged mediastinal nodes as markers of involvement by non-small cell lung cancer. Am Rev Respir Dis 146:1210–1212

[64] Midthun DE, Swensen SJ, Jett JR (1992) Clinical strategies for solitary pulmonary nodules. Annu Rev Med 43:195–208

[65] Minn H, Paul R (1992) Cancer treatment monitoring with fluorine-18 2-fluoro-2-deoxy-D-glucose and positron emission tomography: frustration or future. Eur J Nucl Med 19:921–924

[66] Minn H, Zasadny KR, Quint LE, Wahl RL (1995) Lung cancer: reproducibility of quantitative measurement for evaluating 2-[^{18}F]-fluoro-2-deoxy-D-glucose uptake at PET. Radiology 196:167–173

[67] Minna JD (1991) Neoplasms of the lung. In: Wilson JD, Braunwald E, Isselbacher KJ, Petersdorf RG, Martin JB, Fauci AS, Root RK (eds) Harrison's Principles of Internal Medicine. McGraw-Hill, New York, pp 1102–1110

[68] Miyauchi T, Wahl RL (1996) Regional 2-[^{18}F]fluoro-2-deoxy-D-glucose uptake varies in normal lung. Eur J Nucl Med 23:517–523

[69] Mountain CF, Dresler CM (1997) Regional lymph node classification for lung cancer staging. Chest 111:1718–1723
[70] Nettelbladt OS, Sundin AE, Valind SO, Gustafsson GR, Lamberg K, Langström B, Björnsson EH (1998) Combined fluorine-18-FDG and Carbon-11-methionine PET for diagnosis of tumors in lung and mediastinum. J Nucl Med 39:640–647
[71] Nolop KB, Rhodes CG, Brudin LH, Beaney RP, Krausz T, Jones T, Hughes JMB (1987) Glucose utilization in vivo by human pulmonary neoplasms. Cancer 60:2682–2689
[72] Oriuchi N, Inoue T, Tomiyoshi K, Sando Y, Tsukakoshi M, Aoyagi K, Tomaru Y, Amano S, Endo K (1998) Comparative F-18-fluoro-α-methyl-tyrosine (FMT) and FDG-PET in patients with pulmonary tumors. Eur J Nucl Med 25:1019 (abstr)
[73] Patz EF, Lowe VJ, Goodman PC, Herndon J (1995) Thoracic nodal staging with PET imaging with ^{18}FDG in patients with bronchogenic carcinoma. Chest 108:1617–1621
[74] Patz EF, Lowe VJ, Hoffman JM, Paine SS, Harris LK, Goodman PC (1994) Persistent or recurrent bronchogenic carcinoma: detection with PET and 2-[F-18]-2-deoxy-D-glucose. Radiology 191:379–382
[75] Patz EF, Lowe VJ, Hoffman JM, Paine SS, Burrowes P, Coleman RE, Goodman PC (1993) Focal pulmonary abnormalities: evaluation with F-18fluorodeoxyglucose PET scanning. Radiology 188:487–490
[76] Quint LE, Francis IR, Wahl RL, Gross BH, Glazer GM (1995) Preoperative staging of non-small-cell carcinoma of the lung: imaging methods. AJR 164:1349–1359
[77] Rege SD, Hoh CK, Glaspy JA, Aberle DR, Dahlbom M, Razavi MK, Phelps ME, Hawkins RA (1993) Imaging of pulmonary mass lesions with whole-body positron emission tomography and fluorodeoxyglucose. Cancer 72:82–90
[78] Reske SN, Bares R, Büll U, Guhlmann A, Moser E, Wannenmacher MF (1996) Klinische Wertigkeit der Positronen-Emissions-Tomographie (PET) bei onkologischen Fragestellungen: Ergebnisse einer interdisziplinären Konsensuskonferenz. Nuklearmedizin 35:45–52
[79] Rhodes CG, Hughes JMB (1995) Pulmonary studies using positron emission tomography. Eur Respir J 8:1001–1017
[80] Rigo R, Paulus P, Kaschten BJ, Hustinx R, Bury T, Jerusalem G, Benoit T, Foidart-Willems J (1996) Oncological applications of positron emission tomography with fluorine-18fluorodeoxyglucose. Eur J Nucl Med 23:1641–1674
[81] Sasaki M, Ichiya Y, Kuwabara Y, Akashi Y, Yoshida T, Fukumura T, Murayama S, Ishida T, Sugio K, Masuda K (1996) The usefulness of FDG positron emission tomography for the detection of mediastinal lymph node metastases in patients with non-small cell lung cancer: a comparative study with X-ray computed tomography. Eur J Nucl Med 23:741–747
[82] Sazon DAD, Santiago SM, Soo Hoo GW, Khonsary A, Brown C, Mandelkern M, Blahd W, Williams AJ (1996) Fluorodeoxyglucose-positron emission tomography in the detection and staging of lung cancer. Am Respir Crit Care Med 153:417–421
[83] Scott WJ, Gobar LS, Hauser LG, Sunderland JJ, Dewan NA, Sugimoto JT (1995) Detection of scalene lymph node metastases from lung cancer. Chest 107:1174–1176
[84] Scott WJ, Schwabe JL, Gupta NC, Dewan NA, Reeb SD, Sugimoto JT (1994) Positron emission tomography of lung tumors and mediastinal lymph nodes using [^{18}F]fluorodeoxyglucose. Ann Thorac Surg 58:698–703
[85] Shields AF, Mankoff DA, Link JM, Graham MM, Eary JF, Kozawa SM, Zheng M, Lewellen B, Lewellen TK, Grierson JR, Krohn KA (1998) Carbon-11-thymidine and FDG to measure therapy response. J Nucl Med 39:1757–1762
[86] Slosman DO, Spiliopoulos A, Couson F, Nicod L, Louis O, Lemoine R, Donath A, Junod AF (1993) Satellite PET and lung cancer: a prospective study in surgical patients. Nucl Med Commun 14:955–961
[87] Slosman DO, Spiliopoulos A, Keller A, Lemoine R, Besse F, Couson F, Townsend D, Rochat T (1994) Quantitative metabolic PET imaging of a plasma cell granuloma. J Thorac Imag 9:116–119

[88] Steinert HC, Hauser M, Alleman F, Engel H, Berthold T, von Schulthess GK, Weder W (1997) Non-small cell lung cancer: nodal staging with FDG PET versus CT correlative lymph node mapping and sampling. Radiology 202:441–446

[89] Strauss LG, Conti PS (1991) The applications of PET in clinical oncology. J Nucl Med 32:623–648

[90] Stroobants S, Vansteenkiste J, Dupont P, DeLeyn P, DeWever W, Verbeken E, Deneffe G, Mortelmans L (1998) Value of FDG-PET in the evaluation of downstaging after induction chemotherapy in patients with non-small cell lung cancer (NSCLC). Eur J Nucl Med 25:921 (abstr)

[91] Takahashi N, Fujibayashi Y, Yonekura Y, Welch MJ, Waki A, Tsuchida S, Nakamura S, Sadato N, Sugimoto K, Yamamoto K, Yokoyama TA, Ishii Y (1998) Evaluation of copper-62 ATSM in patients with lung cancer as a hypoxic tissue tracer. J Nucl Med 39:53P (abstr)

[92] Tewson TJ, Krohn KA (1998) PET radiopharmaceuticals: state-of-the-art and future aspects. Sem Nucl Med 28:221–234

[93] Valk PE, Pounds TR, Hopkins DM, Haseman MK, Hofer GA, Greiss HB, Myers RW, Lutrin CL (1995) Staging non-small cell lung cancer by whole-body positron emission tomographic imaging. Ann Thorac Surg 60:1573–1582

[94] Vansteenkiste JF, Stroobants SG, Dupont PJ, De Leyn PR, De Wever WF, Verbeken EK, Nuyts JL, Maes FP, Bogaert JG, and the Leuven Cancer Group (1998) FDG-PET scan in potentially non-small cell lung cancer: do anatometabolic PET-CT fusion images improve the localisation of regional lymph node metastases? Eur J Nucl Med 25:1495–1501

[95] Vansteenkiste JF, Stroobants SG, De Leyn PR, Dupont PJ, Bogaert J, Maes A, Deneffe GJ, Nackaerts KL, Verschakelen JA, Lerut TE, Mortelmans LA, Demedts MG (1998) Lymph node staging in non-small cell lung cancer with FDG-PET scan: a prospective study on 690 lymph node stations from 68 patients. J Clin Oncol 16:2142–2149

[96] Wahl RL, Quint LE, Greenough RL, Meyer CR, White RI, Orringer MB (1994) Staging of mediastinal non-small cell lung cancer with FDG PET, CT, and fusion images: preliminary prospective evaluation. Radiology 191:371–377

[97] Webb WR (1990) Radiologic evaluation of the solitary pulmonary nodule. AJR 154:701–708

[98] Weber W, Voll B, Treumann, Watzlowik P, Präuer H, Schwaiger M (1998) Positronenemissionstomographie mit C-11-Methionin und F-18-Fluorodeoxyglukose in der Diagnostik des Bronchialkarzinoms. Nuklearmedizin 37:A37 (abstr)

[99] Weder W, Schmid RA, Bruchhaus H, Hillinger S, von Schulthess GK, Steinert HC (1998) Detection of extrathoracic metastases by positron emission tomography in lung cancer. Ann Thorac Surg 66:886–893

[100] Wittekind CH, Wagner G (1997) TNM-Klassifikation maligner Tumoren. Springer, Berlin Heidelberg New York

[101] Wolf M, Havemann K, Schneider P, Vogt-Moykopf I, Budach V (1997) Nichtkleinzelliges Bronchialkarzinom. In: Schmoll HJ, Höffken K, Possinger K (eds) Kompendium internistische Onkologie – Teil 2. Springer, Berlin Heidelberg New York, pp 558–600

[102] Zasadny KR, Wahl RL (1993) Standardized uptake values of normal tissues at PET with 2-[fluorine-18]-fluoro-2-deoxy-D-glucose: variations with body weight and a method for correction. Radiology 189:847–850

17 Pancreatic cancer

C. G. Diederichs, P. D. Shreve

17.1 Incidence, etiology, epidemiology

Approximately 50 000 new cases of pancreatic cancer are diagnosed annually in Europe. They represent approximately one-fifth of all gastrointestinal cancers [18]. Mortality is between 96 and 99%. The incidence of pancreatic cancer varies regionally and is between 10/100 000 (i.e., Hungary) and 3/100 000 (Portugal) for unknown reasons [18]. Incidence is highest between ages 55 and 80, men are more likely to develop it than women, and patients from disadvantaged social classes are more frequently affected [1]. It is the fourth largest killer among cancers, in part due to the advanced stage of disease at the time of diagnosis.

The etiology of pancreatic cancer is unclear, but some risk factors have been well known for a long time. Probably the most important risk factor is smoking; the risk is proportional to the amount of tobacco smoked [42]. Experimental animal studies give rise to speculation that an increased ratio of meat, fat and nitrosamines in the patient's diet can favor the development of pancreatic cancer. Studies concerning the influence of alcohol and coffee on the genesis of pancreatic cancer are contradictory. Environmental toxins like DDT can also contribute to the pathogenesis of pancreatic cancer. A higher risk has also been established for patients with chronic pancreatitis. However, the fraction of patients that have pancreatic carcinoma and also chronic pancreatitis is only about 5% [19].

17.2 Histopathologic classification

About 95% of all pancreatic malignancies originates from the exocrine glands. These adenocarcinoma are usually ductal in origin, and 60% to 70% originate in the pancreatic head. Multicentricity is found relatively often with histological work-up. Cystadenocarcinoma originate from acinar cells and macroscopically present as masses with smaller or larger cysts. A histopathologic classification of pancreatic malignancies is summarized in Table 17.1.

Of patients with pancreatic carcinoma 70–80% have elevated levels of mutated K-ras oncogenes and p53 suppressor genes. However, these mutations can also occur with patients who have chronic pancreatitis or hyperplastic cells [46].

Table 17.1. Histological classification of carcinoma.

Malignant
Ductal adenocarcinoma (inclusive mucinous adenocarcinoma)
Mucinous cystadenocarcinoma
Acinar cell carcinoma
Unclassified large-cell carcinoma
Small-cell carcinoma
Pancreatoblastoma
Potentially malignant
Mucine-secreting tumor with ectatic ducts
Mucinous cystadenoma
Papillary-cystic neoplasm
Rapidly growing serous cystadenoma

Table 17.2. UICC and TNM Staging (5th edition 1997).

Primary tumor	
Tx	Primary tumor cannot be assessed
T0	No demonstration of a primary tumor
Tis	Carcinoma in situ
T1	Tumor limited to pancreatic organ, 2 cm or less largest diameter
T2	Tumor limited to pancreatic organ, more than 2 cm largest diameter
T3	Invasion of duodenum, bile duct or peripancreatic tissue
T4	Invasion of stomach, spleen, colon or large vessels
Regional lymph nodes	
Nx	Lymph nodes cannot be assessed
N0	No sign of regional lymph node metastases
N1a	Singular regional lymph node metastasis
N1b	Multiple regional lymph node metastases
Distant metastases	
Mx	Distant metastases cannot be assessed
M0	No sign of distant metastases
M1	Distant metastases
Staging	
Stage 0	Tis, N0, M0
Stage 1	T1–2, N0, M0
Stage 2	T3, N0, M0
Stage 3	T1–3, N1, M0
Stage 4a	T4, every N, M0
Stage 4b	Every T, every N, M1

The extent of the disease can be described as curatively resectable (confined to the pancreas), locally advanced or metastasized. This description is also reflected by the UICC staging classification [43] as illustrated in Table 17.2. Unfortunately, most newly diagnosed pancreatic carcinoma are already locally advanced. Indeed, it is the cancer least likely to be confined to the organ of origin at the time of diagnosis. The pancreas is not surrounded by a tough capsule, and thus extension of a pancreatic cancer into adjacent structures including the stomach, duodenum, colon, and the large vessels are a common presentation influencing resectability. Due to portal venous and lymphatic drainage, pancreatic cancer has a propensity to regional lymph nodes and the liver. Metastases in lung, bone and brain are less common.

17.3 Patient history and clinical exam

Clinical presentation of patients with pancreatic malignancies is not specific. General symptoms like abdominal discomfort, abdominal pain, and loss of weight are most common. More specific symptoms like jaundice, back pain, newly diagnosed diabetes mellitus and/or an elevated alkaline phosphatase possibly in combination with a palpable or sonographically visible abdominal tumor are less common. Seldom, a migratory superficial thrombophlebitis can point to malignant pancreatic disease. Unfortunately, most of these symptoms occur at a relatively late stage of the disease. Tumor marker CA 19-9 is often not markedly elevated, especially if the tumor is small and potentially resectable. On the contrary, high levels of CA 19-9 may also occur with acute inflammatory disease.

17.4 Therapy

A minority of patients are diagnosed at an early stage. Therefore, relatively few patients are potentially curable by surgery. For pancreatic head carcinoma, the surgery of choice is total pancreaticoduodenectomy (Whipple procedure). This is major and difficult surgery with significant morbidity and mortality. Thanks to improved surgical techniques and better intensive care medicine, mortality is below 5% in large centers, and the five-year survival rate for patients with curative surgery has risen to 14–33% [3]. Prognosis for patients with pancreatic tail tumors is worse due to the much later presentation of symptoms and hence more advanced stage at diagnosis. Total pancreatectomy is performed by some centers due to frequent multicentricity of pancreatic carcinoma. However, because of higher complication rates, this procedure is not widely accepted and is reserved for a few special cases. New therapeutic concepts combine radical surgical removal of the tumor with adjuvant region chemotherapy and local radiation therapy. With combined therapies, survival rates are significantly longer for selected patients [38].

Palliative therapy includes procedures for relieving stenotic bile ducts or obstructed intestines. An obstructed bile duct is treated either surgically (biliodigestive anastomoses) or with endoscopic or percutaneous stenting. The latter are less traumatic; however, an occluded stent may lead to later complications, i.e., cholangitis or jaundice. The value of prophylactic gastroenterostomy is subject of debate and is usually reserved for patients with lower tumor stages. Pain that is difficult to treat can be relieved in the majority of patients either by intraoperative or percutaneous ablation of the celiac plexus or by radiation therapy.

17.5 Imaging techniques

Continued dissemination of anatomic cross sectional imaging modalities into routine clinical practice has increased the detection of pancreatic masses both as a finding in response to symptoms relating to pancreatic pathology and as an incidental finding. A pancreatic mass raises two diagnostic issues: 1) is the mass cancer or a benign pseudomass of chronic pancreatitis, and 2) if the mass is cancer, is it resectable? If the mass is not cancer, surgery is avoided, or only a local resection of the mass itself is performed. If the mass represents cancer, staging is crucial. Surgery is not indicated when metastatic spread has already occurred; there will be no survival advantage. The exact nature of local extension of the disease will also determine whether surgery is indicated, and if so, whether the resection will include major extrapancreatic vessels, contiguous solid or hollow organs, and regional lymph nodes.

17.5.1 Computed tomography (CT)

Contrast-enhanced computed tomography continues to be the preferred imaging modality for pancreatic imaging at most centers. Continued advances in scanner technology including spiral and multi-detector spiral CT scanners have improved image quality and detail, especially vascular depiction as thinner section collimation (5 mm or less) and acquisition of the scans during peak arterial and venous phases of the intravenous contrast enhancement are now routinely possible. Diagnostic accuracy for staging and resectability was 73% with a positive predictive value for non-resectability of 90% in a multicenter trial [35], with more recent reports suggesting higher accuracy of 85–95% [5, 16, 34] perhaps in part reflecting the improvements in pancreas and major extrapancreatic vessel depiction afforded by the improved scanner technology. CT still suffers the limitations inherent in anatomic imaging. A pancreatic mass due to cancer is not reliably differentiated from the pseudomass of chronic pancreatitis based on configuration, attenuation, or contrast enhancement characteristics [29, 31, 37]. Acute associated episodes of pancreatitis can result in CT findings which mimic the vessel encasement, neighboring organ infiltration and regional lymph node enlargement usually associated with a malignant neoplasm. The criteria for lymph node involvement from a pancreatic cancer in any case is size (typically > 1 cm), which is non-specific. Finally, diagnosis of hepatic metastases by CT criteria becomes problematic for lesions less than roughly 1 cm, as small hepatic cysts, which are common, are not differentiated reliably from small hepatic metastases [4]. In part due to the inability to detect small liver metastases and spread to non-enlarged lymph nodes, the negative predictive value of CT for non-resectability is less than 30%.

17.5.2 Endoscopic ultrasound (EUS)

Endoscopic ultrasound provides detailed sonographic images of the pancreatic head and body, the associated vascular structures, pancreatic and biliary ducts, and adjacent organs and lymph nodes. The transducer is positioned in the duodenum in close proximity to these structures permitting use of high frequency transducers (and hence high spatial resolution) and providing access to image-guided biopsy devices [23]. In experienced hands, EUS can yield local staging of pancreatic carcinoma (local organ involvement, local lymph node size, presence or absence of vascular encasement) comparable to CT [11, 33]. Differentiation of a pancreatic mass due to cancer and pseudomass of chronic pancreatitis is not possible based on imaging criteria, and like CT, the status of lymph node involvement is based on non-specific size criteria. Finally, the imaging range of EUS is limited; only portions of the liver adjacent to the duodenum can be visualized.

17.5.3 Endoscopic retrograde cholangiopancreaticography (ERCP)

This classic technique has been long regardedas a mainstay of pancreatic diagnosis. Like spiral CT or endosonography, accuracy for differentiation of benign and malignant masses is between 80 and 90% [7, 9, 17]. Also, chronic pancreatitis can be diagnosed due to high resolution imaging of pancreatic ductal structures. ERCP is false negative when the tumor does not originate from the main duct and with inflammatory pseudotumors. Between 3 and 10% of ERCP are not successful technically. One to 8% of patients will have iatrogenic consecutive pancreatitis including fatal complications in about 0.2%. Important advantages, however, are the possibilities to take tissue samples, place stents in obstructed ducts, or acquire duodenal secretions for gene mutation analysis.

17.5.4 Magnetic resonance imaging (MRI)

MRI, like CT, provides detailed anatomy of the pancreas, adjacent organs and vascular structures as well as the liver. Advantages in intravenous contrast material, bowel contrast material, motion artifact compensation techniques and fat suppression pulse sequences have continued to improve MRI of the pancreas, which now includes MRCP or magnetic resonance cholangiopancreaticography, i.e., the depiction and illustration of the pancreatic and bile ducts [5, 6, 32, 44]. Presently, the overall results of MRI for staging of pancreatic cancer and the differential diagnosis of the pancreatic mass remain comparable to CT [11, 28, 48].

17.5.5 Angiography

Prior to the development of cross-sectional anatomic imaging, contrast angiography was the preferred imaging modality for pancreatic diagnosis. The detection of vascular involvement and presence of liver metastases were the major criteria of resectability based on angiographic criteria [20]. In some centers contrast angiography is still part of the evaluation of a pancreatic mass to assess for vascular involvement. Recent advances in CT and MRI have allowed nearly comparable accuracy in the assessment of vascular involvement, although many centers still employ contrast angiography for the preoperative determination of vascular anatomy of patients with a pancreatic cancer resectable by CT criteria and for the further evaluation of equivocal CT, EUS or MRI findings regarding vascular involvement.

17.5.6 Fine needle biopsy

Both CT and ultrasound (transabdominal and endoscopic) allow for image-guided biopsy of a pancreatic mass, liver abnormality or enlarged lymph node as part of the evaluation of suspected pancreatic cancer. A tissue diagnosis has the advantage of specifying the type of cancer as a small fraction of pancreatic masses are lymphoma or metastatic small cell carcinoma, and among pancreatic cancers a small fraction are of endocrine origin. Due to sampling error, the absence of a histological diagnosis of malignancy does not exclude malignancy [8]; however, a positive diagnosis does eliminate the consideration of the pseudomass of chronic pancreatitis. In instances of planned radiation or chemotherapy of a mass presumed to be cancer prior to resection, a tissue diagnosis may be mandatory. The complication rate of fine needle aspiration biopsy is typically very low; however, necrotizing pancreatitis with fatal complications has been reported.

17.6 PET imaging technique

The normal pancreas can be imaged with various tracers, for example with [^{15}O]H_2O due to its high perfusion and with [^{11}C]methionine due to its high rate of protein synthesis. Unfortunately, pancreatic tumors present as unspecific photopenic defects within the parenchyma [41]. With over 300 published patients most clinical experience exists with [^{18}F]fluordeoxyglucose

(FDG) [2, 11, 50]. Pathophysiologically, the reason of the high FDG uptake is an increased expression of glucose transporters and glycolytic key enzymes in pancreatic carcinoma as compared to inflammatory pseudotumor [24, 39].

17.6.1 FDG-PET

As with most other oncologic FDG-PET, patients should be fasted for at least 6, best 12 hours before FDG application. It should be noted that patients may take their medicine and should drink one liter of water in the hours prior to the exam. This leads to lower FDG concentrations in the urine by diuresis and dilution. Artifacts due to high concentrations of FDG in the upper urinary tracts are thereby avoided. Plasma glucose levels should be below 130 mg/dl. Otherwise tumoral uptake of FDG may be reduced [14, 15, 49]. Diabetics should have their glucose levels well adjusted to levels below 130 mg/dl, if possible. The usual administered dose varies between institutions and also depends on the type of scanner employed. For full ring scanners doses commonly used are between 200 and over 600 MBq. Emission should start one to three hours after FDG application. Scanning time is usually between 7 and 15 min per bed position. Therefore, the total scan time is about one hour for the trunk (head to groin). Optional, emission may be done in right lateral positioning following duodenal and gastral distention with water and medical intestinal relaxation (for example: butylscopolamine methylbromide (Buscopan®)). This provides improved visualization of the distended stomach and duodenum for better localization and imaging of the pancreas. The patients should be well hydrated for this. Immediately before emission starts, the patient should drink another 0.4 liters of water and is administered 20–40 mg of Buscopan® (Hydro-PET). Attenuation correction should usually be done. Corrected images are easier to document and easier to interpret. Acceptance by the referring clinicians is higher because the organs are illustrated more homogeneously (like the images in CT and MRI). Another advantage of corrected images is the possibility of a semiquantitative analysis of lesions using standard uptake values (SUV). Clinically, the benefit of SUVs is a matter of debate. Visual interpretation of images was at least equally as accurate as SUV-based interpretation [14, 21]. Also, a comparison of two patient collections that were examined with and without correction yielded no difference in accuracy [12]. The additional diagnostic information of attenuation correction has therefore not been shown yet. If patients are examined using the hydro-technique (right lateral positioning), attenuation correction is not practicable. This may change in the future with simultaneous emission and attenuation scanning. For better interpretation of PET results, inflammatory blood chemistry parameters like C-reactive protein (CRP) should also be assessed at the time of FDG application [13].

17.6.2 Evaluation

The typical finding of pancreatic malignancy is an intensive focally increased uptake within the pancreas (Figs. 17.1 and 17.2). For attenuation-corrected images, standard uptake values (SUV) between 2 and 3 serve as the threshold to differentiate between benign and malignant. Because of some overlap of SUV values with benign and malignant masses, sensitivity is high (> 90%) with a cutoff of 2 at the cost of specificity, and vice versa. With uncorrected images, all lesions that have a higher uptake than the liver must be considered suspicious. Because with uncorrected images the liver seems to have a higher uptake in peripheral segments compared with centrally located segments, a proper liver segment has to be chosen for comparison. A suitable liver segment is best found on coronal images along a longitudinally oriented sight-line that runs through the lesion in question (Figs, 17.2b, 17.3). All extrapancreatic lesions must be considered suspicious for metastasis. Special emphasis should be paid to the liver, the peripancreatic lymph nodes, the abdominal space (peritoneum), the bone marrow, and the lungs (Fig. 17.3). Peritoneal metastases may be difficult to differentiate from unspecific bowel uptake. The latter usually has a linear uptake pattern following the course of the intestines. To reduce unspecific bowel uptake, mechanic and/or medical distention of the bowels prior to FDG application and/or emission is currently under evaluation.

17.6.3 Results

The fact that malignant tumors of the pancreas usually do have a clearly increased FDG uptake has been shown by many groups [2, 10, 14, 15, 21, 25–27, 30, 36, 40, 45, 47, 49, 50]. FDG-PET can differentiate malignant pancreatic tumors from chronic mass forming pancreatitis. While most malignant tumors present with clearly elevated FDG uptake, chronic pancreatitis usually exhibits a low and diffuse FDG uptake pattern or no visible uptake at all. Values for sensitivity and specificity vary between 80 and 100%. A more recent paper found a change of management with 32% of examined patients [10].

Proper patient selection plays an important role. Most false positive findings occur with acute inflammatory conditions [15, 40, 50]. Especially those patients may be false positive with FDG-PET that have acute abdominal illness and elevated blood chemistry parameters like elevated white blood count or elevated C-reactive protein (CRP). Specificity has been reported as low as 50% with that kind of patient selection [40]. Acute bouts of focal pancreatitis and pancreatic abscess are known complications of chronic pancreatitis. However, these patients often have elevated blood chemistry parameters. Therefore, CRP, for example, should be assessed with all patients [13]. False positive focally increased hepatic uptake has also been reported in patients with dilated bile ducts [22].

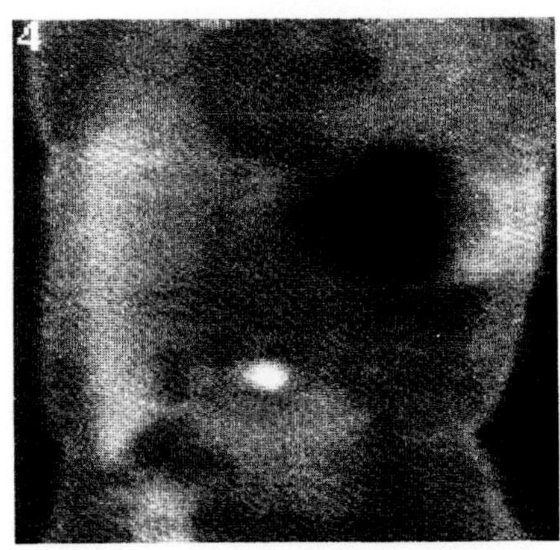

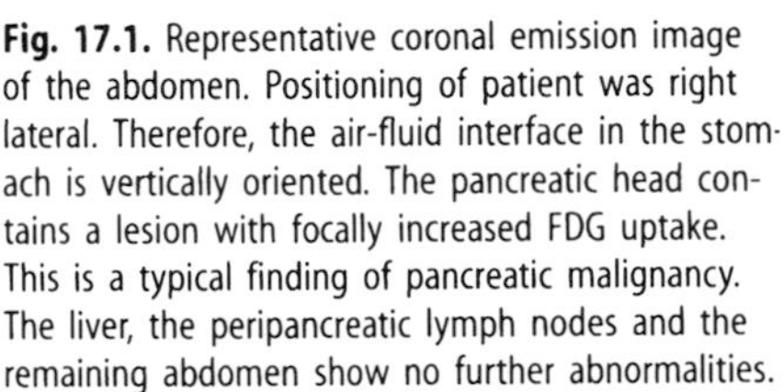

Fig. 17.1. Representative coronal emission image of the abdomen. Positioning of patient was right lateral. Therefore, the air-fluid interface in the stomach is vertically oriented. The pancreatic head contains a lesion with focally increased FDG uptake. This is a typical finding of pancreatic malignancy. The liver, the peripancreatic lymph nodes and the remaining abdomen show no further abnormalities.

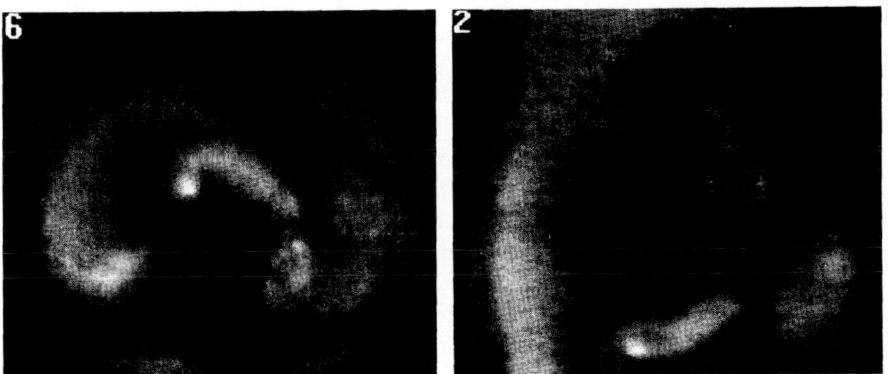

Fig. 17.2 a, b. Transversal and coronal emission image. There is an intensive focally increased uptake in the uncinate process of the pancreas. The diagnosis is pancreatic carcinoma. In addition, the pancreatic segments that are distal to the tumor show diffusely increased uptake. This is secondary post-stenotic pancreatitis.

False negative FDG-PET findings have been found with patients that have very small tumors (< 1 cm). Small tumors are common with ampullary carcinoma and bile duct carcinoma. Also difficult to detect are malignant cystic pancreatic neoplasms, highly differentiated tumors (very seldom) and tumors of patients that have elevated plasma glucose levels [14, 15, 49]. Whether the history of diabetes mellitus or rather the presence of an elevated plasma glucose level is more important is a matter of debate.

Initial results that compare N-staging results to those of endosonography or spiral CT have found no clear advantage over PET. T-staging is a domain of the morphologically oriented imaging test and not usually a question for PET.

There is both retrospective and prospective data now concerning M-staging of pancreatic cancer. Lesions > 1 cm can be detected with PET not only with high sensitivity but also with high specificity. False positive findings

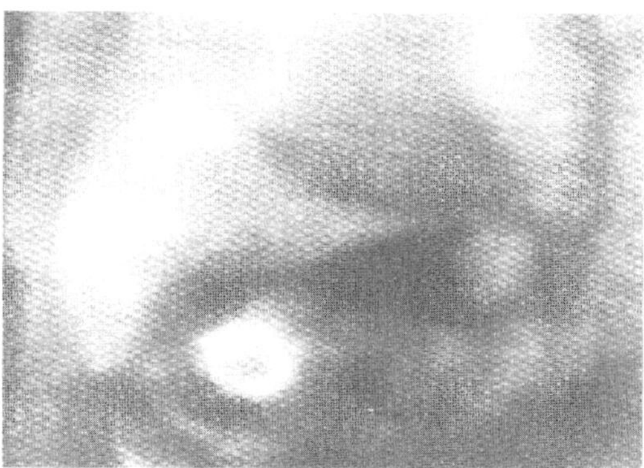

Fig. 17.3. Coronal emission image. The lesion within the pancreatic head shows a large focally increased uptake with a large central photopenic defect. The diagnosis is pancreatic malignancy with central necrosis. Additionally, there are numerous smaller focally increased uptakes in the liver that are hepatic metastases. Of note: improved visualization of stomach and duodenum following oral application of 0.4 liters of water and iv application of 40 mg Buscopan®.

have so far exclusively been found with patients that have dilated bile ducts and concomitant cholangitic granulomata. In the absence of dilated bile ducts FDG-PET's high specificity of near 100% with > 1 cm lesions makes PET distinct from the morphologic tests. In a prospective study, PET detected more distant metastasis than all other conventional imaging [11]; however, numbers are too small, and the difference is not statistically significant. Initial experiences with recurrent pancreatic carcinoma are promising. While CT is often hindered by scar tissue formation, FDG-PET can nicely demonstrate recurrent cancer despite those morphologic limitations.

17.7 Future of PET

Rapid development of modern coincidence cameras and PET scanners with new iterative algorithms, on one hand, and of morphological techniques like multi-detector spiral CT or fast MRI sequences, on the other hand, make it difficult to foresee the future of pancreatic PET. The ability of FDG-PET to differentiate between benign and malignant pancreatic masses has been well documented. FDG-PET is currently finding a niche when other more widely available morphological techniques are technically not successful or if the results of these tests are inconclusive or even contradictory. In the near future it will be shown whether PET is cost effective with whole-body staging with patients who have a high likelihood of pancreatic malignancy. A paucity of results concerning recurrent cancer and therapy monitoring leave this field wide open. It also remains to be seen if new tracers provide PET with a tool to differentiate between acute inflammatory conditions and malignant tumor, an impossible task for static FDG-PET, it seems. Dedicated tracers for endocrine active tumors and special tracers for proliferation, for example, should complete the diagnostic palette of PET.

17.8 Summary

The ability of FDG-PET to differentiate between benign and malignant masses has been well documented. However, patient selection is important. Patients with elevated plasma glucose levels, small tumors < 1 cm, or cystic malignant tumors may be false negative. On the other hand, patients with acute abdominal conditions or elevated blood chemistry parameters may be false positive. T-staging is a morphological domain, N-staging is equally as disappointing as with endosonography or spiral-CT. M-staging appears to provide enough additional information to justify the relatively high cost of FDG-PET in addition to the conventional staging procedures. All other indications (recurrent cancer, therapy monitoring, acute inflammatory pseudotumor versus carcinoma, endocrine tumors, etc.) are experimental to date. FDG-PET is therefore indicated for patients who have a pancreatic mass and indeterminate or contradictory conventional staging results. Patients with suspected pancreatic cancer should receive PET if the detection of (additional) metastases would lead to a change in therapy management.

17.9 Tips and tricks for FDG-PET

- *Indications*
  - Indeterminate pancreatic mass (morphologic tests technically unsuccessful or reports indeterminate or contradictory)
  - Indeterminate abdominal or hepatic mass with suspected pancreatic primary
- *Indications under evaluation*
  - Exclusion of local or distant metastases with negative conventional staging
  - Exclusion of further local or distant metastases with supposed singular or oligofocal metastases
  - Recurrent carcinoma
  - Therapy monitoring
  - Endocrine neoplasms (usually using tracers other than FDG)
- *Patient preparation*: Oral hydration with 1 l of water, otherwise fasted for at least 6 hours. Diabetics with plasma glucose levels below 130 mg/dl. Bladder empty. Optional: Distention of stomach and duodenum with oral water and medically induced hypotony during emission scan.
  Data acquisition: Base of skull to bladder, parameters like with other oncologic studies.
- *Attenuation correction*: Recommended due to easier interpretability and more homogeneous illustration of anatomy. In case of artifacts due to mis-

registration, moving intestinal air bubbles or inadequate noise, additional interpretation of emission scans mandatory.

- *Reconstruction*: Iterated images summed to 1 cm thick slices. Image evaluation using at least two imaging planes (transversal and coronal). Interpretation of non-attenuated images with at least two color-tool settings to compensate for high range of data.
- *Image interpretation*: Any finding with an SUV >2–3 or an intensity greater than the liver must be regarded as probably malignant. Coregistration with CT and/or MRI and/or conference with radiologist is mandatory, if available.
- *False positive*: Acute focal pancreatitis, acute on chronic pancreatitis. Liver: Inflammatory granuloma with marked dilated bile ducts. Acute-phase proteins and white blood count useful for interpretation of positive PET.
- *False negative*: Tumor size <2 times resolution of scanner or malignant cystic tumor with thin septa. Highly differentiated tumors. Endocrine tumors. High plasma glucose levels > 130 mg/dl.

References

[1] American Cancer Society (1995) Cancer Facts and Figures. American Cancer Society, Atalanta, pp 1990

[2] Bares R, Klever P, Hauptmann S, Hellwig D, Fass J, Cremerius U, Schumpelick V, Mittermayer C, Büll U (1994) F-18 fluorodeoxyglucose PET in vivo evaluation of pancreatic glucose metabolism for detection of pancreatic cancer. Radiology 192:79–86

[3] Beger HG, Birk D, Bodner E, Fritsch A, Gall FP, Trede M (1995) Ist die histologische Sicherung des Pankreaskarzinoms Voraussetzung für die Pankreasresektion? Langenbecks Arch Chir 380(1):62–66

[4] Bluemke DA, Cameron IL, Hruban RH, Pitt HA, Siegelman SS, Soyer P, Fishman EK (1995) Potentially resectable pancreatic adenocarcinoma: spiral CT assessment with surgical and pathologic correlation. Radiology 197:381–385

[5] Bluemke DA, Fishman EK (1998) CT and MR evaluation of pancreatic cancer. Surg Oncol Clin N Am 7(1):103–124

[6] Catalano C, Pavone P, Laghi A, et al. (1998) Pancreatic adenocarcinoma: combination of MR imaging, MR angiography and MR cholangiopancreatography for the diagnosis and assessment of resectability. Eur Radiol 8(3):428–434

[7] Cavallini G, Riela A, Angelini GP, et al. (1986) Limitations in the interpretation of endoscopic retrograde pancreatography findings in chronic pancreatitis. In: Malferteiner P, Ditschuneit H (eds) Diagnostic Procedures in Pancreatic Disease. Springer, New York, pp 175–184

[8] Chang KJ, Nguyen P, Erickson RA, Durbin TE, Katz KD (1997) The clinical utility of endoscopic ultrasound-guided fine-needle aspiration in the diagnosis and staging of pancreatic carcinoma. Gastrointest Endosc 45(5):387–393

[9] Costamagna G, Pandolfi M, Mutignani M (1995) Carcinoma of the pancreatic head area. Diagnostic imaging. Direct cholangiography. ERCP. Rays 20(3):269–279

[10] Delbeke D, Chapman WC, Plason CW, Martina WH, Beauchamp DR, Leach S (1998) F-18 Fluorodeoxyglucose imaging with positron emission tomography (FDG-PET) has a significant impact on diagnosis and management of pancreatic ductal adenocarcinoma. J Nucl Med 39:81P (abstr)

[11] Diederichs CG, Sokiranski R, Pauls S, Schwarz M, Guhlmann C, Glatting G, Glasbrenner B, Möller P, Beger HG, Brambs H-G, Reske SN (1999) Preoperative diagnosis of pancreatic tumors: what is the role of FDG-PET following endosonography (ES), ERCP, spiral-CT (CT), and MRI? J Nucl Med 40/5 Suppl: 104P (abstr)
[12] Diederichs CG, Sokiranski R, Pauls S, Schwarz M, Guhlmann CA, Glatting G, Möller P, Beger HG, Reske SN (1998) FDG-PET von pankreatischen Tumoren: Transmission obligat? Nuklearmedizin 37:A83 (abstr)
[13] Diederichs CG, Staib L, Glasbrenner B, Guhlmann A, Glatting G, Pauls S, Beger HG, Reske SN (1999) F-18 Fluorodeoxyglucose (FDG) and C-reactive protein (CRP). Clin Pos Imag 2(3):131–136
[14] Diederichs CG, Staib L, Glatting G, Beger HG, Reske SN (1998) FDG-PET: elevated plasma glucose reduces both uptake and detection rate of pancreatic malignancies. J Nucl Med 39(6):1030–1033
[15] Diederichs CG, Staib L, Vogel J, Glatting G, Glasbrenner B, Brambs H-J, Berger HG, Reske SN (2000) Values and limitations of FDG-PET in pancreatic masses. Pancreas (in press)
[16] Diehl SJ, Lehmann KJ, Sadick M, Lachmann R, Georgi M (1998) Pancreatic cancer: value of dual-phase helical CT in assessing resectability. Radiology 206(2):373–378
[17] DiMagno EP, Malagelada JR, Taylor WF, Go VLW (1977) A prospective comparison of current diagnostic tests for pancreatic cancer. New Engl J Med 297:737–742
[18] Fernandez E, La Vecchia C, Porta M, et al. (1994) Trends in pancreatic cancer mortality in Europe, 1955–1989. Int J Cancer 57:786
[19] Fernandez E, La Vecchia C, Porta M, Negri E, d'Avanzo B, Boyle P (1995) Pancreatitis and the risk of pancreatic cancer. Pancreas 11:185
[20] Freeny PC, Lawson TL (1982) Radiology of the pancreas. Springer, New York
[21] Friess H, Langhans J, Ebert M, Beger HG, Stollfuss J, Reske SN, Büchler MW (1995) Diagnosis of pancreatic cancer by 2[18F]-fluoro-2-deoxy-D-glucose positron emission tomography. Gut 36(5):771–777
[22] Fröhlich A, Diederichs CG, Staib L, Beger HG, Reske SN (1999) FDG-PET in the detection of pancreatic cancer liver metastases. J Nucl Med 40:250–255
[23] Hawes RH, Zaidi S (1995) Endoscopic ultrasonography of the pancreas. Gastrointestinal Endoscopy Clinics of North America 5:61–80
[24] Higashi T, Tamaki N, Honda T, et al. (1997) Expression of glucose transporters in human pancreatic tumors compared with increased FDG accumulation in PET study. J Nucl Med 38(9):1337–1344
[25] Higashi T, Tamaki N, Torizuka T, Inokuma T, Honda T, Magata Y, Yonekura Y, Ohshio G, Hosotani R, Imamura M, Konishi J (1995) Differentiation of malignant from benign pancreatic tumors by FDG-PET: comparison with CT, US, and endoscopic ultrasonography. J Nucl Med 36:224P (abstr)
[26] Ho CL, Dehdashti F, Griffeth LK, Buse PE, Balfe DM, Siegel BA (1996) FDG-PET evaluation of indeterminate pancreatic masses. J Comput Assist Tomogr 20(3):363–369
[27] Inokuma T, Tamaki N, Torizuka T, Fujita T, Magata Y, Yonekura Y, Ohshio G, Imamura M, Konishi J (1995) Value of fluorine-18-fluorodeoxyglucose and thallium-201 in the detection of pancreatic cancer. J Nucl Med 36(2):229–235
[28] Irie H, Honda H, Kaneko K, Kuroiwa T, Yoshimitsu K, Masuda K (1997) Comparison of helical CT and MR imaging in detecting and staging small pancreatic adenocarcinoma. Abdom Imaging 22(4):429–433
[29] Johnson PT, Outwater EK (1999) Pancreatic carcinoma versus chronic pancreatitis: dynamic MR imaging. Radiology 212:213–218
[30] Kato T, Fukatsu H, Ito K, Tadokoro M, Ota R, Ikeda M, Isomura T, Ito S, Nishino M, Ishigaki T (1995) Fluorodeoxyglucose positron emission tomography in pancreatic cancer: an unsolved problem. Eur J Nucl Med 22:32–39
[31] Lammer J, Herlinger H, Zalaudek G, Hofler H (1995) Pseudotumorous pancreatitis. Gastrointest Radiol 10:59–67

[32] Laubenberger J, Buchert M, Schneider B, Blum U, Hennig J, Langer M (1995) Breath-hold projection magnetic resonance-cholangio-pancreaticography (MRCP): new method for the examination of the bile and pancreatic ducts. Magn Res Med 33:18
[33] Legmann P, Vignaux O, Dousset B, et al. (1998) Pancreatic tumors: comparison of dual-phase helical CT and endoscopic sonography. Am J Roentgenol 170(5):1315–1322
[34] Lu DS, Reber HA, Krasny RM, Kadell BM, Sayre J (1997) Local staging of pancreatic cancer: criteria for unresectability of major vessels as revealed by pancreatic-phase, thin-section helical CT. Am J Roentgenol 168(6):1439–1443
[35] Megibow AJ, Zhou XH, Rotterdam H, et al. (1995) Pancreatic adenocarcinoma: CT versus MR imaging in the evaluation of resectability – report of the Radiology Diagnostic Oncology Group. Radiology 195:327–332
[36] Nakata B, Chung YS, Nishimura S, et al. (1997) 18F-fluorodeoxyglucose positron emission tomography and the prognosis of patients with pancreatic adenocarcinoma. Cancer 79(4):695–699
[37] Neff CC, Simeone JF, Wittenberg J, Mueller PR, Ferrucci JT Jr (1984) Inflammatory pancreatic masses: problems in differentiating focal pancreatitis from carcinoma. Radiology 150:35–38
[38] Ozaki H, Hojo K, Kato H, Kinoshita T, Egawa S, Kishi K (1988) Multidisciplinary treatment for resectable pancreatic cancer. Int J Pancreatol 3:249–260
[39] Reske SN, Grillenberger KG, Glatting G, Port M, Hildebrandt M, Gansauge F, Beger HG (1997) Overexpression of glucose transporter-1 and increased FDG-uptake in pancreatic carcinoma. J Nucl Med 38:1344–1347
[40] Shreve PD (1998) Focal fluorine-18-fluorodeoxyglucose accumulation in inflammatory pancreatic disease. Eur J Nucl Med 25(3):259–264
[41] Shreve PD, Gross MD (1997) Imaging of the pancreas and related diseases with PET carbon-11-acetate. J Nucl Med 38(8):1305–1310
[42] Silverman DT, Dunn JA, Hoover RN, et al. (1994) Cigarette smoking and pancreas cancer: a case-control study based on direct interviews. J Natl Cancer Inst 86:1510
[43] Sobin LH, Wittekind C (eds) (1997). TNM classification of malignant tumours, fifth edition. John Wiley & Sons, Inc, New York
[44] Soto JA, Barish MA, Yucel EK, Clarke P, Siegenberg D, Chuttani R, Ferrucci JT (1995) Pancreatic duct: MR cholangiopancreatography with a three-dimensional fast spin-echo technique. Radiology 196:459–464
[45] Staib L, Diederichs CG, Reske SN, Beger HG (1997) PET in pancreatic tumor of unknown origin – luxury or value? Langenbecks Arch Chir Suppl Kongressbd 114:471–473
[46] Tada M, Ohashi M, Shiratori Y, Okudaira T, Komatsu Y, Kawabe T, Yoshida H, Machinami R, Kishi K, Omata M (1996) Analysis of K-ras gene mutation in hyperplastic duct cells of the pancreas without pancreatic disease. Gastroenterology 110:227–231
[47] Teusch M, Buell U (1996) Classification of pancreatic tumors by FDG-PET: comparison of visual and quantitative image interpretation by ROC-analysis. J Nucl Med 37(5):140P (abstr)
[48] Trede M, Rumstadt B, Wendl K, Gaa J, Tesdal K, Lehmann KJ, Meier Willersen HJ, Pescatore P, Schmoll J (1997) Ultrafast magnetic resonance imaging improves the staging of pancreatic tumors. Ann Surg 226:393–405
[49] Zimny M, Bares R, Faß J, Adam G, Cremerius U, Dohmen B, Klever P, Sabri O, Schumpelick V, Buell U (1997) Fluorine-18-fluorodeoxyglucose positron emission tomography in the differential diagnosis of pancreatic carcinoma: a report of 106 cases. Eur J Nucl Med 24:678–682
[50] Zimny M, Buell U, Diederichs CG, Reske SN (1998) False-positive FDG-PET in patients with pancreatic masses: an issue of proper patient selection? Eur J Nucl Med 25(9):1352

18 Hepatobiliary tumors

J. Marienhagen

18.1 Incidence, etiology and epidemiology

Primary hepatobiliary tumors, arising from hepatocytes, liver mesenchyma or biliary tract, are relatively rare in Germany and other western countries, but among the leading causes of death worldwide [1, 3]. Mortality rates in Germany and the USA are comparable: 1.8 for males and 0.6 for females. In contrast, the mortality is much higher in Japan and Hong Kong. Primary liver malignancies have a poor prognosis, because most patients die within one year after diagnosis [17]. Anorexia and cachexia of malignancy are the most frequent causes of death. Age rates of patients with hepatobiliary tumors show a peak between 50 and 69. The geographical distribution of primary liver cancer reflects the different prevalence of hepatitis B virus infection, which is much higher in Asia and Africa. Other well-known risk conditions for the development of primary liver neoplasm are chronic infections with hepatitis C virus, alcoholic liver disease, hemochromatosis, tyrosinemia, oral contraceptives, anabolic steroids and cirrhosis [17]. Food contamination with aflatoxins has been identified as another risk factor for hepatocellular carcinomas. Malignant tumors of the gall bladder exhibit both a higher incidence and mortality in females than in males [1]. The prognosis of gall bladder carcinomas is also poor. Cholelithiasis is a proven risk factor for the development of gall bladder tumors.

18.2 Histopathological classification

Primary hepatobiliary neoplasms show a great histopathological diversity. In principle both epithelial and mesenchymal tumors just as mixed tumors and tumor-like lesions have to be distinguished [2, 3]. Hepatocellular carcinoma is the most common and on the strength of its rapid progression and frequent association with viral hepatitis and cirrhosis the clinically most important malignant epithelial liver tumor. Because of its less specific clinical appearance, early diagnosis of hepatocellular carcinomas is difficult. The determination of serum levels of α-fetoprotein and ultrasound are suitable diagnostic or monitoring methods for patients with known risk factors (hepatitis

Table 18.1. UICC stages of hepatocellular carcinomas and intrahepatic cholangiocellular carcinomas.

Stage I	T1	N0	M0
Stage II	T2	N0	M0
Stage IIIA	T3	N0	M0
Stage IIIB	T1	N1	M0
	T2	N1	M0
	T3	N1	M0
Stage IVA	T4	N0–N4	M0
Stage IVB	T1–T4	N0–N4	M1

and/or cirrhosis). Only biopsy and histological examination of suspected liver lesions provide definite diagnosis and grading of hepatocellular carcinomas (high versus low grade resp. anaplastic variants). Hepatocellular carcinomas exhibit gross invasion into adjacent organs, vessels and bile ducts [2]. A combined occurrence of hepatocellular carcinoma and cholangiocellular carcinoma may happen [19]. Fibrolamellar hepatocellular carcinoma is an important variant, which is found in younger patients without liver cirrhosis. Usually, fibrolamellar hepatocellular carcinomas have a better prognosis [4]. The likewise epithelial cholangiocellular carcinomas originate from the intra- or extrahepatic bile tract. Histologically, most cholangiocellular carcinomas are non-bile producing sclerosing adenocarcinomas. Carcinomas of the gall bladder usually are scirrhoid infiltrating adenocarcinomas with a mean survival of a few months [2, 3]. Well known risk conditions for the development of cholangiocellular carcinomas are liver flukes, carcinogens (nitrosamines, aflatoxins) and predisposing diseases like biliary atresia and sclerosing cholangitis [3]. Jaundice is the cardinal symptom of cholangiocellular carcinomas. The differential diagnosis of the primary hepatobiliary tumors includes secondary malignant liver tumors, especially solitary metastases in a scirrhotic liver or unknown primary tumor. Occasionally, even benign tumors or tumor-like lesions are distinguishable from hepatocellular carcinomas only by histopathological examination. Very rare malignant hepatobiliary tumors are childhood hepatoblastoma as well as the different liver sarcomas (hemangiosarcomas, fibrosarcomas, embryonal rhabdomyosarcomas). Table 18.1 shows the actual TNM classification for primary hepatocellular and intrahepatic cholangiocellular carcinomas [18].

18.3 Diagnostic procedures and treatment strategies

Imaging methods are indispensible for the diagnosis of hepatobiliary malignancies. Beside the determination of the serum level of α-fetoprotein ultrasound is the method of choice for the early detection or screening in patients with risk conditions for hepatocellular carcinomas (chronic hepatitis or cirrhosis). Angiography plays a major role for therapy (operation) planning. Modern computed tomography (CT) procedures are essential for the evaluation of the localization and extent of disease as well as the delineation of the topographic relationship of the tumor and surrounding tissues [8, 25]. Whereas both native and contrast-enhanced CT are pivotal particularly for the detection of liver metastases in colon cancer, the diagnosis of benign liver lesions (hemangiomas, focal nodular hyperplasias, adenomas) requires dynamic incremental (CT) scanning after an intravenous bolus of contrast material or advanced procedures such as triphasic spiral CT. The unmasking of malignant hepatobiliary tumors is the domain of CT-arteriography as well as CT-arterial-portography (CTAP) after injection of contrast material into the hepatic or superior mesenteric artery and obtaining axial CT scans. CTAP has the potential to detect especially small hepatocellular carcinomas (less than 1 cm diameter) with a sensitivity of approximately 66%, whereas greater tumors are detected in up to 95%. CT after intraarterial administration of iodized oil (lipiodol) is another highly sensitive method for the detection of very small hepatocellular carcinomas [8, 25].

Despite the recent developments of imaging technologies, histopathological examination remains the golden standard for the diagnosis of hepatobiliary neoplasms. Therefore, image-guided (CT or ultrasonography) needle biopsy should be mentioned in this context.

Conventional nuclear medicine imaging (blood pool scintigraphy, static colloid as well as hepatobiliary imaging) has proven its value in the differential diagnosis of benign liver lesions, but is not established in the diagnostic algorithms for the detection of hepatobiliary malignancies (e.g., scintigraphy with ^{67}gallium).

Unfortunately, as shown by the epidemiologic (survival) data the development of more effective treatment strategies in hepatobiliary tumors could not keep pace with the progress of the diagnostic procedures. Whenever feasible, surgical resection (partial resection, hemihepatectomy, extended hemihepatectomy) remains the treatment of choice in both hepatocellular and cholangiocellular carcinomas [24]. Liver transplantation can be considered for irresectable hepatocellular carcinomas in the absence of distant metastases, optionally combined with adjuvant immunotherapy [13]. Systemic chemotherapy or percutaneous radiotherapy are less promising [2]. Chemoembolization of irresectable tumors or percutaneous intratumoral ethanol instillation are palliative treatment options [12]. Experimental internal radiotherapy with intraarterial administered [^{131}I]-lipiodol or [^{90}Y]-microspheres in patients with hepatocellular carcinoma is available only in a few centers.

18.4 Positron emission tomography in primary malignant liver and biliary tract tumors

Compared with secondary liver neoplasms (e.g., metastases of colorectal carcinomas) the number of published papers focusing on the diagnostic value of PET in primary hepatobiliary tumors is only small. Therefore, primary hepatobiliary tumors are not mentioned in the consensus paper of the German Society of Nuclear Medicine (1997).

For the first time Fukuda et al. [7] demonstrated an increased uptake of $[^{18}F]$FDG in a rat hepatoma (AH109A) by autoradiography. The first gamma scans (!) of a hepatocellular carcinoma with $[^{18}F]$FDG were published by Paul et al. [16]. Nagata et al. [14] used $[^{18}F]$FDG-PET for the monitoring of liver tumors after therapy. The basic patterns of glucose metabolism of hepatocellular carcinomas, which are essential to understand $[^{18}F]$FDG imaging, were well characterized by the fundamental research papers of Okazumi et al. [15] and Torizuka et al. [21, 22]. The normal liver tissue exhibited a very low hexokinase activity, whereas the glucose-6-phosphatase activity was comparatively high. This ratio was found to be inverse in malignant liver tumors: high hexokinase activity (phosphorylation) combined with a lower rate of dephosphorylation. Okazumi et al. [15] characterized different primary as well as secondary liver tumors in a 3-compartment-model by the metabolic rate constants (k_1, k_2, k_3, k_4) using a dynamic PET protocol. The k_3 constant was found to reflect the hexokinase activity. In 45% of n=20 patients with hepatocellular carcinomas, the k_4 values were similar to the surrounding liver tissue, whereas the k_4 constant was nearly zero in cholangiocellular carcinomas. The k_3 constant was increased in malignant tumors and a cutoff value was found to distinguish between benign and malignant tumors. In static PET scans (60 min. p.i.), three different FDG uptake patterns were described in hepatocellular carcinomas: type-1 lesions showed greater accumulation compared with the surrounding liver (55% of patients), type-2 lesions revealed a liver-like uptake (30%), type-3 lesions demonstrated less FDG accumulation than the liver (15%). The pathobiochemical reason for these different uptake patterns was the particular k_4/k_3 ratio of the hepatocellular carcinomas, which could be used for the assessment of the degree of tumor differentiation. The cholangiocellular carcinomas as well as liver metastases always showed a type-1 tumor (increased uptake). After successful therapy, a decrease of the k_3 constant was observed. Torizuka et al. [21] found a correlation between the degree of the FDG uptake in hepatocellular carcinomas (measured as standardized uptake value, SUV) and the extent of necrosis after therapy. The same authors [22] also showed a correlation of the degree of malignancy with the FDG uptake (SUV 48–60 min. p.i.) as well as the k_3 rate constant in a dynamic model: both SUV and k_3 of the high grade hepatocellular carcinomas were significantly higher than those of the low grade tumors. The findings of Okazumi and Torizuka were essential for a pathobiological understanding of the FDG kinetics in primary hepatobiliary neoplasms. Nevertheless, the calculation of metabolic rate constants as well as dynamic PET protocols are difficult to perform and therefore unsuitable for a clinical routine setting. Recently, Delbeke et al. [5] demonstrated the clinical value of static FDG-PET whole-body imaging in the differential diagnosis of benign and malignant liver lesions. N=110 patients were included in this prospective, blinded comparison clinical cohort study. Histopathological examination served as the golden standard and revealed n=66 secondary liver neoplasms (mostly liver metastases from colon carcinomas), n=8 cholangiocellular carcinomas, n=23 hepatocellular carcinomas and n=13 benign lesions. A static acquisition protocol (68±33 min. p.i.) including thoracic, abdominal and pelvic regions as well as transmission images for the correction of photon attenuation were used. The results of the visual interpretation of the images, the standardized uptake values (SUV) and the lesion to liver ratio were correlated with the histopathological findings. All liver metastases as well as all cholangiocellular carcinomas exhibited a markedly increased FDG uptake. Of the patients with hepatocellular carcinomas 16/23 also showed elevated FDG accumulation. With the exception of one abscess all benign lesions had only poor uptake. The reported absence of FDG accumulation in approximately 30% of the patients with hepatocellular carcinomas corresponds with the results of Okazumi et al. [15]. Nevertheless, this finding should not be interpreted simply as reduced sensitivity, because it possibly provides information of prognostic significance. However, this problem has to be clarified in further studies. In another paper, Vitola et Delbeke [23] proved the value of static FDG-PET imaging in the monitoring after chemoembolization of hepatic lesions. Chronic infection with hepatitis C virus is a well-known risk factor associated with hepatocellular carcinoma making differential diagnosis of focal liver lesions important in this setting. Schroeder et al. [20] found in a small study group of ten patients with hepatitis C associated liver lesions five hepatocellular carcinomas, two metastases and three regenerative nodules. However, only two of the five hepatocellular carcinomas were detectable by FDG-PET. Primary sclerosing cholangitis predisposes to cholangiocellular carcinomas. Keiding et al. [10] found FDG-PET imaging useful for the detection as well as the management of small cholangiocellular carcinomas in patients with concomitant sclerosing cholangitis.

Thus far, we have investigated n=13 patients with primary hepatobiliary tumors (n=11 hepatocellular carcinomas, n=2 hepatocellular carcinoma resp. Klatskin tumor after liver transplantation). In n=4 patients with hepatocellular carcinoma we found a definite FDG uptake in the tumor (Fig. 18.1), which decreased partially after chemoembolization. In n=7 patients the FDG uptake was equal to the surrounding liver, but two patients in this group revealed diabetes mellitus with normal serum glucose levels after treatment. Follow-up investigations after liver transplantation showed additional metastases in two patients, which were previously unknown (Fig. 18.2).

A few papers addressing the use of other positron emitters (^{11}C-ethanol or ^{13}N-ammonia) in liver tumors have been published [6, 9], but these methods have no clinical relevance as yet.

18.5 Perspective

An "evidence-based" assessment of the diagnostic value of [^{18}F]FDG-PET imaging in patients with primary hepatobiliary tumors is not possible as yet.

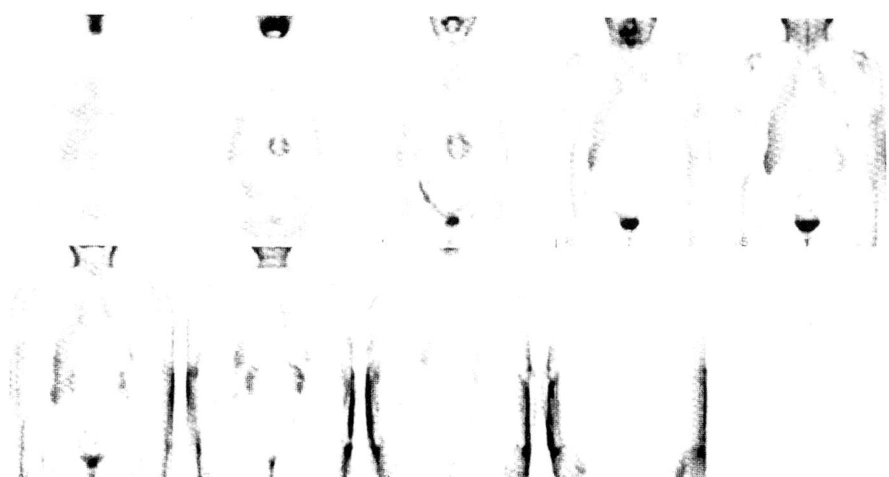

Fig. 18.1. Female patient, 58 years. Hepatocellular carcinoma (segment 3). Static [^{18}F]FDG-PET: tumor with central necrosis and infiltration of duodenum and abdominal wall.

However, ^{18}F-PET could be clinically useful in the differential diagnosis of benign and malignant liver lesions, especially for the early detection of cholangiocellular carcinomas as well as secondary liver neoplasms [5]. Visualization of hepatocellular carcinomas by [^{18}F]FDG-PET will be limited by a relatively high fraction of tumors with low contrast to the surrounding liver. The significance of this not simply "false negative" finding has to be elucidated by further studies. According to the conclusions of Okazumi [15] and Torizuka [21, 22] even the lack of FDG uptake in proven hepatocellular carcinomas could be valuable for the assessment of tumor differentiation and prognosis. Furthermore, FDG-PET seems to be useful in the monitoring after treatment of hepatocellular carcinomas with proven increased FDG uptake. After liver transplantation FDG-PET could provide additional information in the follow-up period (e.g., restaging, detection of metastases). Nevertheless, further work is necessary to determine the role of FDG-PET in the management of primary hepatobiliary malignancies.

18.6 Recommendations for FDG-PET imaging and evaluation in hepatobiliary tumors

- Patient preparation: Fasting period at least 6 h, blood glucose level <120 mg%.
- Data acquisition: Start 50 minutes p.i. (300 MBq [^{18}F]FDG). Static whole body scanning including pelvis, abdomen, chest and cervical regions
- Attenuation correction: Transmission images (before FDG administration) Accurate positioning by the use of laser marks

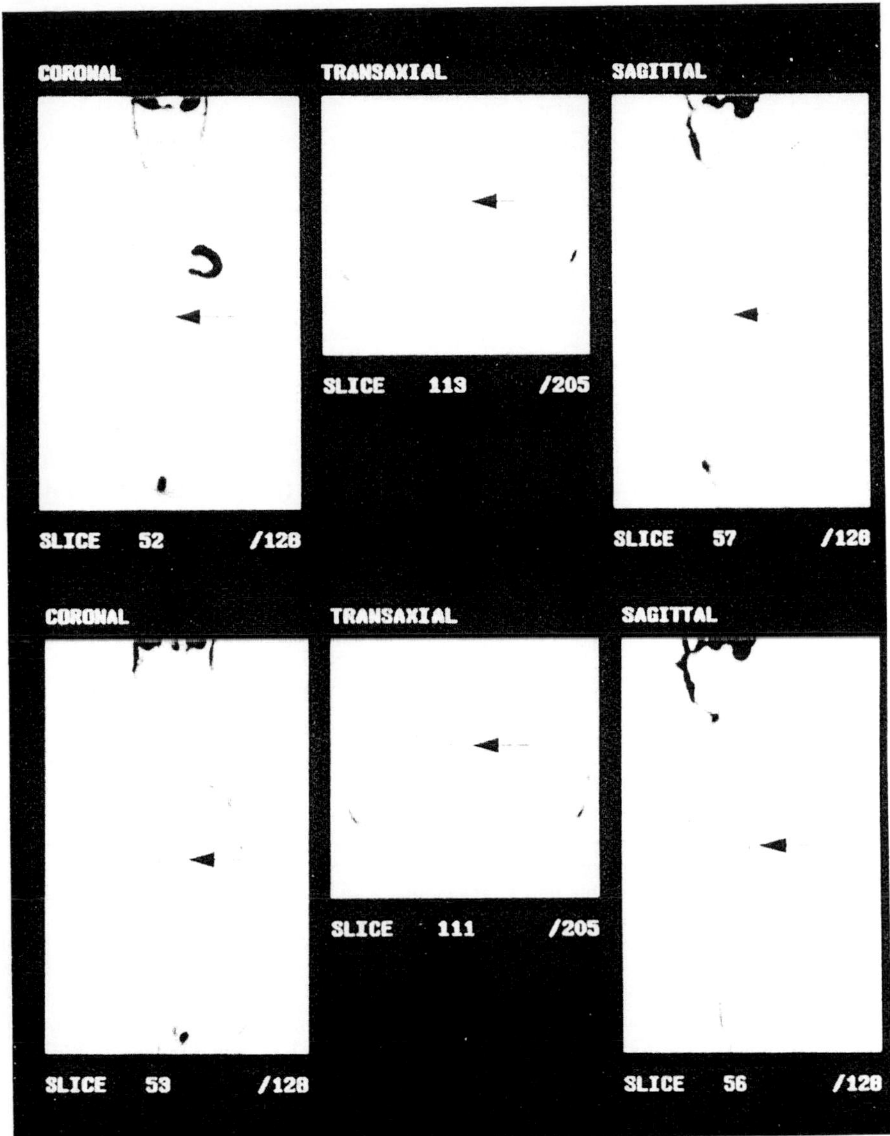

Fig. 18.2. Male patient, 66 years. Follow-up after liver transplantation because of cholangiocellular carcinoma (Klatskin tumor). Static [^{18}F]FDG-PET (upper row: 11/97, lower row: 2/98): progression of mesenteric lymph node metastases.

- Reconstruction: Filtered back projection (optional: iterative reconstruction)
- Dynamic modeling: Calculation of metabolic rate constants not necessary
- Image evaluation: Correlation with CT for lesion localization
  1. Visual analysis:
  Comparison of the tumor uptake with the surrounding liver:
  A: tumor accumulation greater than the liver
  B: tumor accumulation equal to the liver
  C: tumor accumulation lower than the liver
  Central necrosis?
  Additional extrahepatic findings?
  2. Quantitative analysis:
  Calculation of the tumoral SUV for scheduled monitoring after therapy (e.g., chemoembolization, ethanol instillation).

References

[1] Becker N, Wahrendorf J (1998) Atlas of Cancer Mortality in the Federal Republic of Germany. Springer, Berlin Heidelberg New York

[2] Blum HE (1995) Tumoren der Leber und des biliären Systems. In: Gerok W, Blum HE (eds) Hepatologie. Urban & Schwarzenberg, München Wien Baltimore, pp 635–650

[3] Colombo M, Beloqui O, Sangro B (1992) Tumors of the liver and biliary tract. In: Prieto J, Rodés J, Shafritz DA (eds) Hepatobiliary diseases. Springer, Berlin Heidelberg New York, pp 1019–1056

[4] Craig JR, Peters RL, Edmondson HA, Omata M (1980) Fibrolamellar carcinoma of the liver: a tumor of adolescents and young adults with distinctive clinicopathological features. Cancer 40:372–379

[5] Delbeke D, Martin WH, Sandler MO, Chapman WC, Wright Jr JK, Pinson CW (1998) Evaluation of benign vs malignant hepatic lesions with positron emission tomography. Arch Surg 133:510–516

[6] Dimitrakopoulou- Strauss A, Gutzler F, Strauss LG, Irngartinger G, Oberdorfer F, Doll J, Stremmel W, van Kaick G (1996) PET-Studien mit C-11-Äthanol bei der intratumoralen Therapie von hepatozellulären Karzinomen. Radiologe 36:744–749

[7] Fukuda H, Matsuzawa T, Abe Y, et al. (1982) Experimental study for cancer diagnosis with positron-labeled fluorinated glucose analogs: [^{18}F]-2-fluoro-2-deoxy-D-mannose: a new tracer for cancer detection. Eur J Nucl Med 7:294–297

[8] Groß V, Marienhagen J, Feuerbach S (1997) Diagnostische Verfahren: Bildgebende Verfahren einschließlich Laparoskopie. In: Schölmerich J, Bischoff SC, Manns MP (eds) Diagnostik in der Gastroenterologie und Hepatologie. Georg Thieme Verlag, Stuttgart New York, pp 117–123

[9] Hayashi N, Tamaki N, Yonekura Y, Senda M, Saji H, Yamamoto K, Konishi J, Torizuka K (1985) Imaging of the hepatocellular carcinoma using dynamic positron emission tomography with nitrogen-13 ammonia. J Nucl Med 26:254–257

[10] Keiding S, Hansen SB, Rasmussen HH, Gee A, Kruse A, Roelsgaard K, Tage-Jensen U, Dahlerup JF (1998) Detection of cholangiocarcinoma in primary sclerosing cholangitis by positron emission tomography. Hepatology 28:700–706

[11] Konsensus – Onko – PET (1997) Nuklearmedizin 36:45–46

[12] Lee MJ, Mueller PR, Dawson SL, Gazelle SG, Hahn PF, Goldberg MA, Boland GW (1995) Percutaneous ethanol injection for the treatment of hepatic tumors: indications, mechanism of action, technique, and efficacy. AJR 164:215–220

[13] Lygidakis NJ, Kosmidis P, Ziras N, Parissis J, Kyparidou E (1995) Combined transarterial targeting locoregional immunotherapy - chemotherapy for patients with unresectable hepatocellular carcinoma: a new alternative for an old problem. J Interferon Cytokine Res 15:467–472

[14] Nagata Y, Yamamoto K, Hiraoka M et al. (1990) Monitoring liver tumor therapy with [^{18}F]FDG positron emission tomography. J Comput Assist Tomogr 14:370–374

[15] Okazumi S, Isono K, Enomoto K, Kikuchi T, Ozaki M, Yamamoto H, Hayashi H, Asano T, Ryu M (1992) Evaluation of liver tumors using fluorine-18-fluorodeoxyglucose PET: characterization of tumor and assessment of effect of treatment. J Nucl Med 33:333–339

[16] Paul R, Ahonen A, Roeda D, Nordman E (1985) Imaging of Hepatoma with ^{18}F-fluorodeoxyglucose. Lancet 8419:50–51

[17] Schaffer DF, Sorrel MF (1999) Hepatocellular carcinoma. Lancet 353:1253–1257

[18] Sobin LH, Wittekind Ch (1997) UICC (International Union Against Cancer) TNM Classification of Malignant Tumours. Wiley Liss, New York Cichester Weinheim Brisbane Singapore Toronto

[19] Shiomi S, Sasaki N, Kawashima D, Jomura H, Fukuda T, Kuroki T, Koyama K, Kawabe J, Ochi H (1999) Combined hepatocellular carcinoma and cholangiocarcinoma with high F-18 fluorodeoxyglucose positron emission tomographic uptake. Clin Nucl Med 24:370–371

[20] Schroeder O, Trojan J, Zeusem S, Baum RP (1998) Limited value of fluorine-18-fluorodeoxyglucose PET for the differential diagnosis of focal liver lesions in patients with chronic hepatitis C virus infection. Nuklearmedizin 37:279–285

[21] Torizuka T, Tamaki N, Inokuma T, Magata Y, Yonekura Y, Tanaka A,. Yamaoka Y, Yamamoto K, Konisi J (1994) Value of fluorine-18-FDG-PET to monitor hepatocellular carcinoma after interventional therapy. J Nucl Med 35: 1965–1969

[22] Torizuka T, Tamaki N, Inokuma T, Magata Y, Sasayama S, Yonekura Y, Tanaka A, Yamaoka Y, Yamamoto K, Konisi J (1995) In vivo assessment of glucose metabolism in hepatocellular carcinoma with FDG-PET. J Nucl Med 36:1811–1817

[23] Vitola JV, Delbeke D, Meranze SG, Mazer MJ, Pinson CW (1996) Positron emission tomography with F-18-fluorodeoxyglucose to evaluate the results of hepatic chemoembolization. Cancer 78:2216-2222

[24] Weinmann A, Oldhaier KJ, Pichlmayr R (1995) Primary liver cancers. Current Opinion in Oncology 7: 387–396

[25] Yu SCH, Chan MSY, Lau JWY (1999) Diagnostic imaging. In: Leong ASY, Liew CT, Lau JWY, Johnson P (eds) Hepatocellular carcinoma. Arnold, London Sydney Auckland, pp 43–74

19 Colorectal carcinomas

A. Dimitrakopoulou-Strauss

19.1 Incidence

Colorectal cancer is the second most common cancer in the western world [7]. It is the third most common cancer, after prostata carcinoma and lung carcinoma for men and after breast carcinoma and lung carcinoma for women. In the United States colorectal cancer is the second leading cause of cancer-related death, after lung cancer [10].

The incidence of colorectal cancer is high, especially in the United States and in Europe as well in all countries which adopt a typical western diet. The chance of developing this type of cancer increases at 40 years and peaks around 65 to 70 years. Most people who develop colorectal cancer are over the age of 50. However, the disease can occur at any time. Cancer of the large intestine is more common in women, while cancer of the rectum is more frequently observed in men [11].

19.2 Etiology and epidemiology

Several factors influence the development of colorectal cancer, such as dietary components, environmental factors, as well as family history, diet or colon polyps and increase the risk of colorectal carcinoma. The cause is uncertain but diets high in animal fat and low in vegetables, poultry, and fish may contribute to this type of cancer [11].

Several epidemiological studies documented an association between fat consumption and mortality from colorectal cancer. On the other hand, a protective effect of foods with fiber, such as whole grains, fruits and vegetables, has been observed in several epidemiological studies in the past. Recently, Fuchs et al. did not find an important protective effect of dietary fiber against colorectal carcinoma or adenoma in women [21]. Potter tried to analyze the previous and recent data about the role of fiber and colorectal cancer in an editorial and recommended focusing on experimental human biology and better databases of nutritional epidemiology [42]. There is a need for a biologically relevant classification scheme for components and a systemic approach to understanding relevant biology.

Important differences are reported for the sexes. Although, exercise is inversely associated with risk among both women and men, obesity may be a risk factor only among men. Hormonal influences, especially the use of estrogen-replacement therapy by women, appear to reduce risk [42].

Different genetic factors are involved in the development of colorectal cancer. Germline mutations of genes responsible for reparing DNA mismatches may cause hereditary nonpolyposis colorectal cancer (HNPCC) [33]. At least four HNPCC genes have been described: hMSH2, hMLH1, hPMS1, and hPMS2 [43]. Mutations in each of these genes have been found in the germline cells of families with HNPCC. The loss of tumor suppressor genes like p53 gene on the short arm of chromosome 17 as well as the DCC gene (deleted in colorectal cancer) on the long arm of chromosome 18 is associated with a poor prognosis [26].

19.3 Histopathological classification

Approximately 90–95% of the colon carcinomas are adenocarcinomas. A histological classification of primary tumors according to the WHO is presented in Table 19.1 [26]. A classification according to degree of differentiation is given in Table 19.2. TNM classification as well as Dukes classification are used for staging and listed in Table 19.3 [9].

Table 19.1. Histologic classification of the primary colon tumors (according to WHO 1976).

Epithelial tumors:
Adenocarcinoma
Squamous cell carcinoma
Adenosquamous carcinoma
Undifferentiated carcinoma
Unclassified carcinoma
Carcinoids
Non-epithelial tumors (e.g., leiomyosarcoma)
Hematopoetic and lymphoid carcinomas

Table 19.2. Classification according to the degree of differentiation.

G1: well differentiated
G2: intermediate differentiated
G3: least differentiated

Table 19.3. TNM classification of colon and rectal carcinomas [9].

T	Primary tumor
Tx	Primary tumor cannot be assessed
T0	No evidence of tumor in the resected specimen
Tis	Carcinoma in situ
T1	Tumor invades submucosa
T2	Tumor invades muscularis propria
T3	Serosa present: Tumor invades through muscularis propria into subserosa, serosa or pericolic fat within the leaves of the mesentery No serosa: Invades through muscularis propria
T4	Serosa present: Invades through serosa into free peritoneal cavity or through serosa into a contiguous organ No serosa: Invades other organs (vagina, prostate, ureter, kideny)
N	Regional lymph nodes
Nx	Nodes cannot be assessed
N0	No regional node metastases
N1	1–3 positive nodes
N2	4 or more positive nodes
N3	Central nodes positive
M	Distant metastases
Mx	Presence of distant metastases cannot be assessed
M0	No distant metastases
M1	Distant metastases present

Dukes staging system correlated with TNM [26]:

Stage 0	Tis	N0	M0
Stage I	T1–T2	N0	M0 (Dukes A)
Stage II	T3–T4	N0	M0 (Dukes B)
Stage III	any T	any N	M0 (Dukes C)
Stage IV	any T	any N	M1

19.4 Diagnosis of colorectal tumors: a review

Approximately twenty years ago 25–30% of all primary colorectal carcinomas were not curable by surgery [8]. The introduction of screening programs for the general population included the digital rectal examination of the lower rectum. Although, it is difficult to demonstrate a significant improvement in diagnosis, since only 10–15% of the patients without any symptoms and small primary colorectal carcinomas could be diagnosed by digital rectal examination. Recent screening programs recommend the fecal occult blood testing once a year (Hemoccult Test), as well as a sigmoidoscopy every five years for persons above 40 years. Patients with a higher risk due to family history, familial adenomatous polyposis or personal history of cancer or polyps should be screened more often. A cost-effective diagnostic imaging method for the identification of patients with a true positive fecal occult blood test is the air-contrast barium enema examination of the colon, which is a noninvasive technique. Furthermore, a complete colonoscopy together with biopsy is the most direct way to exclude cancer. Computed tomography as well as endosonography are used for the preoperative diagnostics and for staging [8, 48].

Problems exist in the diagnosis of colorectal tumor recurrence, such as recurrence in the anastomosis area, local recurrence as well as lymph node metastases or distant metastases. Local recurrences as well as tumor recurrence in the anastomosis area appear in 75% of the patients during the first two years after surgical resection of the primary tumor, half of them even in the first year after surgical resection [30, 41]. The therapy outcome of these patients is mainly dependent on the very early diagnosis of the recurrence.

Postoperative examination of the tumor markers, particularly of the carcinoembryogenic antigen (CEA) are standard in the follow-up of these patients. Although sensitivity is high, specificity of a tumor marker plasma elevation is low. False-positive results due to a tumor marker elevation cannot be excluded. The best procedure for the diagnosis of a recurrence in the area of the anastomosis is the air-contrast barium enema examination, a diagnostic procedure which allows the diagnosis of polyps, the examination of the anastomosis itself and the assessment of the complete lumen of the colon. Recto-sigmoidoscopy can be used for lesions located accordingly in the sigma or rectum and if final diagnosis is not achieved. The method is not helpful for recurrent tumors located higher than the sigma and in patients with an anus praeter in case of non-continuous resection of the colon. Another procedure which can be used for the diagnosis of tumor recurrence in lesions located in the rectum and sigma is endosonography (EUS). The accuracy of EUS concerning transmural infiltration is in many studies superior to computed tomography (CT) and magnetic resonance imaging (MRI) [3, 22, 35]. CT and MRI are, however, in the context of established postsurgical diagnostic methods, since the limited rectum and sigma range cannot only be judged. Enlarged lymph nodes as well as distant metastases can be diagnosed by both CT and MRI [23, 44, 49]. Diagnostic problems arise with both CT and MRI in the detection of the local recurrence, and the accuracy of both methods is not sufficient. Another procedure for the detection of a local recurrence is the CT-guided biopsy, an invasive procedure, which cannot be used routinely. Although, a positive result is highly correlated with tumor recurrence, a negative result does not exclude a tumor. Another imaging procedure which is still used for the diagnosis of tumor recurrence is immunoscintigraphy (IS). The sensitivity of IS depends mainly on the type of the applied antibody, the physical properties of the applied radionuclide, the labeling technique, the location and size of the suspected tumorous lesion and the examination protocol used by the investigator (planar vs. Single Photon Emission Tomography (SPET)). The sensitivity of IS for the diagnostics of the primary and metastatic colorectal cancer varies from 59 to 70%. Better results have been reported when using an intraoperative probe for the detection of the preoperatively applied antibody, with a sensitivity varying from 70 to 100% and a specificity of 66 to 100% [5]. Bares et al. examined the intratumoral antibody concentration in resected tumor material of 25 patients, who were examined with IS 4–14 days prior to surgery [4]. The authors reported that eleven out of twelve false-negative results were obtained in tumors with a diameter smaller than 4 cm. Furthermore, the authors found both a specific as well as an unspecific uptake of the applied antibodies. The unspecific uptake of the antibodies, high background activity as well as the limited resolution of the SPET technique limited the accuracy of IS in the diagnosis of tumor recurrence. The authors recommend the use of IS in cases with tumor marker elevation and negative conventional diagnosis, as well as in cases with a large lesion located dorsal to the bladder following abdominoperineal extirpation of the primary tumor and a concomitant CEA plasma elevation.

Several imaging techniques are used for the diagnostics of liver metastases, like ultrasound (US), CT and MRI. The sensitivity of ultrasound for the detection of liver metastases depends on the size of the lesion, the location, the contrast of the echo in comparison to the surrounding liver tissue and the experience of the investigator. It is well known that in a clinical environment up to 50% of the metastases may not be detected with US. Approximately 20% of the metastases with a diameter smaller than 1 cm could be diagnosed using US [14]. CT is another morphologic imaging modality used for the diagnosis of liver lesions. In general, CT studies of the liver are performed with the infusion of contrast material, either intravenous or intraarterially via an angiographic placed catheter located in the a. hepatica or the a. mesenterica superior, the so-called angiography-assisted CT (ASCT). ASCT has the highest sensitivity, but is invasive and can be used only in selected cases, e.g., in the preoperative diagnostics. Diagnostic problems can raise in case of vessel anomalies or due to an inhomogeneous enhancement of the normal liver parenchyma. An advantage of helical CT is the ability to image the liver during both the vascular (hepatic arterial-dominant) and redistribution (portal venous-dominant) phase due to its short scan duration. MR studies of the liver have the advantage of multiplanar imaging as compared to CT without the use of x-rays and for patients who cannot receive an iodinated contrast material due to an allergy. The use of contrast material is generally recommended for MR studies of the liver. All these morphologic imaging procedures have a higher resolution than nuclear medicine techniques but a limited specificity. Furthermore, it is generally accepted that immunoscintigraphy has a low sensitivity for the diagnosis of liver metastases and is not the first line technique to detect liver metastases with high accuracy [1, 27, 32, 39].

19.5 PET: current status

PET with different radiopharmaceuticals permits a biological characterization of colorectal tumors. Different parameters, like tissue perfusion, amino acid transport, glucose metabolism as well as the pharmacokinetics of radiolabeled cytostatic agents can be quantitatively assessed by PET.

Different radiopharmaceuticals can be used for tissue perfusion studies, like ^{15}O-labeled water, ^{15}O-labeled CO_2, [^{11}C]butanol, [^{13}N]ammonium as well as [^{62}Cu]PTSM or ^{82}Rb.

Furthermore, PET allows the use of transport markers for the assessment of specific amino acid transport systems. [^{11}C]aminoisobutyric acid (AIB) can be used for measurements of the A-type (alanine-like) amino acid transport and [^{11}C]aminocyclobutancarbon acid (ACBC) for the L-type (leucine-like) transport. Other amino acids, like [^{11}C]methionine, [^{13}N]glutamate and [^{18}F]tyrosine provide important information about the transport and metabolism of amino acids. [^{11}C]thymidine can be used as a proliferation marker.

[^{18}F]Deoxyglucose ([^{18}F]FDG) is the most common tracer for oncological PET studies. [^{18}F]FDG is used not only for the diagnostics, particularly postoperative diagnostics and staging, but also for therapy management. [^{18}F]FDG follow-up studies are used in patients with liver metastases from colorectal cancer prior and during chemotherapy to assess the early therapeutic effect and to predict response to therapy.

[^{18}F]Fluorouracil ([^{18}F]FU) is a dedicated tracer for pharmacokinetic studies of the cytostatic agent, which is identical to the non-labeled substance. 5-FU is the standard cytostatic agent for the chemotherapy of the metastatic colorectal carcinoma. PET with [^{18}F]FU even allows a prediction of the therapeutic effect prior to therapy.

19.5.1 Diagnosis

19.5.1.1 Preoperative diagnosis

Limited data exist about the use of FDG-PET in the preoperative diagnostics of colorectal cancers. Gupta et al. studied 16 patients with FDG-PET and CT and compared the data to the histology [24]. Sensitivity, specificity and accuracy with respect to histology were 90%, 66% and 87% for FDG-PET in comparison to 60%, 100% and 65% for CT accordingly. FDG-PET has a high sensitivity, which can be very helpful even in the preoperative staging.

Abdel-Nabi et al. studied 48 patients with primary colorectal carcinomas using a whole-body protocol and compared the PET data to CT or histology [2]. All intraluminal tumors were correctly classified with FDG-PET; therefore, the sensitivity of this study was 100%. False-positive results were obtained in four of seven patients due to inflammatory processes (three patients) and due to unspecific effects after surgical resection (one patient). Specificity was 43% in this study. FDG-PET indicated true negatives in 35 patients with hyperplastic polyps. The sensitivity of FDG concerning the N-staging was 29% and was comparable to CT. Liver metastases were diagnosed in 7 of 8 patients using FDG in comparison to 3 of 8 patients using CT. FDG-PET was superior to CT for the preoperative staging. A limitation of this study is the use of a whole-body protocol for the [^{18}F]FDG studies, which contributes to the low sensitivity of FDG-PET for the diagnosis of involved lymph nodes.

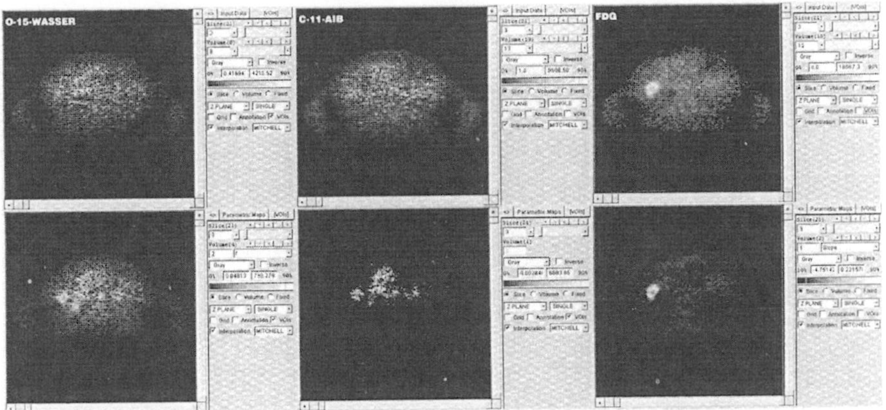

Fig. 19.1. PET image of a patient with an adenoma in the colon ascendens, confirmed by histology after the PET study. The benign process demonstrates an enhanced tissue perfusion, as measured by [^{15}O]water (upper left). The parametric image of the k(2, 1) in the second row left, demonstrates an enhanced influx of the [^{15}O]water. The corresponding images of the alanine-like amino acid transport, as measured with [^{11}C]aminoisobutyric acid ([^{11}C]AIB) are presented in the middle of the figure. The upper image is an SUV cross section acquired 30 min p.i. and the corresponding parametric image of the k(2, 1) is presented in the row below. In particular, the parametric image demonstrates an enhanced [^{11}C]AIB influx in the benign lesion. The FDG transversal SUV image (upper row, right side) demonstrates an enhanced regional FDG metabolism in this benign lesion. In the row below, right side, the corresponding parametric image of the regional metabolic rate for FDG is presented. Analysis and calculation of parametric images were performed with a dedicated software running on PC systems, developed by Burger and Mikolajczyk [6, 36].

False-positive results can be obtained by FDG-PET in some benign diseases and in inflammatory lesions. Adenomas, the most common benign colon tumor, may show an enhanced circumscribed [^{18}F]FDG uptake (Fig. 19.1). Acute abscesses, fistulas or a diverticulitis may also show enhanced [^{18}F]FDG uptake and lead to false-positive results. In this situation the clinical information of the patient is important.

Preliminary data demonstrate that the use of a double tracer approach with an amino acid transport marker, like [^{11}C]AIB, may help to differentiate an abscess from a tumor. Colorectal tumors demonstrate an enhanced AIB uptake (own data), while abscesses show no AIB accumulation. The impact of FDG-PET in the preoperative diagnosis of primary colorectal carcinomas is still open at the moment, because only limited data exist. Larger studies including more patient data are necessary to determine the role of PET.

19.5.1.2 Diagnosis and staging of recurrent tumors

The main reason for a FDG-PET study is the diagnosis of tumor recurrence. In the majority of patients CT or MRI is used for this purpose. Both imaging modalities allow the visualization of a suspicious lesion, but they have low specificity. The main problem of using CT and MRI is the differential diagnosis of tumor recurrence and scar tissue following surgical resection. The first

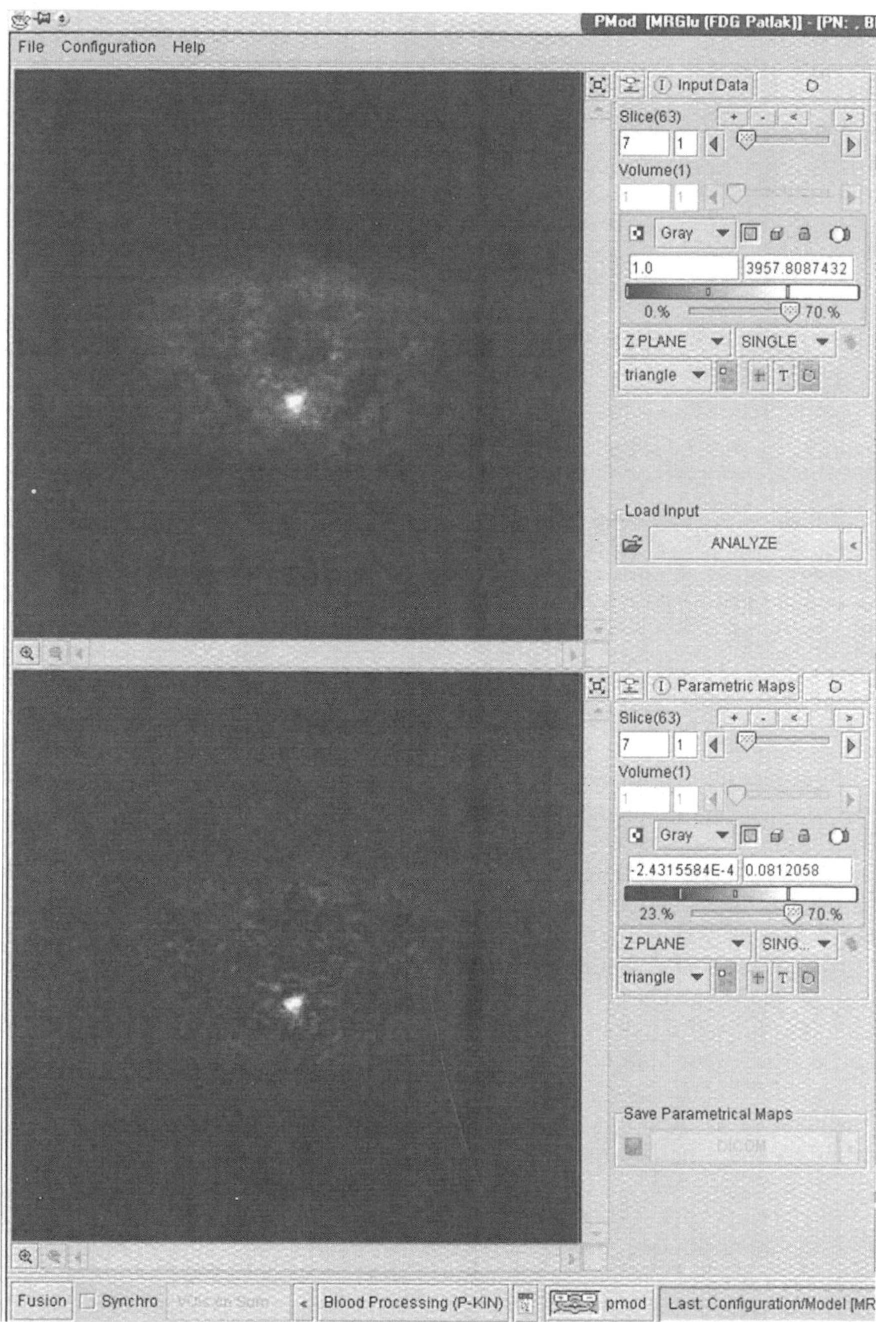

Fig. 19.2. Iterative reconstructed transversal FDG-PET image (upper row: SUV image, below: parametric influx image) of a patient with a recurrence in the anastomosis area, following anterior resection of the primary tumor. Enhanced FDG uptake as well as enhanced FDG influx in the anastomosis are indicative for tumor recurrence.

results with FDG-PET in patients with colorectal recurrences were published in 1989 [47]. This first study included 29 patients who had undergone an abdominoperineal rectum extirpation and where a suspicious lesion was noted in CT. All suspicious lesions had a tumor diameter of at least 1.5 cm. Histological data were used as reference for the PET data. 20/21 tumor recurrences were true positive in FDG-PET. One recurrence showed low $[^{18}F]$FDG uptake and was false negative. Eight patients had a scar and were true negative on FDG-PET. $[^{18}F]$FDG uptake varied in the tumor recurrences between 1.14 and 4.17 SUV and in the scar tissue between 0.56 and 1.15 SUV. The median value for the ratio lesion to muscle was 2.08 for tumors and 0.96 for scar tissue.

Double tracer studies with $[^{15}O]$water and $[^{18}F]$FDG were performed in 18 of the patients in this study. Thirteen of these patients had a tumor recurrence and five of them scar tissue. The results demonstrate that the perfusion data alone did not allow differentiation between tumor recurrence and scar tissue. There was no statistically significant correlation between the tissue perfusion and the $[^{18}F]$FDG uptake in tumors ($r=0.674$, for $p=0.01$ not significant). All PET images used in this study were iteratively reconstructed, so that the high activity in the bladder did not cause any problems in the visualization and evaluation of the retrovesical area. Furthermore, all PET images were corrected for scatter and attenuation (Fig. 19.2). The results were confirmed by other groups. Keogan et al. studied 18 patients with questionable local recurrence following abdominoperineal rectum extirpation. The authors found a sensitivity of 92.3% (12/13 tumor recurrences true positive) and a specificity of 80% (4/5 scars true negative). The authors report a mean $[^{18}F]$FDG uptake of 6.89 SUV for the recurrences and 1.96 for the scar tissue [28]. The higher $[^{18}F]$FDG uptake values for tumor and scar tissues are caused by the missing scatter correction.

PET images in the pelvic area require high image quality, which is presently a problem due to the lack of the iterative reconstruction for routine use. Some new software permits the iterative reconstruction of the PET data. Due to the lack of the software for iterative reconstruction on a routine basis, several authors, e.g., Miraldi et al., used a Foley catheter in the bladder to avoid artifacts caused by the $[^{18}F]$FDG activity [37]. This procedure is invasive and not required if iterative reconstruction is used.

Ogunbiyi et al. examined 58 patients with recurrent (40 patients) or metastatic (11 patients) colorectal carcinoma and compared FDG-PET and CT [40]. Sensitivity and specifity of FDG-PET [40] were 91% and 100% for the detection of the local recurrence in contrast to 52% and 80% for CT.

Some authors used the whole-body imaging technique; Valk et al. reported about 68 patients with suspected colorectal recurrence [50]. The study demonstrated a higher accuracy of FDG-PET in comparison to CT. Therefore, the authors recommend a combination of both CT and FDG-PET for the diagnosis and follow-up of patients with colorectal tumors as the best cost-effective diagnostic approach.

Delbeke et al. examined the value of PET for staging colorectal recurrences and compared FDG-PET data with CT. In the case of liver metastases the CT portography was used for reference [13]. The study includes 52 patients and 61 PET examinations, performed as a static acquisition and using a transmission measurement in several positions (thorax, abdomen, pelvic area). Histology (44 examinations) or the clinical as well as radiological follow-up data (17 examinations) were used for reference. FDP-PET demonstrated an accuracy of 92% in the detection of liver metastases in comparison to 78% for CT and 80% for CT portography. The accuracy of FDG-PET in the detection of extrahepatic metastases was 92% in comparison to 71% for CT. Unknown metastases were diagnosed for the first time with FDG-PET in 17 patients. This was important for the therapy management of these patients and led to a change of the planned surgical procedure in 28% of the examined patients.

Lai et al. studied 34 patients with a suspicious recurrent colorectal carcinoma. FDG-PET data were compared to CT or other conventional, radiological imaging procedures (X-ray of the thorax, MRI) [31]. Histology or radiological and clinical follow-up data were used for reference. FDG-PET diagnosed unknown extrahepatic metastases first in 11 patients (32%) and the results were true positive. Therapeutic management was changed in a total of 10 patients (29%) based on the PET results.

19.5.1.3 Diagnosis of liver metastases

In the preoperative diagnosis of liver metastases from colorectal carcinoma, methods like ultrasound, CT, MRI are primarily used and nuclear medicine procedures in the second line. However, it is known that untreated liver metastases show a high contrast to normal liver parenchyma, and the delineation of the lesions with [^{18}F]FDG is not a problem.

In 1982 Yonekura et al. reported on the enhanced [^{18}F]FDG uptake in three patients with liver metastases from colorectal cancer [52]. Delbeke et al. examined 110 patients with liver lesions with a diameter greater than 1 cm in CT and compared FDG-PET data to histological data [12]. The authors correctly identified all liver metastases from primary adenocarcinoma due to the enhanced FDG uptake. Benign lesions, like adenomas and focal nodular hyperplasia, did not show an enhanced [^{18}F]FDG uptake. False-positive results were obtained in one patient with an abscess. The data demonstrate that FDG-PET is a reliable diagnostic procedure for the differential diagnosis of liver lesions. Ogunbiyi et al. report a sensitivity of 95% and a specificity of 100% in the detection of liver metastases, in comparison to a sensitivity of 74% and a specificity 85% for CT [40]. The authors conclude that PET is superior to CT for the detection of liver metastases and that in 43% (10/23) of the patients the PET data changed the therapy management (10/23).

Problems may exist in the diagnosis of treated liver metastases. We analyzed the FDG-PET data in 31 patients with recurrent colorectal cancer and 52 histologically proven liver metastases after onset of chemotherapy. Approximately 17.5% of the metastases were hypometabolic in FDG-PET and revealed a metastasis/liver (M/L) ratio lower than 1.0, 51% of the metastases revealed a M/L ratio between 1.0 and 2.0, and 31.5% of the metastases had a M/L ratio greater than 2.0. The data demonstrated that approximately one third of the treated metastases were well delineated in FDG-PET [34].

19.5.2 Therapy management

19.5.2.1 [^{18}F]FDG follow-up studies after radiation therapy

Changes of the FDG metabolism can reflect early as well as late effects of a therapeutic intervention. In colorectal carcinomas, PET-FDG studies were performed in 21 patients with unresectable presacral recurrences after combined photon-neutron therapy and the data were compared to CT follow-up examinations as well as to the tumor marker follow-up [19]. All patients demonstrated a well-delineated lesion in the CT study prior to radiation therapy and showed elevated tumor markers as well as an enhanced FDG uptake in the presacral lesions. The median FDG uptake was 2.3 SUV (1.1 to 5.0 SUV) and decreased three months after radiation therapy to 1.9 SUV. Constant or elevated FDG uptake values were not always associated with tumor progression. A differentiation between viable proliferating tumor cells and cells undergoing repair processes after radiation therapy was not possible according to these data.

Haberkorn et al. reported about FDG follow-up studies in patients with unresectable colorectal cancer that was examined prior to radiation therapy, after photon-therapy and after the end of the combined photon-neutron therapy (40 Gy photons followed by 10 Gy neutrons) [25]. Eleven of twenty patients examined prior to and after photon therapy demonstrated a decrease in FDG uptake, two showed an increase and seven constant values. Twelve of these patients were examined in a triple follow-up protocol, including a baseline study prior to radiation therapy, a study after the end of the photon therapy and a study after the end of the neutron therapy. The comparison of the FDG uptake prior to therapy and after the combined photon-neutron therapy revealed an FDG increase in three patients, constant FDG uptake in further three patients and a FDG decrease in six patients. The comparison of the FDG uptake after photon and after neutron therapy revealed an increase in five patients, constant values in two patients and a decrease in three patients. The data gave evidence that PET is a sensitive method for the assessment of early therapeutic effects. The interpretation of the FDG data is not yet conclusive. Most of the patients demonstrated the maximum effect (FDG decrease) after the photon therapy. The FDG uptake in patients with colorectal recurrences examined with PET shortly after the completion of radiation therapy reflects primarily not only viable tumor tissue but also unspecific benign processes, e.g., due to repair mechanisms. A differentiation between viable tumor tissue and unspecific benign reactions with FDG is not possible shortly after ending radiation therapy. To minimize unspecific reactions with

FDG it is recommended to perform the FDG study at least six months after the completion of radiation therapy. The value of short-term follow-up FDG studies for the individualization and optimization of radiation therapy should be examined further in larger studies.

19.5.2.2 [^{18}F]FDG follow-up studies after chemotherapy

FDG follow-up studies in patients with liver metastases of colorectal carcinoma were first reported in 1992. Smith et al. examined five patients prior, during and after a combined chemotherapy with interleucin-2 (IL2) and fluorouracil [45]. The liver metastases demonstrated a nearly constant FDG uptake after the application of IL2 followed by a rim-like FDG uptake in the peripheral parts of the metastases and a hypometabolic center after the end of the combined therapy with FU.

Vitola et al. performed FDG follow-up studies in four patients with liver metastases prior to and after chemoembolization [51]. Of 34 liver metastases 25 demonstrated a decrease of the FDG uptake in the follo-wup and this was associated with a decrease of the tumor markers. Six of 34 metastases revealed a FDG increase, which was associated with a non-response to chemotherapy.

Findlay et al. examined the value of the FDG follow-up studies in patients with liver metastases from colorectal carcinomas, who received a combined fluorouracil/interferon-alpha therapy [20]. The study included 20 patients with 27 liver metastases. All patients had been studied prior to onset to chemotherapy, 1–2 weeks and 4–5 weeks after beginning therapy. The pretherapeutic tumor/liver (T/L) ratio showed no correlation to the therapeutic result. Metastases which responded to the applied FU chemotherapy demonstrated a higher decrease of the FDG uptake (67% versus 99%). Furthermore, the authors reported that only the T/L ratio 4–5 weeks after onset of chemotherapy was predictive for therapy response. The data gave evidence of an association between the change in the FDG uptake and the response to chemotherapy.

The value of FDG follow-up studies is still being examined and should be evaluated in larger studies. The best time interval for performing a FDG-PET study is dependent on the type of therapy. Short-term follow-up FDG studies are very interesting for scientific purposes, because they provide information about even small changes in tumor metabolism shortly after initiation of chemotherapy. For clinical application, a baseline study prior to therapy and a follow-up study prior to onset of the next cycle are adequate and may help to predict the therapeutic outcome provided that the therapeutic protocol remains unchanged.

19.5.2.3 PET studies with labeled cytostatic agents

[^{18}F]Fluorouracil ([^{18}F]FU) is the most frequently used tracer for studies with radiolabeled cytostatic agents for therapy monitoring. [^{18}F]FU is identical to the non-labeled FU and can be used for pharmacokinetic studies.

Dynamic PET studies of the FU pharmacokinetics were performed in 78 liver metastases (50 patients) following the intravenous application of the radiopharmaceutical and demonstrated a relatively low [^{18}F]FU uptake in the metastases two hours after the infusion of the radiopharmaceutical [15]. The mean [^{18}F]FU uptake in the metastases was 1.3 SUV 2 h p.i. in comparison to 3.9 SUV for the normal liver parenchyma. The mean transit time was 68.2 min for the liver and 83.7 min for the metastases. The elimination half-life was 22.0 min for the liver parenchyma and 29.9 min for the metastases. The individual variation of the [^{18}F]FU uptake values for the metastases was high, although the metastases did not reach the maximum uptake in comparison to the normal parenchyma. Normal liver parenchyma achieved the maximum [^{18}F]FU uptake at 30 min p.i. (25 to 40 min) with a mean value of 11.3 SUV.

Double studies after intravenous (i.v.) and intraarterial (i.a.) application of [^{15}O]water and [^{18}F]FU were performed in patients with surgically implanted catheters in the a. gastroduodenalis, who were scheduled for intraarterial chemotherapy [17]. The evaluation included 15 patients with 24 histologically proven liver metastases. Twenty-one of 24 metastases (87.5%) demonstrated improved access using the i.a. application and 20 lesions (83.3%) an improved FU influx. The maximum [^{18}F]FU concentration was measured after the intraarterial application with a maximum uptake of 18.75 SUV for the FU influx and 5.03 SUV for FU trapping. Only 33.3% (8/24) of the metastases demonstrated improved FU trapping using the intraarterial application. Cluster analysis revealed two different transport systems. An energy-dependent transport system, which is saturable even after the i.v. application of FU, was observed in 6/24 metastases. However, most metastases revealed a perfusion-dependent transport system. Double tracer studies with [^{15}O]water and [^{18}F]FU can be used for the identification of the transport system of FU in the metastases and to select those patients who are more likely to profit from intaarterial chemotherapy. The data demonstrate that rapid elimination of FU as well as a saturable, energy-dependent transport mechanism are likely to be limiting factors for successful chemotherapy, because they reduce the benefit of the enhanced dose in the target area.

Modulation of the FU chemotherapy using folinic acid is still used to improve the response rate, because folinic acid enhances the ability of the fluorinated nucleotide to inhibit the activity of thymidilate synthetase and therefore more FU should be incorporated into DNA and RNA. However, more side effects are observed in comparison to the FU monotherapy. Double studies with [^{18}F]FU-PET with and without folinic acid application were performed in 10 patients and the [^{18}F]FU kinetics in the metastases were evaluated [16]. Six of 14 metastases demonstrated an enhanced trapping of

[^{18}F]FU after folinic acid pretreatment. However, a statistically significant enhancement of the [^{18}F]FU uptake was achieved in only one of ten patients after folinic acid pretreatment. [^{18}F]FU studies with and without folinic acid pretreatment may be used to select those patients who are most likely to profit from a modulated FU chemotherapy.

An important aspect for the application of [^{18}F]FU for therapy management is the prediction of therapy outcome. [^{18}F]FU trapping, as measured by [^{18}F]FU-PET prior to onset of chemotherapy, correlates with the growth rate of the metastases as measured by CT follow-up studies under FU chemotherapy [18]. This was shown in 17 patients with 25 liver metastases from colorectal carcinomas. The authors report a significant correlation of 0.86 ($p < 0.001$) between the [^{18}F]FU uptake prior to therapy and the tumor growth rate. Furthermore, the data gave evidence that only metastases with a high FU trapping exceeding 3.0 SUV (120 min p.i.) achieve a negative growth rate following chemotherapy. Möhler et al. examined the prognostic value of [^{18}F]FU-PET in 14 patients with liver metastases and found a significant correlation of 0.65 ($p < 0.012$) between the FU trapping and the survival of the patients after FU chemotherapy [38].

19.6 Outlook

[^{18}F]FDG is the most important radiopharmaceutical for the diagnosis and the therapy monitoring of patients with colorectal cancer. Other radiopharmaceuticals, like ^{11}C-labeled amino acids, can be used in combination with FDG to provide information about tumor biochemistry and may help in the differentiation, for example, of tumor vs. abscess [46]. PET studies with labeled cytostatic drugs like [^{18}F]FU provide important information about the individual biokinetics of a cytostatic agent in the target area. Studies with [^{18}F]FU have shown that the rapid elimination of the cytostatic agent is a major limiting parameter for a sufficient cytostatic effect. Furthermore, [^{18}F]FU-PET data gave evidence of at least two different transport mechanisms of FU, which lead to a different trapping of the tracer.

FDG follow-up studies are more often used in a clinical environment to assess therapeutic effects of different treatment protocols. Chemotherapy, radiation therapy or even gene therapy may be evaluated by quantifying differences in the regional FDG metabolism.

19.7 Recommendations for the performance and interpretation of PET studies

It is recommended that PET studies of the pelvic area and of the liver should be iteratively reconstructed to reduce artifacts, particularly in the pelvic area due to the excreted FDG activity in the bladder. A bladder catheterization as recommended by some authors is not required if iterative reconstruction is used. A cost-effective alternative is the use of iterative reconstruction programs which run on PC systems and are very efficient [29]. We use routinely an iterative reconstruction program based on a Pentium system and a web-interface (Javascript) for the reconstruction parameters.

Attenuation-corrected static emission measurements at several bed positions (pelvic area, abdomen, lung) are helpful and should be performed also for staging studies. Only attenuation-corrected PET slices and the quantification of the uptake data help to achieve reliable results. The use of short measurement intervals for the transmission and emission (5–10 min for each measurement if iterative reconstruction is provided) allow the examination of different regions of the body in a reasonable time.

In selected cases, like in patients who are scheduled for surgical intervention, a correlation of morphological tomographic imaging procedures, like CT or MRI, is important and supports a correct interpretation of PET images.

19.7.1 Protocol for a staging study with [^{18}F]FDG (static acquisition)

- Patient preparation: fasting for at least 4–6 h prior to the FDG study; measurement of blood glucose level
- Positioning: lowest level for studies of the pelvic area approximately 2 cm below the symphysis
- Radiopharmaceutical: i.v. injection of [^{18}F]FDG (185–370 MBq)
- Data acquisition: 30 min p.i. transmission measurement (5–10 min) followed by an emission measurement (5–10 min) of the pelvic area
  further bed positions accordingly to the same acquisition protocol if required up to the lung
- Reconstruction: iterative reconstruction of transmission and emission (e.g., OS-EM, 6 iterations, 4 segments, 256 × 256 matrix)
- Quantification: ROIs in the target area (tumor, metastasis) and in the reference tissue (muscle, vessel), SUV calculation
- *Alternatively:* Whole-body protocil with or without transmission measurement
  Begin of the emission measurement 30 min p.i. (important: voiding of the bladder prior to onset of the measurement)
  first bed position in the pelvic area to avoid artifacts in the retrovesical region

19.7.2 Protocol for a therapy monitoring study with [^{18}F]FDG (dynamic)

- Patient preparation: see 19.7.1
- Positioning: pelvic area (see 19.7.1)
  liver: identification of the liver dome with US or CT
- Data acquisition: 5–10 min transmission measurement of the target area (pelvic region or liver)
- Radiopharmaceutical: i.v. injection of [^{18}F]FDG (185–370 MBq), dynamic measurement for 60 min (5×120 s, 10×300 s)
- Reconstruction: see 19.7.1
- Quantification: ROIs for tumor, surrounding tissue (liver, gluteal muscle)
  calculation of SUV
  in selected cases calculation of parametric images of the [^{18}F]FDG influx according to the Patlak procedure or use of a two-compartment model; input function for the compartment analysis: a vessel volume-ROI (VOI) obtained from the image (positioning of the vessel VOI in the early phase)

19.7.3 Protocol for a therapy monitoring study with [^{18}F]FDG (static)

- Patient preparation: see 19.7.1
- Radiopharmaceutical: i.v. injection of [^{18}F]FDG (185–370 MBq)
- Positioning: see 19.7.2
- Data acquisition: 30 min p.i. transmission measurement (5–10 min) of the target area emission measurement (5–10 min)
- Reconstruction: see 19.7.1
- Quantification: calculation of SUV for the tumor, surrounding tissue (liver, gluteal muscle), vessel
- *Alternatively:* see 19.7.1

19.7.4 Protocol for a study with [^{18}F]FU (dynamic)

- Patient preparation: no chemotherapeutic treatment at the time of the PET study
- Positioning: see 19.7.2
- Data acquisition: 5–10 min transmission measurement in the target area (pelvic area or liver)
- Radiopharmaceutical: i.v. short infusion (12 min) of [^{18}F]FU (370 MBq) together with 500 mg unlabeled FU

dynamic measurement for 120 min (12 × 120 s, 7 × 300 s, 6 × 600 s)

- Reconstruction: see 19.7.1
- Quantification: SUV 120 min p.i. for tumor, vessel, surrounding tissue
  ratio 20/120 min SUV, estimation of the growth rate [18]

19.7.5 Protocol for a study with [^{18}F]FU (static)

- Patient preparation: see 19.7.4
- Radiopharmaceutical: see 19.7.4
- Positioning: see 19.7.2
- Data acquisition: 90 min p.i. transmission measurement (5–10 min) of the target area
  110–120 min p.i. emission measurement of the target area
- Reconstruction: see 19.7.1
- Quantification: SUV for tumor, surrounding tissue, vessel
  estimation of the growth rate [18]

References

[1] Abdel-Nabi HH, Dörr RJ (1992) Multicenter clinical trials of monoclonal antibody B72.3-GYK-DTPA 111In (111In-CYT-103; OncoScint CR 103) in patients with colorectal carcinoma. Targeted Diagn Ther 6:73–88

[2] Abdel-Nabi HH, Dörr RJ, Lamonica DM, Cronin VR, Galantowicz PJ, Carbone GM, Spaulding MB (1998) Stating of primary colorectal carcinomas with fluorine-18 fluorodeoxyglucose whole-body PET: correlation with histopathologic and CT findings. Radiology 206:755–760

[3] Barbaro B, Valentin V, Manfredi R (1995) Combined modality staging of high risk rectal cancer. Rays 20:165–181

[4] Bares R, Fass J, Hauptmann S, Braun J, Grehl O, Reinartz R, Büll U, Schumpelick V, Mittermayer C (1993) Quantitative analysis of anti-CEA antibody accumulation in human colorectal carcinomas. Nuklearmedizin 32:65–72

[5] Brzezinski W (1992) Monoclonal antibodies – why should surgeons be interested? Mater Med Pol 24:271–272

[6] Burger C, Buck A (1997) Requirements and implementation of a flexible kinetic modeling tool. J Nucl Med 38:1818–1823

[7] Cancer and the Immune System: The Vital Connection, http://www.cancerresearch.org

[8] Cappel J, Blum U, Ungeheuer E (1983) Bedeutung der Vorsorgeuntersuchung für die Prognose des Dickdarmkarzinoms. Schweiz Med Wochenschr 113:550–552

[9] Cohen AM, Minsky BD, Schilsky RL (1997) Cancer of the Colon staging and prognostic features. In: DeVita VT, Hellman S, Rosenberg SA (eds) Cancer: Principles and Practice of Oncology, 5th edition. Lippincott-Raven Publishers, Philadelphia, pp 1155–1156

[10] Colorectal Cancer, http://www.medicare.gov

[11] Colon Cancer, http://www.health-center.com

[12] Delbeke D, Martin WH, Sandler MP, Chapman WC, Wright JK Jr, Pinson CW (1998) Evaluation of benign vs malignant hepatic lesions with positron emission tomography. Arch Surg 133:510–515

[13] Delbeke D, Vitola JV, Sandler MP, Arildsen RC, Powers TA, Wright KJ Jr, Chapman WC, Pinson CW (1997) Staging recurrent metastatic colorectal carcinoma with PET. J Nucl Med 38:1196–1201

[14] Delorme S (1995) Sonographische Diagnostik in der Onkologie III-4. In: Zeller J, zur Hausen H (eds) Onkologie: Grundlagen-Diagnostik-Therapie-Entwicklungen, 1st edition. ecomed, Landsberg/Lech, pp 1–11

[15] Dimitrakopoulou A, Strauss LG, Clorius JH, Ostertag H, Schlag P, Heim M, Oberdorfer F, Helus F, Haberkorn U, van Kaick G (1993) Studies with positron emission tomography after systemic administration of fluorine-18-uracil in patients with liver metastases from colorectal carcinoma. J Nucl Med 34:1075–1081

[16] Dimitrakopoulou A, Strauss LG, Knopp MV, Haberkorn U, Helus F, Maier-Borst W (1992) Evaluation of modulated fluorouracil chemotherapy with positron emission tomography in patients with metastatic colorectal cancer. In: Breit (ed) Advanced Radiation Therapy Tumor Response Monitoring and Treatment Planning. Springer, Berlin Heidelberg, pp 227–230

[17] Dimitrakopoulou-Strauss A, Strauss LG, Schlag P, Hohenberger P, Irngartinger G, Oberdorfer F, Doll J, van Kaick G (1998) Intravenous and intra-arterial oxygen-15-labeled water and fluorine-18-labeled fluorouracil in patients with liver metastases from colorectal carcinoma. J Nucl Med 39:465–473

[18] Dimitrakopoulou-Strauss A, Strauss LG, Schlag P, Hohenberger P, Möhler M, Oberdorfer F, van Kaick G (1998) Fluorine-18-fluorouracil to predict therapy response in liver metastases from colorectal carcinoma. J Nucl Med 39:1197–1202

[19] Engenhart R, Kimmig BN, Strauss LG, Höver KH, Romahn J, Haberkorn U, van Kaick G, Wannenmacher M (1992) Therapy monitoring of presacral recurrences after high-dose irradiation: value of PET, CT, CEA and pain score. Strahlenther Onkol 168:203–212

[20] Findlay M, Young H, Cunningham D, Iveson A, Cronin B, Hickish T, Pratt B, Husband J, Flower M, Ott R (1996) Noninvasive monitoring of tumor metabolism using fluordeoxyglucose and positron emission tomography in colorectal cancer liver metastases: correlation with tumor response to fluorouracil. J Clin Oncol 14:700–708

[21] Fuchs CS, Giovannucci EL, Colditz GA, Hunter DJ, Stampfer MJ, Rosner B, Speizer FE, Willet WC (1999) Dietary fiber and the risk of colorectal cancer and adenoma in women. N Engl J Med 340:169–176

[22] Golfieri R, Giampalma E, Leo P, Colecchia A, Selleri S, Poggioli G, Gozzetti G, Trebbi F, Russo A et al. (1993) Comparison of magnetic resonance (0.5 T), computed tomography, and endorectal ultrasonography in the preoperative stating of neoplasms of the rectum-sigma. Correlation with surgical and anatomopathologic findings. Radiol Med Torino 85:773–783

[23] Grabbe E, Winkler R (1985) Local recurrence after sphincter-saving resection for rectal rectosigmoid cancer. Value of diagnostic methods. Radiology 155:305–310

[24] Gupta NC, Falk PM, Frank AL, Thorson AM, Frick MP, Bowman B (1993) Pre-operative staging of colorectal carcinoma using positron emission tomography. Nebr Med J 78:30–35

[25] Haberkorn U, Strauss LG, Dimitrakopoulou A, Engenhart R, Oberdorfer F, Ostertag H, Romahn J, van Kaick G (1991) PET studies of fluorodeoxyglucose metabolism in patients with recurrent colorectal tumors receiving radiotherapy. J Nucl Med 32:1485–1490

[26] Heim ME (1995) Gastrointestinale Tumoren V-2.5. In: Zeller J, zur Hausen H (eds) Onkologie: Grundlagen-Diagnostik-Therapie-Entwicklungen, 1st edition. ecomed, Landsberg/Lerch, pp 1–23

[27] Imdahl A, Bräutigam P, Hauenstein KH, Eggstein S, Waninger J, Farthmann EH (1994) The value of CEA immunoscintigraphy for diagnosis of colorectal cancer and its metastases: results of a prospective study. Zentralbl Chir 119:17–22

[28] Keogan MT, Lowe VJ, Baker ME, McDermott VG, Lyerly HK, Coleman RE (1997) Local recurrence of rectal cancer: evaluation with F-18 fluordeoxyglucose PET imaging. Abdom Imaging 22:327–332

[29] Kontaxakis G, Tzanakos GS, Strauss LG, Dimitrakopoulou-Strauss A, Mantaka P, van Kaick G (1997) Characteristics of the local convergence behavior of the iterative ML-EM image reconstruction algorithms for PET. J Nucl Med 38:202P (abstr)

[30] Kummer D, Bertsch G, Breucha G, Domers B, Müller GE, Sommer (1997) Die Bedeutung der Krebsnachsorge beim Magen-, Dick- und Mastdarmoperierten. Med Welt 28:1920–1925

[31] Lai DT, Fulham M, Stephen MS, Chu KM, Solomon M, Thompson JF, Sheldon DM, Storey DW (1996) The role of whole-body positron emission tomography with 18F-fluorodeoxyglucose in identifying operable colorectal cancer metastases to the liver. Arch Surg 131:703–707

[32] Leitha T, Baur M, Steger D, Dudczak R (1990) Anti-CEA immunoscintigraphy in post-operative follow-up of tumor patients. Differentiated use of various monoclonal antibody preparations. Wien Klin Wochenschr 102:503–509

[33] Lynch HT, Smyrk TC (1998) Identifying hereditary nonpolyposis colorectal cancer. N Engl J Med 338:1537–1538

[34] Mantaka P, Dimitrakopoulou-Strauss A, Gutzler F, Kontaxakis G, Schlag P, Oberdorfer F, van Kaick G, Strauss LG (1997) Evaluation of PET-FDG for the detection and differential diagnosis of liver lesions. J Nucl Med 38:137P (abstr)

[35] Meyenberger C, Wildi S, Kulling D, Bertschinger P, Zala GF, Klotz HP, Krestin GP (1996) Tumor staging and follow-up care in rectosigmoid carcinoma: colonoscopic endosonography compared to CT, MRI and endorectal MRI. Schweiz Rundsch Med Prax 85:622–631

[36] Mikolajczyk K, Szabatin M, Rudnicki P, Grodzki M, Burger C (1998) A JAVA environment for medical image data analysis: initial application for brain PET quantitation. Med Inform 23:207–214

[37] Miraldi F, Vesselle H, Faulhaber PF, Adler LP, Leisure GP (1998) Elimination of artifactual accumulation of FDG in PET imaging of colorectal cancer. Clin Nucl Med 23:3–7

[38] Möhler M, Dimitrakopoulou-Strauss A, Gutzler F, Räth U, Strauss LG, Stremmel W (1998) 18F-labeled fluorouracil positron emission tomography and the prognoses of colorectal carcinoma patients with liver metastases to the liver treated with 5-fluorouracil. Cancer 83:245–253

[39] Muxi Pradas MA, Pons-Pons F, Huguet-Planella M, Novell-Capilla F, Garcia-Romero RH, Trias-Fo Ich M (1996) Immunogammagraphy with anti-CEA and anti-TAG-72 monoclonal antibodies in the diagnosis of colorectal carcinoma. Med Clin Barc 107:601–607

[40] Ogunbiyi OA, Flanagan FL, Dehdashti F, Siegel BA, Trask DD, Birnbaum EH, Fleshman JW, Read TE, Philpott GW, Kodner IJ (1997) Detection of recurrent and metastatic colorectal cancer: comparison of positron emission tomography and computed tomography. Ann Surg Oncol 4:613–620

[41] Polk HC, Spratt JS (1971) Recurrent colorectal carcinoma: detection, treatment and other considerations. Surgery 69:9–13

[42] Potter JD (1999) Fiber and colorectal cancer. N Engl J Med 340:223–224 (editorial)

[43] Sancar A (1994) Mechanisms of DNA excision repair. Science 266:1954–1956

[44] Scharling ES, Wolfman NT, Bechtold RE (1996) Computed tomography evaluation of colorectal carcinoma. Semin Roentgenol 31:142–153

[45] Smith FW, Heys SD, Evans NTS, Roeda D, Gvozdanovic D, Eremin O, Mallard JR (1992) Pattern of 2-deoxy-2-18F-fluoro-D-glucose accumulation in liver tumours: Primary, metastatic, and after chemotherapy. Nucl Med Comm 13:193–195

[46] Strauss LG (1996) Fluorine-18 deoxyglucose and false-positive results: a major problem in the diagnostics of oncological patients. Eur J Nucl Med 23:1409–1415

[47] Strauss LG, Clorius JH, Schlag P, Lehner B, Kimmig B, Engenhart R, Marin-Grez M, Helus F, Oberdorfer F, Schmidlin P, van Kaick G (1989) Recurrence of colorectal tumors: PET evaluation. Radiology 170:329–332

[48] Thoeni RF, Rogalla P (1995) CT for evaluation of carcinomas in the colon and rectum. Semin Ultrasound CT MR 16:112–126

[49] Thompson WM, Halvorsen RA, Foster WL, Roberts L, Gibbons R (1987) Computed tomography of the rectum. RadioGraphics 7:773–807

[50] Valk PE, Pounds TR, Tesar RD, Hopkins DM, Haseman MK (1996) Cost-effectiveness of PET imaging in clinical oncology. Nucl Med Biol 23:737–743

[51] Vitola JV, Delbeke D, Meranze SG, Mazer MJ, Pinson CW (1996) Positron emission tomography with F-18-fluorodeoxyglucose to evaluate the results of hepatic chemoembolization. Cancer 78:2216–2222

[52] Yonekura Y, Benua RS, Brill AB, Som P, Yeh SD, Kemeny NE, Fowler JS, MacGregor RR, Stamm R, Christman DR, Wolf AP (1982) Increased accumulation of 2-deoxy-2-18F-fluoro-D-glucose in liver metastases from colon carcinoma. J Nucl Med 23:1133–1137

20 Hodgkin and Non-Hodgkin lymphoma

F. Moog

20.1 Etiology, epidemiology, histopathologic classification

The incidence of malignant lymphomas stands at about five new cases per 100 000 persons per year. These include instances both of Hodgkin's disease (HD) and the heterogeneous group of non-Hodgkin lymphomas (NHL), with a relative frequency of about 1:3. Lymphomas originate from cells of the pulpal tissue of the lymph nodes. Hodgkin's lymphomas are characterized by a very small proportion of specific tumor cells (Hodgkin cells, Reed-Sternberg giant cells) surrounded by numerous nonneoplastic cells. This is distinct from the histological picture of NHL, whose pathognomonic cells constitute the main mass of the tumor.

The etiology of HD remains uncertain. An infectious agent has been suspected, but never confirmed. Viral infections appear causative in a few subtypes of NHL (e.g., adult T-cell lymphoma, Burkitt's lymphoma), but in most instances the etiology is also unknown. Prognostic criteria include the extent of disease spread and the histological subtype, though the latter factor is of subordinate importance in cases of HD.

The individual types and subtypes differ significantly in terms of age distribution, pattern of involvement, therapeutic options and prognosis. At present, there are several competing, but mutually incompatible classifications. Low-grade malignant NHL manifests itself most frequently in later life. While often showing a protracted clinical course, curative therapy is possible only in exceptional cases. High-grade forms resemble acute leukemias and require aggressive management. Of the frequently encountered types of high-grade HD and NHL, all show two periods of peak incidence: one in the earlier decades of life, with a second observed in advancing age. Advances in lymphoma therapy have increased the survival chances for patients with early-stage HD to 90%, with remission rates of about 50% even in cases of advanced disease. Of patients with high-grade NHL, up to 60% experience complete remission, with as many as 50% of these patients remaining free of disease recurrence.

20.2 Conventional diagnostic features in malignant lymphoma

The introduction of computed tomography (CT) and, later, magnetic resonance imaging (MRI) resulted in significant advances in the diagnostic imaging of both HD and NHL [14, 29, 45, 61, 70]. Despite improvements in methodology, these leaps have become smaller. The primary reason may be inherent limitations in the capabilities of conventional cross-sectional imaging technologies. Criteria employed for the evaluation of diagnostic imaging results are based on morphological changes, which may represent a problem in the interpretation of normal sized or only slightly enlarged lymph nodes, in the case of parenchymal organs or of residual tissues remaining after therapy. Limitations affecting other diagnostic methods, such as ultrasound, have resulted in the staging of malignant lymphomas being dependent today on a growing number of organ-system-specific methods. Beside the considerable discomfort to the patient undergoing, for example, liver and bone marrow punctures, this battery of tests is associated with significant expenditure in terms of time, logistics and costs.

20.3 PET

20.3.1 Technical aspects

20.3.1.1 The PET "signal"

Differences of opinion still exist with regard to the correct pathophysiologic interpretation of the [^{18}F]FDG signal. Cytometric studies by Higashi et al. showed a highly significant correlation between cellular [^{18}F]FDG uptake and the number of viable tumor cells [28]. Earlier studies had shown a correlation between [^{18}F]FDG uptake and the rate of cell proliferation, not, however, with the number of viable lymphoma cells [56]. A significant relationship of [^{18}F]FDG uptake and the cell proliferation rate was also identified by Lapela et al. [40], who also reported a close correlation with the degree of malignancy of the disease. Findings by Dimitrakopoulou-Strauss et al. suggest that [^{18}F]FDG also accumulates in non-proliferating cells in the G_0 phase; hence, [^{18}F]FDG is primarily a marker of tumor viability [18]. It remains uncertain to what degree non-malignant cells are responsible for the intratumoral [^{18}F]FDG uptake. Microautoradiographic studies in animal models show that up to 29% of intratumoral glucose utilization takes place in non-malignant granulation tissue or in other tumor-associated cell groups [39]. While NHLs recruit predominantly from malignant cells, the proportion of characteristic Hodgkin and Reed-Sternberg cells in some subtypes of HD is quite small: in fact, the main tumor mass consists of reactive accompanying cells, such as lymphocytes, histiocytes and fibroblasts. These histomorphological differences must be considered in the interpretation of PET findings.

20.3.1.2 Transmission

The diagnostic relevance of quantifying [^{18}F]FDG metabolism is controversial. It is generally believed helpful in the differentiation of [^{18}F]FDG uptake in non-malignant malignant processes such as inflammation, aspergillosis and some granulomatous disease entities which may lead to false-positive [^{18}F]FDG-PET findings [44, 59, 75]. Although the rate of [^{18}F]FDG metabolism of many malignancies is greater than in benign entities, the standard deviations in the individual case are too large for this difference to be useful as a definite criterion of malignancy. Overlapping is particularly common in tumors with relatively discrete [^{18}F]FDG uptake, such as prostate carcinoma [71]. Malignant lymphomas, on the other hand, are characterized by a very intense glucose metabolism; SUV values are quite variable, however, in relation to the degree of malignancy of the individual subtypes, ranging from 3.5 to 31.0 (median 8.5) [40]. As a rule, however, the contrast is sufficient to permit a definitive differentiation from benign processes [31, 47]. Questionable findings are infrequent, particularly in untreated patients, in whom, despite adequate history and knowledge of the common sites for lymphomatous disease, the differential diagnosis may be problematic. The clinical experience of the examiner remains of utmost importance in the differentiation of the manifestations of lymphoma from benign processes or artifacts.

Non-transmission-corrected scans are characterized by a relative overemphasis of the skin ('hot skin') and the lung. This may interfere with the evaluation of small lymph nodes in the vicinity of the skin (e.g., cervical and inguinal nodes), and anatomical delineation of lung parenchyma from the hilus or mediastinum may be difficult. Studies on models have demonstrated a relative object distortion in non-corrected scans [6]. A direct comparison of corrected and non-corrected scans obtained in 51 lymphoma patients by Kotzerke et al. found differences in visualization in only five of 187 findings which were sufficient to complicate the differentiation of benign from malignant processes [38].

The principal arguments against transmission correction include, among others, the increased time requirement, the poor reproducibility, the unfavorable target-background relationship and the "snowy" image quality at inadequate transmission rates.

It appears useful to quantify glucose metabolism as part of therapy monitoring. It is known, however, that the simple serial calculation of the tumor-background ratio, which does not require transmission correction, correlates closely with the kinetics of glucose metabolism [56]. This simple technique may actually be suitable for evaluation of therapeutic efficacy, though there is still a paucity of confirmatory data.

20.3.1.3 Tracer

At the present time, [^{18}F]FDG is the tracer of choice in the diagnosis of lymphomas. Other positron-emitting radiopharmaceuticals, such as [^{11}C]methionine or $[^{11}C]$thyrosine, or $[^{15}O]H_2O$, which have significantly shorter half-lives, are only suitable for use with PET units possessing their own cyclotrons. In comparison with other researchers, Rodriguez et al. have shown equally good results in the imaging of lymphomatous tissue with both $[^{11}C]$methionine and $[^{18}F]$FDG; however, unlike $[^{18}F]$FDG, the intensity of tumor uptake of $[^{11}C]$methionine did not prove useful in differentiating between high- and low-grade lymphoma types [43, 65]. Double tracer studies with both $[^{15}O]H_2O$ and $[^{18}F]$FDG show a significant, nonlinear correlation between perfusion and glucose metabolism. Estimation of tumor metabolism based on perfusion could be of use at treatment follow-up, since it remains to be determined to what extent tumor metabolism during chemotherapy is controlled by the perfusion [17].

20.3.2 Primary staging

20.3.2.1 Nodal disease

At morphologic imaging, it is usual to regard cervical and mediastinal lymph nodes not occurring in groups to be unremarkable up to a diameter of 10 mm. Generally recognized is a gradual, caudally directed size increase in retroperitoneal lymph nodes: thus, the upper limit for retrocrural nodes stands at 6 mm, increasing to 8 mm in the upper retroperitoneum and 10 mm at the level of the aortic bifurcation. Pelvic nodes with diameters in excess of 8 mm are considered suspicious [19, 22]. It has been shown, however, that, depending on tumor type, between 7% and 70% of macroscopically normal lymph nodes actually contain malignant cells [2, 13, 21, 27, 37]. Conversely, there are also instances in which lymph nodes are enlarged but not affected by malignant disease [33]. Secondary signs of malignancy such as necroses or pathological patterns of contrast medium enhancement are to be expected only in those nodes with diameters above 15 mm, but are rather unusual in lymphomas [25].

The interpretation of lymph node size exerts an immediate influence on the sensitivity of morphologic imaging techniques. The lower the size selected as a criterion of suspected malignancy, the higher the sensitivity of the method; at the same time, however, there is a corresponding decrease in specificity. This diagnostic dilemma is probably one reason for the fact that mesenteric and retrocrural lymph nodes, for example, are diagnosed corrected at CT in only 57–75% of cases [12, 45, 51]. MRI appears to be equivalent to CT without, however, demonstrating any superiority in the interpretation of patient lymph node status [29, 72].

Modern PET scanners are able to detect objects with diameters significantly under 1 cm. There have been several published case reports in patients with metastatic otolaryngeal tumors as well as with malignant lymphomas in which microscopic tumor infiltration in non-enlarged lymph nodes has been detected using $[^{18}F]$FDG-PET [7, 18]. Considering all currently available reports in the literature, [^{18}F]FDG-PET remains a potential imaging technique for evaluation of nodal involvement in patients with lymphomas. Depending on the threshold for lymph node diameter selected as a criterion of malignancy, [^{18}F]FDG-PET returns up to 18% more suspicious findings than CT [5, 9, 32, 47, 52]. These results are not, however, directly comparable, because definitive verification of the additional nodes detected at PET was made only in a few cases. Therefore the true sensitivity, specificity and accuracy cannot be evaluated. False-positive findings, due mostly to unspecific or inflammatory changes, were described [18, 47].

The degree to which significant limitations in the interpretation of low-grade malignant lymphomas do exist, or whether they only affect certain subtypes of the disease is unclear. It is known that low-grade malignancies exhibit lower rates of [^{18}F]FDG metabolism; this rate, however, is usually sufficient to provide a significant contrast to the lesion's surroundings [47]. The risk of underestimating the uptake intensity or of overlooking suspicious sites altogether because of resolution or contrast effects is particularly acute in the immediate vicinity of structures with physiologically high tracer uptake, such as the renal hilus. In some cases, cervical lymph nodes may be difficult to differentiate from the salivary glands, which also may exhibit significant tracer uptake. Erroneous findings may also be caused by increased muscle activity of the speech-associated musculature of the larynx: hence, patients should be instructed to refrain from speaking for 10 min prior to and at least 20 min following tracer application. In the case of simple emission measurements, the uptake intensity of deep lymph nodes around the splenic and hepatic hili may be underestimated [38]. One must also not overlook the influence of the so-called 'partial volume effect,' which, in the case of small tumors (less than two times the spatial resolution of the scanner), may lead to underestimation of glucose metabolism.

The recognition of characteristic patterns of involvement for individual lymphoma subtypes can be of importance in the evaluation of a patient's PET findings. For example, in HD, there is frequent involvement of the cervical and supraclavicular lymph nodes; the latter, in turn, may be associated with mediastinal disease manifestation. Spread of the disease follows the contiguity model with continuous progression of disease to neighboring lymph node stations. In such patients, 'leap-frogging' of lymph node stations is unusual and, if it is detected, can be an important factor in the differential diagnosis. Conversely, the pattern of involvement in NHL is rather haphazard with generalized metastasis detectable at the time of first diagnosis.

20.3.2.2 Organ involvement

Organ involvement is a frequently encountered feature of both HD and NHL in untreated patients. For example, liver involvement is found in about 3% of patients with HD, and up to about 23% in those with NHL. The spleen is affected in about 15% of HD patients and 22% of NHL patients. The gastrointestinal (GI) tract is almost never affected in HD, but in up to 40% of patients with NHL. Similarly, bone marrow involvement in MH is found in only about 15% of patients; this is significantly less frequent than in NHL, in some subtypes of which bone marrow involvement is observed practically as a rule. Because of its less favorable prognosis, each instance of organ involvement is assigned to stages III or IV, depending on the patient's pattern of disease spread [36, 67].

Spleen, liver, lung

Lymphomatous involvement of the spleen and liver is often associated with a microscopic or micronodular pattern of infiltration which frequently escapes detection with CT [25]. Clinical and laboratory parameters are of no diagnostic efficacy in these cases. Organ enlargement cannot be used as definitive evidence of infiltration since about 60% of cases of lymphoma-associated hepatomegaly represent benign, usually lymphocytic infiltrates. Similarly, up to 30% of instances of splenic enlargement in patients with lymphomas are due to benign causes [11, 73]. The sensitivity and specificity of CT stand at 38% and 61%, respectively, when the size of the spleen is used as a criterion for lymphomatous involvement. Other studies report similarly disappointing findings with sensitivities of 15–37% for the spleen and 19–33% for the liver [1, 13, 45]. The value of diagnostic ultrasound seems to be equivalent to that of CT, while data published for one study suggest that it may actually be superior to CT [51]. In up to 30% of patients, in whom only supradiaphragmatic involvement was detected using conventional methods, exploratory laparotomy reveals the presence of infradiaphragmatic disease in which the spleen is affected in a majority of cases [42, 60]. MRI is affected by similar problems, though its accuracy may be increased by the use of supraparametric iron oxide, whose uptake is observed only in normal tissues [82]. Because of the weakening of the immune system in later life and the recently observed increase in the rate of secondary malignancies, the use of the staging laparotomy has been generally abandoned. In order to detect liver involvement, current practice relies on blind percutaneous puncture of the liver; this procedure, however, may miss up to 50% of cases of involvement demonstrated at open biopsy [3].

The hepatic and splenic parenchyma in healthy subjects shows a homogeneous pattern of [^{18}F]FDG uptake with comparable signal intensity. If transmission correction is not done, areas of both organs near the thorax wall may be associated with higher signal intensities and thus be somewhat more difficult to evaluate. Corresponding to the variable patterns of involvement seen in lymphomas, there may be homogeneous or focal areas or mixed forms of enhanced [^{18}F]FDG uptake. The anatomic differentiation of lesions located in the vault of the liver from those at the base of the lung may not always be possible with complete certainty.

Similarly, pulmonary disease may present as an isolated focal lesion or as a diffuse pattern of increased tracer uptake, the latter of which may exhibit comparatively low signal intensity. The topographic differentiation between a lesion near to the pleura and a costal lesion or thorax wall infiltration is often difficult. Furthermore, when transmission correction is not done, it may be difficult to delineate the pulmonary parenchyma from hilar tissues. Sometimes it may be necessary to obtain orientational findings from another morphologic imaging methods.

Only a few [^{18}F]FDG-PET studies published to date have differentiated between nodal and extranodal lymphomas; those that have, moreover, included relatively small numbers of patients [32, 77]. Our review of the literature discovered one PET/CT comparative study performed on 81 patients with newly diagnosed lymphomas. In these patients, PET and conventional CT returned 42 concurring findings of extranodal disease manifestation [48]. Splenic involvement was detected most frequently, followed by lung, skeletal system, liver and diverse other locations. Compared with CT, PET visualized an addition 24 suspicious focal lesions, mostly in the bone (marrow), followed by spleen and lung. Of these, further work-up revealed that 13 were correctly diagnosed as positive for disease involvement, with one instance of false-positive findings in a patient with focal autonomy of the thyroid gland. The dignity of the remaining ten lesions could not be determined. On the other hand, five of seven lesions detected only at CT were later identified as benign entities. Based on the findings of [^{18}F]FDG-PET, re-evaluation of the disease stage was required in 16% of patients examined. Other researchers, however, found FDG-PET to have disadvantages for assessing extranodal lymphoma (HD) compared to conventional imaging procedures [81].

GI tract

Unlike HD, cases of NHL often manifest themselves in the GI tract. Here, we distinguish primary forms, which originate in the lymphoid cells of the lamina propria or the submucosa, from secondary forms, which infiltrate the GI tract from adjacent lymph nodes. The stomach is the organ most commonly involved (ca. 50%) [64]. Although relatively little data has been published to date, [^{18}F]FDG-PET seems to be a promising method for diagnosis of gastric lymphomas. Rodriguez et al. found intense [^{18}F]FDG metabolism with SUVs between 6.2 and 38.7 (mean 25.5) in seven of eight patients with confirmed NHL. CT detected these disease manifestations in only six of eight cases [64]. In the eighth patient, who suffered with a low-grade MALT lymphoma, PET failed to detect the presence of disease due to a very discrete increased uptake of [^{18}F]FDG. This is remarkable in view of findings published by Reske et al., who reported pronounced [^{18}F]FDG uptake in cases of this lymphoma subtype which is usually limited to the stomach [63].

Several factors complicate the evaluation of the abdominal and retroperitoneal organs. Tracer uptake in the urinary tract may cause artifacts which mask adjacent lesions. In most cases, this can be controlled by the intravenous administration of furosemide with simultaneous adequate hydration. In many patients, there may be a prominent, though usually inhomogeneous uptake pattern in the colon, which usually reaches a maximum in the ascending colon. The rectum and anal canal may also exhibit enhanced signal intensities. The reasons for this phenomenon, whose extent varies from patient to patient, remain unclear. Vesselle et al. have suggested that these artifacts can be reduced by adequate bowel preparation using isoosmotic laxatives [78]. One further restriction affecting PET is its limited capacity for topographic orientation of focal abdominal lesions. Interpretation often requires findings from an additional morphologic imaging technique.

Cerebrum

An important new indication for [^{18}F]FDG-PET is the work-up of cerebral processes in patients with acquired immunodeficiency syndrome (AIDS). Immunosuppressed patients represent a particular challenge to diagnostic imaging, since opportunistic infections of the brain often cannot be differentiated from high-grade NHL, both of which occur at a higher incidence in these patients. Especially problematic is the differentiation from toxoplasmosis, which may show identical findings at both CT and MRI. [^{18}F]FDG metabolism differs so greatly between the two diseases that certainty in differentiation is possible even using only visual criteria. In these patients, malignant lymphomas exhibit signal intensities equal to or higher than the cerebral cortex, while the intensity of toxoplasmosis lesions is significantly lower [31]. Similarly, there are significantly higher SUVs for lymphomatous disease manifestations; overlap with the SUVs of benign entities is rare [55, 79].

Bone and bone marrow

The conventional method for evaluation of the bone marrow is the uni- or bilateral puncture biopsy of the iliac crest. Positive findings often influence primary staging. Because bone marrow involvement is a criterion for stage IV disease, positive findings in a patient with a clinical status suggestive of low-grade disease may result in a change in that patient's management [61]. Bone marrow biopsy, however, is not a definitive method since many lymphoma forms are characterized by a more focal pattern of involvement. A few types tend to include early osteodestruction, but remain in sharply demarcated lesions, while other, less aggressive forms do not attack the trabecular structure of the bone but rapidly spread through large areas of bone marrow [8, 46]. Biopsies, of course, represent only a tiny section of bone marrow; hence, it is understandable that there may be errors in tissue sampling [15, 23].

Recent studies have shown that MRI is capable of detecting focal bone marrow involvement in up to 33% of patients with negative biopsy findings, though, on the other hand, diffuse infiltrations are often overlooked [29, 70].

Earlier studies, however, have shown less promising results, with sensitivity and positive predictive values of 55.6% and 38.5% respectively [76, 83].

Normal bone marrow in patients who have not yet undergone chemotherapy or radiation shows a relatively discrete and homogeneous [^{18}F]FDG metabolism with SUV values of 0.7 to 1.3 [84]. Manifestations of lymphoma can present as uni- or multifocal lesions or diffuse areas of increased [^{18}F]FDG uptake in the marrow. Because of the typically intense pattern of tracer uptake, disease manifestation is easy to diagnose. It seems redundant in these cases to quantify the glucose metabolism. Modern PET scanners permit a visual differentiation of cortical from medullary portions of the vertebral column, femora and humeri and, to a lesser extent, of the central sections of the bony pelvis. Here, our own experience suggests that iterative data reconstructions provide the best image quality. Evaluation of the vertebral column is best done in the sagittal plane, which permits visualization of the entire bone marrow (Fig. 20.1). The femora are the individual bones most often exhibiting lymphomatous involvement. Hence, the proximal segments with the highest marrow content should lie within the measurement field [20, 58]. Here, the best overview is obtained in the longitudinal plane. Following chemotherapy, there is sometimes a nonhomogeneous uptake pattern, particular-

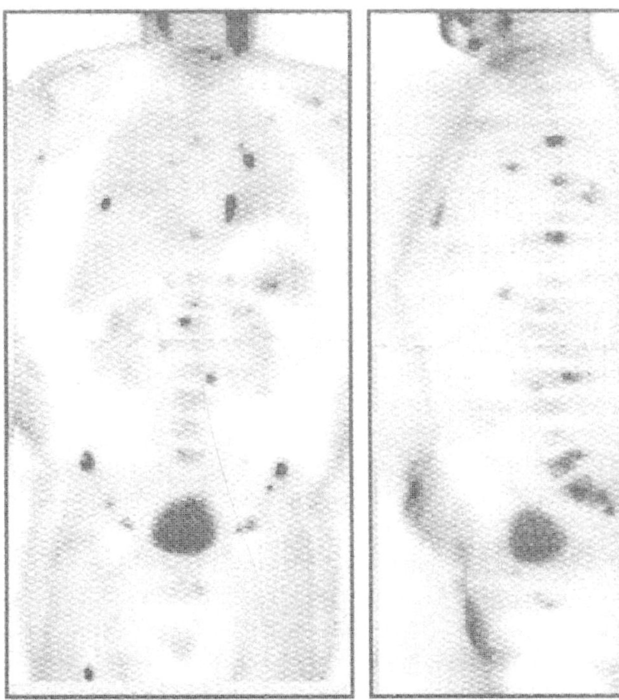

Fig. 20.1. Bone (marrow) involvement in non-Hodgkin lymphoma in sagittal and coronal planes. There is multifocal [^{18}F]FDG uptake in the vertebral column, bony pelvis, sternum and the right proximal femur. In addition, PET visualized several pulmonary and one splenic lesion.

ly following application of a bone marrow-stimulating agent, which is associated with more intense uptake. This may complicate evaluation.

Clinical studies published to date suggest that [^{18}F]FDG-PET could establish itself as an adjunct to bone marrow biopsy. The method is also capable of detecting the osseous manifestations of plasmocytoma, an NHL of the B-cell line [69]. Beside those patients in whom CT and PET return concordant findings suggestive for high- or low-grade malignant lymphomas, [^{18}F]FDG-PET may reveal areas with suspicious levels of glucose metabolism in 15–25% of all patients with normal findings at bone marrow biopsy of the iliac crest. In up to 11.5% of patients, this results in upgrading of their tumor stage with corresponding changes to their therapeutic management [10, 49]. The majority of these cases include higher-grade NHL subtypes or Hodgkin's disease. The pattern of tracer uptake is focal or nonhomogeneous, with involvement seen in the vertebral column (sometimes only individual vertebrae) and less commonly in the pelvis or femora.

As a rule, the findings are apparent with generally intense patterns of uptake. Characteristic histologic findings include a tightly joined pattern of infiltration pushing back the normal bone marrow, often with significant destruction of the trabecular structure [49]. False-positive findings are almost never observed. It is possible that the diffuse pattern of increased glucose metabolism in Hodgkin's disease may be caused by a reactive myeloid hyperplasia [10]. Conversely, bone marrow involvement may escape detection with PET, particularly in low-grade subtypes of NHL. The instances of false-negative findings described to date had in common a very loose pattern of infiltration with only slight displacement of normal bone marrow. The trabecular structure of the spongiosa was intact. Apparently, the relatively low [^{18}F]FDG metabolism seen in low-grade forms and a low concentration of tumor cells does not provide for sufficient [^{18}F]FDG accumulation to permit visualization.

The blood supply of bone and bone marrow is usually provided by a common vascular system [24]. Consequently, lymphomas may also arise as primary entities within cortical structures and only at a later date infiltrate the marrow. More commonly, however, there is direct infiltration from adjacent bone marrow manifestations. Bone scintigraphy, despite its only moderate sensitivity, remains an established technique used to exclude osseous involvement in cases of lymphomatous disease [58, 68]. Tracer uptake is often quite discrete and the osteolytic lesions predominantly seen in NHL regularly escape detection [34]. That the method continues to occupy its place in lymphoma diagnostics is primarily related to the fact that there is no suitable alternative.

One important advantage of PET over skeletal scintigraphy is found in the obligatory tomography data visualization. SPECT imaging of the entire skeleton, on the other hand, is not practicable as a routine clinical procedure and is performed only in cases of suspected disease. With [^{18}F]FDG-PET, both the osseous and medullary compartment of the skeletal system can be visualized in a single examination. This was confirmed by preliminary examinations of 56 patients using [^{18}F]FDG-PET which showed a significantly higher sensitivity in comparison with conventional bone scintigraphy [50]. Beside the higher uptake intensity, there were almost twice as many sites of focal [^{18}F]FDG uptake in comparison to those with diphosphonate uptake. All correctly identified positive findings at bone scintigraphy also showed [^{18}F]FDG uptake; hence, no additional information was provided by bone scintigraphy in comparison with [^{18}F]FDG-PET.

20.3.3 Therapy control

20.3.3.1 Residual tumor

Involvement of the mediastinum is encountered in about 60% of all patients with HD and in about 20% of those with NHL. This localization is often the site of bulky disease, representing particularly large tumor mass. Bulks represent a risk factor and, should persistent tumor mass be identified following conclusion of chemotherapy, are the target for additional chemotherapy or radiation. The diagnostic dilemma consists of the fact that up to 88% of all patients exhibit residual tissue of varying size following completion of therapy

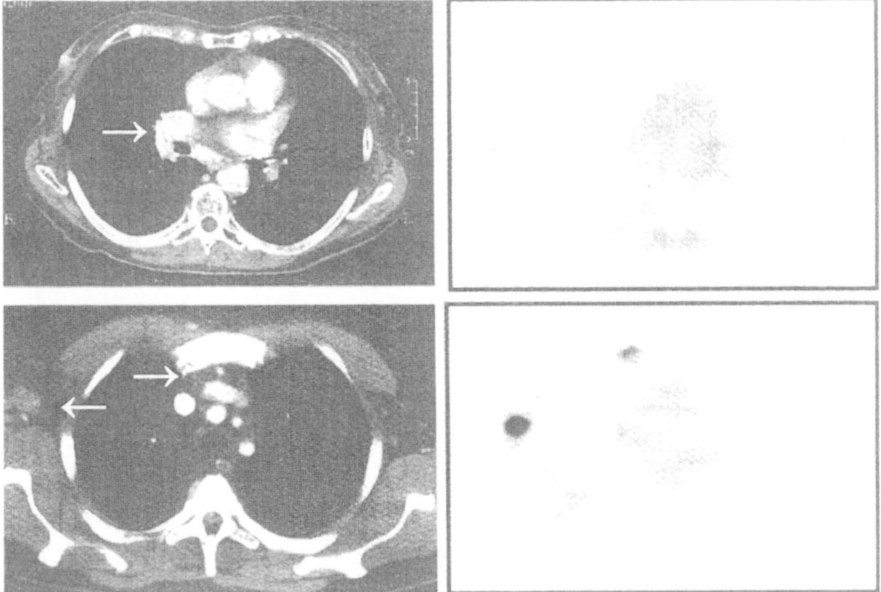

Fig. 20.2. 'Residual' lesions of unknown dignity in the area of the pulmonary hilus (upper row) and axilla (lower row) following therapy of Hodgkin's disease. The unremarkable [^{18}F]FDG metabolism in the upper row suggests scar tissue formation (complete remission for longer than three years), while the pronounced [^{18}F]FDG uptake in the lower row is evidence for residual, viable lymphomatous tissue (confirmed at histology). In addition, there is evidence for a newly recognized parasternal manifestation on the right.

[53, 62]. The proportion of connective tissue varies greatly between lymphoma types with correspondingly large differences in the degree of scar tissue formation [74]. The devitalization of lymphoma cells occurs more rapidly than their removal; this leads to regression over a period of months [54]. Conventional imaging is usually unable to differentiate between regressive scar tissue and viable lymphomatous tissue (Fig. 20.2). Because of the restricted therapeutic options in recurrent lymphomas, it is of the utmost importance to detect recurrence in the stage of 'minimal disease'. Scintigraphy using ^{67}Ga as a marker is often able to differentiate lymphomatous from scar tissue, though the usefulness of the method is reduced in low-grade lymphoma subtypes [41]. In addition, use of the method for evaluating abdominal findings is complicated by hepatic excretion of the radiopharmaceutical.

Findings published to date confirm [^{18}F]FDG-PET's capabilities for overcoming these difficulties. In a series of 17 patients with posttherapeutic residual tumor but normal findings at [^{18}F]FDG-PET, Wit et al. found that all patients remained in complete remission over a relatively short follow-up period of a median 62.6 weeks (1–25 months). Conversely, seven of ten patients with positive PET findings experienced disease recurrence [16]. Bangerter et al. studied 36 patients with residual tumors > 1 cm, 27 of whom had normal findings at PET. After a median follow-up of 25 months (range: 7–60 months), only two patients experienced disease recurrence, corresponding to a negative predictive value (NPV) of 93%. Conversely, of nine patients with positive PET findings, five experienced recurrence within seven months, while the remaining four remained clinically in remission within a follow-up period of at least 24 months. This corresponds to a relatively disappointing positive predictive value (PPV) of 56% [4].

Two of these inadequate interpretations could have been avoided with the experience possessed today. In both cases, a cap-shaped pattern of enhanced [^{18}F]FDG uptake was noted in a high, retrosternal localization. Biopsy revealed hyperplastic thymus tissue [26]. This is sometimes noted in young patients following completion of chemotherapy. The constellation of a more or less flat, immediately retrosternal area of tracer uptake following completion of chemotherapy should always suggest the possibility of this phenomenon. As already explained, intratumoral glucose utilization is influenced by active granulation tissue and other tumor-associated cells. A discrete [^{18}F]FDG metabolism may persist in lymphoma patients with posttherapeutic scar tissue: this has been ascribed to inflammatory cell infiltrations into necrotic tissue or to the forming granulation tissue [57]. Immediately following therapy, [^{18}F]FDG uptake may mathematically be two to three times higher than that of surrounding tissue [26]; using visual criteria, however, it does not reach the typical uptake intensity of viable lymphomatous tissue. These therapy-induced inflammatory effects disappear over time, but may still be detected for months following radiation therapy. While there are still no generally accepted recommendations regarding the length of the period following chemotherapy or radiation during which [^{18}F]FDG-PET may return equivocal findings, a period of at least four weeks is advisable. A characteristic pattern

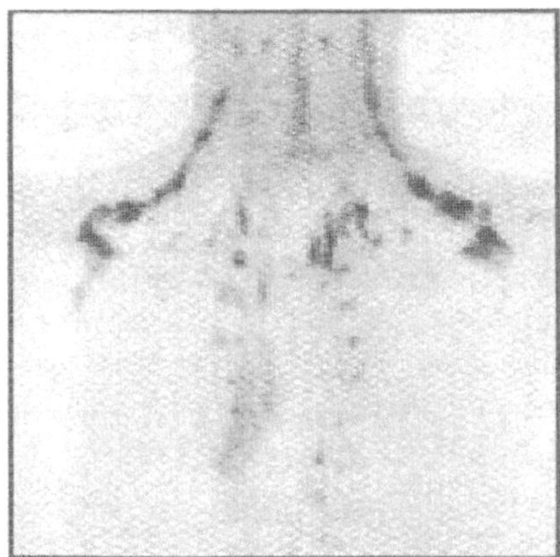
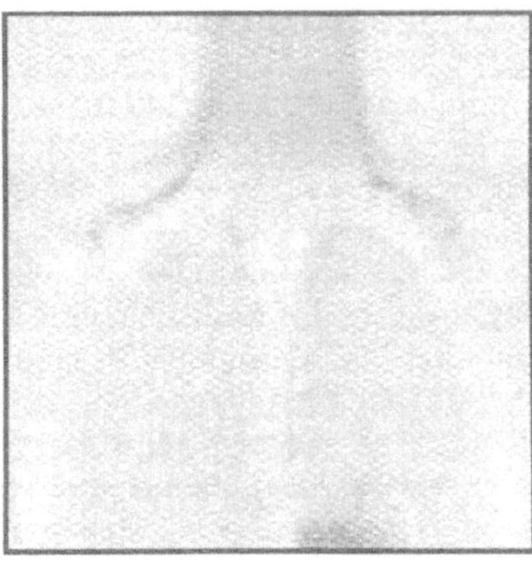

Fig. 20.3. Symmetrical patterns of [^{18}F]FDG uptake in the cervical, clavicular and paratracheal lymph node groups three weeks after chemotherapy. There is also a scattered pattern of unspecific findings in the area of the paravertebral muscles of the thoracic spine. Two months later, there was significant normalization in the patient's findings.

of [^{18}F]FDG uptake is noted in some patients following chemotherapy and manifests as a symmetrical, chain-like enhanced visualization of cervical, clavicular and paratracheal lymph node chains. The pathophysiology underlying this phenomenon, which takes weeks or months to disappear, is unclear (Fig. 20.3). Hyperventilation may induce uptake in diaphragm and stress-induced muscle tension is often seen in trapezius and paraspinal muscle. Relaxants such as benzodiazepines may be helpful in these patients. Also difficult to evaluate are the nonhomogeneous sites of increased uptake in the area of the pulmonary hili or along the trachea. These are probably unspecific changes, though, in the individual case, the persistence of lymphoma cannot be excluded. Hence, one must remain cognizant of the limitations of the method: the persistence of isolated tumor cells can never be excluded; hence, false-negative findings will still occur in the future. Furthermore, when evaluating small tissue masses, one must remember the influence of 'partial volume effects,' which may result in an underestimation of the uptake intensity.

20.3.3.2 Monitoring

Although the majority of all lymphomas can be induced to undergo a presumed remission, up to 80% of patients, depending on subtype, will experience recurrent disease. Clinically speaking, it would be very helpful to be able to evaluate the efficacy or non-efficacy of a therapy form at as early a date as possible such that any necessary changes in the therapeutic regimen can be promptly made. PET is, in principle, a technique which can detect functional changes in the tumor at an early date and long before a macroscopic, morphological correlate has had time to form.

In patients with mammary and soft-tissue carcinomas, average reductions in [^{18}F]FDG uptake of 22% and 37%, respectively, were observed in the group of therapy responders as early as one to three weeks following the initiation of therapy. In non-responders or in those with progressive disease, on the other hand, there was no change in uptake or even an increase in [^{18}F]FDG metabolism [35, 80]. The exact mechanism of changes in glucose metabolism during therapy is not known. Immediately after beginning of therapy, there is sometimes a paradoxical increase in [^{18}F]FDG uptake; hence, measurements on solid tumors seem unsuitable at very early stages [80].

Whether these observations also pertain to malignant lymphomas is unknown. Preliminary studies carried out in patients with various subtypes also showed a significant decrease in [^{18}F]FDG uptake during the first chemotherapy cycle [30]. Double measurements, before and after chemotherapy, point to a correlation between [^{18}F]FDG accumulation and patients' prognoses [17]. Römer et al. observed a decrease in [^{18}F]FDG uptake of 62–72% within seven days of beginning therapy in patients with high-grade NHL. After 42 days, there was a drop of 79–90% as compared with baseline values. There was a close correlation between [^{18}F]FDG uptake on day 42 and the prognosis of the patients examined. A cut-off point of $SUV_{max} = 2.5$ was able to differentiate patients with stable complete remission from those who would later suffer recurrent disease with a PPV of 100% and a NPV of 80% [67]. Because of the great heterogeneity of the various subtypes of lymphoma, it is not yet possible to transfer these findings to other subtypes.

As a rule, follow-up examinations should be performed using an intra-individually constant examination protocol. In particular, factors such as the blood glucose level and the time interval between application and commencing measurement are important parameters influencing the pattern of tracer uptake by the tumor.

References

[1] Ahmann DL, Kiely JM, Harrison EG et al. (1966) Malignant lymphoma of the spleen: a review of 49 cases in which the diagnosis was made at splenectomy. Cancer 19:461–469

[2] Arita T, Kuramitsu T, Kawamura M et al. (1995) Bronchogenic carcinoma: incidence of metastases to normal sized lymph nodes. Thorax 50:1267–1269

[3] Bagley CM, Roth JA, Thomas LB et al. (1972) The liver biopsy in Hodgkin's disease. Clinicopathologic correlation in 127 patients. Ann Int Med 76:219–225

[4] Bangerter M, Moog F (1998) Role of whole body FDG-PET in predicting relapse in residual masses after treatment of malignant lymphoma. Brit J Hematol 102 (abstr)

[5] Bangerter M, Kotzerke J, Griesshammer M et al. (1999) PET with 18-fluorodeoxyglucose in the staging and follow-up of lymphoma of the chest. Acta Oncol 38:799–804

[6] Bengel FM, Ziegler S, Avril N et al. (1997) Whole body PET in clinical oncology: comparison between attenuation-corrected and uncorrected images. Eur J Nucl Med 24:1091–1098

[7] Braams JW, Pruim J, Freling NJM et al. (1995) Detection of lymph node metastases of squamous-cell cancer of the head and neck with FDG-PET and MRI. J Nucl Med 36:211–216

[8] Braunstein EM, White SJ (1980) Non-Hodgkin lymphoma of bone. Radiology 135:59–63
[9] Bumann D, de Wit M, Beyer W et al. (1998) CT and F-18-FDG-PET in staging of malignant lymphoma. RöFo 168:457–465
[10] Carr R, Barrington SF, Madan B et al. (1998) Detection of lymphoma in bone marrow by whole-body positron emission tomography. Blood 91:3340–3346
[11] Castellino RA (1982) Imaging techniques for staging abdominal Hodgkin's disease. Cancer Treat Rep 66:697–700
[12] Castellino RA (1992) Diagnostic imaging studies in patients with newly diagnosed Hodgkińs disease. Annals of Oncology 3 (Suppl 4):45–47
[13] Castellino RA, Blank N, Hoppe RT et al. (1986) Hodgkin's disease: contribution of chest CT in the initial staging evaluation. Radiology 160:603–605
[14] Castellino RA, Hoppe R, Blank N et al. (1984) Computed tomography, lymphography, and staging laparatomy: correlations in initial staging of Hodgkin's disease. AJR 143:37–41
[15] Coller BS, Chabner BA, Gralnick HR et al. (1977) Frequencies and patterns of bone marrow involvement in non-Hodgkin lymphoma: observations on the value of bilateral biopsies. Am J Pathol 3:105–119
[16] De Wit M, Bumann D, Beyer W et al. (1997) Whole-body PET for diagnosis of residual mass in patients with lymphoma. Ann Oncol 8 Suppl 1:57–60
[17] Dimitrakopoulou-Strauss A, Strauss LG, Goldschmidt H et al. (1995) Evaluation of tumour metabolism and multidrug resistance in patients with treated malignant lymphomas. Eur J Nucl Med 22:434–442
[18] Dimitrakopoulou-Strauss A, Strauss LG, Goldschmidt H et al. (1997) Die Positronenemissionstomographie (PET) bei der Diagnostik und Therapieplanung von malignen Lymphomen. Radiologe 37:74–80
[19] Dorfman RE, Alpern MB, Gross BH et al. (1991) Upper abdominal lymph node size determined with CT. Radiology 180:319–322
[20] Edeiken-Monroe B, Edeiken J, Kim E (1990) Radiologic concepts of lymphoma of bone. Radiol Clin North Am 28:841–864
[21] Eichhorn T, Schroeder HG, Glatz H et al. (1987) Histologisch kontrollierter Vergleich von Palpation und Sonographie bei der Diagnose von Halslymphknotenmetastasen. Laryngol Rhinol Otol 66:266–274
[22] Einstein DM, Singer AA, Chilcote WA et al. (1991) Abdominal lymphadenopathy: spectrum of CT findings. RadioGraphics 11:457–472
[23] Ellis ME, Diehl LF, Granger E et al. (1989) Trephine needle bone marrow biopsy in the initial staging of Hodgkin's disease: sensitivity and specificity of the Ann Arbor staging procedure criteria. Am J Haematol 30:115–120
[24] Ferrant A, Rodhain J, Michaux JL et al. (1975) Detection of skeletal involvement in Hodgkin's disease: a comparison of radiography, bone scanning, and bone marrow biopsy in 38 patients. Cancer 35:1346–1353
[25] Fishman EK, Kuhlman LE, Jones RJ et al. (1991) CT of lymphoma: spectrum of disease. RadioGraphics 11:647–669
[26] Glatz S, Kotzerke J, Moog F et al. (1996) Vortäuschung eines mediastinalen Non-Hodgkin-Lymphomrezidivs durch diffuse Thymushyperplasie. RöFo 165:309–310
[27] Gross BH, Glatzer GM, Orringer MB et al. (1988) Bronchogenic carcinoma metastatic to normal-sized nodes: frequency and significance. Radiology 166:71–74
[28] Higashi K, Clavo A, Wahl RL (1993) Does FDG uptake measure proliferative activity of human cancer cells? In vitro comparison with DNA flow cytometry and tritiated thymidine uptake. J Nucl Med 34:414–419
[29] Hoane BR, Shields AF, Porter BA et al. (1991) Detection of lymphomatous bone marrow involvement with magnetic resonance imaging. Blood 78:728–738
[30] Hoekstra O, Ossenkoppele GJ, Golding R et al. (1993) Early treatment response in malignant lymphoma, as determined by planar fluorine-18-fluorodesoxyglucose scintigraphy. J Nucl Med 34:1706–1710

[31] Hoffman JM, Waskin HA, Hanson MW et al. (1993) FDG-PET in differentiating lymphoma from nonmalignant central nervous system lesions in patients with AIDS. J Nucl Med 34:567–575

[32] Hoh CK, Glaspy J, Rosen P et al. (1997) Whole-body FDG-PET imaging for staging of Hodgkin's disease and lymphoma. J Nucl Med 38:343–348

[33] Jabour BA, Choi Y, Hoh C et al. (1993) Extracranial head and neck: PET imaging with 2-(F^{18}-)fluoro-2-deoxy-glucose and MR imaging correlation. Radiology 186:27–35

[34] Jánoskuti L, Szilvási I, Papp G et al. (1988) Bone scanning and radiography in the evaluation of patients with malignant lymphoma. Fortschr Röntgenstr 149:427–428

[35] Jones DN, McCovage GB, Sostman HD et al. (1996) Monitoring of neoadjuvant therapy response of soft-tissue and muskuloskeletal sarcoma using F-18-FDG. J Nucl Med 37:1438–1444

[36] Kaplan HS (1973) Staging laparatomy and splenectomy in Hodgkin's disease: analysis of indications and patterns of involvement in 285 consecutive, unselected patients. Nat Canc Inst Monogr 36:291–298

[37] Kaplan HS (1980) Hodgkin's Disease, 2nd ed. Harvard University Press, Cambridge, MA

[38] Kotzerke J, Guhlmann A, Moog F et al. (1998) Role of attenuation correction for FDG-PET in the primary staging of malignant lymphoma. Eur J Nucl Med (in press)

[39] Kubota R, Yamada S, Ishiwata K et al. (1992) Intratumoral distribution of fluorine-18-fluorodeoxyglucose in vivo: high accumulation in macrophages and granulation tissues studied by microautoradiography. J Nucl Med 33:1972–1980

[40] Lapela M, Leskinen S, Minn H et al. (1995) Increased glucose metabolism in untreated non-Hodgkin's lymphoma: a study with positron emission tomography and fluorine-18-fluorodeoxyglucose. Blood 9:3522–3527

[41] Larcos G, Farlow DC, Antico VF et al. (1994) The role of high dose 67-gallium scintigraphy in staging of untreated patients with lymphoma. Aust N Z J Med 24:5–8

[42] Leibenhaut MH, Hoppe RT, Efron B et al. (1989) Prognostic indicators of laparatomy findings in clinical stage III supradiaphragmatic Hodgkin's disease. J Clin Oncol 7:81–91

[43] Leskinen-Kallio S, Ruotsalainen U, Någren K et al. (1991) Uptake of carbon-11-methionine and fluorodeoxyglucose in non-Hodgkin's lymphoma: a PET study. J Nucl Med 32:1211–1218

[44] Lowe VJ, Hoffman JM, DeLong DM et al. (1994) Semiquantitative and visual analysis of FDG-PET images in pulmonary abnormalities. J Nucl Med 35:1771–1777

[45] Mansfield C, Fabian C, Jones S et al. (1990) Comparison of lymphangiography and CT scanning in evaluating abdominal disease in stages III and IV Hodgkin's disease. Cancer 66:2295–2299

[46] McKenna RW, Hernandez JA (1988) Bone marrow in malignant lymphoma. Haematol/Oncol Clin North Am 2:617–635

[47] Moog F, Bangerter M, Diederichs C et al. (1997) Lymphoma: role of whole-body FDG-PET in nodal staging. Radiology 203:795–800

[48] Moog F, Bangerter M, Diederichs C et al. (1998) Detection of extranodal malignant lymphoma with PET using FDG: comparison with computed tomography. Radiology 206:475–481

[49] Moog F, Bangerter M, Kotzerke J et al. (1998) FDG-PET as a new approach to detect lymphomatous bone marrow. J Clin Oncol 16:603–609

[50] Moog F, Kotzerke J, Reske SN (1999) FDG PET can replace bone scintigraphy in primary staging of malignant lymphoma. J Nucl Med 40:1407–1413

[51] Munker R, Stengel A, Stäbler A et al. (1995) Diagnostic accuracy of US and CT in the staging of Hodgkin's disease. 76:1460–1466

[52] Newman JS, Francis IR, Kaminski MS et al. (1994) Imaging of lymphoma with PET with 2-(F-18)-fluoro-2-deoxy-d-glucose: correlation with CT. Radiology 190:111–116

[53] North LB, Fuller LM, Sullivan-Halley JA et al. (1987) Regression of mediastinal Hodgkin's disease after therapy: evaluation of time interval. Radiology 164:599–602

[54] North LB, Fuller LM (1982) Importance of initial mediastinal adenopathy in Hodgkin's disease. AJR 138:229–235

[55] O'Doherty MJ, Barrington SF, Campell M et al. (1997) PET scanning and the human immunodeficiency virus-positive patient. J Nucl Med 38:1575–1583

[56] Okada J, Yoshikawa K, Imazeki K et al. (1992) Positron emission tomography using fluorine-18-fluorodeoxy-glucose in malignant lymphoma: a comparison with proliferative activity. J Nucl Med 33:325–329

[57] Okada J, Oonishi I, Yoshikawa K et al. (1994) FDG-PET for the evaluation of tumor viability after anticancer therapy. Ann Nucl Med 8:109–113

[58] Orzel J, Sawaf NW, Richardson (1988) Lymphoma of the skeleton: scintigraphic evaluation. AJR 150:1095–1099

[59] Patz EF (1993) Focal pulmonary abnormalities: evaluation with F^{18}-fluorodeoxyglucose PET scanning. Radiology 188:487–490

[60] Pendlebury SC, Koutts J, Boyages J et al. (1994) Hodgkin's disease: clinical and radiological prognostic factors in a laparatomy series. Australasian Radiology 38:123–126

[61] Pond GD, Castellino RA, Horning S et al. (1989) Non-Hodgkin lymphoma: influence of lymphography, CT, and bone marrow biopsy on staging and management. Radiology 170:159–164

[62] Radford JA, Cowan RA, Flanagan M et al. (1988) The significance of residual mediastinal abnormality on the chest radiography following radiation therapy for Hodgkin's disease. J Clin Oncol 6:940–946

[63] Reske SN, Guhlmann A, Schirrmeister H et al (1998) PET in the diagnosis of abdominal tumors. Schweiz-Med-Wochenschr 128:96–108

[64] Rodriguez M (1998) CT, MRI, and PET in non-Hodgkin's lymphoma. Acta Radiol Suppl 417:1–36

[65] Rodriguez M, Rehn S, Ahlström H et al. (1995) Predicting malignancy grade with PET in non-Hodgkin's lymphoma. J Nucl Med 36:1790–1796

[66] Römer W, Hanauske AR, Ziegler S et al. (1998) PET in non-Hodgkin's lymphoma: assessment of chemotherapy with FDG. Blood 91:4464–4471

[67] Rosenberg SA, Berard CW, Brown BW et al. (1982) National Cancer Institute sponsored study of classification of non-Hodgkin's lymphomas: summary and description of a working formulation for clinical use. Cancer 49:2112–2135

[68] Schechter JP, Jones SE, Woolfenden JM et al. (1976) Bone scanning in lymphoma. Cancer 38:1142–1146

[69] Schirrmeister H (1998) Nachweis eines ossären Befalls beim Plasmozytom mit F-18-FDG-PET. Nuklearmedizin 37:43–82 (abstr)

[70] Shields AF, Porter BA, Churchley S et al. (1987) The detection of bone marrow involvement by lymphoma using magnetic resonance imaging. J Clin Oncol 5:225–230

[71] Shreve PD, Grossman HB, Gross MD et al. (1996) Metastatic prostate cancer: initial findings of PET with 2-deoxy-2-(F-18)fluoro-D-glucose. Radiology 199:751–756

[72] Skillings JR, Bramwell V, Nicholson RL et al. (1991) A prospective study of MRI in lymphoma staging. Cancer 67:1838–1843

[73] Skovsgaard T, Brinckmeyer M, Vesterager L et al. (1982) The liver in Hodgkin's disease-II. Histopathologic findings. Eur J Cancer Clin Oncol 18:429–435

[74] Specht L (1992) Tumor burden as the main indicator of prognosis in Hodgkin's disease. Eur J Cancer 12:1982–1985

[75] Taylor IK, Hill AA, Hayes M et al. (1996) Imaging allergen-invoked airway inflammation in atopic asthma with [^{18}F]-fluorodeoxyglucose and positron emission tomography. Lancet 347:937–940

[76] Tesoro-Tess JD, Balzarini L, Ceglia E et al. (1991) Magnetic resonance imaging in the initial staging of Hodgkin's disease and non-Hodgkin lymphoma. Eur J Rad 12:81–90

[77] Thill R, Neuerburg J, Fabry U et al. (1997) Comparison of findings with F-18-FDG PET and CT in pretherapeutic staging of malignant lymphoma. Nuklearmedizin 36:234–239

[78] Vesselle HJ, Miraldi FD (1998) FDG PET of the retroperitoneum: normal anatomy, variants, pathologic conditions, and strategies to avoid diagnostic pitfalls. RadioGraphics 18:805–823
[79] Villringer K, Jager H, Dichgans M et al. (1995) Differential diagnosis of CNS lesions in AIDS patients by FDG-PET. J Comput Assist Tomogr 19:532–536
[80] Wahl RL, Zasadny K, Helvie M et al. (1993) Metabolic monitoring of breast cancer chemohormonotherapy using PET: initial evaluation. J Clin Oncol 11:2101–2107
[81] Weidmann E, Baican B, Hertel A et al. (1999) PET for staging and evaluation of response to treatment in patients with Hodgkin's disease. Leuc and Lymph 34:545–551
[82] Weissleder R, Elizondo G, Stark DD et al. (1989) The diagnosis of splenic lymphoma by MR imaging: value of supraparamagnetic iron oxide. AJR 152:175–180
[83] Widding A, Smolorz J, Franke M et al. (1989) Bone marrow investigation with technetium-99m microcolloid and magnetic resonance imaging in patients with malignant myelolympho-proliferative diseases. J Nucl Med 15:230–238
[84] Zasadny K, Wahl RL (1993) Standardized uptake values of normal tissues at PET with 2-(fluorine-18)-fluoro-2-deoxy-D-glucose: variations with body weight and a method for correction. Radiology 189:847–850

21 Testicular cancer

M. Reinhardt

21.1 Incidence, etiology, epidemiology

With an incidence of 3.7 per 100000 males, testicular cancer (TC) is a rare disease. Each year 5500 new cases can be expected in the US. TC is the most frequent malignant disease of 20 to 34 year old men (42% of all malignant tumors in this age group in Germany); 70% of patients are 20 to 40 years old. The peak incidence of nonseminomatous TC is at the age of 28 years, whereas the peak incidence of seminomas is from 35 to 39 years of age.

The incidence of TC varies between different ethnic groups and countries (American white 4, American black 1, Chinese 0.4, African black 0.3 per 100000 males). These variations are interpreted to be due to genetic or ethnic differences. The incidence of TC increases with higher social status and declines from town to countryside. This indicates a socioeconomic influence. Proven risk factors are cryptorchidism, Caucasian race and unilateral TC. Multiple other possible risk factors have been discussed, such as urogenital abnormalities, testicular atrophy, mumps associated atrophy, genetic factors, low birth weight, inguinal hernias and high social state [20].

21.2 Histology

Different benign and malignant tumors can arise from testicular tissue. Typical tumors are germ cell tumors that originate from totipotential germ cells that are thought to undergo malignant transformation. The histological classification of testicular tumors is of high therapeutic and prognostic value.

Seminomas are the most frequent testicular tumors (40%). Testicular tumors with other histologies are summarized in the group of nonseminomatous germ cell tumors (NSGCT) because of similar clinical, therapeutical and prognostic criteria. The most frequent NSGCT are embryonal carcinomas, teratocarcinomas, teratomas and pure choriocarcinomas. Combined histological patterns are frequent (15%). Teratomas exist in different degrees of differentiation: mature teratomas show a high differentiation with organ-like histology and immature teratomas are undifferentiated [20, 26].

21.3 Metastases

At the time of diagnosis only 49% of patients present with TC limited to the testes, 38% of patients already show regional lymph node metastases, and 13% distant metastases. Of patients with seminomas 30% have metastases at the time of primary diagnosis, whereas 70% of patients with NSGCT show metastatic disease. Regional lymph nodes of the testes are the retroperitoneal lymph nodes due to testicular embryology. As a consequence 75% of patients with lymph node metastases have metastases in the paraaortal lymph nodes, 15% in the iliac lymph nodes. Distant metastases are most frequently found in the lung (60% of cases) followed by hepatic, pleural, and cerebral metastases [21].

21.4 Clinical staging

The TNM system describes the primary tumor (T), the staging of the lymph nodes (N) and possible distant metastases (M). The disadvantage of the TNM system is the limited consideration of treatment strategies and prognosis. Most clinical staging systems are modifications of the system proposed by Boden and Gibb in 1951, which defines three stages: stage I, tumor limited to the testis; stage II, tumor extension beyond the testis, but contained within the regional lymph nodes; stage III, spread beyond the regional lymph nodes. The Lugano staging system [3] is a widely accepted modification of the Boden/Gibb staging system. The advantage of the Lugano staging system is that distant metastases and pulmonary tumor mass that significantly influence prognosis are taken into consideration (Table 21.1).

Table 21.1. Lugano staging system

I	**No metastases**	
I A	Tumor limited to testis	
I B	Tumor with infiltration of the epididymis or in cryptorchidism	
I C	Tumor infiltrates scrotum or was resected transscrotally or rose after inguinal or scrotal surgery	
I X	Extent of the primary tumor can not be determined	
II	**Infradiaphragmatic lymph node metastases**	
II A	All lymph nodes <2 cm	
II B	At least 1 lymph node 2-5 cm	
II C	Retroperitoneal lymph nodes >5 cm	
II D	Palpable abdominal tumor or fixed inguinal tumor	
III	**Mediastinal or supraclavicular lymph node metastases, distant metastases**	
III A	Mediastinal and / or supraclavicular lymph node metastases (no distant metastases)	
III B	Lung metastases	
	minimal pulmonary disease:	less than 5 nodules per lung <2 cm
	advanced pulmonary disease:	more than 5 nodules per lung or 1 pulmonary nodule >2 cm or pleural effusion
III C	Extrapulmonary distant metastases	
III D	Persistent tumor markers after orchiectomy without detectable metastases	

21.5 Diagnosis and therapy

21.5.1 Primary tumor

Most primary tumors are recognized by palpation. Ultrasonography is used to identify not palpable testicular tumors. In suspicious cases surgical exploration of the testis is necessary. The tumor and testis are removed by unilateral radical or inguinal orchiectomy to provide histological diagnosis with local staging information (pT category) and allows local control of the disease in nearly 100% of patients [10].

21.5.2 Staging of metastases

Besides clinical examination with palpation of the abdomen and lymph node sites, chest x-rays, abdominal CT, chest CT and tumor markers are recommended for staging. Pedal lymphangiography and intravenous urography were replaced by abdominal CT due to high error rates. The new diagnostic method FDG-PET will be discussed below. Staging is usually carried out after surgical removal of the primary tumor with histological diagnosis. Restaging is undertaken after chemotherapy or radiation therapy.

21.5.3 Abdominal CT

Abdominal CT and chest CT are used for staging of retroperitoneal, retrocrural and mediastinal lymph nodes and for evaluation of liver and lung. Whereas the chest CT is very sensitive for the evaluation of lungs and pleura, the accuracy of abdominal CT for the evaluation of retroperitoneal lymph nodes is limited. The accuracy of abdominal CT depends on the size of the enlarged lymph nodes [24]. If lymph nodes with diameters above 5 mm in the abdominal CT are diagnosed as metastases, the sensitivity is 88%, but the specificity is only 44%. At a minimum diameter of 15 mm, the sensitivity decreases to 58% but specificity increases to 76%. At retroperitoneal lymph node diameters above 25 mm, the specificity of abdominal CT is close to 100%, but the sensitivity is as low as 33%. Even newer generation CT scanners generation with higher resolution show false-negative results in 33% of patients with testicular cancers in clinical stage I [5]. The consequence of a false-positive abdominal CT scan will be overtreatment of the patient with unnecessary retroperitoneal lymph node dissection or chemotherapy. A false-negative CT scan may cause insufficient therapy.

21.5.4 Tumor markers

Alpha-fetoprotein (AFP), human chorionic gonadotropin (β-hCG), lactic acid dehydrogenase (LDH) and placental alkaline phosphatase (PLAP) are tumor markers with diagnostic relevance in TC. In nonseminomatous TC, AFP and β-hCG are the most important markers. The sensitivity of tumor markers for detection of metastases depends on the size of the metastases. For metastases with diameters below 2 cm, the sensitivities of AFP and β-hCG are 44% and 23%, respectively, if the primary tumor is marker positive [2]. Negative tumor markers do not exclude viable tumor tissue or metastases. Additionally, LDH and PLAP are applied in seminomas. LDH is used as an unspecific tumor marker for monitoring therapeutic response and follow-up in advanced seminomas [8].

21.5.5 Retroperitoneal lymph node dissection

Patients with NSGCT in clinical stages I and II A/B undergo a retroperitoneal lymph node dissection (RPLND) after orchiectomy. In clinical stage I a diagnostic RPLND is necessary because 17 to 38% of patients have retroperitoneal metastases even though clinical staging is negative [7, 22]. Only in patients with a low risk of metastases or relapse has a surveillance therapy without diagnostic RPLND been proposed. In more advanced NSGCT, the RPLND is made after two to four cycles of combination chemotherapy for restaging and removal of residual retroperitoneal tumor masses [20].

In most cases the modified RPLND, which protects the sympathetic chains, is the procedure of choice because of the better preservation of ejaculation function as compared to the standard techniques [6].

21.5.6 Therapy

21.5.6.1 Seminoma

In stages I, II A and II B standard therapy is primary infradiaphragmatic radiation therapy that covers the inguinal, iliac and paraaortic lymphatics [26]. An alternative therapeutic regimen in clinical stage I is chemotherapy with Carboplatin [13]. In advanced seminomas, patients receive combination chemotherapy [9].

21.5.6.2 Nonseminomatous germ cell tumors (NSGCT)

In clinical stage I, patients with a negative RPLND histology are observed without additional therapy. An alternative is a surveillance strategy without

RPLND and careful follow-up [14]. Standard therapy for patients with NSGCT in clinical stages II A/B is a RPLND followed by chemotherapy [27]. Alternatively chemotherapy can be given first followed by a RPLND to remove residual retroperitoneal tumor [15]. In more advanced NSGCT (stages II C, II D and III) patients receive chemotherapy first and the RPLND is made afterwards for restaging and removal of residual retroperitoneal tumor masses. For patients with pulmonary metastasis alone and complete remission after chemotherapy, surveillance without RPLND is possible but these patients have to be followed carefully because of an increased risk for relapse [20].

21.6 Prognosis

Most patients with testicular tumors have a good prognosis due to good tumor response to chemotherapy and radiation therapy. Risk factors for a bad prognosis are large lymph node metastases, existence of distant metastases and excessive tumor marker levels. Patients with a good prognosis achieve complete remissions in 98 to 100%. This is reduced to 55 to 86% for patients in the poor prognosis category [26].

21.7 Positron emission tomography

21.7.1 Radiopharmacy

PET studies of patients with testicular cancers have been published by several groups. In nearly all studies [^{18}F]FDG has been used. There is enough data to judge the diagnostic potential of FDG-PET in testicular cancers. Little data based on other radiopharmaceuticals, for example [^{11}C]thymidine, is available and not conclusive.

21.7.2 Methods

After at least 5 hours fasting to achieve plasma glucose levels below 100 mg/dl [^{18}F]FDG (185–370 MBq depending on the PET scanner) is injected intravenously. Due to suppression of tumor glucose metabolism by chemotherapy the PET scan should be done before the start of chemotherapy or in case of follow-up after chemotherapy as late as possible after the last chemotherapy (own unpublished data and [4].) Emission data is measured 40 min to 90 min after injection of [^{18}F]FDG. Later measurements are possible because the tumor to background ratio improves with time, even though the measurement time must be longer because of the decay of FDG. Usually emission data is corrected for attenuation by transmission data that is measured in a transmission scan. Whole-body scans are indicated in advanced stages if metastases are expected at sites other than the retroperitoneal lymph nodes. Iterative image reconstruction is preferred to image reconstruction by filtered backprojection because of better image quality, and fewer artifacts, especially in the lower urinary tract, can be achieved with the latter method. Semiquantitative estimation of FDG uptake in tumor tissue by calculation of the SUV (*s*tandardized *u*ptake *v*alue) allows comparisons of tumor glucose metabolism and follow-up during chemotherapy. Attenuation correction of emission data is essential for the estimation of tumor SUV.

21.7.3 Indications for FDG-PET in testicular cancer

In testicular cancers there are several possible applications for FDG-PET:

- Diagnosis of the primary tumor
- Staging at time of diagnosis
- Therapy control during chemotherapy
- Restaging after chemotherapy
- Staging at relapse
- Follow-up

Due to different biological behavior, prognostic factors and therapies of seminomas and NSGCTs, the FDG-PET indications for the two tumor groups are discussed separately. Most publications dealing with FDG-PET in TC present very limited patient numbers and lack precise data about clinical stage and clinical course. The data presented in this chapter are mostly unpublished data from our group. We made a prospective study to analyze the diagnostic potential of FDG-PET in TC that was supported by the "Deutsche Krebshilfe", Bonn. A total of 72 patients with TC were examined during 1992 and 1998 in this study. Multicenter studies with larger numbers are still in progress.

21.7.3.1 Evaluation of the primary tumor

The testis of patients with suspected TC is usually evaluated surgically and a histological diagnosis is obtained. Thus, in only a few cases is an examination of the testis by FDG-PET possible. The differentiation of inflammations of testis or epididymis and TC by FDG-PET is not promising because FDG is also accumulated in inflammations.

21.7.3.2 Staging at time of diagnosis

Seminomas

We examined the largest patient group with seminomas by FDG-PET so far, a group of 26 patients [11]. In 21 patients with clinical stage I, FDG-PET and abdominal CT showed no indications of metastases. A correlation with histology was not possible in these patients because they received radiation therapy or monochemotherapy with carboplatin and the retroperitoneal lymph nodes were not resected. In the follow-up (2 to 72 months), these 21 patients in stage I remained free of relapse of metastases. Five patients were in clinical stage II because of enlarged retroperitoneal lymph nodes in the abdominal CT. In 4/5 patients, FDG-PET showed retroperitoneal lesions that also indicated for metastases. One patient with a retroperitoneal mass (diameter 6 cm) at the time of diagnosis, interpreted to be a metastasis of the seminoma, had a normal FDG-PET scan. The retroperitoneal mass remained unchanged during chemotherapy and turned out to be a benign tumor not originating from the testes (histology: ganglioneuroma), so FDG-PET was truly negative. Other studies show similar results, but patient groups are smaller [4]. FDG-PET in high grade seminomas has been reported only in few single cases.

The data does not prove an advantage of using FDG-PET over abdominal CT in staging retroperitoneal lymph nodes in seminomas with clinical stage I and II, but in stage II a more accurate characterization of a retroperitoneal mass by FDG-PET may be possible.

Nonseminomatous germ cell tumors (NSGCT)

We studied 28 patients with NSGCT in clinical stage I, II and III by FDG-PET at the time of diagnosis of the primary tumor. In 17/28 patients, FDG-PET detected retroperitoneal foci with increased FDG uptake (2.9 to 14.1 SUV) that indicated metastases, whereas abdominal CT showed enlarged lymph nodes only in 13/28 patients. In 7 patients in clinical stage I, correlation of FDG-PET, CT and histology was possible because retroperitoneal lymph nodes were resected by primary RPLND. Micrometastases were found in 6/7 patients, only one patient was free of metastases. FDG-PET detected metastatic foci in 2/6 patients with micrometastases and was true negative in the patient without metastases, but was false negative in four other patients. CT was false negative in all 6/7 patients in clinical stage I failing to detect any of the micrometastases. Similar results have been reported recently [1, 4]. Cremerius et al. postulate a higher accuracy for FDG-PET as compared to CT in clinical stage I.

The data show that FDG-PET is more accurate than abdominal CT for staging of retroperitoneal lymph nodes in patients with NSGCT at the time of diagnosis due to its better sensitivity.

21.7.3.3 Therapy control during chemotherapy

Patients with seminomas in clinical stage III and NSGCT in stages II and III receive chemotherapy. Monitoring of chemotherapy by CT is difficult because of persistent or even growing metastatic masses. In cases with marker negative tumors, monitoring by tumor markers is not possible and an additional biological indicator of tumor response to chemotherapy besides CT is desirable. Measurement of FDG uptake in tumor tissue by FDG-PET could become an additional indicator of tumor response. Because chemotherapy significantly suppresses tumor glucose metabolism, a baseline FDG-PET has to be made prior to chemotherapy and follow-up scans should be as late as possible after the last application of chemotherapy. FDG-PET has to be corrected for attenuation to allow calculation of SUV for estimation of tumor response to chemotherapy.

We examined 13 patients with retroperitoneal metastases from TC before and after chemotherapy by FDG-PET. Scans after chemotherapy were acquired at least 21 days after the last application of chemotherapeutics. All 13 patients showed increased FDG uptakes in the metastases before therapy (3.4–14.1 SUV). After chemotherapy FDG uptake was normal in 12/13 patients. In one patient with an increased FDG uptake before chemotherapy (12.3 SUV), a small focus was found after chemotherapy (3.3 SUV) and interpreted as residual malignant tumor tissue (Fig. 21.1). Similar observations have been reported for other tumors as well [16]. These results show that FDG-PET is promising as an additional indicator of tumor response. Especially in cases where other means are not able to estimate therapeutic effect, for example, large residual tumors after chemotherapy or in growing teratomas (Fig. 21.2), additional data from FDG-PET can be of great clinical impor-

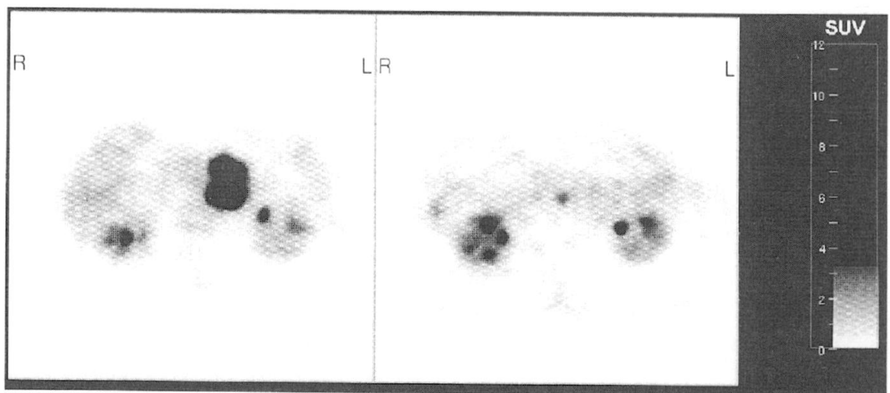

Fig. 21.1. FDG-PET in nonseminomatous testicular cancer before (left) and after (right) chemotherapy. Before chemotherapy, FDG uptake is increased up to 12.2 SUV in the large retroperitoneal tumor mass. After chemotherapy FDG uptake is reduced; only a small focus with a slightly increased FDG uptake of 3.3 SUV remains. Histology revealed an inflammatory lymph node but no residual tumor cells.

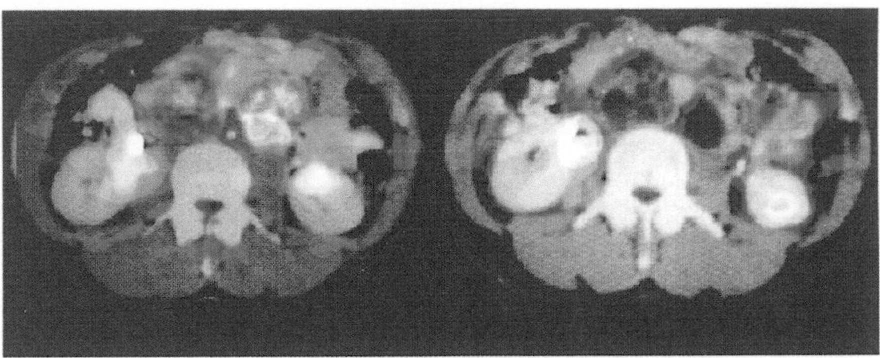

Fig. 21.2. Overlay of FDG-PET (color) and CT (black and white) of a mixed testicular tumor before (left) and after (right) chemotherapy. Before chemotherapy a bulky paraaortal tumor mass is found with irregular x-ray absorption in CT. In FDG-PET the mass shows inhomogeneous FDG uptake with areas of FDG uptake increased up to 10.7 SUV and regions without any FDG uptake. After chemotherapy the tumor mass has grown, but FDG-PET shows normalization of FDG uptake to the value at the background level. A pure mature teratoma was found at histology.

tance. FDG-PET may help to decide whether a second line chemotherapy or the resection of a residual tumor mass is required [17].

21.7.3.4 Restaging after chemotherapy

After chemotherapy about one third of patients have residual retroperitoneal masses in the abdominal CT. The potential of CT for differentiation of necrosis and viable tumor is limited. On the other hand, relatively often viable tumor tissue is found in retroperitoneal lymph nodes at RPLND in NSGCT cases in stage II with negative abdominal CT after chemotherapy [25]. With more accurate restaging methods, unnecessary surgery or chemotherapy could be avoided. We examined 19 patients with TC in stages II and III after chemotherapy by FDG-PET and CT to study whether FDG-PET is superior to CT for restaging. All patients received RPLND after imaging. FDG-PET, CT and histology were correlated [18]. In six patients with NSGCT, mature teratomas without any undifferentiated tumor tissue were found at RPLND. FDG-PET was negative in all six patients whereas CT showed retroperitoneal masses indicative of metastases in 2/6 patients (max. diameters 3 cm and 11 cm) and negative or inconclusive results in the other four patients with teratomas. In one patient with a micrometastasis of an embryonal cell carcinoma (max. diameter 4 mm), FDG-PET was negative and CT inconclusive. One patient with an inflammatory lymph node but free of metastases by histology had false-positive CT and FDG-PET scans consisting of an enlarged lymph node with increased FDG uptake (3.3 SUV) that was indicative of a metastasis (Fig. 21.1). In 10/11 patients that were free of metastases by histology, FDG-PET was true negative whereas CT was true negative in only 7/11 patients and inconclusive in 3 patients. A study from Stephens et al. [23] reported similar results in 30 patients with NSGCT. Mature teratomas found at histology in 15 patients were not detected by FDG-PET due to their low FDG uptake. A false-positive FDG-PET during post-chemotherapy restaging of TC caused by inflammatory lymph nodes has been observed [12].

It is concluded that FDG-PET is more accurate than CT for restaging of TC after chemotherapy and should be applied. Because mature teratomas and micrometastases are not detected safely, FDG-PET can not replace resection of residual retroperitoneal tumor masses. FDG-PET should be applied to differentiate residual viable tumor requiring additional chemotherapy from necrosis or mature teratoma requiring surgical resection or follow-up. In cases with increased surgical risk, FDG-PET may also be helpful. TC patients free of residual tumor masses and with negative tumor markers after chemotherapy are not recommended for FDG-PET because data shows no advantage over CT.

21.7.3.5 Diagnosis and staging at relapse

Few FDG-PET scans have been reported for patients suffering a relapse of TC [4]. We examined a recurrent seminoma with increased FDG uptake (10.7 SUV). In suspected relapse (for example, elevated tumor markers) with unknown localization whole-body FDG-PET is promising for tumor localization. This is particularly the case where chemotherapy is undesirable and local therapy (surgery or radiation therapy) is the treatment of choice. In this case accurate staging of the entire body is useful. However, the accuracy of whole-body FDG-PET in cases of tumor relapse remains to be evaluated by further studies.

21.7.3.6 Follow-up

Follow-up in TC includes physical examination, tumor markers and CT. FDG-PET is a promising tool, but prospective clinical studies have not yet been published. Radiation dose is not a problem because 370 MBq FDG results in an exposure of 8–10 mSv, which is significantly less than an abdominal CT (20 mSv). Replacement of CT scans by FDG-PET could reduce radiation dose, especially in patients under a surveillance strategy (stage I) or at high tumor grades who receive abdominal CTs every 2–6 months. It is likely that FDG-PET will be mainly applied due to high costs in patients with a high risk of tumor relapse. Further studies have to establish when FDG-PET is of benefit in the follow-up of TC.

21.8 Conclusions

FDG-PET is an accurate diagnostic tool for detection of testicular tumor tissue. Mature teratomas are not visualized due to their low glucose metabolism. Because chemotherapy suppresses FDG uptake in TC, FDG-PET has to take place before or as late as possible after chemotherapy.

According to the presented data, FDG-PET in TC is indicated in the following clinical settings:

- staging of metastases at primary diagnosis in nonseminomatous testicular cancers
- control of tumor response to chemotherapy
- evaluation of residual tumor masses after chemotherapy

Future studies will show whether additional applications for FDG-PET in TC exist, for example, staging of retroperitoneal lymph nodes in seminomas, staging at tumor relapse or in the follow-up [19].

21.9 Recommendations for performing FDG-PET and interpretation

- Patient preparation: Overnight fast, at least for 5 h, plasma glucose < 100 mg/dl.
- Data acquisition: Emission scans start 30 min after injection of 185–370 MBq [^{18}F]FDG (depending on sensitivity of the PET camera). Measurement of the abdomen (groin to diaphragm) and regions suspicious for metastases, whole-body scan in advanced tumor stages.
- Attenuation correction: Measurement of transmission scans for attenuation correction of emission data because of inhomogeneous attenuation in abdomen and thorax is mandatory.
- Image reconstruction: Iterative reconstruction is preferred to filtered backprojection because of higher image quality.
- Quantification: Semiquantitative analysis with calculation of SUV (standardized uptake value) to reduce influence of body weight and injected FDG dose. Sampling of blood for determination of input function to allow quantification of glucose metabolism is not necessary in clinical setting.
- Image interpretation: Foci with FDG uptake above 2.5 SUV are suspicious for metastases. Problem: increased FDG concentration in urinary tract and bowels, especially the ureters may cause misinterpretations.

References

[1] Albers P, Bender H, Yilmaz H, et al. (1999) Positron emission tomography in the clinical staging of patients with stage I and II testicular germ cell tumors. Urology 53:808–811

[2] Bussar-Maatz R, Weißbach L (1993) Retroperitoneal lymph node staging of testicular tumours. TNM study group. Br J Urol 72:234–240

[3] Cavalli F, Monfardini S, Pizzocaro G (1980) Report on the international workshop on staging and treatment of testicular cancer. Eur J Cancer 16:1367–1372

[4] Cremerius U, Effert PJ, Adam G, et al. (1998) FDG PET for detection and therapy control of metastatic germ cell cancer. J Nucl Med 39:815–822

[5] Fernandez EB, Moul JW, Foley JP, et al. (1994) Retroperitoneal imaging with third and fourth generation computed axial tomography in clinical stage 1 nonseminomatous germ cell tumors. Urology 44:548–552

[6] Hartlapp JH, Weißbach L (1988) Therapie nichtseminomatöser Hodentumoren im Stadium IIA/B: Lymphadenektomie ± adjuvante Chemotherapie vs. primäre Chemotherapie. In: Schmoll HJ, Weißbach L (eds) Diagnostik und Therapie von Hodentumoren. Springer, Berlin Heidelberg New York, pp 179–187

[7] Klepp O (1989) Risk indicators in stage I testicular teratoma. Lancet II:506

[8] Lippert MC, Javadpour N (1981) Lactic dehydrogenase in the monitoring and prognosis of testicular cancer. Cancer 48:2274–2278

[9] Loehrer PJ, Elson P, Williams SD, et al. (1987) Chemotherapy in metastatic seminoma: the Southeastern Cancer Study Group experience. J Clin Oncol 5:1212–1220

[10] Morse MJ, Whitmore WF (1984) Neoplasms of the testis. In: Walsh PC, Gittes RF, Perlmutter AD, et al. (eds) Campbell's Urology. Saunders Company, Philadelphia, pp 1535–1582

[11] Müller-Mattheis V, Reinhardt M, Gerharz CD (1998) Die Bedeutung der Positronenemissionstomographie mit [18F]-2-fluoro-2-deoxy-D-glukose (18FDG-PET) bei der Diagnostik retroperitonealer Lymphknotenmetastasen von Hodentumoren. Kann die Staging-RLA in Zukunft durch 18FDG-PET ersetzt werden? Urologe [A] 37:609–620

[12] Nuutinen JM, Leskinen S, Elmoaa I, et al. (1997) Detection of residual tumours in postchemotherapy testicular cancer by FDG-PET. Eur J Cancer 33:1234–1241

[13] Oliver RTD (1989) Alternatives to radiotherapy in patients with seminoma. Proc ECCO 5:No P-0836

[14] Peckham MJ, Brada M (1987) Surveillance following orchiectomy for stage I testicular cancer. In J Androl 10:247

[15] Peckham MJ, Hendry WF (1985) Clinical stage II non-seminomatous germ cell testicular tumors. Results of management by primary chemotherapy. Br J Urol 57:763–768

[16] Price P, Jones T (1995) Can positron emission tomography (PET) be used to detect subclinical response to cancer therapy? Eur J Cancer 31A:1924–1927

[17] Reinhardt MJ, Müller-Mattheis VG, Gerharz CD, et al. (1997) FDG-PET evaluation of retroperitoneal metastases of testicular cancer before and after chemotherapy. J Nucl Med 38:99–101

[18] Reinhardt MJ, Müller-Mattheis VG, Waltemath HG, et al. (1998) Staging of retroperitoneal lymph nodes in nonseminomatous germ cell cancer by FDG-PET. Eur J Nucl Med 25:943 (abstr)

[19] Reske SN (1998) Positronen-Emissions-Tomographie in der Onkologie. Dt Ärzteblatt 95:B1495–B1497

[20] Richie JP (1992) Neoplasms of the testis. In: Walsh PC, Retik AB, Stamey TA Vaughan ED (eds) Campbell's Urology. Saunders Company, Philadelphia, pp 1222–1263

[21] Schultz HP, Arends J, Barblebo H, et al. (1984) Testicular carcinoma in Denmark 1986–1980. Stage and selected clinical parameters at presentation. Acta Radiol Oncol 23:249–253

[22] Seppelt U (1988) Validierung verschiedener diagnostischer Methoden zur Beurteilung des Lymphknotenstatus. In: Weißbach L, Bussar-Maatz R (eds) Die Diagnostik des Hodentumors und seiner Metastasen. Karger, Basel, pp 154–169

[23] Stephens AW, Gonin R, Hutchins GD, et al. (1996) Positron emission tomography evaluation of residual radiographic abnormalities in postchemotherapy germ cell tumor patients. J Clin Oncol 14:1637–1641

[24] Stomper PC, Fung CY, Socinski MA, et al. (1987) Detection of retroperitoneal metastases in early-stage nonseminomatous testicular cancer: analysis of different CT criteria. Am J Rad 149:1187–1190

[25] Stomper PC, Kalish LA, Garnick MB, et al. (1991) CT and pathologic predictive features of residual mass histologic findings after chemotherapy for nonseminomatous germ cell tumors: can residual malignancy or teratoma be excluded? Radiology 180:711–714

[26] Weißbach L, Bussar-Maatz R (1994) Hodentumoren. In: Rübben H (ed) Uro-Onkologie. Springer, Berlin Heidelberg New York London Paris Tokyo Hongkong Barcelona Budapest, pp 275–359

[27] Weißbach L, Hartlapp JH (1991) Adjuvant chemotherapy of metastatic stage II nonseminomatous testis tumor. J Urol 146:1295–1298

22 Prostate cancer

N. Avril, W. Weber, J. Breul

22.1 Incidence and etiology

The normal adult prostate weighs approximately 20 grams, is located below the base of the bladder and transversed by the first portion of the urethra. The prostate has three anatomic regions, an inner periurethral zone (transition zone) composed of short glands, the central zone located around the ejaculatory ducts and an outer peripheral zone composed of longer, branched glands. Prostatic carcinoma may occur anywhere in the prostate but has a predilection for the peripheral zone. It presents with variable biological behavior and may persist for long periods without causing significant problems [3]. Carcinoma of the prostate is extremely common in men in the western countries with approximately 317000 newly diagnosed cases in the United States in 1996 and more than 33000 cancer-related deaths [1]. The disease is rare before the age of 40, but the incidence subsequently increases in aging men [18]. Autopsy results show that prostate cancer is found in about 30% of men at the age of 50 and in approximately 60–70% at the age of 70 years. It is important to note that only about one third are clinically manifest [29]. The US has nearly 17.5 deaths per 100,000 men per year compared with 22 for Sweden and 3.7 for Japan. However, Japanese immigrants to the US develop prostatic cancer in the next generation at a frequency similar to other men in that country, supporting the influence of environmental factors. Some studies have shown a relationship between fat intake or being overweight and the development of prostate cancer, and the protective effect of fruits and green or yellow vegetables has been described [4].

22.2 Histopathology

Adenocarcinomas account for the majority (> 95%) of prostate cancer. Pathologically, adenocarcinomas originate from the prostatic acini and are frequently multifocal. The remaining tumors consist of squamous cell carcinomas, transitional cell carcinomas, undifferentiated carcinomas and sarcomas [5]. Development of benign prostatic hyperplasia (BPH) occurs in the majority of men over 50 years. With increasing frequency more than 90% of men have BPH by the age of 80 at autopsy. Histology shows nodular hyperplasia of prostate tissue composed of varying amounts of glandular epithelium, stroma and smooth muscle. BPH typically occurs within the transition zone and, therefore, accounts for the most common cause of obstruction to urinary outflow in men. Prostatic intraepithelial neoplasia (PIN) found in the peripheral zone has been identified as the most likely preinvasive stage of adenocarcinoma [2, 14]. It is present in up to 16.5% of cases undergoing needle biopsies. Microscopic findings are dysplastic tissue mimicking cancer, including nuclear and nucleolar enlargement. Low grade PIN has no clinical consequence, whereas high grade PIN is often associated with invasive cancer, occurring in about 80% of patients under 60 and about 50% in older patients [29]. Identification of high grade PIN in biopsy specimens justifies further search for concurrent invasive carcinoma, including close surveillance and follow-up biopsies.

Clinically manifest prostate cancer is either palpable in digital rectal examination and confined or unconfined to the organ or detected by elevated serum prostate-specific antigen (PSA) level. *Incidental, non-palpable prostate cancer* is found by histological tissue analysis after surgery for apparently benign prostatic hyperplasia. *Occult prostate cancer* presents with metastases while the primary tumor may not be detected. *Latent prostate cancer* is very common but clinically unapparent during a person's life time and only found at autopsy. Prostate cancer often shows wide morphologic heterogeneity within tumor specimens including cellular size, nuclear shape and glandular differentiation. The histologic grade of prostate cancer is important for prognosis and subsequent aggressiveness of treatment. The most poorly differentiated area of the tumor appears to determine the biologic behavior. To address differences in histopathological appearance, the Gleason grading scheme is commonly used assigning the glandular histologic patterns to numbers between 1 (best differentiated) and 5 (least differentiated). These numbers are summed providing a score ranging from 2 to 10 for each tumor [8]. Combining such grading with the clinical stage of disease correlates with the course of disease and with patient survival [9]. All information available prior to the first definitive treatment may be used for clinical staging. Primary tumor assessment includes digital rectal examination of the prostate, transrectal ultrasound (TRUS) and cytologic or histologic tissue analysis. Histopathology following total prostatovesiculectomy, including regional lymph node specimens, are required for pathologic TNM classification [26]. All clinically unapparent tumors that are not palpable and not visible by anatomical imaging procedures are classified as T1. Stage T1a includes incidental histologic findings of prostate cancer accounting for 5% or less of tissue resected and T1b for more than 5%. Nonpalpable tumor found in one or both lobes by needle biopsy performed due to elevated PSA level is classified as T1c. This tumor stage gains increasing clinical relevance by PSA screening. Tumor confined within the prostate is classified as T2 and invasion beyond the prostatic capsule is classified as T3.

The treatment of prostate cancer is predicated largely on the stage of disease (Table 22.1 and 22.2), emphasizing the need for accurate staging. The

Table 22.1. Clinical TNM classification (only adenocarcinoma).

Tx	Primary tumor cannot be assessed
T0	No evidence of primary tumor
T1	**Clinically inapparent tumor (not palpable nor visible by imaging)**
T1a	Tumor incidental histologic finding < 5% of tissue resected
T1b	Tumor incidental histologic finding > 5% of tissue resected
T1c	Tumor identified by needle biopsy
T2	**Tumor confined within the prostate**
T2a	Tumor involves one lobe
T2b	Tumor involves both lobes
T3	**Tumor extends through the prostate capsule***
T3a	Extracapsular extension without infiltration of the seminal vesicle(s)
T3b	Tumor invades seminal vesicle(s)
T4	**Tumor is fixed or invades adjacent structures other than seminal vesicle(s)**

* Invasion into the prostatic apex or into (but not beyond) the prostatic capsule is classified as T2

Table 22.2. Pathologic TNM classification (only adenocarcinoma).

Primary tumor (pT)	
	There is no pathologic T1 classification
pT2	**Tumor confined to the prostate**
pT2a	Unilateral (tumor involves one lobe)
pT2b	Bilateral (tumor involves both lobes)
pT3	**Extraprostatic extension**
pT3a	Extracapsular extension without infiltration of the seminal vesicle(s)
pT3b	Tumor invades seminal vesicle(s)
pT4	**Invasion of adjacent structures** (bladder, rectum, muscles, pelvis)
Regional lymph nodes (N)	
Nx	Regional lymph nodes cannot be assessed
N0	No regional lymph node metastasis
N1	Metastasis in regional lymph node or nodes
Distant metastasis (M)	
Mx	Distant metastasis cannot be assessed
M1	Distant metastasis
M1a	Nonregional lymph node(s)
M1b	Bone(s)
M1c	Other site(s)

disease most commonly metastasizes to the pelvic lymph nodes and the skeleton, especially the pelvis and lumbar spine. Visceral metastases, which occur later in the course of disease, are less common and frequently involve the lungs, liver, and adrenals. Distant spread through lymphatic routes involves primarily the regional pelvic nodes including the iliac, obturator, and sacral nodes. Distant lymph node metastases to the aortic lymphatic tissue without involvement of the regional lymph nodes are rarely seen. According to the current TNM classification from 1997, patients without regional lymph node metastases are classified as stage N0 and with positive lymph nodes as N1. Involvement of distant lymphatic tissue is classified as M1a [26]. The presence of lymph node metastases is greatly dependent on the extension of the primary tumor and the histopathologic grade. In our patient population we found no lymphatic involvement in 192 patients presenting in stage pT2a, whereas 11 (3.4%) out of 327 were positive in stage pT2b, 22 (9.1%) out of 241 in stage pT3a, 34 (28.1%) out of 120 in stage pT3b and 12 (38.7%) out of 31 in stage pT4. The presence of lymph node metastases increases with the loss of differentiation and is reported for well-differentiated tumors (Gleason score 2–4) up to 5%, for moderately differentiated tumors (Gleason score 5–6) between 20 and 30% and for poorly differentiated tumors (Gleason score > 7) about 50%.

22.3 Diagnosis

Early stage carcinoma of the prostate is asymptomatic. Although most adenocarcinomas occur in the peripheral region, invasion of the periurethral tissue is common and can eventually cause urethral obstruction. Leading symptoms such as hesitancy in initiating voiding, diminution of the urinary flow and incomplete emptying of the urinary bladder are indistinguishable from those produced by BPH. On the other hand, uremia, urinary retention, skeletal pain and pathologic fractures may be initial symptoms of advanced disease. The diagnosis of prostatic cancer is based on digital rectal examination, transrectal ultrasound (TRUS), serum prostate-specific antigen (PSA) and biopsy of the prostate [15]. Digital rectal examination allows one to determine size, consistency and shape of the prostate. Characteristic findings of carcinoma are hard and irregular shaped nodular changes. Since the posterior surfaces of the lateral lobes, where carcinomas most often begin, are easily assessable, digital rectal examination allows sensitive detection of all stages of disease other than stage T1. Transrectal digital examination also reveals local extraprostatic extension into the seminal vesicles. Elevation of serum prostate-specific antigen (PSA) level (normal, < 4.0 ng per milliliter) is the most sensitive marker for early detection of prostatic cancer. PSA was initially discovered in seminal plasma and is a 34 kDa serine protease produced by the prostatic epithelium. It is detectable in the serum of all men with functioning prostate. PSA can also be elevated in patients with BPH, acute prostatitis and after digital rectal examination. However, it has been found that prostate cancer contributes about 10 times more to the serum PSA than does the same volume of BPH [25]. Approximately 25% of patients with PSA between 4 and 10 ng/ml have prostatic cancer and more than 65% with levels above 10 ng/ml [29]. Determination of free PSA versus protein-bound PSA has been found to aid in the differentiation between BPH and prostatic carcinoma [11]. In cancer patients, the PSA level correlates with the size or tumor volume as well as with the degree of malignancy. However, in individual patients the PSA level does not allow one to distinguish organ-confined from more advanced disease. Determination of PSA allows assessment of treatment response and should fall below the level of detection after successful surgical excision of the entire gland. Raising PSA levels following radical prostatectomy or radiotherapy is generally the first indication of progression.

Transrectal sonography (TRUS) provides visualization of the internal architecture and the entire contour of the prostate [28]. TRUS is an important modality in staging of prostate cancer. Diagnosis is based on the shape, capsular echoes and internal echoes of the prostate. Typical sonographic findings of cancer are hypoechoic lesions; however, some carcinomas may appear hyperechoic or with mixed echogenicity. TRUS is sensitive enough to detect hyperechoic prostatic cancer but its use as a screening test is affected by its limited specificity. In contrast to digital rectal examination, which is limited to the side facing the rectum, transrectal sonography provides information about the entire prostate margin and the extent of disease including invasion of the seminal vessel. TRUS is recommended if either the digital rectal examination is positive or the PSA level is elevated. The combined use of these modalities increases early detection of prostatic cancers in a localized and potentially curable stage. Ultrasound-guided biopsy is clearly superior to finger-guided biopsy, not only in targeting the prostate but also in decreasing side effects such as bleeding. The increasing use of the PSA test has resulted in an increasing number of patients with negative digital rectal examination and negative TRUS. For further evaluation, random biopsy of the prostate is necessary, e.g., by applying systematic sextant biopsies [24].

Computed tomography (CT) and magnetic resonance imaging (MRI) have also been used for evaluation of the prostate. Similarities in the physical density and CT attenuation of prostatic carcinoma, BPH and normal prostate tissue, even with intravenous contrast agents, do not allow the use of CT in the routine evaluation of localized prostate cancer [17]. Early MR studies used body coil imaging that resulted in poor image resolution. The development of endorectal coil MRI resulted in high resolution images around the rectum, in the mid and posterior aspects of the prostate but poor evaluation of the anterior margin. Recently, phased-array, pelvic surface coil combined with endorectal coil has been shown to produce a more homogeneous signal throughout the prostate [19]. However, 35–52% of pathologically proven cancer is undetected by MR imaging. The use of paramagnetic contrast agent does not provide additional information; however, it may be helpful in the detection of seminal vesicle invasion in some cases. Evaluation of the regional lymph node status using noninvasive imaging methods is extremely difficult. MRI, CT, as well as sonography and lymphangiography provide an unacceptable low sensitivity and specificity to detect tumor-involved lymph nodes. However, in patients with gross lymphadenopathy, ultrasound- and CT-guided fine-needle aspiration biopsies may be helpful. Currently, histopathological evaluation of surgically removed lymphatic tissue serves as the gold standard for therapeutic decisions. The value of pelvic node dissection is most likely not therapeutic, and in some centers patients with positive nodes may not undergo prostatectomy. New insights in the development and progression of prostate cancer, as well as the predictive value of clinical staging as determined by biopsy material, transrectal ultrasound and PSA levels are reducing the number of patients undergoing pelvic lymphadenectomy. Patients age, histologic grade, Gleason score, PSA level, disease confined to organ, surgical margin status and co-morbid diseases have been identified as independent prognostic indicators for survival in addition to pathologic stage.

The following questions and demands are raised from urologists towards noninvasive imaging procedures:

- (Early) diagnosis of prostate cancer
  - Differentiation between BPH and prostate cancer
  - Identification of prostate cancer among men with elevated PSA
- Staging of prostate cancer
  - Local extent of disease (tumor volume and confined or unconfined to organ)
  - Involvement of seminal vesicles
  - Involvement of regional lymph nodes
  - Distant metastases
- Evaluation of therapy response.

22.4 Positron emission tomography

Since the most commonly used PET tracer for oncological studies, [^{18}F]fluorodeoxyglucose (FDG), is eliminated via the kidneys, evaluation of the pelvic regions is often difficult. To study the prostate it is mandatory to reduce the excreted radioactivity in the bladder, e.g., by placing a urine catheter. In addition, it may be necessary to rinse the bladder with sterile sodium chloride solution; however, there are risks of urinary tract infection and in handling the radioactive waste. It has been shown useful to increase the urinary flow by intravenous application of diuretic agents. In all patients undergoing FDG-PET scans that include the abdomen, we routinely administer 20 mg furosemide i.v. at the time of tracer injection. For imaging the prostate patients also received a saline infusion of 500–1000 ml to clear bladder radioactivity. Following an uptake period of at least 60 min most patients have only little radioactivity remaining in the bladder when the emission scan is started. The blocking balloon of a urine catheter may serve as anatomical landmark and can easily be identified as tracer defect surrounded by little amounts of radioactive urine.

In 1996 Effert and colleagues reported on 64 patients studied with FDG-PET including 48 patients with primary prostate cancer and 16 with benign disease [6]. They found increased FDG uptake in the prostate region in only 9 cases with cancer and only 4 showed markedly increased tracer uptake. Most of the tumors displayed only little tracer accumulation, comparable to that in the normal prostate. No relationship was found between glucose metabolism and extension of the disease or histologic grading. On the other hand, 13 out of 16 patients with benign disease had increased FDG uptake in the prostate. Additionally, one patient with chronic granulomatous prostatitis and 2 patients with benign prostate hyperplasia (BPH) had markedly increased tracer uptake. Quantification of tracer uptake using standardized uptake values (SUV) showed a wide overlap between benign and malignant prostatic lesions. In our experience zero out of 11 patients with advanced prostate cancer prior to prostatectomy exhibited increased FDG uptake in the tumor region [10]. In general, prostate cancer showed very low FDG uptake including 3 cases with local recurrence. The tracer kinetics using dynamic PET scanning revealed no difference between primary tumors, local recurrence and scar tissue after radical prostatectomy. Seltzer et al. compared helical CT, FDG-PET and monoclonal antibody scanning in patients with elevated PSA levels for detection of local recurrence and lymph node metastases [20]. Forty-five patients underwent CT and PET imaging and 21 patients monoclonal antibody scanning. CT and PET were positive for local recurrence or distant disease in 50% of the patients and monoclonal antibody scanning was only true-positive in 1 out of 6 patients with histologically proven metastases. An explanation for the observed low glucose metabolism of most prostatic carcinomas is not known. Presently, results from FDG-PET imaging are not sufficient to differentiate between BPH and prostate cancer, or to detect local recurrence. Therefore, PET imaging with FDG cannot be recommended in patients with prostate cancer.

22.5 Distant metastases

Distant metastases of prostate cancer are predominately found in bone and lung. Chest x-ray is therefore included in the diagnostic work-up of prostate cancer patients. Bone metastases occur via hematological spread of cancer cells to the bone marrow. Magnetic resonance imaging (MRI) is more sensitive than bone scanning to visualize bone marrow infiltration; however, bone scans are highly sensitive to detect increased osteoblastic activity and, therefore, serve as a screening test. The classic patterns often found in advanced disease are multiple, small, occasionally congruent metastases involving the axial skeleton. It has to be considered that patients with PSA levels below 10 ng/ml are unlikely to have distant metastases.

Shreve et al. studied metastatic prostate cancer using FDG-PET compared to conventional diagnostic procedures including bone scanning, computed tomography (CT) and follow-up findings [22]. In 22 patients with untreated bone metastases, only 65% (131 out of 202) were identified by FDG-PET. Even in large metastases the average SUV was low, ranging between 2.5 and 3.5. Some lymph node metastases had higher FDG uptake (SUV up to 5.7) and in four patients with SUV values above 5.0 they found rapid progression in disease suggesting higher glucose metabolism in undifferentiated tumors. An important finding is that positive PET scans had a high positive predictive value (98%) to represent metastases. Yeh and colleagues from the Memorial Sloan Kettering Cancer Center found in 13 patients, with extensive bony metastases shown in bone scans, only about 18% corresponding increased FDG uptake [30]. Positive FDG uptake was not related to the duration of illness, level of PSA or extent of disease suggesting that prostate cancer is preferentially metabolizing other substrates as primary energy source rather than glucose.

Very promising results have been reported for the use of [^{18}F]PET to detect skeleton metastases. Fluorine-18 is a bone seeking agent that has been first used almost 30 years ago [23]. Recent developments in PET scanner technologies have led to a reappraisal for using this radionuclide. Schirrmeister et al. compared conventional planar bone scanning with [^{18}F]PET imaging for detection of bone metastases in 44 patients including 20 patients with prostate cancer. A combination of scintigraphy, planar radiography, CT, and MRI served as gold standard. [^{18}F]PET identified 67 bone metastases of prostate carcinoma compared to 33 with conventional bone scanning. The area under the ROC curve was 0.99 for [^{18}F]PET and 0.64 for bone scanning. [^{18}F]PET was more sensitive to detect benign as well as malignant lesions of the skeleton and the higher spatial resolution of PET resulted in an increased accuracy for differentiation between benign and malignant lesions. It is important to note that [^{18}F]PET had a detection rate comparable to MRI and spiral CT. Currently, PET imaging is still too expensive to serve as a screening method: however, the increasing use and availability of this technique will also result in lower costs in the future.

22.6 New tracer developments

The naturally occurring polyamine putrescine (1,4-diaminobutane) is known to be associated with cell division. ^{11}C-labeled putrescine has been used to study the higher proliferation rate of prostate cancer compared to surrounding tissue [27]. In eight patients with advanced disease and three normal controls, ^{11}C-labeled putrescine rapidly accumulated in prostate, bone and rectum. Since the tracer uptake was higher in normal prostate and normal bone compared to prostate cancer and its metastasis, [^{11}C]putrescine cannot be used for clinical staging. Recently, Hara et al. published a study using [^{11}C]choline. Phosphatidylcholine is an abundant phospholipid predominantly in cell membranes. A rapid tissue uptake was observed after intravenous injection and urinary excretion was found to be negligible. In 10 patients studied, a higher [^{11}C]choline uptake was found in primary prostate tumors and local metastasis compared to [^{18}F]FDG. However, significant uptake of [^{11}C]choline in the normal prostate tissue does not allow to differentiate benign disease from prostate cancer. [^{11}C]5-hydroxytryptophan was studied in 10 patients with hormone-refractory metastatic disease [12]. A moderate tracer uptake was found in skeletal metastases with an initial increase during

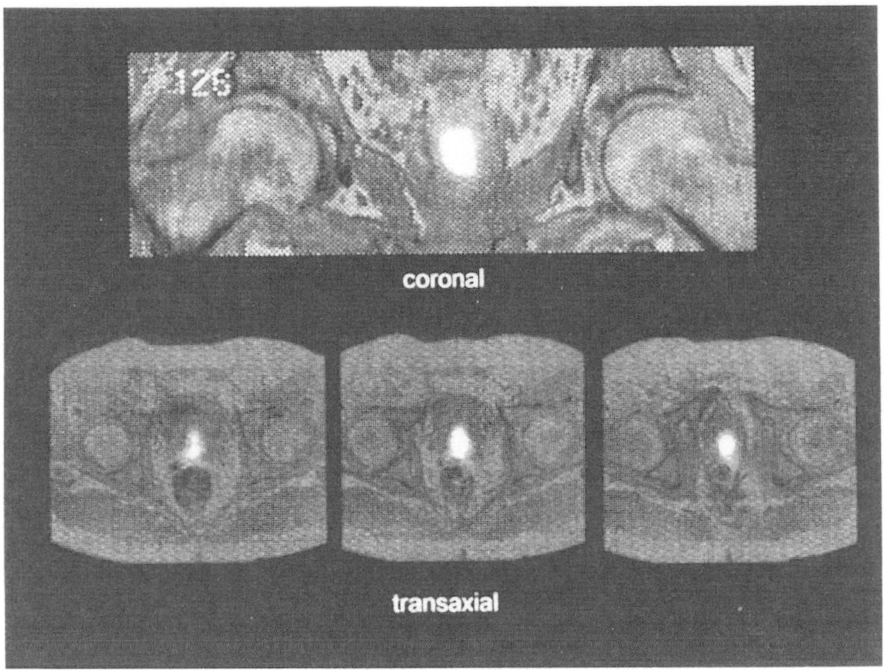

Fig. 22.1. An image fusion between MR imaging of the pelvis and [^{11}C]acetate PET scanning is shown. The patient presented with elevated PSA level and PET demonstrates focally increased tracer uptake in the prostate. Ultrasonographic guided biopsy turned out to be positive for prostate cancer.

the first few minutes followed by a wash-out period. Low accumulation of radiolabeled hydroxytryptophan in metastatic disease may impair the application of this tracer. Various androgens labeled with ^{18}F have been studied in animal experiments as imaging agents for prostatic cancer [13]. Most of the fluorine-substituted androgens show high affinity for the androgen receptor, although fluorine substitution lowers their affinity. A group from Denmark studied 16-β-[^{18}F]fluoro-5-α-dihydrotestosterone as a PET ligand for androgen receptors in 12 prostate cancer patients [7]. They found a positive binding to the prostate but no bone metastases. This very interesting approach needs further evaluation to determine the potential use in prostatic imaging. [^{11}C]acetate is also currently being studied for its application to visualize prostate cancer (Fig. 22.1). Radiolabeled acetate is commonly used to study oxidative metabolism of the heart. Acetate has a rapid blood clearance and after metabolism through the citrate cycle the label is mainly found in [^{11}C]CO_2 exhaled over the lungs. Recently, Shreve from the University of Michigan reported on 18 patients with local, recurrent, or regional metastatic disease [21]. SUV for prostate cancer ranged from 2.8 to 10.6 (mean 5.9) compared to 1.6 to 2.5 (mean 1.9) for normal prostate tissue. Regional tumor involved lymph nodes as small as 8 mm were visualized. A Japanese group from the Fukai Medical School studied 12 patients with histologically proven prostate cancer and one patient with

BPH [16]. All tumors were positive in the ^{11}C-acetate scan and the patient with BPH showed only faint tracer uptake. The underlying biochemical explanation for the observed trapping of the radioactive label by prostate cancer is unknown and needs further evaluation. However, due to the negligible tracer excretion in the urinary tract this tracer may be promising for detection of primary tumors and recurrent prostate cancer.

22.7 Summary and outlook

It has been shown that PET using FDG has a low detection rate to identify prostate cancer. There is also no evidence that staging of regional and distant (lymph node) metastases as well as detection of recurrent cancer can be accomplished with sufficient accuracy by FDG-PET. With respect to the high sensitive detection of bone metastasis using conventional bone scanning, FDG-PET is also not useful for the evaluation of distant tumor involvement to the skeleton. Currently, there is no indication for FDG-PET scanning in patients with prostatic cancer.

There are promising developments using PET tracers other than [^{18}F]FDG. Specifically [^{11}C]acetate has been reported to provide a highly sensitive detection of prostatic cancer. Further studies are needed that include benign diseases of the prostate for assessment of specificity. However, the limited spatial resolution and partial volume effects may effect image quality to a degree that visualization of the extent of disease including capsular and extracapsular infiltration or involvement of the seminal vesicles is not possible. Further technical developments in scanner technology and overlay techniques may help to overcome these problems. The challenge in the future will not be to diagnose advanced stages of disease but to visualize non-palpable prostatic carcinoma (stage T1) and to aid therapeutic decisions by differentiating insignificant prostate cancer from significant disease.

References

[1] Black RJ, Bray F, Ferlay J, Parkin DM (1997) Cancer incidence and mortality in the European Union: cancer registry data and estimates of national incidence for 1990. Eur J Cancer 33:1075–1079

[2] Bostwick DG (1995) Clinical utility of prostatic intraepithelial neoplasia. Mayo Clin Proc 70:395–396

[3] Chodak GW, Thisted RA, Gerber GS, Johansson JE, Adolfsson J, Jones GW, Chisholm GD, Moskovitz B, Livne PM, Warner J (1994) Results of conservative management of clinically localized prostate cancer. N Engl J Med 330:242–248

[4] Denis LJ, Morton MS, Griffiths K (1999) Diet and its preventive role in prostatic disease. Eur Urol 35:377–387

[5] Denis LJ, Murphy GP, Schröder FH (1995) Report of the Consensus Workshop on screening and global strategy for prostate cancer. Cancer 75:1187–1209

[6] Effert PJ, Bares R, Handt S, Wolff JM, Bull U, Jakse G (1996) Metabolic imaging of untreated prostate cancer by positron emission tomography with 18fluorine-labeled deoxyglucose. J Urol 155:994–998
[7] Eigtved A, Jensen M, Holm S, Foder B, Larsen P, Hoejgaard L, Iversen P, Friberg L (1999) 16beta-F-18-fluoro-5-alpha-dihydrotestosterone as a PET ligand for androgen receptors in prostate cancer. Eur J Nucl Med 26:1118P (abstr)
[8] Gleason DF (1992) Histologic grading of prostate cancer: a perspective. Human Pathology 23:273–279
[9] Gleason DF, Mellinger GT (1974) Prediction of prognosis for prostatic adenocarcinoma by combined histological grading and clinical staging. J Urol 111:58–64
[10] Hofer C, Laubenbacher C, Block T, Breul J, Hartung R, Schwaiger M (1999) Fluorine-18-fluorodeoxyglucose positron emission tomography is useless for the detection of local recurrence after radical prostatectomy. Eur Urol 36:31–35
[11] Hofer C, Sauerstein P, Wolter C, Scholz M, Hartung R, Breul J (1999) The value of free prostate-specific antigen PSA (Hybritech Tanden E) in symptomatic patients consulting the urologist. Urol Internat (in press)
[12] Kalkner KM, Ginman C, Nilsson S, Bergstrom M, Antoni G, Ahlstrom H, Langstrom B, Westlin JE (1997) Positron emission tomography (PET) with 11C-5-hydroxytryptophan (5-HTP) in patients with metastatic hormone-refractory prostatic adenocarcinoma. J Nucl Med 38:1215–1221
[13] Liu A, Carlson KE, Katzenellenbogen JA (1992) Synthesis of high affinity fluorine-substituted ligands for the androgen receptor. Potential agents for imaging prostatic cancer by positron emission tomography. J Urol 148:1457–1460
[14] McNeal JE, Bostwick DG (1986) Intraductal dysplasia: a premalignant lesion of the prostate. Hum Pathol 17:64–71
[15] Mettlin C, Murphy GP, Babaian RJ, Chesley A, Kane RA, Littrup PJ, Mostofi FK, Ray PS, Shanberg AM, Toi A (1996) The results of a five-year early prostate cancer detection intervention. Investigators of the American Cancer Society National Prostate Cancer Detection Project. Cancer 77:150–159
[16] Muranoto S, Yamamoto K, Ohyama N, Takahashi N, Nakamura S, Ishizu K, Sugimoto K, Waki A, Sadato N, Yonekura Y, Okada K, Ishii Y (1999) Positive Imaging of Prostate Cancer with Carbon-11 Acetate and PET. J Nucl Med 40:60P (abstr)
[17] Platt JF, Bree RL, Schwab RE (1987) The accuracy of CT in the staging of carcinoma of the prostate. AJR Am J Roentgenol 149:315–318
[18] Sakr WA, Haas GP, Cassin BF, Pontes JE, Crissman JD (1993) The frequency of carcinoma and intraepithelial neoplasia of the prostate in young male patients. J Urol 150:379–385
[19] Schiebler ML, Schnall MD, Pollack HM, Lenkinski RE, Tomaszewski JE, Wein AJ, Whittington R, Rauschnig W, Kressel HY (1993) Current role of MR imaging in the staging of adenocarcinoma of the prostate. Radiology 189:339–352
[20] Seltzer MA, Barbaric Z, Belldegrun A, Naitoh J, Dorey F, Phelps ME, Gambhir SS, Hoh CK (1999) Comparison of helical computerized tomography, positron emission tomography and monoclonal antibody scans for evaluation of lymph node metastases in patients with prostate specific antigen relapse after treatment for localized prostate cancer. J Urol 162:1322–1328
[21] Shreve PD (1999) Carbon-11 acetate PET imaging of prostate cancer. J Nucl Med 40:60P (abstr)
[22] Shreve PD, Grossman HB, Gross MD, Wahl RL (1996) Metastatic prostate cancer: initial findings of PET with 2-deoxy-2-[F-18]fluoro-D-glucose. Radiology 199:751–756
[23] Silberstein EB, Saenger EL, Tofe AJ, Alexander GW Jr, Park HM (1973) Imaging of bone metastases with 99m Tc-Sn-EHDP (diphosphonate), 18 F, and skeletal radiography. A comparison of sensitivity. Radiology 107:551–555
[24] Stamey TA (1995) Making the most out of six systematic sextant biopsies. Urology 45:2–12

[25] Stamey TA, Yang N, Hay AR, McNeal JE, Freiha FS, Redwine E (1987) Prostate-specific antigen as a serum marker for adenocarcinoma of the prostate. N Engl J Med 317:909-916

[26] UICC (1997) TNM Classification of Malignant Tumors. John Wiley & Sons, New York

[27] Wang GJ, Volkow ND, Wolf AP, Madajewicz S, Fowler JS, Schlyer DJ, MacGregor RR (1994) Positron emission tomography study of human prostatic adenocarcinoma using carbon-11 putrescine. Nucl Med Biol 21:77-82

[28] Watanabe H, Kaiho H, Tanaka M, Terasawa Y (1971) Diagnostic application of ultrasonotomography to the prostate. Invest Urol 8:548-559

[29] Wirth M, Otto T, Rübben H (1998) Prostatakarzinom. W. Zuckschwerdt Verlag, Munich, pp 92-126

[30] Yeh SD, Imbriaco M, Larson SM, Garza D, Zhang JJ, Kalaigian H, Finn RD, Reddy D, Horowitz SM, Goldsmith SJ, Scher HI (1996) Detection of bony metastases of androgen-independent prostate cancer by PET-FDG. Nucl Med Biol 23:693-697

23 Malignant melanoma

M.H. Thelen, R. Bares

23.1 Incidence, etiology and epidemiology

The malignant melanoma belongs to the group of malignant tumors of the skin or mucous membrane. The global incidence of malignant melanomas has risen continuously over the past few years. In Europe, the incidence of malignant melanomas among the white population is 8 in 100 000, rising with greater proximity to the equator to 20 in 100 000. In the Federal Republic of Germany, the frequency of new cases has doubled every 12 to 15 years [11]. A main cause is said to be the changing exposure of the population to ultraviolet light, primarily as a result of changing living habits (brief exposure to high doses of UV light during leisure hours as against former exposure patterns which were chronic but not lower in cumulative terms) [20, 23]. Alongside exposure to UV light, skin type, hair color and the number of melanocytic naevi are all considered to constitute risk factors for the development of a malignant melanoma [2, 12]. Alongside race and gender (more favorable prognosis for women despite higher incidence), other prognostic factors include the anatomic localization of the primary tumor [13, 14, 34].

Given the improvements which have been achieved in early detection over recent years, despite increasing incidence it has been possible to observe a reduction in mortality [17]. In particular where tumors have not reached an advanced stage, therapeutic intervention in the form of surgery or radiotherapy offers an approach for curative treatment [1].

23.2 Manifestation of the malignant melanoma

The course of a malignant melanoma is chronic and progressive in character, with gradual malignization of the tumor through disturbance of melanocyte growth regulation, loss of identical reduplication, clonal evolution and the creation of malignant tumor cells. Malignant melanomas are characterized by potent metastatic spread; in frequent cases and at an early juncture, lymphogenous migration occurs. Particularly in the case of advanced primary tumors, a hematogenous metastatic spread is observed. The following symptoms are indicative of the existence of a malignant melanoma: fast increase in the size of a naevus, generation of a rough surface, increase of pigmentation, blue-black discoloration, a reddish inflamed areola around a naevus, tendency to bleed, ulceration, regional metastatic spread in the form of small satellite nodes, swelling of the relevant lymph nodes and possibly also subjective symptoms of pain and itchiness. The peak of metastasis formation is reached in the first and second year after diagnosis, although late metastases also occur [26].

23.3 Histopathological classification

In clinical and histopathological terms, four different forms of cutaneous melanoma can be identified, whose differentiation is of major importance with regard to therapy planning and estimation of the prognosis. A difference is drawn between the superficially spreading melanoma (SSM), the acrolentiginous melanoma (ALM), the primary nodular melanoma (NMM) and the lentigo malignant melanoma (LMM) [32].

With the onset of vertical growth and diminishing horizontal growth in the skin, the nodular melanoma demonstrates increasingly aggressive behavior.

Classification of the malignant melanoma stage based upon invasion depth in the cutis and thickness of the tumor, as well as upon existence of regional, lymph node or distant metastases (Table 23.1) [7, 8].

23.4 Conventional staging

Alongside clinical methods of examination, during primary staging a variety of imaging methods are applied. In the staging of regional lymph nodes, high resolution sonography is the most predominantly used method. Chest X-rays and sonography of the abdomen are also used. Where findings are inconclusive or pathological, computer tomography (CT) of the chest, abdomen and if applicable also the skull is carried out. At present it is not possible to conclusively assess the value of molecular biological methods such as RT-PCR (reverse transcriptase-polymerase chain reaction) in tracing tyrosinase in the blood or lymph nodes.

Table 23.1. Clinical stages (DDG 1994).

UICC	Stage
pT 1	I a
pT 2	I b
pT 3	II a
pT 4	II b
pT a/b	III a
N 1/2 (each T)	III b
M 1 (each T, each N)	IV

23.5 Diagnosis using nuclear medicine

Over recent years, endeavors have been under way in the field of nuclear medicine to develop methods permitting the specific scintigraphic detection of the malignant melanoma. Despite the fact that a wide variety of links with a varying degree of affinity to melanoma cells have been described within the framework of immunoscintigraphy or receptor scintigraphy, to date none of these methods have become an established feature of routine clinical examinations [6, 10, 19].

Conversely, a number of non-specific methods have succeeded in gaining significance in routine diagnostic procedures. These include skeletal scintigraphy with [^{99m}Tc]-marked phosphates for verifying or excluding the presence of osseous metastases.

But predominantly it is the lymph outflow scintigraphy method with subsequent intraoperative gamma probe-supported sentinel node detection which is enjoying ever more frequent use. This method has become the established standard over recent years for primary lymph node staging of the malignant melanoma in stage 1, despite the fact that no major multicenter studies on the value of this method have yet been published [15, 25].

23.6 PET

Positron emission tomography (PET) with [^{18}F]fluorodeoxyglucose (FDG) makes use of the fact that the majority of malignant tumors demonstrate increased glucose metabolism and consequently absorb greater quantities of glucose or its analogs. This permits depiction of the three-dimensional tumor extension and a metabolic characterization of the investigated tumor. PET represents an addition to established methods of examination such as sonography, X-ray and computer tomography, as it does not use morphological criteria such as size or shape to verify the existence of malignant tumors, but bases its findings on metabolic tumor characteristics which are independent of the size of a malignant lesion.

The fact that a change in the glucose metabolism is not specific to a particular tumor entity and that reactive or inflammatory processes can also lead to enhanced FDG absorption limits the value of this method. For the diagnosis of lymph node metastases in particular, these represent an important differential diagnosis.

23.6.1 PET examination method

After fasting for 12 h, the patients are injected intravenously with 300–400 MBq [^{18}F]FDG. After an uptake time of 60 min, an emission scan is obtained. In particular in the event of tumor localization at the distal extremities, whole-body examination is necessary, otherwise it is sufficient to image torso, skull and proximal upper thigh. Examinations should be performed using a whole-body PET scanner (axial face area of at least 15 cm) in order to avoid unnecessarily long periods of measurement. Good hydration of the patient should also be aimed for with enforced diuresis to reduce urinary and bladder activity.

SUV scaling (SUV: 0–8) in the documentation has proven to be useful to standardize image quality and interindividual comparisons.

Although no systematic comparative studies have as yet been carried out on the value of attenuation correction, it appears to be advisable particularly in the case of metastases localized close to the skin surface which are typical findings in malignant melanoma. A fast procedure ideal for this purpose is segmented iteration, for which transmission measurements of 2–4 min duration per field of view are sufficient.

23.6.2 Results

From the author's own case material, a total of 51 patients (20 women, 31 men) with known metastatic spread on whom a FDG-PET and a CT had been performed within a period of 3 weeks were retrospectively evaluated. The mean age of the patients was 56.3 years, with the range spanning 16 to 79 years. In order to exclude therapeutic effects, only patients in which no chemotherapy, immunotherapy or radiotherapy had been performed during the 8 weeks previous to the PET were included. Suspended metastasis findings were confirmed either bioptically or by means of other imaging techniques such as X-ray, sonography, MRT or bone scintigraphy.

Of the total of 64 confirmed lymph node metastases, 63 (98%) were verified by PET and 59 (92%) by CT. Of liver metastases 88% (30/34) were verified by PET and 100% by CT (34/34). Of a total of 179 lung metastases, computer tomography revealed 172 (96%). PET succeeded in recognizing only 43% (77/179) of lung metastases, of which the large majority were, however, only a few millimeters in size.

The minimum detectable tumor size was between 2 mm in the lung and 10 mm in the liver in the case of CT, and 3 mm in the lung and 15 mm in the liver for PET.

In four examinations, PET produced false positive lymph node findings, of which three were due to infections and to a post-operative condition. False positive lung findings occurred in five patients. In two of these cases, changes brought about by inflammation were the cause. In the remaining three cases, no explanation has yet come forth. A post-examination observation period of at least four months has not produced any morphological tumor identification in these cases.

In one case involving a 15 mm large axillary lymph node, PET and CT both produced false positive results. The histological findings were reactively inflammatory changes. With eight of the lung metastases traced in CT, it was

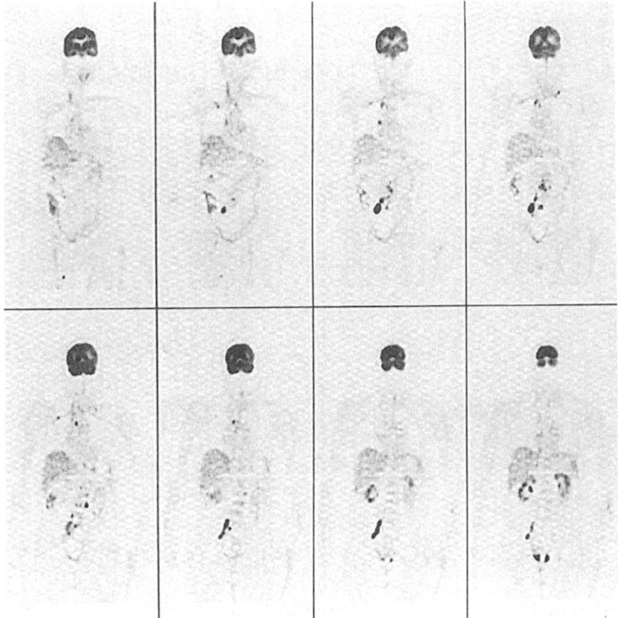

Fig. 23.1. FDG-PET (coronal sections) from a 67-year-old female patient with known malignant melanoma (FD 1990, stage 4, left lower thigh) after three local recurrences in the inguinal and parailiacal lymph nodes. Now sonographically hyperperfused lymph nodes in the groin (right side) and questionably enlarged lymph nodes ventrally to the iliac vein in the MRI. The PET indicates multiple hypermetabolic foci, right inguinal, right parailiacal, mediastinal, right supra- and infraclavicular, and left cervical (histology right supraclavicular: melanoma metastasis). On the basis of the PET finding, the planned surgical treatment was abandoned and systemic therapy initiated.

impossible to confirm these using any other method including clinical course, and must be assessed as incorrect positive diagnoses.

A further prospective study since carried out on the use of PET in primary staging in patients with high-risk melanomas and a tumor thickness of at least 1.5 mm registered a total of 33 patients (15 female, 18 male). In this case, pathological findings identified using PET or computer tomography have been confirmed both histologically and by clinical follow-up. At the time of primary staging, 28 patients were free of metastases. In five patients, metastatic spread was confirmed. Twenty-two patients (79%) were correctly staged negative by PET, and CT produced a correct negative diagnosis in 24 patients (86%). The false positives produced by both PET and CT were due to inflammatory changes in the lymph nodes; in one case the patient was found to be suffering with sarcoidosis with multiorgan manifestation.

The rate of correct positive diagnosis was 4/5 with PET and 3/5 with CT. Both PET and CT produced a false negative diagnosis in the case of a sentinel node in which metastasis formation was verified histologically. CT produced another false negative in the case of a melanoma metastasis in the cardia which was registered by PET and gastroscopically confirmed.

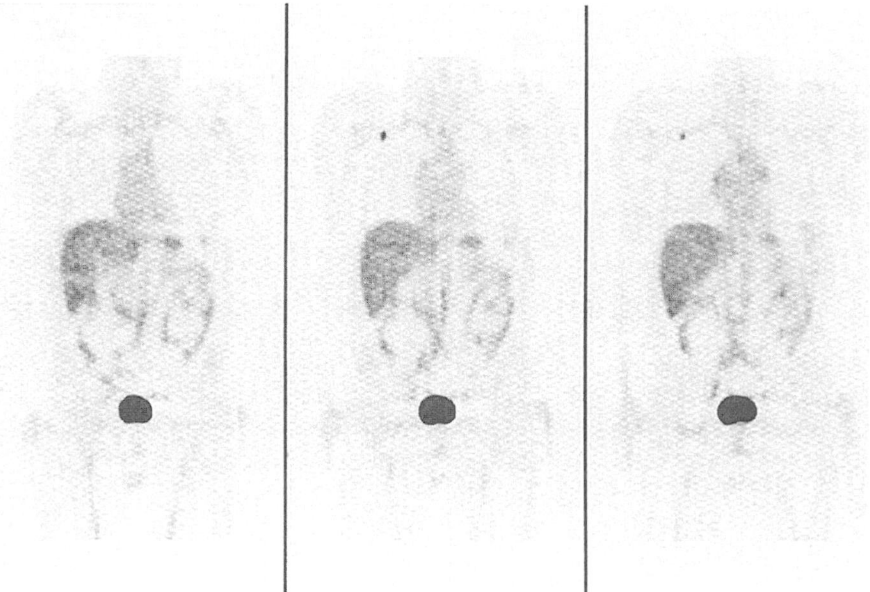

Fig. 23.2. FDG-PET in a 58-year-old patient four weeks after excision of a malignant melanoma (Clark level IV, TD 3.4 mm) on the right side. A hypermetabolic focus has been detected in the right axilla which corresponds in computer tomographic terms to an enlarged lymph node. Sonographic examination of this area produced no findings. (A melanoma metastasis was histologically confirmed).

Given the overall low number of positive findings among this patient group, this study indicates a sensitivity rate of 80% for PET and 60% for CT, and specificity of 79% and 86%, respectively.

23.7 Discussion

The detection of individual metastases or scattered metastatic spread at the time of initial diagnosis or during restaging is of decisive prognostic significance in the treatment of malignant tumors. Frequently, as with malignant melanoma, however, no curative treatment approach exists in the case of disseminated metastatic spread. Conventional diagnostic methods, in which a decision between pathological and normal findings is based exclusively on morphological changes, involve distinct disadvantages, as here a finding can only be assessed as pathological from a certain size of tumor. Smaller lesions which fall below this limit cannot be diagnosed for methodological reasons. The early detection of metabolic changes, which can in many cases precede morphological deviations by a long period of time, represents a major advantage of positron emission tomography. Another benefit of PET is the possibility to perform a whole-body scan and to assess all organ systems for tumor invasion.

Table 23.2. Results of the Consensus Conference Oncological PET, 1997.

Malignant melanoma	Category
Lymph node staging, distant metastases in stage 2	1a
Therapy control	2b
Lymph node staging, distant metastases in stage 1	3a

Initial systematic studies on the use of positron emission tomography in the detection of malignant melanoma indicate major benefits with this method within the framework of primary staging and where tumor metastasis is known to have taken place [5, 9, 16, 29]. While sensitivity in the detection of lymph node metastases has been shown to be as high as 100% [28, 35], due to its limited spatial resolution PET proved insufficiently sensitive for the detection of micrometastases [18, 22]. Although the sensitivity of PET is greater than that of CT in the detection of superficial lymph node metastases, it offers no benefits above sonography. False positive diagnoses due to reactively inflammatory processes place a limitation on its usefulness here [3]. Conversely, in adipose patients, PET has proven markedly superior to sonography in the detection of retroperitoneal or paraaortal lymph node metastases.

The detection of metastases in the brain is impeded by the physiologically high level of cerebral FDG uptake. Small metastases with only slightly increased FDG uptake, in particular, can escape detection. For this reason, an additional MRI of the cerebrum is recommended by a number of working groups [28].

Follow-up examinations have shown that PET has a higher sensitivity and specificity in the detection of lymph node and abdominal metastases in comparison with conventional diagnostic methods, in particular CT. Conversely, smaller lung metastases are detected earlier by CT than by PET [28]. However, in many cases the dignity of small, isolated lung foci (<5 mm) remains open and can only be successfully evaluated with further progress of the disease.

In detecting the primary tumor and diagnosing local recurrence, PET is less effective than conventional diagnostic methods, making PET unsuitable as a sole means of local diagnosis.

Compared to established methods, the costs of positron emission tomography are much higher. One way to reduce the costs of clinical oncology is by cutting back on therapeutic measures which have proven to be ineffective [4, 33]. From the economic viewpoint, there appears to be little sense in the systematic use of PET in patients with high-risk melanoma. Cost savings could accordingly only be achieved by further selection of patients with increased risk of metastasis [30]. Nor does replacing classical PET by coincidence techniques offer good perspectives for success at present. Results to date indicate massively reduced sensitivity of the coincidence technique, which affects primarily very small tumor foci and lesions in regions with high background activity [31].

Due to the described limitations, at the present time PET is not yet capable of replacing the conventional staging examinations applied in primary staging of a malignant melanoma despite its high degree of sensitivity and specificity. More particularly, it is not suitable for the detection or exclusion of micrometastases. As a result, it is not possible to dispense with surgery in clarifying lymph node stages, where use of sentinel node dissection has now become the accepted method [36]. However, the use of PET can be helpful in clarifying questionable lymph node findings identified by CT, where these are of relevance for further therapeutic measures (such as surgical removal).

More recent studies involving positron-emitting radiopharmaceuticals such as [^{11}C]methionine or [^{18}F]DOPA analogs have opened up some interesting approaches for diagnostic research and possibly also therapy of malignant melanoma [21, 24]. However, as yet any concrete clinical benefit is not in sight and will necessitate systematic prior evaluation.

23.8 Tips on practical use and image interpretation

- *Patient preparation:*
  Empty stomach (12 h fast), sufficient oral or, in the case of tumor localization in the lower extremities, i.v. hydration, enforced diuresis, miction prior to start of the examination, if necessary use of a catheter.
- *Data acquisition:*
  Whole-body scan, only in case of tumor localization in the thorax area can scanning of the extremities be dispensed;
  Emission measurements starting 60 min after i.v. injection of appr. 300–400 MBq [^{18}F]FDG.
- *Attenuation correction:*
  Transmission measurements depending on the design of the PET scanner used before or after emission measurement. Scan duration depending on equipment; adequate statistics are of decisive importance for the resulting image quality.
- *Reconstruction:*
  Where available, segmented iteration of the whole-body scan.
- *Documentation:*
  Coronal layers (5–10 mm thickness), with SUV scaling (SUV 0–8);
  Optionally also transversal layers for examination of the brain or improved allocation of focal findings.
- *Image interpretation:*
  Primary visual image analysis at the workstation;
  Followed by standardized documentation and quantification of detected foci.

References

[1] Allen RE, Epstein WL (1992) Melanoma therapy. Clin Dermatol 10:317–325
[2] Autier P, Dore JF, Schifflers E (1995) Melanoma and the use of sunscreens: an EORTC case-control study in Germany, Belgium and France. Int J Cancer 61:749–755
[3] Blessing C, Feine U, Geiger L, Carl M, Rassner G, Fierlbeck G (1995) Positron emission tomography and ultrasonography – a comparative retrospective study assessing the diagnostic validity in lymph node metastases of malignant melanoma. Arch Dermatol 131:1394–1398
[4] Böni R, Huch Böni RA, Steinert H, Burg G, Buck A, Marincek B, Berthold T, Dummer R, Voellmy D, Ballmer B, von Schulthess GK (1995) Staging of metastatic melanoma by whole-body positron emission tomography using 2-fluorine-18-fluoro-2-deoxy-D-glucose. Br J Dermatol 132:556–562
[5] Böni R, Huch Böni RA, Steinert H, von Schulthess GK, Burg G (1996) Early detection of melanoma metastasis using fluorodeoxyglucose F-18 positron emission tomography. Arch Dermatol 132:875–876
[6] Böni R, Steinert H, Huch Böni RA, von Schulthess GK, Meyer J, Dummer R, Burg G, Westera G (1997) Radioiodine-labelled alpha-methyl-tyrosine in malignant melanoma: cell culture studies and results in patients. Br J Dermatol 137:96–100
[7] Breslow A (1970) Thickness, cross sectional areas and depth of invasion in the prognosis of cutaneous melanoma. Ann Surg 172:902–908
[8] Clark WH, From L, Bernardino EA, Mihm MC (1969) The histogenesis and biologic behavior of primary human malignant melanoma of the skin. Cancer Res 29:705–726
[9] Damian DL, Fulham MJ, Thompson E, Thompson JF (1996) Positron emission tomography in the detection and management of metastatic melanoma. Melanoma Res 6:325–329
[10] Divgi CR, Larson SM (1989) Radiolabelled monoclonal antibodies in the diagnosis and treatment of malignant melanoma. Semin Nucl Med 19:252–261
[11] Garbe C, Büttner B, Weiß J, et al (1994a) Risk factors for developing cutaneous melanoma and criteria for identifying persons at risk: multicenter case-control study of the central malignant melanoma registry of the German dermatological society. J Invest Dermatol 102:695–699
[12] Garbe C, Büttner B, Weiß J, et al (1994b) Associated factors in the prevalence of more than 50 common melanocytic nevi, atypical melanocytic nevi and actinic lentigines: multicenter case-control study of the central malignant melanoma registry of the German dermatological society. J Invest Dermatol 102:700–705
[13] Garbe C, Büttner B, Bertz J, et al (1995a) Primary cutaneous melanoma: identification of prognostic groups and estimation of individual prognosis for 5093 patients. Cancer 75:2484–2491
[14] Garbe C, Büttner B, Bertz J, et al (1995b) Primary cutaneous melanoma: prognostic classification of anatomic location. Cancer 75:2492–2498
[15] Goydos JS, Ravikumar TS, Germino FJ, Yudd A, Bancila E (1998) Minimally invasive staging of patients with melanoma: sentinel lymphadenectomy and detection of the melanoma-spezific proteins MART-1 and tyrosinase by reverse transcriptase polymerase chain reaction. J Am Coll Surg 187:182–188
[16] Gritters LS, Francis IR, Zasadny KR, Wahl RL (1993) Initial assessment of positron emission tomography using 2-fluorine-18-fluoro-2-deoxy-D-glucose in the imaging of malignant melanoma. J Nucl Med 34:1420–1427
[17] Hoffmeister H, Bertz J, Garbe C (1990) Mortality and incidence of malignant melanoma in Germany 1970–1986. In: Orfanos CE, Garbe C (eds) Malignant melanoma of the Skin: New Results of Epidemiology, Diagnosis, Experimental Research, Therapy and After-care. Zuckschwerdt Verlag GmbH, Munich, pp 3–12
[18] Holder WD Jr, White RL, Zuger JH, Easton EJ Jr, Greene FL (1998) Effectiveness of positron emission tomography for the detection of melanoma metastases. Ann Surg 227:764–769

[19] Kagan R, Witt T, Bines S, Mesleh G, Economou S (1988) Gallium-67 scanning for malignant melanoma. Cancer 61:272–274

[20] Katsambas A, Nicolaidou E (1996) Cutaneous malignant melanoma and sun exposure – recent developments in epidemiology. Arch Dermatol 132:444–450

[21] Lindholm P, Leskinen S, Nagren K, Lehikoinen P, Ruotsalainen U, Teras M, Joensuu H (1995) Carbon-11-methionine PET imaging of malignant melanoma. J Nucl Med 36:1806–1810

[22] Macfarlane DJ, Sondak V, Jahnson T, Wahl RL (1998) Prospective evaluation of 2-[18F]-2-deoxy-D-glucose positron emission tomography in staging of regional lymph nodes in patients with cutaneous malignant melanoma. J Clin Oncol 16:1770–1776

[23] MacKie RM, Hole DJ (1996) Incidence and thickness of primary tumours and survival of patients with cutaneous malignant melanoma in relation to socioeconomic status. BMJ 312:1125–1128

[24] Mishima Y, Imahori Y, Honda C, Hiratsuka J, Ueda S, Ido T (1997) In vivo diagnosis of human malignant melanoma with positron emission tomography using specific melanoma-seeking 18F-DOPA analogue. J Neurooncol 33:163–169

[25] Morton DL (1997) Sentinel lymphadenectomy for patients with clinical stage I melanoma. J Surg Oncol 66:267–269

[26] Rassner G (1992) Dermatology. In: Rassner G, Steinert U (eds) Dermatology. Textbook and Atlas. Urban & Schwarzenberg, München Wien Baltimore

[27] Reske SN, Bares R, Büll U, Guhlmann A, Moser E, Wannenmacher MF (1996) Clinical value of positron emission tomography (PET) in oncologic questions: results of an interdisciplinary consensus conference. Under the patronage of the German Society of Nuclear Medicine. Nuklearmedizin 35:42–52

[28] Rinne D, Baum RP, Hör G, Kaufmann R (1998) Primary staging and follow-up of high risk melanoma patients with whole-body 18F-fluorodeoxyglucose positron emission tomography: results of a prospective study of 100 patients. Cancer 82:1664–1671

[29] Steinert HC, Huch Böni, RA, Buck A, Böni R, Berthold T, Marincek B, Burg G (1995) Malignant melanoma: staging with whole-body positron emission tomography and 2-[F-18]-fluoro-2-deoxy-D-glucose. Radiology 195:705–709

[30] Steinert HC, Ullrich SP, Böni R, von Schulthess GK, Dummer R (1998a) Cost-effectiveness of staging in malignant melanoma: whole body PET vs. conventional staging methods. Nuklearmedizin 37:A37, V 136 (abstr)

[31] Steinert HC, Voellmy DR, Trachsel C, Bicik I, Buck A, Huch RA, von Schulthess GK (1998b) Planar coincidence scintigraphy and PET in staging of malignant melanoma. J Nucl Med 39:1892–1897

[32] Stolz W, Landthaler M (1994) Classification, diagnosis and differential diagnosis of malignant melanoma. Chirurg 64:145–152

[33] Valk PE, Pounds TR, Tesar RD, Hopkins DM, Haseman MK (1996) Cost-effectiveness of PET imaging in clinical oncology. Nucl Med Biol 23:737–743

[34] Vollmer RT (1989) Malignant melanoma: a multivariate analysis of prognostic factors. Pathol Ann 24:383–407

[35] Wagner JD, Schauwecker D, Hutchins G, Coleman JJ 3rd (1997) Initial assessment of positron emission tomography for detection of nonpalpable regional lymphatic metastases in melanoma. J Surg Oncol 64:181–189

[36] Wagner JD, Schauwecker D, Davidson D, Coleman JJ 3rd, Saxman S, Hutchins G, Love C, Hayes JT (1999) Prospective study of fluorodeoxyglucose-positron emission tomography imaging of lymph node basins in melanoma patients undergoing sentinel node biopsy. J Clin Oncol 17:1508–1515

24 Musculoskeletal tumors

M. Schulte, D. Brecht-Krauss, J. Kotzerke

24.1 Incidence, etiology, epidemiology

Musculoskeletal sarcomas are relatively rare tumors compared to carcinomas and other neoplasms. The overall annual incidence rate is approximately 2 per 100 000 for soft tissue sarcomas, and 1 per 100 000 for malignant primary bone tumors [3]. Except for secondary tumors such as radiation-induced sarcoma, pathogenesis of most lesions is still unknown.

Soft tissue sarcomas may occur anywhere in the body, but the majority arise from the muscles of the extremities, the retroperitoneum, the chest wall, and the mediastinum. Individuals of any age can be affected; about 15% develop in children younger than 15 years, and about 40% in patients older than 55 years [8]. Various types of soft tissue sarcomas show a characteristic age distribution (Table 24.1). For instance, embryonal rhabdomyosarcoma predominantly occurs in children, whereas malignant fibrous histiocytoma represents a lesion typically occurring in advanced age [8].

Similarly, *osseous sarcomas* display a typical age preference as well as characteristic predilection sites (Table 24.2). Osteosarcomas and Ewing's sarcomas preferentially occur in the first and second decade, whereas chondrosarcomas predominantly can be observed after the third decade [3].

In comparison to primary osseous neoplasms *secondary bone tumors* occur frequently. About 50% of patients suffering from a carcinoma develop clinically apparent bone metastases, for example, the rate of skeletal dissemination confirmed by autopsy is about 70% in breast cancer [9].

Cancers of the breast, prostate, lung, thyroid and kidney represent a group of primary tumors, which cause about 80% of all skeletal secondaries. Predilection sites for bone metastases are the spine, proximal femur, pelvis, ribs, sternum, and proximal humerus [9]. The age peak for manifestation of osseous metastases is in the sixth decade.

24.2 Histopathologic classification

Soft tissue sarcomas comprise a multitude of entities with heterogeneous biological behavior. The grade of malignancy has a high prognostic relevance and is determined by the entity a priori in certain cases [8]. For instance,

Table 24.1. Classification of soft tissue sarcomas.

Histologic type	M:F	Relative incidence	Typical age distribution	Preferential site
Malignant fibrous histiocytoma (MFH)	60:40	~20–30%	50–70	Proximal portions of the extremities; retroperitoneum
Fibrosarcoma	50:50	~10%	30–50	Extremities; trunk (rare in childhood); preferentially thigh, knee region
Liposarcoma	55:45	15–18%	40–60	70% lower extremities and buttocks; retroperitoneum
Leiomyosarcoma	40:60	~7%	50–60	Retroperitoneum; cutis and subcutis of the lower extremities
Embryonal rhabdomyosarcoma	60:40	~14%	7–11	35–60% head and neck region; 20% urogenital region; retroperitoneum
Alveolar rhabdomyosarcoma	55:45	~4%	15–25	Extremities; head and neck region; urogenital region; retroperitoneum
Pleomorphic rhabdomyosarcoma	55:45	1%	40–60	33% extremities; 24% urogenital region; 7% head and neck region
Angiosarcoma	55:45	< 1%	50–70	Cutis and subcutis of the head; lower extremities
Synovial sarcoma	55:45	8–10%	20–35	Joints of the lower extremities, but preferentially extraarticular
Malignant schwannoma (MPNST)	56:44	5–10%	25–50	Trunk; proximal portions of extremities
Neuroblastoma	53:47	10–12%*	1–2	40% adrenal gland; sympathetic ganglia; mediastinum; retroperitoneum
Primitive neuroectodermal tumor (PNET)		1%	15–35	Trunk; lower extremities
Extraskeletal Ewing's sarcoma	55:45	rare	10–30	30% extremities, preferentially lower extremities; 30% paravertebral region; 15% chest wall

* In children

rhabdomyosarcoma, neuroblastoma and extraskeletal Ewing's sarcoma as a rule belong to the high-grade sarcomas, whereas myxoid liposarcoma is a low-grade lesion exclusively.

Problems concerning tumor grading may be caused by morphological variations in different parts of the same tumor: well differentiated and poorly differentiated portions can be encountered, for instance, in leiomyosarcomas, dedifferentiated liposarcomas, and malignant schwannomas [8].

Apart from the necessity of obtaining a second opinion by a specialized pathologist in many cases, a reliable diagnosis of primary bone tumors requires careful consideration of clinical (age, sex, site), radiologic and histologic findings. For instance, differentiation of central, periosteal, or parosteal osteosarcoma implicating different treatment strategies is based on clinical and radiologic rather than on histopathologic criteria alone [25].

Table 24.2. Classification of malignant bone tumors.

Histologic type	M:W	Relative incidence	Typical age distribution	Preferential site
Central classic osteosarcoma	61:39	24%	10–20	80% in long bones, predominantly metaphysis; 45% knee region; 10% humerus
Periosteal osteosarcoma	45:55	0.2%	10–20	Diaphysis of tibia and femur
Parosteal osteosarcoma	51:49	1%	15–40	Metaphysis of lower extremities, preferentially knee region; 65% femur
Chondrosarcoma	62:38	13%	30–60	Trunk, preferentially pelvis; proximal portions of extremities; facial bones, jaw bones
Dedifferentiated chondrosarcoma	64:36	1%	50–80	See chondrosarcoma
Clear-cell chondrosarcoma	72:28	Rare	30–40	Epiphysis of long bones; preferentially femur
Mesenchymal chondrosarcoma	50:50	Rare	20–40	Entire skeleton; increased number in the jaw bones
Malignant giant cell tumor	48:52	0.5%	20–40	Epiphyses of long bones; preferentially knee region
Fibrosarcoma	56:44	3.3%	15–60	Entire skeleton; preferentially knee region
Malignant fibrous histiocytoma	54:46	1.6%	10–70	Long bones
Ewing's sarcoma	63:37	6.6%	10–20	Entire skeleton; preferentially diaphyses of long bones
Malignant lymphoma of bone	62:38	6.6%	20–70	Entire skeleton; preferentially lower extremities and trunk
Plasmacytoma	59:41	40%	40–70	Skull; spine; pelvis; proximal portions of extremities

24.3 Clinical classification

Musculoskeletal sarcomas metastasize hematogeneously with preference for the lung. Lymphatic spread is rarely seen and bears the same significance as hematogeneous metastases concerning the prognosis of disease. Furthermore, nodules separated from the main tumor mass, known as "skip lesions", represent a typical, but infrequent modality of tumor spread in the same or an adjacent anatomical compartment. Therefore, the TNM system, while being the standard classification for carcinomas, has only minor importance for the staging of sarcomas. Since biology of sarcomas displays specific features and because treatment results of tumor centers can only be compared when they rely on a standardized classification, a comprehensive staging system covering benign and malignant skeletal and soft tissue lesions was established by Enneking [7]. This classification is of relevance for the prognosis as well as the therapeutic regime. It reflects the histologic grade (low-grade or high-grade lesion, stage I vs. II), regional or distant metastatic spread (stage III) and the anatomical situation of the neoplasm (intra- or extracompartmental, A vs. B). Using the same system, *benign tumors* can be classified as latent (stage 1), active (stage 2), and aggressive (stage 3) lesions.

Secondary bone tumors are classified regarding stage of disease – solitary, polytopic or diffuse affection of the skeleton – and morphology of the lesion – osteolytic, osteoplastic or mixed type of metastasis. Furthermore, differentiation of bone metastases without impairment of stability, with impending instability and with manifest pathological fracture has major therapeutic relevance.

24.4 Local recurrence, metastasis

The incidence of local recurrences is influenced by a number of factors: tumor type and grade, surgical margins, and response behavior of the tumor after neoadjuvant chemotherapy or preoperative radiotherapy all have an impact on the rate of local relapse. Some investigators recommend the grade of tumor response after neoadjuvant chemotherapy to be taken into consideration when planning the adequate degree of surgical radicality [23]. Local recurrence of sarcoma is frequently associated with both synchronous or metachronous metastatic spread and a deterioration in the histologic grade. The prime target organ of a dissemination is the lung, exhibiting 70–80% of all sarcoma secondaries, followed by the skeleton.

24.5 Standard diagnostic procedures

Treatment of sarcomas require subtle imaging techniques. Evaluation of the local and systemic tumor spread is mandatory, especially if a limb sparing procedure is intended. Because of possible difficulties with the histopathologic diagnosis and the estimation of the grade of malignancy, which are frequently based on a limited biopsy specimen, all radiologic findings should be matched with the histologic assessments. In sarcomas undergoing neoadjuvant chemotherapy, tumor regression has to be evaluated by a second preoperative staging procedure.

Established imaging modalities for the investigation of musculoskeletal lesions comprise conventional radiography, ultrasound, CT scanning and contrast-enhanced MRI. Additionally, tumor staging in sarcomas requires chest CT and bone scintigraphy in order to exclude pulmonary and skeletal metastases, respectively.

In carcinomas, bone scintigraphy represents the commonly used screening method for the detection of bone metastases. Suspected lesions have to be clarified by conventional radiography, whereas in the spine by an additional CT or MRI. Since therapy of skeletal metastases implicates an exclusively palliative treatment goal in the vast majority of patients concerned, diagnostic procedures should be restricted to investigations with immediate therapeutic consequences.

24.6 Basics of therapy

Multimodal treatment protocols comprising chemotherapy, radiotherapy, and surgery have been established in some musculoskeletal sarcomas, such as osteosarcoma, Ewing's sarcoma or rhabdomyosarcoma. Multimodal therapy is reserved for high-grade lesions, whereas surgery remains the mainstay in treatment of low-grade sarcomas. Certain tumors, such as chondrosarcoma, are regarded as resistant to chemotherapy or irradiation, irrespective of their individual grade of malignancy. In contrast, excellent response of Ewing's sarcoma to combined chemoradiotherapy opens a relevant chance of survival even in patients with unresectable tumor mass.

24.7 FDG-PET

First investigations concerning the usefulness of FDG-PET in the diagnosis of malignant musculoskeletal tumors started more than 10 years ago [13]. Recently, some studies have shown that glucose metabolism can be used for distinguishing benign and malignant lesions, for grading, for detection of local recurrences and distant metastases, and for the assessment of neoadjuvant chemotherapy response.

Patients have to fast for at least eight hours before the PET examination; at FDG administration, plasma glucose levels should not exceed 130 mg/dl in order to prevent a reduction of intratumoral FDG uptake [32]. If transmission scans are required, precise repositioning of the patient using laser-guided landmarks is essential before emission scans are performed. The necessity of an attenuation correction is not yet proven, and absorption must be regarded as low in extremities. Since FDG uptake of muscles varies with activity, patients should rest before and after FDG administration. The injection should not be performed at the affected limb. A reduction of radiation exposure can be achieved by supplying plenty of liquid, which leads to an accelerated elimination of FDG with the urine. Emission scans of the tumor site and the corresponding contralateral area start from 60 min after intravenous administration of a body mass-dependent dose of FDG.

Positioning of the patient has to consider axial symmetry. Movement artifacts due to pain are reduced, e.g., by suitable cushions. In order to detect tumor satellites, skip lesions and regional lymphatic metastases not only the suspected lesion, but the entire skeletal or muscular compartment with the adjacent joints should be included in the scan. Reliable calculation of emission data requires consideration of injected activity, time interval before emission scans are acquired, sensitivity of the scanner, and time of acquisition. Image reconstruction using a multiplicative iterative reconstruction algorithm should be preferred. Findings are documented in coronal, transaxial, and sagittal planes with consideration of an axial symmetric reconstruction, which permits improved distinction of soft tissue, bone and medullary canal.

Interpretation of PET findings requires knowledge of the anatomical imaging, which must be available for direct comparison. Follow-up studies should aim at an identical documentation and quantification technique, preferentially using tumor background ratios (TBRs).

24.7.1 Assessment criteria

Areas with a long-drawn FDG uptake mostly can be correlated with muscle activity or blood vessels. Any focal hypermetabolism has to be explained, for instance, by elevated uptake at a venous valve or caused by an insertion tendinosis. Lesions with a TBR exceeding 3.0 are suspicious of being malignant. Comparison to FDG uptake of the liver as a reference organ is not suitable for extremity tumors. The extension of each lesion has to be characterized regarding involvement of soft tissue, bone or medullary canal. Increased FDG uptake of the growth plates must be considered in children. Following chemotherapy an activation of the blood-forming bone marrow may be observed. Since unspecific peritumoral inflammatory processes can be confused with neoplastic activity [18], FDG accumulations should be localized anatomically as precisely as possible in follow-up studies.

24.7.2 Quantification

The most commonly used quantification technique describes regional activity in correlation to both total amount of activity administered and body volume, the latter generally substituted by body weight. The significance of these "standardized uptake values" (SUV) is not undisputed [14]. Calculation of SUVs requires attenuation correction of the emission data creating problems, such as increased examination time, elevated exposure to radiation, and methodological failures due to repositioning of the patient. The discussion concerning the necessity of transmission scanning is not yet finished [17]. A comparison of the tumoral FDG accumulation to the activity of a corresponding reference area in the contralateral, healthy extremity ("tumor background ratio", TBR) seems to be more practicable. TBR calculation can be performed with or without attenuation correction. Changes of TBR could be shown to provide improved correlation to the neoadjuvant chemotherapy response compared to SUV [28, 29]. Assessment of the regional metabolic rate requires dynamic monitoring of arterial supply and tumoral FDG uptake followed by an analysis using Patlak plots [22]. Though regional metabolic rates appeared superior to SUVs regarding estimation of the grade of malignancy in musculoskeletal tumors [21], an unequivocal distinction of benign and malignant lesions could not be achieved by this method [15], which also can not be recommended as a routine procedure because of its high methodological demands.

24.7.3 Results

Early studies disclosed a correlation of glucose consumption with the grade of malignancy in musculoskeletal tumors [13] and the possibility of distinguishing well-differentiated from undifferentiated liposarcoma [2]. Results could be confirmed by more extensive investigations in soft tissue tumors [1] and bone lesions [5]. While some authors claimed a precise discrimination of benign and malignant lesions [10], an overlap of these tumors was reported from other studies [15, 21]. Distinction of high-grade malignancies and benign tumors could be obtained without exception [6, 21]. In addition, transformation of Paget's disease as a primarily benign lesion with moderate FDG uptake into a Paget's sarcoma with highly elevated glucose utilization could be diagnosed [4]. A

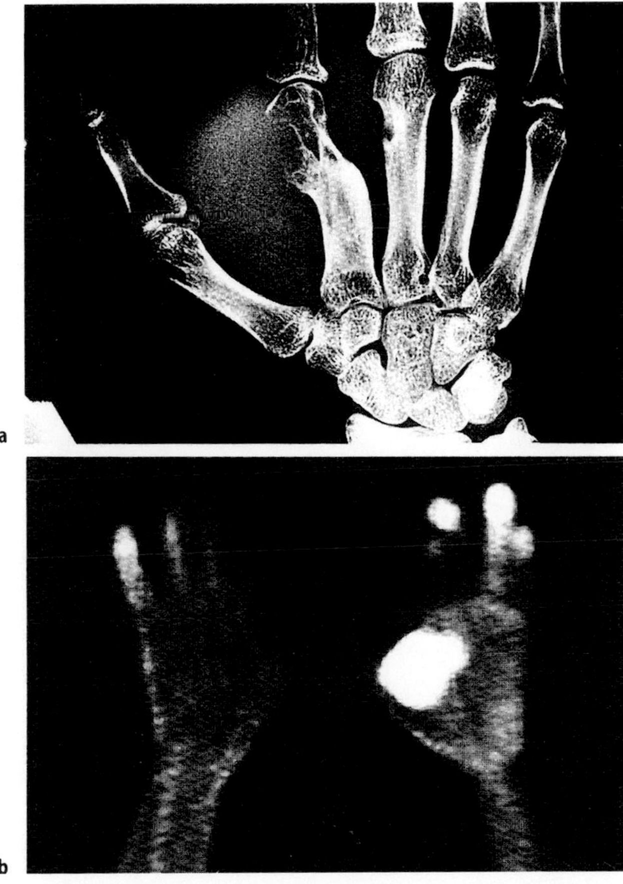

Fig. 24.1. Thirteen-year-old girl with a indolent progressive swelling of the right metacarpus. **a** Plain radiograph shows a circumscribed osteolytic destruction of the second and third metacarpal bone. **b** FDG-PET reveals a homogenous hypermetabolic lesion (TBR 4.6) extending from the first to the third ray. Histologic diagnosis: nodular fasciitis. Therapy: wide resection with disarticulation of the second and third ray.

high sensitivity of FDG-PET for the detection of malignancy in musculoskeletal tumors was demonstrated in our own series [26, 27] amounting to 95% for skeletal neoplasms (Table 24.3) and 97% for soft tissue sarcomas (Table 24.4) using a TBR of 3.0 as the cut-off level for suspected malignancy. Due to false-positive findings in aggressive benign tumors and pseudotumoral inflammatory lesions, specificity of the method must be regarded as comparatively low. In the group of sarcomas, the degree of hypermetabolism reflects the grade of malignancy. A high sensitivity also can be observed in the diagnosis of a local relapse [16]; FDG-PET offers a particular diagnostic advantage in patients, in whom follow-up CT or MRI investigations are restricted due to the method of surgical bone defect reconstruction [19]. For the detection of lung metastases, accuracy of FDG-PET is comparable to spiral CT. Whether the sensitivity in detecting osseous secondaries of musculoskeletal sarcomas is superior to bone scintigraphy is still unresolved [24, 30]. The histologic response to neoadjuvant chemotherapy represents an important prognostic indicator for disease-free survival following multimodal treatment of osteogenic sarcoma and Ewing's sarcoma [20]. The risk of local recurrence which drastically

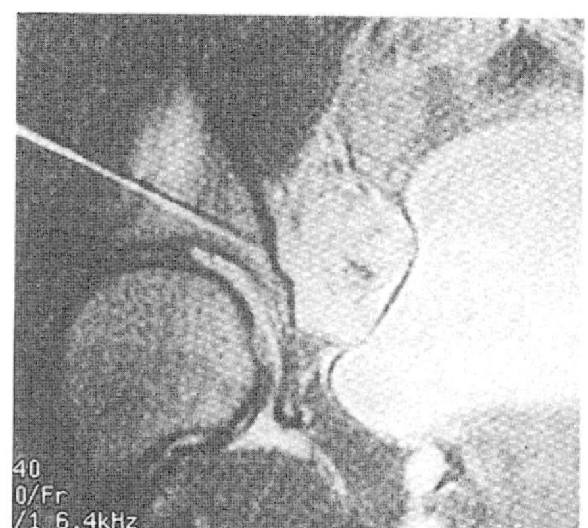

b

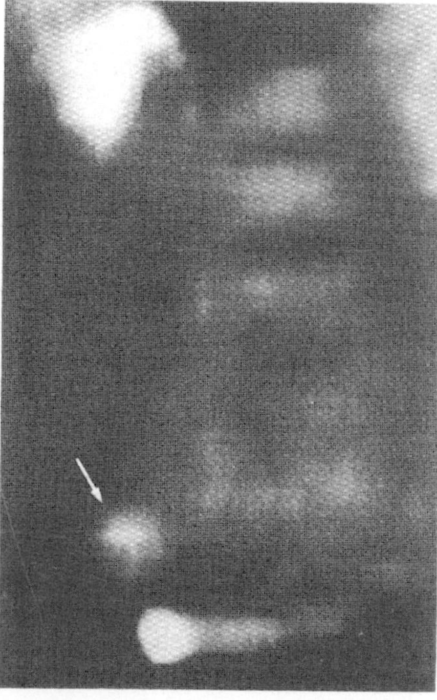

a

Fig. 24.2. Thirty-three-year-old woman suffering from uncharacteristic moderate pain in the right pelvic region. **a** Detection of a parosteal paravesical mass infiltrating the iliac muscle by contrast-enhanced MRI. **b** FDG-PET displays a focal elevated glucose utilization (TBR 3.2, arrow); visualization of the lesion requires empty urinary bladder. Because of suspected malignancy incisional biopsy is indicated. Histologic diagnosis: well-differentiated extraskeletal chondrosarcoma. Therapy: wide resection.

Table 24.3. Histologic diagnosis and distribution of TBR values in 243 skeletal lesions. A TBR value of 3.0 is used as the cut-off level for suspected malignancy.

Diagnosis	N	TBR	Median	False negative	False positive
Osteosarcoma	49	3.3–33.2	9.5	–	
Ewing's sarcoma	12	4.1–31.0	4.7	–	
Primitive neuroectodermal tumor	3	4.0–8.4	5.6	–	
Chondrosarcoma	16	1.5–11.8	2.7	69%	
Dedifferentiated chondrosarcoma	3	7.0–73.0	10.0	–	
Clear-cell chondrosarcoma	1	5.6		–	
Malignant fibrous histiocytoma	6	3.3–26.0	14.6	–	
Angiosarcoma	4	3.5–31.0	15.2	–	
Leiomyosarcoma	1	27.2		–	
Epithelioid sarcoma	1	20.5		–	
Chordoma	6	2.7–12.5	5.4	17%	
Giant cell tumor	5	10.1–35.0	19.1		100%
Aneurysmatic bone cyst	15	1.1–5.9	2.3		40%
Simple bone cyst	11	1.0–3.5	1.5		9%
Chondroma	9	1.4–4.0	2.3		11%
Periosteal chondroma	4	1.0–2.7	2.1		–
Osteochondroma	10	1.0–4.7	2.1		10%
Chondroblastoma	2	6.5–33.6			–
Chondromyxoidfibroma	1	2.9			–
Fibrous dysplasia	4	5.2–11.5	6.5		100%
Non-ossifying fibroma	9	1.2–18.6	3.6		56%
Desmoplastic fibroma	2	2.2–7.0			50%
Osteoidosteoma	3	1.4–2.9	2.4		–
Eosinophilic granuloma	3	4.5–6.3	4.6		100%
Osteofibrous dysplasia	1	2.8			–
Parathyroid osteopathy	1	5.1			100%
Osteomyelitis	12	1.1–24.1	2.0		25%
Other tumor-like lesions	9	1.0–2.3	1.7		–
Bone metastasis	25	1.8–34.0	7.8	12%	
Malignant lymphoma of bone	7	3.5–49.2	17.7	–	
Plasmacytoma	8	1.3–15.1	6.1	25%	

reduces the chances for survival is linked to both the response to preoperative therapy and the type of surgery. The overall local failure rate rises in patients with poor response (defined as less than 90% tumor destruction) when treated by a limb salvage procedure instead of an amputation [23].

Since PET directly assesses active glucose metabolism, viable sarcoma tissue and tumor necrosis can be discerned by FDG uptake [31]. Therefore, the efficiency of chemotherapy can be estimated by measuring tumoral glucose utilization [12]. In our experience, the decrease of FDG uptake in osteosarcomas and Ewing's sarcomas expressed as ratio of post- and pretherapeutic TBRs correlates closely with the amount of tumor necrosis induced by polychemotherapy. A decrease in FDG uptake of at least 40% can be used to reliably identify responders with a tumor necrosis rate of more than 90%. Based on semiquantitative analysis using TBRs, an accuracy of better than 90% was attained for distinguishing responders and non-responders [28, 29].

Table 24.4. Histologic diagnosis and distribution of TBR values in 125 soft tissue lesions. A TBR value of 3.0 is used as the cut-off level for suspected malignancy.

Diagnosis	N	TBR	Median	False negative	False positive
Malignant fibrous histiocytoma	29	2.6–51.4	12.3	3%	
Liposarcoma	11	1.5–24.5	4.4	36%	
Rhabdomyosarcoma	9	4.6–27.3	14.9	–	
Malignant schwannoma	6	5.8–20.0	11.0	–	
Extrasekeletal chondrosarcoma	5	3.2–18.4	15.0	–	
Leiomyosarcoma	4	3.4–7.2	5.5	–	
Synovial sarcoma	4	5.1–39.2	10.3	–	
Fibrosarcoma	3	6.4–8.3	7.1	–	
Primitive neuroectodermal tumor	2	7.0–11.1		–	
Angiosarcoma	2	6.2–8.8		–	
Extraskeletal Ewing's sarcoma	1	14.1		–	
Extraskeletal osteosarcoma	1	23.0		–	
Epithelioid sarcoma	1	3.1		–	
Non-Hodgkin lymphoma	1	39.0		–	
Hemangioendothelioma	1	3.1		–	
Hemangioma	9	1.1–3.9	2.1		11%
Aggressive fibromatosis	7	1.5–12.0	2.8		43%
Lipoma	5	1.0–1.7	1.0		–
Pigmented villonodular synovitis	2	2.7–6.9			50%
Nodular fasciitis	2	4.6–15.9			100%
Schwannoma	2	1.9–2.9			–
Neurofibroma	2	2.5–2.7			–
Intramuscular glomangioma	2	3.0–10.7			100%
Hemangiopericytoma	2	1.8–2.2			–
Myxolipoma	2	1.4–2.8			–
Angiolipoma	1	2.2			–
Spindle-cell lipoma	1	2.4			–
Lymphangioma	1	1.9			–
Langerhans' cell histiocytosis	1	6.7			100%
Aneurysm	1	1.0			–
Spontaneous myositis ossificans	6	3.1–20.8	4.2		100%

24.7.4 Oncological consensus conference

The relevance of FDG-PET for staging of musculoskeletal tumors was discussed at the second Consensus Conference in Ulm, Germany, in 1997. Due to the lack of published data at that time, a definitive assessment of the diagnostic importance in sarcomas had not been established. Recommendations based on currently published studies are expected to be given by the third Consensus Conference, which will be held in 2000.

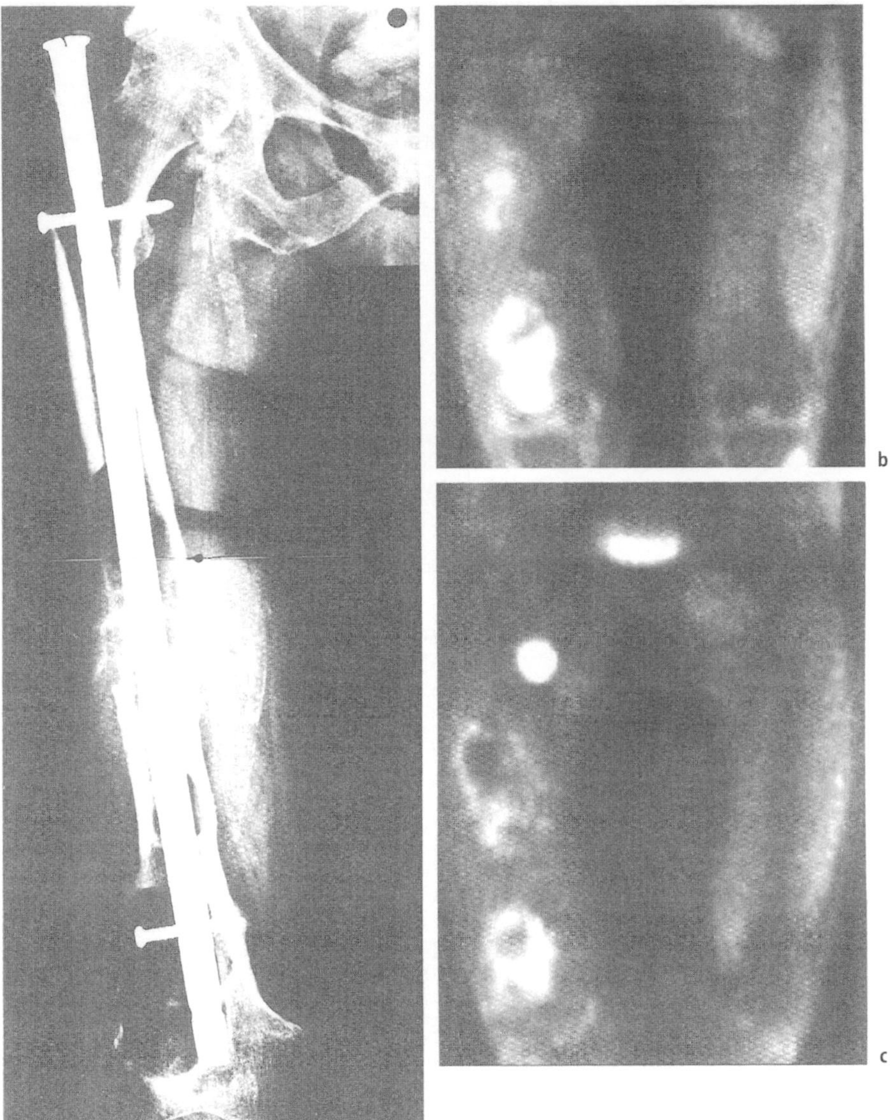

Fig. 24.3. Seventy-six-year-old woman with histologically ascertained epithelioid angiosarcoma of right femur; intralesional resection and intramedullary nailing because of pathologic fracture one year before. **a** Plain radiograph revèals a bifocal local recurrence in the middle and distal portion of femur. Due to artifacts caused by the implant, CT scans or MRI can not be used for the estimation of soft tissue infiltration and local staging. **b** FDG-PET confirms a bifocal recurrent tumor within the bone with considerable hypermetabolism (TBR of the distal lesion 31.0). **c** Detection of a satellite lesion (TBR 8.2) in the soft tissues of the proximal thigh, corresponding to an infrainguinal lymph node metastasis. In whole-body PET, no evidence of further distant metastases. Therapy: wide tumor resection including lymph node dissection, total femur replacement by megaprosthesis.

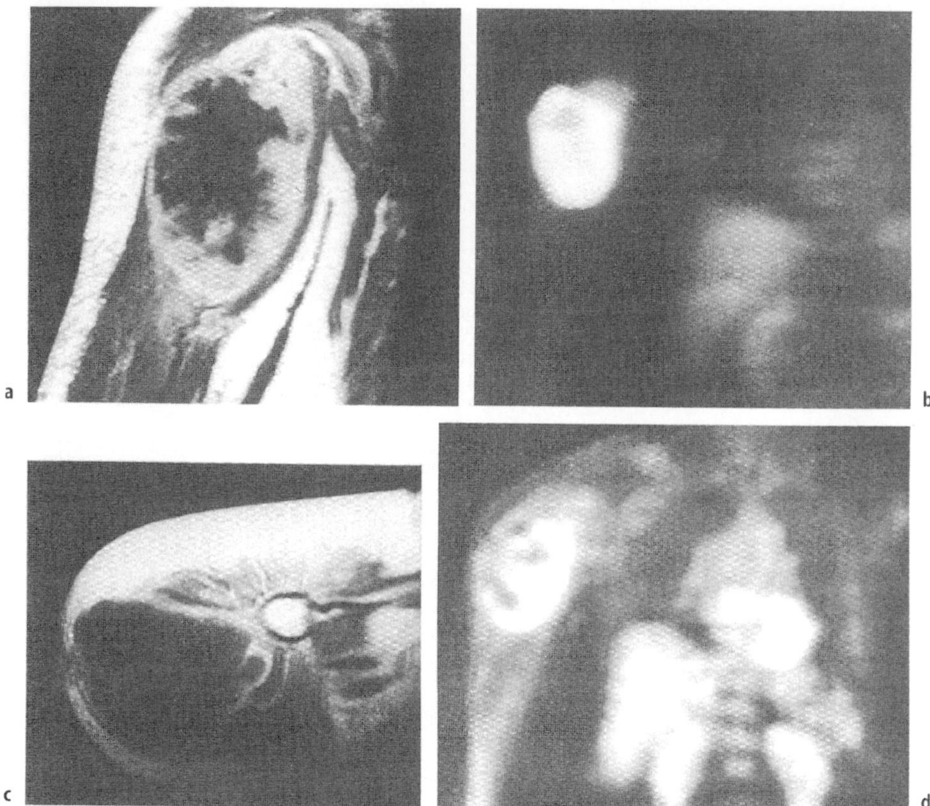

Fig. 24.4. Seventy-two-year-old woman with malignant fibrous histiocytoma G3 of the right proximal upper arm. **a** Contrast-enhanced MRI reveals an intramuscular lesion with peripheral gadolinium uptake and central necrotic areas. **b** PET displays an inhomogeneous lesion with considerable FDG uptake (TBR 6.7). **c** Following preoperative radiotherapy (55 Gy), a predominantly necrotic transformation of the sarcoma is visualized by MRI. **d** Significant decrease of glucose consumption (TBR 2.8) in follow-up PET. Therapy: wide tumor resection; histologically only minute fraction of viable tumor cells within the specimen.

24.8 Future aspects

Grading of musculoskeletal neoplasms using FDG-PET can be helpful in equivocal tumors, in particular in lesions with a discrepancy between histopathological and clinical diagnosis or with inconclusive radiologic findings. Sarcomas and aggressive benign tumors, which both have to be resected with wide surgical margins, show a markedly elevated glucose metabolism as compared to latent or active benign lesions. Preoperative analysis of glucose metabolism can, therefore, help to choose the most appropriate surgical procedure. In bone tumors, if the character of an asymptomatic lesion is questionable on standard radiograms, the level of metabolic activity can be used to decide whether a histologic evaluation is required. This holds particularly true, if a biopsy is difficult as for instance in the pelvis. From the data currently available, a malignant or aggressive benign lesion can be safely excluded if TBR values are low (< 1.5). An intermediate TBR value (between 1.5 and 3) can be consistent with a low-grade sarcoma at most, while all high-grade sarcomas and the vast majority of both low-grade sarcomas and aggressive benign lesions disclose markedly increased TBR values (> 3). Furthermore, the high sensitivity of PET in detecting malignant musculoskeletal primaries implicates a similar relevance for diagnosing skip lesions as well as occult lymph node, skeletal, lung, and visceral metastases; this aspect of tumor staging deserves further evaluation including comparison to standard procedures, such as CT and bone scintigraphy [24].

A combined visualization of the tumor and the skeleton after simultaneous application of ^{18}F-fluoride ion and ^{18}F-FDG may improve the anatomical orientation in isolated cases [11]; in this subject sufficient experience is not yet available. Since current treatment protocols for osteosarcoma and Ewing's sarcoma require a monitoring of preoperative chemotherapy response prior to surgical removal of the tumor, particularly if a limb salvage procedure is intended, FDG-PET should be established as a non-invasive tool to identify responders after neoadjuvant treatment as a standard procedure for the assessment of tumor regression. Reliable prediction of response behavior could implicate consequences for the choice of surgical strategy, because a limb salvage procedure cannot be recommended in patients non-responsive to preoperative chemotherapy unless wide surgical margins can safely be achieved. In addition, an inhomogeneous distribution of the viable tumor fraction in different parts of a neoplasm as visualized by FDG-PET might have an influence on the surgical procedure in sarcomas amenable to a preoperative treatment (chemotherapy, radiotherapy).

24.9 [^{18}F]FDG-PET: practical use and image interpretation

Patient preparation: fasted > 12 h; plasma glucose level < 130 mg/dl; resting during waiting period to avoid FDG uptake in muscles; no tracer injection in the extremity to be investigated; cannula removal before starting acquisition

Data acquisition: 60 min after injection of 370 MBq FDG, multi-static acquisition of the extremity including the adjacent joints, additionally imaging of the lung to exclude metastasis

Attenuation correction: transmission scans dispensable for staging studies due to minor absorption from the extremities

Reconstruction: iterative reconstruction is preferred, image reangulation for optimal display of the long bones in coronal and sagittal view

Imaging interpretation: always considering the morphologic imaging (X-ray, MRI, CT, ultrasound)
1. Qualitative analysis: assessment of the lesion's intensity; assigning to bone, medullary cavity, or soft tissue; beware of moderate uptake of the epiphyseal growth plates in children up to 10 years
2. Quantitative analysis: calculation of tumor background ratio (TBR) with outlining the region of interest (ROI) using a transversal scan at the center of the lesion (necrotic areas without metabolism should be excluded) and transcription of the ROI to the opposite site; in very large tumors logical reduction of the background ROI to reasonable size. TBR > 3.0 is suspicious for malignancy.

References

[1] Adler LP, Blair HF, Makley JT et al. (1991) Noninvasive grading of musculoskeletal tumors using PET. J Nucl Med 32:1508–1512
[2] Adler LP, Blair HF, Williams RP et al. (1990) Grading liposarcomas with PET using [18F]FDG. J Comput Assist Tomogr 14:960–962
[3] Campanacci M (1990) Bone and Soft Tissue Tumors. Springer, Wien New York
[4] Cook GJ, Maisey MN, Fogelman I (1997) Fluorine-18-FDG PET in Paget's disease of bone. J Nucl Med 38:1495–1497
[5] Dehdashti F, Siegel BA, Griffeth LK, Fusselman MJ, Trask DD, McGuire AH, McGuire DJ (1996) Benign versus malignant intraosseous lesions: discrimination by means of PET with 2-[F-18]fluoro-2-deoxy-D-glucose. Radiology 200:243–247
[6] Eary JF, Conrad EU, Bruckner JD, Folpe A, Hunt KJ, Mankoff DA, Howlett AT (1998) Quantitative [F-18]fluorodeoxyglucose positron emission tomography in pretreatment and grading of sarcoma. Clin Cancer Res 4:1215–1220
[7] Enneking WF (1986) A system of staging musculoskeletal neoplasms. Clin Orthop 204:9–24
[8] Enzinger FM, Weiss SW (1995) Soft Tissue Tumors. Mosby, St. Louis Baltimore Berlin
[9] Galasko CSB (1986) Skeletal Metastases. Butterworths, London
[10] Griffeth LK, Dehdashti F, McGuire AH, McGuire DJ, Perry DJ, Moerlein SM, Siegel BA (1992) PET evaluation of soft-tissue masses with fluorine-18 fluoro-2-deoxy-D-glucose. Radiology 182:185–194
[11] Hoegerle S, Juengling F, Otte A, Moser EA, Nitzsche EU (1998) Combined FDG and [F-18]fluoride whole-body PET: a feasible two-in-one approach to cancer imaging? Radiology 209:253–258
[12] Jones DN, McCowage GB, Sostman HD et al. (1996) Monitoring of neoadjuvant therapy response of soft-tissue and musculoskeletal sarcoma using fluorine-18-FDG PET. J Nucl Med 37:1438–1444
[13] Kern KA, Brunetti A, Norton JA et al. (1988) Metabolic imaging of human extremity musculoskeletal tumors by PET. J Nucl Med 29:181–186
[14] Keyes JW (1995) SUV: standard uptake or silly useless value? J Nucl Med 36:1836–1839
[15] Kole AC, Nieweg OE, Hoekstra HJ, van Horn JR, Koops HS, Vaalburg W (1998) Fluorine-18-fluorodeoxyglucose assessment of glucose metabolism in bone tumors. J Nucl Med 39:810–815

[16] Kole AC, Nieweg OE, van Ginkel RJ et al. (1997) Detection of local recurrence of soft-tissue sarcoma with positron emission tomography using [18F]fluorodeoxyglucose. Ann Surg Oncol 4:57–63
[17] Kotzerke J, Guhlmann A, Moog F, Reske SN (1999) Role of attenuation correction for FDG-PET in the primary staging of malignant lymphoma. Eur J Nucl Med 26:31–38
[18] Kubota R, Yamada S, Kubota K, Ishiwata K, Tamahashi N, Ido T (1992) Intratumoral distribution of fluorine-18-fluorodeoxyglucose in vivo: high accumulation in macrophages and granulation tissues studied by microautoradiography. J Nucl Med 33:1972–1980
[19] Lucas JD, O'Doherty MJ, Wong JC, Bingham JB, McKee PH, Fletcher CD, Smith MA (1998) Evaluation of fluorodeoxyglucose positron emission tomography in the management of soft-tissue sarcomas. J Bone Joint Surg Br 80:441–447
[20] Meyers PA, Heller G, Healey J et al. (1992) Chemotherapy for nonmetastatic osteogenic sarcoma: the Memorial Sloan-Kettering experience. J Clin Oncol 10:5–15
[21] Nieweg OE, Pruim J, van Ginkel RJ et al. (1996) Fluorine-18-fluorodeoxyglucose PET imaging of soft-tissue sarcoma. J Nucl Med 37:257–261
[22] Patlak CS, Blasberg RG, Fenstermacher JD (1983) Graphical evaluation of blood-to-brain transfer constants from multiple-time uptake data. J Cereb Blood Flow Metab 3:1–7
[23] Picci P, Sangiorgi L, Rougraff BT, Neff JR, Casadei R, Campanacci M (1994) Relationship of chemotherapy-induced necrosis and surgical margins to local recurrence in osteosarcoma. J Clin Oncol 12:2699–2705
[24] Sasaki M, Ichiya Y, Kuwabara Y et al. (1993) Fluorine-18-fluorodeoxyglucose positron emission tomography in technetium-99m-hydroxymethylenediphosphate negative bone tumors. J Nucl Med 34:288–290
[25] Schajowicz F (1994) Tumors and Tumor like Lesions of Bone. Springer, Berlin Heidelberg New York
[26] Schulte M, Brecht-Krauss D, Heymer B, Guhlmann A, Hartwig E, Sarkar MR, Diederichs CG, v. Baer A, Kotzerke J, Reske SN (2000) Grading of tumors and tumor like lesions of bone: evaluation by 2-(fluorine-18)-fluoro-2-deoxy-d-glucose positron emission tomography. J Nucl Med (in press)
[27] Schulte M, Brecht-Krauss D, Heymer B, Guhlmann A, Hartwig E, Sarkar MR, Diederichs CG, Schultheiss M, Kotzerke J, Reske SN (1999) Fluorodeoxyglucose positron emission tomography in soft tissue neoplasms: is a non-invasive estimation of biological activity possible? Eur J Nucl Med 26:599–605
[28] Schulte M, Brecht-Krauss D, Werner M, Hartwig E, Sarkar MR, Keppler P, Kotzerke J, Delling G, Reske SN (1999) Evaluation of neoadjuvant therapy response of osteogenic sarcoma using 2-(fluorine-18)-fluoro-2-deoxy-D-glucose positron emission tomography. J Nucl Med 40:1637–1643
[29] Schulte M, Brecht-Krauss D, Hartwig E, Guhlmann A, Sarkar MR, Kotzerke J, Reske SN (1999) Tumour regression monitoring in osteosarcoma and Ewing's sarcoma following neoadjuvant chemotherapy using FDG positron emission tomography (PET). Eur J Nucl Med 26:980 (abstr)
[30] Tse N, Hoh C, Hawkins R, Phelps M, Glaspy J (1994) Positron emission tomography diagnosis of pulmonary metastases in osteogenic sarcoma. Am J Clin Oncol 17:22–25
[31] van Ginkel RJ, Hoekstra HJ, Pruim J et al. (1996) FDG-PET to evaluate response to hyperthermic isolated limb perfusion for locally advanced soft-tissue sarcoma. J Nucl Med 37:984–990
[32] Zimny M, Bares R, Fass J et al. (1997) Fluorine-18 fluorodeoxyglucose positron emission tomography in the differential diagnosis of pancreatic carcinoma: a report of 106 cases. Eur J Nucl Med 24:678–682

25 Metastatic bone disease

H. Schirrmeister

25.1 Incidence, etiology, epidemiology

Bone metastases are common in the most prevalent cancers in Western Europe and the USA. Carcinomas of the breast (45–85%), prostate (33–85%) and lung (33–50%) are most commonly associated with metastatic bone disease. Bone metastases are also very common in renal carcinoma (33–40%) and follicular thyroid cancer (28–60%). After primary diagnosis of metastatic bone disease the average length of survival is reported 20 months for breast cancer, 17 months for prostate cancer and only a few months for lung cancer [21].

25.2 Pathophysiology, distribution, pattern of metastatic bone disease

Bone remodeling is a continuous process controlled by osteoclasts, which are derived from the macrophage and monocyte system and by osteoblasts, derived from the fibroblast system. Osteoblasts are concerned with bone formation while osteoclasts are involved in bone resorption. The rates of bone formation and bone resorption are balanced in healthy persons. In patients with metastatic bone disease, bone remodeling is influenced by several paracrine factors secreted from metastatic tumor cells. Osteolytic metastases deposits cause bone resorption by the local release of cytokines and growth factors which stimulate osteoclastic bone resorption [17]. Osteolytic metastases are frequently observed in most cancers (e.g., lung cancer, thyroid cancer, renal carcinoma). Osteosclerosis is typical of prostate cancer and is a result of local release of osteoblast stimulating factors. A mixed pattern of osteosclerotic/osteolytic metastases is often observed in breast cancer. The vertebral column is the most common site of metastatic bone disease [2, 17, 24, 25, 32]. This is due to tumor spread via the Batson's plexus which surrounds the vertebrae [2]. This venous plexus is connected extensively with the veins of the caval, portal and pulmonary venous system. Hematogenous spread of metastases is most likely to co-occur via arterial and venous vessels entering anterior and posterior parts of the vertebral bodies. Metastases are therefore most likely to be localized at the ventral or posterior edge of the vertebral body [1]. Metastases usually extend into the medullary cavity but cannot affect the adjacent bone because of the natural barrier established by the cortex [14].

25.3 Assessment of metastatic bone disease

Skeletal scintigraphy is widely regarded as a routine procedure for initial staging of patients with tumors associated with a high prevalence of bone metastases. Metastatic bone disease must be excluded in these patients before initiation of a potentially curative therapy. Bone scintigraphy (BS) is also useful in patients with previously known bone metastases for evaluation of systemic therapy and in order to exclude metastases at critical anatomical sites, such as the long bones (risk of pathological fractures) or at the vertebral column (risk of spinal cord compression). The attributes required of diagnostic methods for screening for metastatic bone disease are as follows: 1) high specificity to avoid the need of further examinations. 2) High sensitivity to exclude/detect bone metastases at primary staging and for the accurate description of extent of metastatic bone disease for later therapy control. 3) The possibility of whole-body surveys allows assessment of the entire skeleton in practicable examination times.

25.3.1 Comparison of bone scintigraphy, magnetic resonance imaging, bone marrow scintigraphy, planar x-ray and computed tomography

Several comparative studies have shown that bone scintigraphy using ^{18}F-sodium fluoride is clearly more sensitive than planar x-ray in detection of metastatic bone disease in tumors with a high incidence of bone metastases. Between 1962 and 1973 planar bone scintigraphy was considered the most sensitive imaging method for primary staging as well as for follow-up examinations [3, 10, 11]. Bone scintigraphy using ^{99m}Tc-labeled polyphosphonates is approximately twofold more sensitive and offers a better spatial resolution than ^{18}F-fluoride bone scans because conventional gamma cameras respond better in terms of sensitivity and resolution to the 140 keV photons of ^{99m}Tc than to the 511 keV photons of ^{18}F [21, 28, 31]. Since the 1970s, gamma camera bone scans have therefore been performed with ^{99m}Tc-labeled polyphosphonates. Bone scanning is considered less sensitive in osteolytic than in osteosclerotic metastases [16]. In detection of osteolytic metastases, bone marrow scintigraphy (BMS), computed tomography (CT) and magnetic resonance imaging (MRI) bone scanning were shown to be clearly more sensitive [9, 10, 20, 29, 30]. Although BS is commonly regarded as highly sensitive in osteosclerotic metastases, false-negative BS have been previously reported even in osteosclerotic metastases from prostate cancer [30]. When indeterminate vertebral lesions are present on planar BS, SPECT is currently used as a complementary method for differentiating between benign and malignant lesions due to its more precise anatomical localization [14]. In a study performed by Kosuda et al. [13] routine SPECT was as sensitive as MRI in detection of vertebral metastases. In a further study, planar BS was 80–90% sensitive in the detection of metastases present at the peripheral skeleton but as low as 20–40% sensitive in the detection of vertebral metastases [25]. The results of these two studies suggest that SPECT of the entire vertebral column might be useful in all patients with a high risk of metastatic bone disease even when there is no sign of metastasis in planar BS. MRI was shown to be superior to CT in detecting bone metastases [9]. Both MRI and CT are, however, impracticable for whole-body imaging. At present MRI is therefore used to clarify indeterminate lesions detected with BS. Planar x-ray and CT are not useful for the screening of metastatic bone disease but are adequate for estimating fracture risk and for confirmation of metastases detected with BS [9].

25.3.2 PET

Examination of metastatic bone disease with PET is possible using 2-[^{18}F] fluoro-2-deoxy-D-glucose (FDG-PET) or ^{18}F-sodium fluoride (^{18}F-PET) alternatively. The principles of tracer accumulation are quite different in these two radiotracers. FDG accumulates in tumor cells and is therefore a marker for metastatic cell metabolism. By contrast bone metastases are shown indirectly with ^{18}F-sodium fluoride as altered bone mineralization is made visible. Uptake of ^{18}F-sodium fluoride into bone is two-fold higher and its blood clearance is faster than the blood clearance of technetium polyphosphonates [6–8]. This results in a superior bone to background ratio using ^{18}F-sodium fluoride instead of [^{99m}Tc]-polyphosphonates. Due to its pharmacological properties ^{18}F-sodium fluoride can be regarded as optimal radiotracer for bone imaging.

25.3.2.1 Imaging technique (^{18}F-PET)

As with conventional bone scanning procedures, patients do not have to fast before the PET scan but should be well hydrated. All drugs can be taken. Quantitative measurement of fluoride uptake into bone is not useful since there is a wide range in tracer uptake in both benign and malignant lesions (Fig. 25.1–25.4). For examination in typical full-ring scanners, the injected activity of ^{18}F-sodium fluoride is 370 MBq. For 370 MBq ^{18}F-sodium fluoride, the whole-body equivalent-dose is 9.9 mSv (BS with 740 MBq [^{99m}Tc] MDP: 5.5 mSv). Stimulation of diuresis or transmission scanning is not recommended. The time interval between application and emission scanning should be at least one hour and should be increased to at least two hours in older patients. The required imaging time per bed position is 10–12 min. The uptake into bone and the soft tissue clearance of ^{18}F-sodium fluoride is much faster

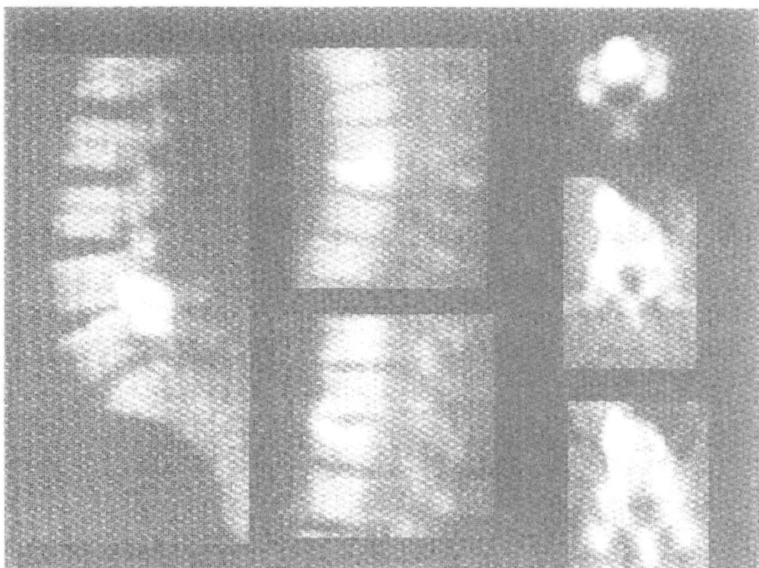

Fig. 25.1. ^{18}F-PET, commonly observed benign lesions. Left: Arthritis of the intervertebral joint L4/L5. Center: (sagittal sections) endplate fractures. Right: osteophytes appearing with different tracer uptake.

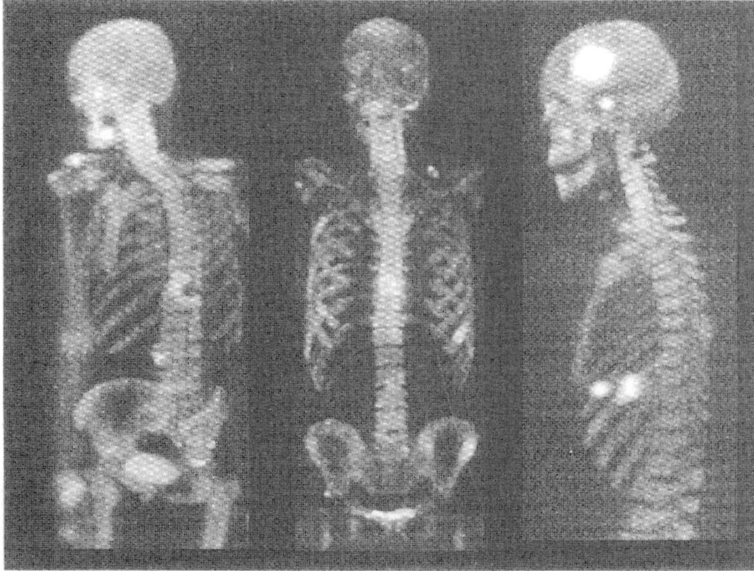

Fig. 25.2. Whole-body images (maximum intensity projections, MIP). Bone metastases in thyroid cancer (left), lung cancer (center), breast cancer (right). The rib lesions in the patient with breast cancer are corresponding to rib fractures.

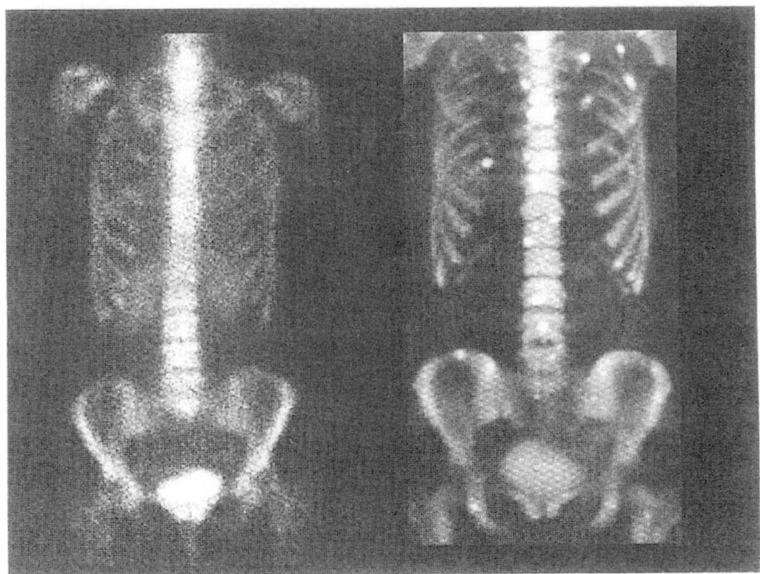

Fig. 25.3. The extent of metastatic bone disease in a breast cancer patient is significantly underestimated with the conventional planar bone scan (left: [^{99m}Tc]MDP, right: ^{18}F-PET, MIP).

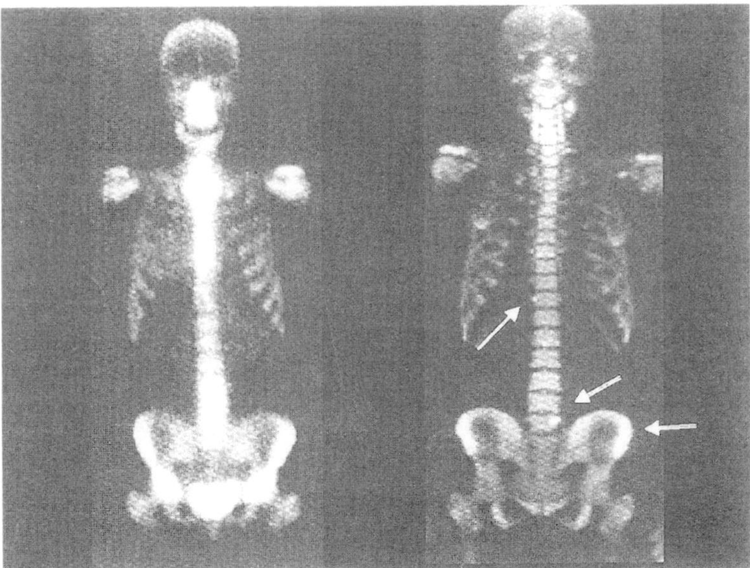

Fig. 25.4. False-negative bone scintigraphy in breast cancer (left). ^{18}F-PET shows metastases in the thoracic and lumbar spine and in the pelvis (→).

than that of technetium-labeled polyphosphonates. Therefore there is no prominence of soft tissue in ^{18}F-PET images. Imaging quality of the PET scans may be limited in patients with decreased renal function or when renal elimination or the osseous uptake of ^{18}F-sodium fluoride is decreased due to patient-independent parameters such as silver ion from the target material.

25.3.2.2 Criteria for image interpretation

With ^{18}F-PET osteolytic metastases often appear as photopenic lesions surrounded by a rim of increased activity. This pattern was observed exclusively in metastases but never in benign lesions [22–24]. In contrast, lesions showing focally increased uptake can not only be observed in osteosclerotic and osteolytic metastases but also in benign lesions [18, 19, 22–26]. Malignant lesions appear with a wide range of tracer uptake (Fig. 25.2). Interpretation of these lesions is therefore independent of tracer uptake but dependent on exact anatomical localization [12, 22, 23]. The interpretation criteria are the same as commonly employed for the interpretation of conventional biphosphonate bone scans [22]. The superior spatial resolution of modern PET scanners allows exact anatomical localization of lesions and better differentiation between benign and malignant lesions. Metastases are suspected when lesions are neither located at joints nor show the typical pattern of endplate fractures or serial rib fractures [24]. In contrast to benign lesions (Fig. 25.1) the spongious bone is commonly affected by metastases [24].

Similar to conventional bone scanning, differentiation between single rib metastases and rib fractures remains difficult with ^{18}F-PET [24]. Endplate fractures show up as linear tracer uptake at the endplates and are therefore easy to differentiate from metastases [23]. As in the well-known pattern of radiographs, osteophytes appear as lesions with variable tracer uptake located at the upper and lower edges of adjacent endplates (Fig. 25.1). The spongiose bone is commonly excluded from the tracer uptake in these lesions. An increased uptake located at the juxtaarticular surfaces of intervertebral joints is typical of intervertebral arthritis. The joint space is often made visible with ^{18}F-PET (Fig. 25.1). Arthritis of the acromeoclavicular joints or of the intervertebral joints as well as endplate fractures account for more than 80% of all benign lesions detected with ^{18}F-PET. These lesions have a very characteristic pattern of uptake so that they are easy to distinguish from metastases even when single areas of increased uptake are present on ^{18}F-PET scans [23].

25.3.2.3 Results

FDG-PET has been reported to be more sensitive than planar bone scintigraphy in detecting metastases of lung cancer and also in detecting lymphomatous bone marrow [4, 15]. Other studies have indicated that FDG-PET is less sensitive in detecting osteoblastic metastases from cancer of the prostate or the breast [5, 27]. Cook et al. [5] suggested therefore that FDG-PET might be less sensitive in detecting osteosclerotic metastases and more sensitive in osteolytic metastases in general. Due to the lack of studies comparing FDG-PET with an adequate reference method such as MRI, there is currently no sufficient data for calculating the sensitivity of FDG-PET in screening for bone metastases.

By contrast ^{18}F-PET has been shown to be clearly more sensitive than BS and as sensitive as MRI in detecting both osteosclerotic and osteolytic metastases [25]. The sensitivity of ^{18}F-PET has been compared with BS in two studies which included patients with cancer of the prostate, thyroid or lung. One important finding of the first study is that the sensitivity in detecting benign and malignant bone lesions with planar bone scintigraphy is highly dependent on their anatomical localization but independent thereof with ^{18}F-PET [25]. Uptake of ^{18}F-sodium fluoride or Tc-labeled polyphosphonates depends on the degree of bone remineralization and also on blood supply. Focally increased tracer uptake is therefore also present in benign lesions with ^{18}F-PET [22-24]. ^{18}F-PET scans offer more anatomical detail compared with conventional gamma camera systems [22]. Superior anatomical localization of bone lesions with ^{18}F-PET is therefore related to superior specificity compared with planar bone scans [25]. Due to its higher sensitivity, disseminated metastatic bone disease is often observed in patients with single metastases on planar bone scans. In a further study, ^{18}F-PET was performed in addition to conventional bone scintigraphy in patients with breast cancer and a high risk of metastatic bone disease [26]. Extent of metastatic bone disease was underestimated in 11 of 17 patients with BS but was interpreted correctly with ^{18}F-PET (Fig. 25.3). Three patients presented a normal bone scan but had metastases with ^{18}F-PET (Fig. 25.4). In a further patient with known metastases, an osteolytic metastasis that had been missed with bone scintigraphy was detected with ^{18}F-PET. Because of the risk of fracture, this metastasis was stabilized by surgery. Due to intensive focal tracer uptake bone scans were interpreted false positive in two patients. In conclusion, clinical management was influenced in six patients (17.6%) because of the use of ^{18}F-PET in this study.

25.3.2.4 Guidelines for clinical use

At present ^{18}F-PET remains time consuming, costly and often not available for routine use. Therefore, ^{18}F-PET can not currently replace the conventional BS as a screening method. Between 1995 and 1999 more than 150 ^{18}F-PET scans were carried out in different studies at the University Hospital of Ulm [22-26]. The experiences obtained during that time were helpful to determine when ^{18}F-PET imaging can be effective in improving patient management. One indication is screening for metastatic bone disease in patients with increased tumor markers and unsuspicious findings with all other imaging methods. ^{18}F-PET is also useful in patients with unclear solitary lesions on bone scans since higher sensitivity of ^{18}F-PET may reveal disseminated small skeletal metastases and since superior spatial resolution allows better anatomical localization. Due to the possibility of whole body imaging, ^{18}F-PET should be used on further studies instead of MRI or in combination with MRI when highly accurate and non-invasive references for metastatic bone disease are needed.

25.4 Outlook

Looking at the increasing number of PET scanners and cyclotron units, ^{18}F-PET should become more cost effective in the future than it is today. Based on the encouraging results previously reported by Kosuda et al. [13], whole-body SPECT might be a practicable and cost-effective alternative to ^{18}F-PET. Currently, the use of coincidence imaging with double-headed gamma camera systems is still increasing. It is unclear whether ^{18}F-PET imaging using coincidence gamma cameras is as sensitive as using full-ring scanners. For these reasons, further studies comparing the accuracy of whole-body bone SPECT and the accuracy of coincidence gamma cameras with the accuracy of full-ring PET as well as studies examining whether there is a benefit to patients when metastatic bone disease is detected earlier are required before a definite conclusion on the routine use of ^{18}F-PET can be made.

25.5 Summary – guidelines for practical use of [^{18}F]PET and image interpretation

- Imaging technique: 370 MBq sodium fluoride intravenously, 10–12 min per bed position, no attenuation correction, emission scanning 1–2 h p.i., no quantification of tracer uptake
- Interpretation of findings: quantification of tracer uptake is not useful for differentiating between benign and malignant lesions
  - normal variations of increased tracer uptake are often observed at the sutures of the skull, at the manubriosternal joint or at the orbita
  - typical signs of degenerative disease are hot spots at corresponding articulation surfaces, hot spots at the ventral or lateral vertebral bodies without involvement of the spongiosa, homogeneously increased tracer uptake at the endplates (endplate fracture)
  - rib fractures or benign bone tumors are often not distinguishable from bone metastases.

References

[1] Algra PR, Heimans JJ, Valk J, Nauta JJ, Lachniet M, Van Kooten (1992) Do metastases in vertebrae begin in the body or the pedicles? Imaging study in 45 patients. Am J Roentgenol 158:1275–1279

[2] Batson OV (1995) The function of the vertebral veins and their role in the spread of metastases. Clin Orthop 312:4–9

[3] Blau M (1972) 18F-Fluoride for bone imaging. Semin Nucl Med 21:31–33

[4] Bury T, Barreto A, Daenen F, Barthelemy N, Ghaye B, Rigo P (1998) Fluorine-18 deoxyglucose positron emission tomography for detection of bone metastases in patients with non-small cell lung cancer. Eur J Nucl Med 25:1244–1247

[5] Cook GJ, Houston S, Rubens R, Maisey MN, Fogelman I (1998) Detection of bone metastases in breast cancer by 18FDG PET: differing metabolic activity in osteoblastic and osteolytic lesions. J Clin Oncol 16:3375–3379

[6] Creutzig H, Creutzig A, Gerdts KG, Greif E, Eckhardt W (1975) Vergleichende Untersuchungen mit osteotropen Radiopharmaka. I. Tierexperimentelle Untersuchungen zur Anreicherung von ^{18}F, ^{85}Sr und ^{99m}Tc-EHDP. Fortschr Röntgenstr 123:137–143

[7] Creutzig H (1975) Vergleichende Untersuchungen mit osteotropen Radiopharmaka. II. Plasmaclearance von ^{18}F und ^{99m}Tc-EHDP. Fortschr Röntgenstr 123:313–318

[8] Creutzig H (1975) Vergleichende Untersuchungen mit osteotropen Radiopharmaka. III. Szintigraphie mit ^{18}F und ^{99m}Tc-EHDP bei malignen und nicht malignen Erkrankungen. Fortschr Röntgenstr 123:462–467

[9] Frank JA, Ling A, Patronas NJ, Carrasquillo JA, Horvath K, Hickey AM, Dwyer AJ (1990) Detection of malignant bone tumors: MR imaging vs scintigraphy. Amer J Roentgenol 155:1043–1048

[10] Gosfield E, Alavi A, Kneeland B (1993) Comparison of radionuclide bone scans and magnetic resonance imaging in detecting spinal metastases. J Nucl Med 34:2191–2198

[11] Green D, Jeremy R, Towson J, Morris J (1973) The role of fluorine 18 scanning in the detection of skeletal metastases in early breast cancer. Aust N Z J Surg 43:251–254

[12] Hoh CK, Hawkins RA, Dahlbom M, Glaspy JA, Seeger LL, Choi Y, Schiepers CW, Huang SC, Satyamurthy N, Barrio JR, Phelps ME (1993) Whole body skeletal imaging with [18F] fluoride ion and PET. J Comput Assist Tomogr 17:34–41

[13] Kosuda S, Kaji T, Jokawa H et al. (1996) Does bone SPECT actually have a lower sensitivity for detecting vertebral metastases than MRI? J Nucl Med 37:975–978

[14] Krasnow AZ, Hellman RS, Timins ME (1997) Diagnostic bone scanning in oncology. Semin Nucl Med 27:107–141

[15] Moog F, Bangerter M, Kotzerke J, Guhlmann A, Frickhofen N, Reske SN (1998) 18-F-fluorodeoxyglucose-positron-emission tomography as a new approach to detect lymphomatous bone marrow. J Clin Oncol 16:603–609

[16] Munz DL (1994) Ist die Skelettszintigraphie zum Metastasenscreening noch erforderlich? Nuklearmedizin 32:5–10

[17] Orr FW, Sanchez OH, Kostenuik P, Singh G (1995) Tumor interactions in skeletal metastasis. Clin Orthop 312:19–33

[18] Petren-Mallmin M (1994) Clinical and experimental imaging of breast cancer metastases in the spine. Acta Radiol Suppl 391:1–23

[19] Petren-Mallmin M, Andreasson I, Ljunggren O, Ahlstrom H, Bergh J, Antonini G, Langstrom B, Bergstrom M (1998) Skeletal metastases from breast cancer: uptake of 18-fluoride measured with positron emission tomography in correlation with CT. Skeletal Radiol 27:72–76

[20] Reske SN, Karstens JH, Glöckner WM, Ammon J, Büll U (1990) Nachweis des Knochenmarksbefalls beim Mammakarzinom und bei malignen Lymphomen durch Immunszintigraphie des hämatopoetischen Knochenmarks. Fortschr Röntgenstr 152:60–66

[21] Rubens RD, Fogelman I (1991) Bone Metastases. Springer, London Berlin Heidelberg New York Tokio Hongkong

[22] Schirrmeister H, Rentschler M, Diederichs CG, Kotzerke J, Reske SN (1998) Darstellung des normalen Skelettsystems mit ^{18}FNa-PET im Vergleich zur konventionellen Skelettszintigraphie. Fortschr Röntgenstr 168:451–456

[23] Schirrmeister H, Diederichs CG, Rentschler M, Kotzerke J, Reske SN (1998) Die Positronenemissionstomographie des Skelettsystems mit ^{18}FNa: Häufigkeit, Befundmuster und Verteilung benigner Veränderungen. Fortschr Röntgenstr 169:310–314

[24] Schirrmeister H, Guhlmann CA, Elsner K, Nüssle K, Träger J, Kotzerke J, Reske SN (1999) Die Positronenemissionstomographie des Skelettsystems mit ^{18}FNa: Häufigkeit, Befundmuster und Verteilung von Skelettmetastasen. Röntgenpraxis 52:19–25

[25] Schirrmeister H, Guhlmann CA, Diederichs CG, Träger H, Reske SN (1999) Planar bone imaging vs. 18F-PET in patients with cancer of the prostate, thyroid and lung. J Nucl Med 40:1623–1629

[26] Schirrmeister H, Guhlmann CA, Kotzerke J, Santjohanser C, Kühn T, Kreienberg R, Messer P, Nüssle K, Elsner K, Glatting G, Träger H, Neumaier B, Diederichs CD, Reske SN (1999) Early detection and accurate description of extent of metastatic bone disease in breast cancer with 18F-fluoride ion and positron emission tomography. J Clin Oncol 17:2381–2389

[27] Shreve PD, Grossman HB, Gross MD, Wahl RL (1996) Metastatic prostate cancer: Initial findings of PET with 2-deoxy-2[F-18]fluoro-D-glucose. Radiology 199:751–756

[28] Silberstein ER, Saenger EL, Tofe AJ, Alexander GW, Park HM (1973) Imaging of bone metastases with ^{99m}Tc-Sn-HEDP (diphosphonate), ^{18}F and skeletal radiography. Radiology 107:551–555

[29] Traill Z, Richards MA, Moore N (1995) Magnetic resonance imaging of metastatic bone disease. Clin Orthop 312:76–88

[30] Venz S, Hosten N, Friedrichs R, Neumann K, Nagel R, Felix R (1994) Osteoplastische Knochenmetastasen beim Prostatakarzinom: Magnetresonanztomographie und Knochenmarkszintigraphie. Fortschr Röntgenstr 161:64–69

[31] Weber DA, Keyes JW, Landmann S, Wilson GA (1974) Comparison of Tc-polyphosphate and F18 for bone imaging. Am J Roentgen Rad Ther Nucl Med 121:184–190

[32] Wilson MA, Calhoun FW (1981) The distribution of skeletal metastases in breast and pulmonary cancer: concise communication. J Nucl Med 22:594–597

26 Renal cell and urothelial cancer

A. R. Börner, M. Hofmann, V. Müller-Mattheis

26.1 Incidence, etiology and epidemiology

Renal cell cancer (RCC) has an incidence similar to differentiated thyroid cancer or Hodgkin's disease and comprises approx. 2% of all cancers. More than 90% of these tumors are found in adults with a preference for the 7th and 8th decade of life. The male gender displays an increased incidence of about twice that of females. Over the last 40 years, mortality due to renal cell cancer has been rising at a rate of 2% per year in the developed countries in Europe and North America. This rise and the sex predilection are attributed to the use of tobacco products, the packaging (cardboard) industry, other environmental factors in petroleum and leather industries and exposure to cadmium, asbestos and trichlorethylene [3]. Obesity and chronic kidney failure are other contributing factors which are frequently observed in female renal cell cancer patients. The pathogenesis of renal cell cancer is still largely unclear. The prognosis of this tumor type in adults is rather poor with 5 year survival rates between 36 and 54%. If widespread tumor manifestations are present at admission, the 5-year survival rate decreases to virtually zero. All renal cell cancers are insensitive to chemotherapy with conventional cytostatic drugs and are primarily radiation resistant. Therefore, radical surgical removal of the tumor and solitary metastases are the only ways to achieve full remission. In particular, with lymph node and lung metastases, the eventual prognosis is critically dependent on the radicality of the primary surgical intervention. Additional determinants of prognosis are the size and number of metastases. Current therapeutic options for bone and liver metastases are limited and usually consist of palliation.

26.2 Histopathological classification

Renal cell cancers were previously divided into clear-cell, granular, spindle-cell or oncocytic tumors according to their histologic appearance. Another classification divides renal cell tumors on the basis of their growth patterns into acinous, papillary and sarcomatoid types. However, these classifications do not clearly describe the clinical behavior of these tumors. In 1986 a new

Table 26.1. The five types of renal cell cancer based on cyto- and molecular-genetic criteria (adapted from [27]).

Tumor type	Incidence (%)	Number (unpublished)	Characteristics	Typical genetic defects	Cell of origin
Clear-cell renal cancer	75–85	11		deletion of one or both copies 3p	proximal tubule
Chromophilic (papillary) cancer	12–14	5	multifocal or bilateral good prognosis	Y-monosomy, trisomy 7 or 17	proximal tubule
Chromophobic cancer	4–6	2	good prognosis	hypoploid	intercalated cell of cort. collecting duct
Oncocytic renal cancer	2–4	2	non-metastastic	undetermined	intercalated cell of cort. collecting duct
Collecting duct cancer (Bellini)	1%	–	extremely aggressive	undetermined	medullary collecting duct

histopathological classification of renal cell cancer was developed describing five types of renal cell cancer based on cyto- and molecular-genetic criteria (Table 26.1).

26.3 [^{18}F]FDG-PET

Na^+/glucose co-transporters are expressed in the proximal tubular epithelium of the kidney and are supposed to play a substantial role in the active reabsorption of glucose from the glomerular filtrate of the apical membrane. The glucose analogue 2-fluoro-deoxy-D-glucose (FDG) is a substrate for facilitated diffusion by Na^+ independent glucose transporters in the renal basolateral membrane. Differentiation of malignant from benign renal tumors is not easily accomplished with current non-invasive methods. Metabolic imaging using FDG-PET resulted in large inter- and intra-individual variances of tumor-to-non-tumor ratios rendering negative PET scans non-diagnostic. These variances are largely caused by variances in the expression of the enzyme glucose-6-phosphatase (G-6-Pse) which is responsible for the efflux of [^{18}F]FDG from the metabolic tissue compartment. Relative mRNA levels of G-6-Pse ranged from 1% to 840% in primary RCC and from 48% to 315% in RCC metastases. Thus, relative differences of up to 800% in primary tumors and of >60% in metastases were observed [18]. This large variability in G-6-Pse expression in clear cell renal cancers contributes to the poor utility of FDG-PET in this tumor. Another reason might be variances in the expression of glucose transporters (Glut 1–7) which are still under investigation. Model-based parametric imaging should improve the potential of FDG-PET for tissue characterization. A three compartment model is sufficient to describe the relation of intravascular glucose, intracellular glucose and glucose-6-phos-

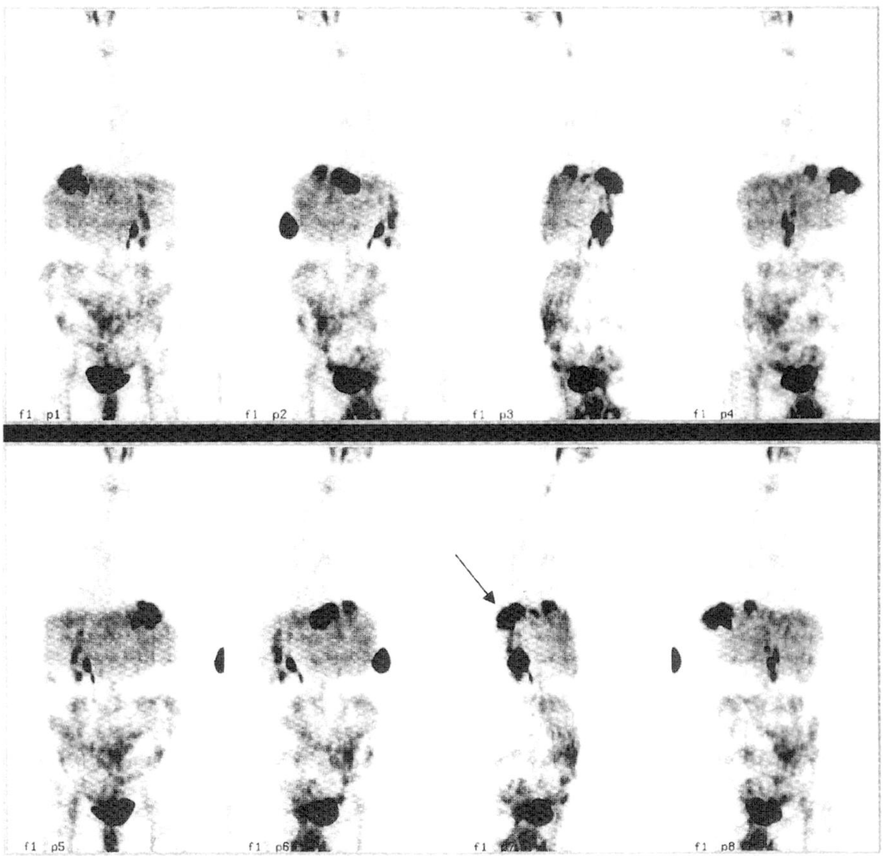

Fig. 26.1. Diplogenesis of the right kidney in a female patient. The patient was followed up because of an ovarian cancer three years prior to this PET scan. Maximum intensity projection images, acquisition time 1 h At surgery, extensive scarring but no viable tumor tissue was detected.

phate 'trapped' in the cell. The tumor-typical and tissue-specific characteristics of the enzyme pattern expressed cause variations in the "lumped constant" describing the relation between glucose and FDG metabolism. Thus, quantitation using an overall "glucose metabolic rate" is not useful.

The most common type of renal cell cancer, clear-cell renal cancer, usually displays a distinct hyperperfusion pattern but FDG hypermetabolism is observed in only 60% of patients. FDG accumulation is seen more frequently in rarer tumors of the kidneys but does not correlate to differentiation, stage nor size of the cancer. In large tumors, urine retention due to obstruction is frequently observed and sometimes resists forced diuresis resulting in these lesions being judged as pathological by FDG-PET due to the intense physiological urine concentration of FDG. Especially in the early phase, glucose transport in renal cell cancers is supposed to be similar to normal kidney tissue. Inflammatory lesions may also cause intensive glucose hypermetabolism

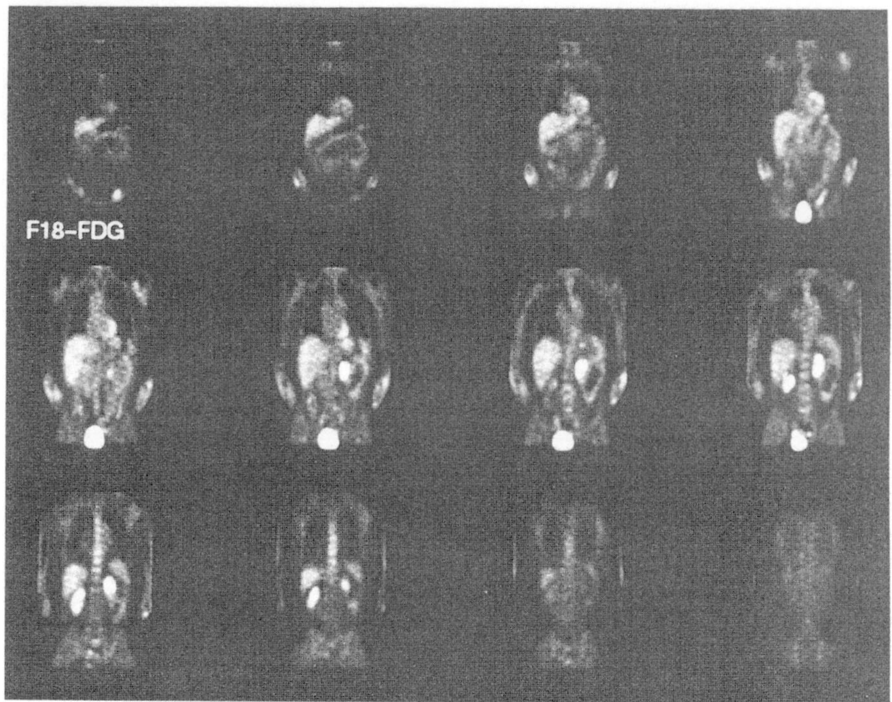

Fig. 26.2. Coronal slices of a patient with a renal mass in the middle of the left kidney. The surgical removal and histological evaluation revealed clear-cell renal cancer with a maximum diameter of 4.3 cm. In the FDG-PET study, the tumor presented at both 1 and 3 h after the injection as a cold lesion compared to the normal kidney (arrow). There was no focal accumulation of the tracer within the area of the primary tumor, the regional lymph nodes nor in the entire abdominal region. No metastatic disease was found either at surgery or by histopathology.

[23] so that a cancer in the rim of an inflammatory cyst cannot be identified while bland cysts or necroses tend to show glucose hypometabolism. The FDG-PET method is not capable of making an effective contribution to the primary diagnosis and differentiation of renal cell cancer. Masses of the kidney are usually diagnosed by abdominal ultrasound. Currently, further differentiation is the domain of CT and, in some cases, MRI while angiography is rarely of any use. In cases of lymph node or distant metastases of renal cell cancer, the accuracy of [^{18}F]FDG whole-body PET imaging increases substantially and independently of the primary histological tumor classification (Fig. 26.2). Still, this fact does little to improve individual prognosis and overall survival.

26.3.1 Acquisition

Preparation: Patient fasting for at least 12 hours, transmission measurement (10 million counts per bed position), intravenous injection of approx. 300–400 MBq [^{18}F]FDG. In selective cases, immediate dynamic acquisition is performed according to the following protocol:

- 12 × 10 s
- 12 × 15 s
- 10 × 30 s
- 4 × 300 s

Total scan duration: 30 min with arterialized venous blood sampling. Start of the static acquisition (900 s per bed position) 1 to 3 h after injection, and, if possible, comparison of early and late scans, e.g., 1 and 3 h after injection. Reconstruction is preferably iterative because of low count rates and high in-plane contrast. Visual evaluation in transverse, sagittal and coronal slices. Specialized investigations require that a blood activity curve be derived for an input function followed by calculation of the local regional glucose consumption as well as for the determination of the kinetic constants (modeling). The radiation exposure is moderate with 21–29 µSv/MBq equating to 10 mSv whole-body absorbed dose per investigation with injection of 370 MBq [^{18}F]FDG.

26.3.2 Perfusion markers

26.3.2.1 [^{15}O]H_2O

The oxygen isotope ^{15}O, with its short radioactive half-life of 123 s, is frequently used for the measurement of the regional cerebral blood flow (rCBF) and for the determination of the regional blood volume and oxygen consumption in the form of H_2O, $C^{15}O$ (linkage to hemoglobin) and O_2-saturated blood. It may also be employed to measure renal tumor perfusion and vascularization.

26.3.2.2 [^{15}O]Butanol

Compared to water, ^{15}O-butanol displays better tissue extraction and is preferred as a blood flow tracer. Repetitive intravenous injections are necessary in each case consisting of 1500 MBq [^{15}O]butanol followed by PET measurements for 2 min. An arterial puncture is necessary in order to determine the arterial time activity curve (input function) of the [^{15}O]butanol by repeated blood sampling.

26.3.3 Labeled amino acids

26.3.3.1 Amino acid metabolism

Quantitation of amino acid metabolism via labeled amino acids represents the challenge of all scintigraphic methods for competitive measurements. In vivo protein metabolism remains an unknown factor because unlabeled amino acids are produced by endogenous protein catabolism or re-synthesis from non-essential amino acids. The determination of an absolutely quantified regional protein synthesis rate is therefore problematic using PET. Increased amino acid accumulation has been demonstrated in many tumors including lung, prostate, pancreatic and breast cancer. In patients with renal cell cancer, slightly increased amino acid turnover and metabolism are common. The application of a combination of different PET tracers promises better preoperative differentiation of various tumor types. In the follow-up of many tumors, including RCC, a non-invasive diagnostic method is needed for the differentiation between scar and relapse. The early evaluation of therapeutic effects is possible using a PET method yielding higher accuracy than either CT or MRI. Anatomically based imaging procedures are more valuable for the evaluation of tumor extension and position relative to other organs while tumor spread is observed more easily with functional imaging using whole-body PET.

26.3.3.2 [^{11}C]Methionine

The in vivo metabolic fate of [^{11}C]methionine may follow different pathways (Fig. 28.3):

- Up to approximately 90% is incorporated into structural proteins,
- part of the remainder into secreted proteins (enzymes, proteo-hormones) and
- the rest deaminated and transfered to the metabolic protein pool with subsequent degradation to CO_2.

The protein incorporation takes place very fast (within 20 min) such that these faster kinetics compared to FDG must be considered during the imaging procedure, which limits its clinical application.

26.3.3.3 [^{18}F]Fluorotyrosine and [^{18}F]fluoroproline

[^{18}F]Fluorotyrosine is a typical tracer used for the determination of protein synthesis while [^{18}F]fluoroproline is used in studies of amino acid transport. [^{18}F]Fluorotyrosine occurs in both a free and a protein-bound state in blood. Further metabolites have not been identified using both HPLC and the physiological distribution in benign and malignant tissue.

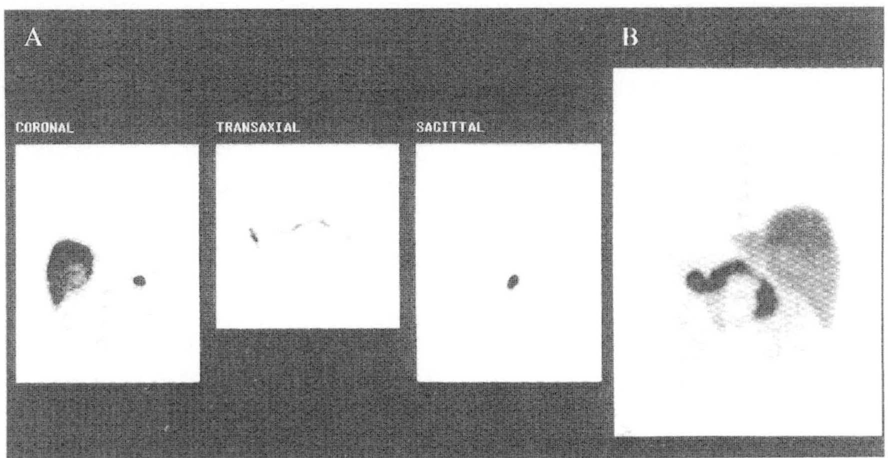

Fig. 26.3. Normal distribution of [^{11}C]methionine in the abdomen and kidneys of a patient with a sarcoma of the left forearm. Cross-sectional slices (A) and maximum intensity projection image (B) at acquisition time 20 min p.i.

Summary

Renal cancer is a major cause of death in adults in developed countries. Differentiation of malignant versus benign renal tumors still represents a problem for current diagnostic methods. Renal cancer occurs frequently making up approximately 2% of all malignant tumors. Virtually all patients presenting with disseminated tumor die of the disease within 5 years. The prognosis is more favorable for patients who develop local tumor involvement more than 2 years after primary surgery and the 5-year survival amounts to approximately 20%. Radical surgical intervention is the most important component of therapy. With lymph node and lung metastases present at admission, the eventual prognosis essentially depends on the radicality of surgery, but palliation is most common. Numerous adjuvant therapies have been proposed but proven little effect on the progress of the disease and patient survival. Renal cancer is still a fatal disease for the vast majority of these patients.

References

[1] Bachor R, Kotzerke J, Gottfried HW, Brandle E, Reske SN, Hautmann R (1996) Positron emission tomography in diagnosis of renal cell carcinoma. Urolog A 35 (2):146–150
[2] Balfe DM, McClennan BL, Stanley RJ, Weymann PJ, Sagel SS (1982) Evaluation of renal masses considered indeterminate on computed tomography. Radiology 142:421–428
[3] Bell ET (1950) Renal Diseases, 2nd ed. Lea and Felbiger, Philadelphia
[4] Bender H, Schomburg A, Albers P, Ruhlmann J, Biersack HJ (1997) Possible role of FDG-PET in the evaluation of urologic malignancies. Anticancer Res 17:1655–1660

[5] Brock CS, Meikle SR, Price P (1997) Does fluorine-18 fluorodeoxyglucose metabolic imaging of tumours benefit oncology? Eur J Nucl Med 24:691–705
[6] Budinger TF, Brennan KM, Moses WW, Derenzo SE (1996) Advances in positron emission tomography for oncology. Nucl Med Biol 23:659–667
[7] Campbell SC, Novick AC, Herts B, Fischler DF, Meyer J, Levin HS, Chen RN (1997) Prospective evaluation of fine needle aspiration of small, solid renal masses: accuracy and morbidity. Urology 50:25–29
[8] Chaiken L, Rege S, Hoh C, Choi Y, Jabour B, Juillard G, Hawkins R, Parker (1993) Positron emission tomography with fluorodeoxyglucose to evaluate tumor response and control after radiation therapy. Int J Radiat Oncol Biol Phys 27:455–464
[9] Coleman RE (1991) Single photon emission computed tomography and positron emission tomography in cancer imaging. Cancer 67:1261–1270
[10] Cremerius U, Fabry U, Kroll U, Zimny M, Neuerburg J, Osieka R, Büll U (1999) Klinischer Wert der FDG PET im Therapiemonitoring bei malignen Lymphomen – Resultate einer retrospektiven Studie an 72 Patienten. Nuklearmedizin 38:24–30
[11] Figlin RA, Belldegrun A (1995) Introduction: renal-cell carcinoma. Seminars in Oncology 22:1–2
[12] Fischman AJ, Alpert MN (1993) FDG-PET in oncology: there's more to it than looking at pictures. J Nucl Med 34:1–6
[13] Francois C, Decaestecker C, Petein M, van Ham P, Peltier A, Pasteels JL, Danguy A, Salmon I, van Velthoven R, Kiss R (1997) Classification strategies for the grading of renal cell carcinomas, based on nuclear morphometry and densitometry. J Pathol 183: 141–150
[14] Glaspy JA, Hawkins R, Hoh CK, Phelps ME (1993) Use of positron emission tomography in oncology. Oncology 7:41–46
[15] Goldberg MA, Mayo-Smith WW, Papanicolaou N, Fischman AJ, Lee MJ (1997) FDG PET characterization of renal masses: preliminary experience. Clin Radiol 52 (7):510–515
[16] Hartman, DS, Aronson S, Frazer H (1991) Current status of imaging indeterminate renal masses. Radiol Clin North Am 29:475–496
[17] Hawkins RA, Hoh C, Glaspy J, Rege S, Choi Y, Phelps ME (1994) Positron emission tomography scanning in cancer. Cancer Invest 12:74–87
[18] Hofmann M, Börner AR, Kühnel G, Knoop BO, Binder L, Dölting J, Knapp WH (2000) Interindividual variance of glucose-6-phosphatase (G-6-Pse) expression in renal cell cancer. Eur J Nucl Med 27(1):104 (abst)
[19] Henschler D, Vamvacas S, Lammert M, Decant W, Kraus B, Thomas B, Ulm K (1995) Increased incidence of renal cell tumors in a cohort of cardboard workers exposed to trichloroethene. Arch Toxicol 69:291–299
[20] Hoh CK, Seltzer MA, Franklin J, deKernion JB, Phelps ME, Belldegrun A (1998) Positron emission tomography in urological oncology. J Urol 159:347–356
[21] Klingel R, Dippold W, Störkel S, Meyer-zum Büschenfelde KH, Köhler H (1992) Expression of differentiation antigens and growth-related genes in normal kidney, autosomal dominant polycystic kidney disease, and renal cell carcinoma. Am J Kidney Dis 19:22–30
[22] Kovacs G, Akhtar M, Beckwith BJ, Bugert P, Cooper CS, Delahunt B, Eble JN, Fleming S, Ljungberg B, Medeiros LJ, Moch H, Reuter VE, Ritz E, Roos G, Schmidt D, Srigley JR, Störkel S, van den Berg E, Zbar B (1997) The Heidelberg classification of renal cell tumours. J Pathol 183:131–133
[23] Kubota R, Yamada S, Kubota K, Ishiwata K, Tamahashi N, Ido T (1992) Intratumoral distribution of fluorine-18-fluorodeoxyglucose in vivo: high accumulation in macrophages and granulation tissues studied by microautoradiography. J Nucl Med 33: 1972–1980
[24] Mankoff DA, Thompson JA, Gold P, Eary JF, Guinee Jr DG, Samlowski WE (1997) Identification of interleukin-2-induced complete response in metastatic renal cell carcinoma by FDG PET despite radiographic evidence suggesting persistent tumor. Am J Roentgenol 169:1046–1050

[25] Miyauchi T, Wahl RL (1996) Regional 2-[18F]fluoro-2-deoxy-D-glucose uptake varies in normal lung. Eur J Nucl Med 23:517–523

[26] Moon DH, Maddahi J, Silverman DH, Glaspy JA, Phelps ME, Hoh CK (1998) Accuracy of whole-body fluorine-18-FDG PET for the detection of recurrent or metastatic breast carcinoma. J Nucl Med 39:431–435

[27] Motzer RJ, Bander NH, Nanus DM (1996) Renal-cell carcinoma. N Engl J Med 335 (12):865–875

[28] Müller-Mattheis V, Reinhardt M, Müller-Gärtner HW, Ackermann R (1995) Differenzierung von Raumforderungen der Niere durch die Positronen-Emissionstomographie mit 2-[18F]-2-deoxy-D-glucose (18FDG-PET). Urologe[A](Suppl) 34:103

[29] Reske SN, Bares R, Büll U, Guhlmann A, Moser E, Wannenmacher MF (1996) Clinical value of positron emission tomography (PET) in oncology: results of an interdisciplinary consensus conference. Nucl Med 35:42–52; Update: Moser E, Krause Th (1997) Konsensus Onko-PET. Nucl Med 36:45–46

[30] Shinohara N, Ogiso Y, Tanaka M, Sazawa A, Harabayashi T, Koyanagi T (1997) The significance of Ras guanine nucleotide exchange factor, son of sevenless protein, in renal cell carcinoma cell lines. J Urol 158:908–911

[31] Silver DA, Morash C, Brenner P, Campbell S, Russo P (1997) Pathologic findings at the time of nephrectomy for renal mass. Ann Surg Oncol 4:570–574

[32] Stöckle M, Steinbach F, Schweden F, Hohenfellner R (1992) Klinik des Nierenzellkarzinoms – Stellenwert der bildgebenden Diagnostik. Radiologe 32:95–103

[33] Störkel S, Jacobi GH (1989) Systematik, Histogenese und Prognose der Nierenzellkarzinome und des Onkozytoms. Verh Dtsch Ges Pathol 73:321–328

[34] Strauss LG (1996) Fluorine-18 deoxyglucose and false positive results: a major problem in the diagnostics of oncological patients. Eur J Nucl Med 23:1409–1415

[35] Wahl RL, Cody R, Hutchins G, Mudgett E (1991) Positron-emission tomographic scanning of primary and metastatic breast carcinoma with the radiolabeled glucose analogue 2-deoxy-2-[18F]fluoro-D-glucose. N Engl J Med 324:200

[36] Yao WJ, Hoh CK, Hawkins RA, Glaspy JA, Weil JA, Lee SJ, Maddahi J, Phelps ME (1994) Quantitative PET imaging of bone marrow glucose metabolic response to hematopoietic cytokines. J Nucl Med 36:794–799

[37] Zasadny KR, Wahl RL (1993) Standardized uptake values of normal tissues at PET with 2-[fluorine-18]-fluoro-2-deoxy-D-glucose: variations with body weight and a method for correction. Radiology 189:847–850

27 Endocrine/neuroendocrine tumors

P. Reuland, S.M. Larson

27.1 Introduction

Development of nuclear medicine is closely related to examinations of endocrine active organs. ^{128}Iodine was one of the first artificially produced radioisotopes by Fermi in the year 1934. This isotope had already been used for studies of iodine metabolism and for experiments on the physiology of the thyroid, in 1938. In 1939 ^{131}iodine was applied in humans for the first time [14] and basic research on scintigraphic application had already been reported in 1951 [6]. While ^{131}iodine is still used in nuclear medicine because of its property as a β-emitter, it has lost its importance for diagnosis.

Two other areas of scintigraphy in endocrinology should be stressed. In the 1960s radiotracers for testing adrenal function had already been developed. Wieland et al. [38] suggested meta-iodobenzylguanidine labeled with ^{131}iodine to be an important radiotracer which is still used today for detection and therapy for, e.g., pheochromocytomas and neuroblastomas. Increasing interest is directed to analogs of somatostatine, such as octreotide for detection of endocrine active tumors, including gastrinomas, insulinomas, glucagenomas, paragangliomas, small cell bronchogenic carcinoma, Merkel cell tumors, and tumors of various origin of the pituitary gland [4]. This chapter will stress the importance of 'conventional' or 'single photon' nuclear medicine for diagnosis of endocrine/neuroendocrine active tumors. The role of positron emission tomography in this field is still not well defined; but 2-[^{18}F]fluoro-2-deoxy-D-glucose (FDG) has already shown some interesting perspecitves.

27.2 Overview on endocrine/neuroendocrine tumors

Although experiences with PET tracers are not reported in the literature for all endocrine/neuroendocrine active tumors, for completeness we will give an overview over the whole spectrum of these tumors, because especially PET tracers as kinetically identical radioactive chemical compounds are ideal vehicles for testing hormonal precursors. In the future, PET tracers will probably take a prominent role in the diagnosis of these tumors.

The numerous endocrine/neuroendocrine tumors have led to classification of tumors as concerning total organs, substructures of organs or disseminated cell groups. This subdivision is also used in this chapter.

27.2.1 Endocrine and neuroendocrine organs

- Thyroid (endocrine function): the different types of thyroid tumors are presented in chapter 15.
- Parathyroid (neuroendocrine function): the most frequent tumor of the parathyroid is the benign adenoma of the parathyroid, which has to be differentiated from hyperplasia. Causal reasons led to classification into primary hyperparathyroidism (incidence 30/100 000 inhabitants, females are involved 2–3 as often as males, a peak is found in the 5th and 6th decade), secondary and tertiary hyperparathyroidism (caused by other underlying diseases, especially by malnutrition and renal failure). Carcinoma of the parathyroid is rare and often difficult to differentiate from a benign tumor.
- Pituitary gland: the prolactinoma is one of the frequent tumors of the pituitary glands and is diagnosed by elevated serum levels of prolactine.
  Rare tumors include adenomas which produce adrenocorticotropic hormone thyroid stimulating hormones, gonadotropine hormone or somatotropine. Endocrine active tumors have to be differentiated from edocrine inactive tumors like craniopharyngeoma, metastases of brochogenic carcinomas, breast cancer, or cancer of the stomach, cysts, gliomas, meningeomas, chondromas, and germinomas.
  Very rare tumors are thyreotrope adenomas and gonadotrope adenomas.

27.2.2 Endocrine and neuroendocrine parts of organs

- Cortex of adrenal glands: location of mesodermal adrenocortical tumors leading to hypercortisolism, adrenogenital syndrome or feminine phenotype.
- Medullary part of adrenal glands (and paraganglia): location of adrenal paragangliomas, pheochromocytomas (mostly benign, arising from chromeaffine cells of the adrenal medulla, less often arising from extraadrenal sympathetic nerve cells (paraganglia), especially found in middle-aged patients; incidence is 3–4 per million inhabitants; a rare malignant type metastasizes in liver, lungs and bone. Pheochromocytomas may occur in cases of multiple endocrine neoplasia (MEN II a and b), the benign type involves females in 55% and males in 45% of cases, and the malignant type involves females in 70% and males in 30% of cases), and neuroblastomas (the most frequent solid, extracranial tumor in childhood, is found 96% of the time in children under 10 years, the incidence is 1–1.4 per 10 000 inhabitants, and the ratio of involved males to females is 1.2:1). Sympathetic and parasympathetic paraganglia may give rise to paragangliomas and neuroblastomas.

- Endocrine part of the pancreas: location of insulinoma, glucagonoma, vipoma, gipoma.
- Medullary part of thyroid (C-cells): location of medullary or c-cell carcinoma (see chapter 15).

27.2.3 Disseminated endocrine/neuroendocrine system

Locations are
- Gastro-intestinal tract. Examples for pancreatic-gastrointestinal tumors are carcinoids and gastrinomas.
- Bronchial system. Tumors include the carcinoid and the small cell bronchogenic carcinoma (partly with paraneoplastic syndrome).
- Liver, kidneys, gonads, breast, and larynx are also locations where carcinoids may develop.

27.3 PET tracer for detection of endocrine/neuroendocrine tumors

2-Fluoro-deoxy-D-glucose (FDG) labeled with ^{18}fluorine has become the most important PET tracer for the detection of tumors. There are two reasons for this: tumor related increased metabolism of glucose [35] followed by the cellular trapping mechanism of FDG after phosphorilation and the well-established, automated production of the stable tracer FDG, including the fact that ^{18}fluorine has a sufficiently long half-life of 110 min. FDG is now widely available at reasonable cost throughout Europe and North America.

On the other hand FDG is not of special importance for endocrine/neuroendocrine tumors. The importance of PET is based on the development of tracers, which are precursors of hormonally active compounds, formed in endocrine cells, and maintin their biokinetic behavior. These specific tracers may not only localize endocrine tumors, but may also demonstrate their endocrine activity and changed biological behavior after therapy.

The following PET tracers (beside FDG) have been reported for application in enodcrine/neuroendocrine tumors: [^{11}C]5-HTP (hydroxytryptophane) [2], [^{11}C]L-DOPA [2], [^{11}C]methionine [21], [^{11}C]L-deprenyl [3], [^{11}C]raclopride [3], [^{11}C]N-methylspiperone [3], [^{11}C]hydroxyephedrine [30], [^{18}F]fluoroiodobenzylguanidine [35].

27.3.1 Principle of tumor visualization with 2-[^{18}F]fluoro-2-deoxy-D-glucose

Already in 1920, Warburg was the first to report on highly increased metabolism of glucose in tumor cells [36, 37]. The transport system of glucose is changed in tumor cells compared to normal somatic cells. Glucose transport in tumor cells is increased in cases of low and high blood levels of glucose and is not changed by different inhibitors which block glucose transport and metabolism in normal somatic cells [15, 19].

Transport channels in the cell membrane are increased in number [8] and the effect is boostered by raised induction of cytosolic transporters [20]. GLUT1 and GLUT3 have been found to be especially increased in number and basic for increased glucose uptake in tumor cells [23]. The trapping mechanism of 2-FDG in tumors cells is effected by fast types of isoenzymes of the hexokinase, especially in the mitochondria [5], and by strongly reduced dephosphorilation via glucose-6-phosphatase [10] caused by chemical properties of 2-FDG.

Kinetic aspects of 2-FDG [32] are reported in detail in chapter 6; thus a rough overview on some aspects may be sufficient here.

27.3.2 Experiences with 2-[^{18}F]fluoro-2-desoxy-D-glucose

On FDG-PET scanning, the thyroid shows strong variation in uptake of glucose [27]. However incidental focal uptake in the thyroid gland should not be ignored and may reflect undiagnosed thyroid cancer (Larson et al., personal communication). In primary malignant tumors of the thyroid, uptake of glucose is also variable. As a rule, glucose uptake in well-differentiated papillary carcinoma of the thyroid is not increased compared to normal thyroid tissue [16]. Metastases and tumor recurrence with low or absent uptake of iodine seem to take up more glucose than iodine positive tumor tissue [17]. Thus, staging with FDG is of special value for therapeutic decisions in the follow-up of patients with thyroid cancer. PET with FDG may possibly play a role also for primary staging in cases with higher probability of metastasizing [12].

Glucose uptake in medullary carcinomas of the thyroid seems to be very variable. Because there are still no criteria for cases with a higher probability of tumor detection with FDG, PET with FDG is not indicated in patients with medullary carinoma at this time [11, 27]. Glucose uptake in adenomas and hyperplasia of epithel bodies is uncertain; thus PET with FDG is diagnostically not adequate in these cases [31]. PET studies with FDG in patients suffering from pheochromocytomas showed increased glucose uptake in these tumors, so that FDG plays a major role especially in pheochromocytomas with no uptake of mIBG or octreotide. Another PET tracer for pheochromocytomas is meta-iodobenzylguanidine labeled with ^{18}F instead of radioactive iodine [4, 28, 33].

FDG seems to become of special value for detection of malignancy of incidental adrenal tumors [1, 4]. Some research groups report high detection rates for carcinoids with FDG [9]. Also, the small cell bronchogenic carcinoma seems to be detected with FDG with a sufficiently high probability, but the value for therapeutic decisions is not yet established. Single reports exist about detection of other tumors of the disseminated neuroendocrine system, e.g., in the case of a gastrinoma, but no final statements are possible [27].

Adenomas of the pituitary gland regularly show high uptake rates of glucose, allowing for differentiation from meningeomas. However, conventional diagnostic tools are normally sufficient for a clear diagnosis, so that PET is of additional use only in single cases [3, 21]. Our own experiences confirm the role of FDG for primary and secondary staging of neuroblastomas which show no accumulation of mIBG. FDG is of special value for detection of lymph node metastases in these cases [26, 29]. Concurrent with this aspect are anti-ganglioside antibodies [25], which also detect mIBG negative neuroblastomas. Other diagnostic tools with high sensitivity for detection of lymph node metastases of neuroblastomas are ultrasound and CT.

27.3.3 Principle of tumor detection with other PET tracers

Endocrine active tumor cells incorporate substrates which are natural precursors for the production of endocrine active compounds. An example is mIBG, which was developed in the early 1960s. mIBG is norepinephrine analog, and as such is incorporated by tumor cells arising from the neural crest via channels and stored in the cytosol in vesicular storage. Thus, catecholamines and their precursors are suitable tracers for detection of tumors of this type. Other important precursors for tumor cells include amino acids and nucleic acids. These precursors are also incorporated into the cell and metabolized in different parts of the cell.

Endocrine active tumors are also characterized by receptors on the cell surface. Some of these receptors include somatostatine receptors, which could be characterized in many endocrine tumors with the help of octreotide or pentreotide labeled with ^{111}In or ^{99m}Tc. Other receptor ligands important in these tumors are neuropeptides, such as, the vasoactive intestinal peptide (VIP), substance P, bombesin, gastrin, cholecystokinin, gonadotropine, endothelin, alpha-melanocyte stimulating hormone and growth factors [24].

27.3.4 Experiences with PET tracers other than FDG

Most experiences in the field of PET and endocrine/neuroendocrine tumors have been made with the 'working horse' FDG. This is not caused by a special role of glucose metabolism in endocrine tumors, but is just due to the fact that FDG is the best available PET tracer and that endocrine tumors also may show increased uptake of FDG like other tumors. Only endocrine/neuroendocrine tumors, however, present special properties so that precursors of physiologic compounds can be used as tumor markers.

The importance of mIBG and ligands of somatostatine receptors in conventional nuclear medicine have been mentioned already. PET tracers can also be used for labeling of these compounds. Only PET tracers can be used to label compounds without changing their biochemical properties. However experiences with radiochemical processes for these special tracers are limited and no automated, routine processing has been developed. Thus, only a few reports from single research centers exist in this field and most are of the basic theoretical type.

Bergström et al. started to use [^{11}C]raclopride [7], [^{11}C]N-methylspiperone [34], and later [^{11}C]C-bromocriptin and [^{11}C]methionine [22] to diagnose adenomas of the pituitary gland. While MRI shows high sensitivity for primary detection of tumors of the pituitary gland, these types of radiotracers show endocrine activity. Thus increased uptake of [^{11}C]methionine demonstrates residual, vital tumor tissue posttherapeutically with high accuracy in differential diagnosis to fibrosis, cyst or hematoma. Rapid blood clearance allows for good discrimination between parasellar blood volumes and aneurysms [3].

In the case of normal or slightly elevated hormone levels, differential diagnoses of endocrine-active adenomas of the pituitary gland are non-secreting pituitary adenomas, craniopharyngeomas, meningeomas, neurinomas, chordomas, metastases, sarcoidosis and aneurysms. In secreting adenomas of the pituitary gland, ^{11}C-methionine shows a ratio of tumor-to-brain uptake above 2, while benign tumors, for example, neurinomas show a value below 2 [3].

Strong uptake of ^{11}C-L-deprenyl in secreting adenomas of the pituitary gland is caused by high concentrations of monoaminooxidase, while low concentrations in meningeomas are combined with low uptake values. ^{11}C-methionine, however, shows increased uptake in both tumor types [3]. Taking advantage of different uptake values of glucose and methionine in chordomas (higher uptake of glucose compared to the brain than methionine) can also for this tumor type result in differentiation from secreting adenomas of the pituitary gland [3].

Prior to therapy of prolactinomas with bromocriptine, whether a sufficient number of D2-dopamine receptors are present, can be tested by application of the dopamine antagonist [^{11}C]raclopride or [^{11}C]N-methylspiperone [7, 34]. Raclopride has the advantage of higher specificity and fewer problems with metabolites. While high serum levels of prolactine indicate a sufficient number of D2-dopamine receptors in most prolactinomas, only 30% of GH-secreting tumors can be treated with dopamine receptor antagonists, thus, justifying the preceding receptor test. Some initial results have been also reported with [^{11}C]somatostatine applied in these tumors [3].

The therapeutic effect of bromocriptine on prolactinomas and of somatostatine analogs on GH-secreting adenomas may be assessed early by measuring the uptake of ^{11}C-methionine. Uptake of the D_2-dopamine receptor binding agent indicates that a therapeutic trial with bromocriptin is indicated, and it sufficient drug is used to block tumor activity, uptake of the radiotracer should be greatly diminished post treatment. The demand of higher therapeutic doses or of a change of therapy can easily be detected [3]. Interesting results have been reported on the use of [^{11}C]L-DOPA and [^{11}C]5-hydroxytryptophane for the detection of functional active pancreatic and intestinal tumors [2, 9, 13]. The lack of uptake in non-secreting tumors, however, is a relevant disadvantage. Other PET tracers like [^{11}C]hydroxyephedrine [30] and [^{18}F]fluoroiodobenzylguanidine [33] have been discussed as effective compounds for detecting neuroendocrine tumors by different research groups, but sufficient experience in patients is lacking.

27.4 Outlook

Like in other tumors, use of FDG to detect endocrine/neuroendocrine tumors is based on generally increased metabolism of glucose in tumorous lesions. The special property of these tumors, to produce endocrine/neuroendocrine effective messenger substances, is not taken advantage of. By using different precursors of these messenger substances, these tumors can be specifically detected as has been discussed above for single tumor types. Moreover, the possibility or effect of specific therapeutic concepts can be tested in advance. At the moment, most of these specific tracers are still labeled with ^{11}C. The short half-life of ^{11}C limits these examinations to diagnostic institutes placed in the direct neighborhood of a cyclotron and a radiochemical laboratory. The aim of broader application of PET and also of these specific PET tracers may be reached by using ^{18}fluorine or ^{124}iodine for labeling. In the field of PET, ^{18}fluorine may occupy the same place as ^{99m}technetium in the field of conventional nuclear medicine. This aspect is a challenge for radiopharmaceutical research institutes. As an example of an interesting PET tracer, which is availiable for satellite PET sites, [^{18}F]DOPA should be mentioned. Initially only used for diagnosing metabolic disorders of the brain, now [^{18}F]DOPA is also applied in patients with other disorders, e.g., an initial study has been started in Freiburg for diagnosing endocrine/neuroendocrine tumors (Fig. 27.1).

27.5 Practical hints for acquisition and interpretation of PET examinations in endocrine/neuroendocrine tumors

- Patient preparation: in the case of FDG: patient should be examined after overnight fasting, serum level of glucose should not exceed 110 mg%; sufficient hydration; continuous rinsing of the bladder, when tumor is expected in this area; in the case of precursors: care of cross-reactions with other drugs, in some special cases tracer uptake may be increased by stimulation of the tumor via drugs.
- Acquisition of data: imaging 90 min p.i. in the case of FDG, different times with other PET tracers, depending on radionuclides used and on biokinetics of the

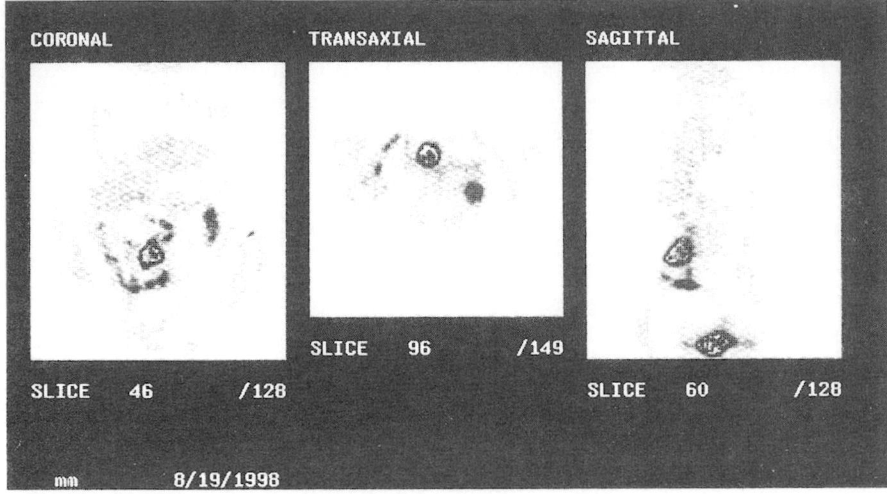

Fig. 27.1. A 64 year old patient with an endocrine active tumor. After injection with [^{18}F]DOPA, a large tumor conglomerate ventral in the middle of the abdomen as well as an extended part of the ileum show increased uptake of L-DOPA. An additional site is localized in the upper part of the descending colon. Diagnosis: cancer of the large and small intestine with abdominal metastasis. (This figure is printed with kind permission from the University PET Center, Freiburg.)

tracer in the tumor cell; amount of activity: 400 MBq in the case of FDG, different with other tracers, administration of furosemide is optional for improved renal clearance.

- Absorption correction: via transmission data ('hot' transmission when possible in order to avoid artifacts).
- Type of reconstruction: iterative reconstruction including transmission data.
- Functionalizing: in most cases of FDG not necessary; experience with other tracers is lacking.
- Interpretation: regularly visual interpretation of PET images, 3-dimensional, rotating views may be helpful for interpretation of anatomical structures; SUV may be helpful in single tumors for better discrimination from benign lesions (data are inconclusive); interpretation is complicated when metabolites occur, kinetic modeling and possibly exact quantification via arterial blood sampling will be necessary; morphological tomographic images should be available for localizing and interpreting tumors and anatomical structures.

References

[1] Abrams HL, Spiro R, Goldstein N (1950) Metastases in carcinoma: analysis of 1000 autopsied cases. Cancer 3:74–85

[2] Ahlstrom H, Eriksson B, Bergstrom M, et al. (1995) Pancreatic neuroendocrine tumors: diagnosis with PET. Radiology 195:333–337

[3] Bergstrom M, Muhr C, Lundberg PO, Langstrom B (1991) PET as a tool in the clinical evaluation of pituitary adenomas. J Nucl Med 32:610–615

[4] Boland GW, Goldberg MA, Lee MJ, et al. (1995) Indeterminate adrenal mass in patients with cancer: evaluation at PET with 2-(F-18)-fluoro-deoxy-D-glucose. Radiology 194:131–134

[5] Bustamante E, Morris HP, Pederson PL (1981) Energy metabolism of tumor cells: requirement for a form of hexokinase with a propensity for mitochondrial binding. J Biol Chem 256:8699–8704

[6] Cassen B, Curtis L, Reed C, Libby R (1951) Instrumentation for 131I use in medical studies. Nucleonics 9:46

[7] Farde L, Ehrin E, Eriksson L, et al. (1985) Substituted benzamides as ligands for visualization of dopamine receptor binding in the human brain by positron emission tomography. Proc Natl Acad Sci 82:3863–3867

[8] Flier JS, Mueckler MM, Usher P, Lodish HF (1987) Elevated levels of glucose transport and transporter messenger RNA are induced by ras or src oncogenes. Science 235: 1492–1495

[9] Foidart-Willems J, Depas G, Vivegnis D, et al. (1995) positron emission tomography and radiolabelled octreotide scintigraphy in carcinoid tumors. Eur J Nucl Med 22:635

[10] Gallagher BM, Fowler JS, Gutterson NI, MacGregor RR, Wan CN, Wolf AP (1978) Metabolic trapping as a principle of radiopharmaceutical design. Some factors responsible for the biodistribution of (18-F) 2 deoxy-2-fluoro-D-glucose. J Nucl Med 19: 1154–1161

[11] Gasparoni P, Rubello D, Ferlin G (1997) Potential role of fluorine-18-deoxyglucose (FDG) positron emission tomography (PET) in the staging of primitive and recurrent medullary thyroid carcinoma. J Endocrinol Invest 20:527–530

[12] Grunwald F, Schomburg A, Bender H, et al. (1996) Fluorine-18 fluorodeoxyglucose positron emission tomography in the follow-up of differentiated thyroid cancer. Eur J Nucl Med 23:312–319

[13] Gupta N, Bradfield H (1996) Role of positron emission tomography scanning in evaluating gastrointestinal neoplasms. Sem Nucl Med 26:65–73

[14] Hamilton, JG, Soley MH (1939) Studies in iodine metabolism by the use of a new radioactive iodine. Amer J Physiol 127:557

[15] Hatanaka M (1974) Transport of sugars in tumor cell membranes. Biochem Biophys Acta 355:77–104

[16] Joensuu H, Ahonen A, Klemi PJ (1988) 18F-Fluorodeoxyglucose imaging in preoperative diagnosis of thyroid malignancy. Eur J Nucl Med 13:502–506

[17] Joensuu H, Ahonen A (1987) Imaging of metastases of thyroid carcinoma with fluorine-18 fluorodeoxyglucose. J Nucl Med 1987:910–914

[18] Krenning EP, Kwekkeboom DJ, Bakker WH, et al. (1993) Somatostatin receptor scintigraphy with (In-111-DTPA-D-Phe)- and (J-123-Tyr)-Oktreotide: The Rotterdam experience with more than 1000 patients. Eur J Nucl Med 20:716–731

[19] Martineau R, Kohlbacher M, Shaw SN, Amos H (1972) Enhancement of hexoses entry into chick fibroblasts by starvation: differential effect on galactose and glucose. Proc Natl Acad Sci USA 69:3407–3411

[20] Mueckler MM (1994) Facilitative glucose transporters. Eur J Biochem 219:713–725

[21] Muhr C, Bergstrom M (1991) Positron emission tomography applied in the study of pituitary adenomas. J Endocrinol Invest 14:509–528

[22] Muhr C, Lundberg PO, Antoni G, et al. (1984) The uptake of 11C-labeled bromocriptine and methionine in pituitary tumors studied by positron emission tomography

(PET). In: Lamberts, Tilders, van der Veen, et al. (eds) Trends in Diagnosis and Treatment of Pituatary Adenomas. Amsterdam: Free University Press, pp 151–155
[23] Murakami T, Nishiyama T, Shirotani T, et al. (1992) Type 1 glucose transporter from the mouse which are responsive to serum, growth factor, and oncogenes. J Biol Chem 267:9300–9306
[24] Pauwels EKJ, McCready VR, Stoot JHMB, van Deurzen FP (1998) The mechanism of accumulation of tumour-localising radiopharmaceuticals. Eur J Nucl Med 25:277–305
[25] Reuland P, Handgretinger R, Smykowsky H, et al. (1991) Application of the murine anti-Gd-2 antibody 14.Gd-2a for diagnosis and therapy of neuroblastoma. Nucl Med Biol 18:121–125
[26] Reuland P, Geiger L, Klingebiel Th, Laniado K, Feine U, Bares R, Niethammer D, Handgretinger R (1996) Clinical impact of the different diagnostic tools for neuroblastoma. Adv Neuroblastoma Res 5:23
[27] Rigo P, Paulus P, Kaschten BJ, Hustinx R, Bury T, Jerusalem G, Benoit T, Foidart-Willems J (1996) Oncological applications of positron emission tomography with fluorine-18 fluorodeoxyglucose. Eur J Nucl Med 23:1641–1674
[28] Shulkin BL, Koeppe RA, Francis IR, et al. (1993) Pheochromocytomas that do not accumulate metaiodobenzylguanidine: localization with PET and administration of FDG. Radiology 186:11–15
[29] Shulkin BL, Sisson JC, Hutchinson RJ (1994) PET FDG studies of neuroblastoma. J Nucl Med 35:135 (abstr.)
[30] Shulkin BL, Wieland DM, Schwaiger M (1992) PET scanning with hydroxyephedrine: an approach to the localization of pheochromocytoma. J Nucl Med 33:1125–1131
[31] Sisson JC, Thompson NW, Ackerman RJ, Wahl RL (1994) Use of 2-(F-18)-fluoro-2-deoxy-D-glucose PET to locate parathyroid adenomas in primary hyperparathyroidism. Radiology 192:280
[32] Sokoloff L, Reivich M, Kennedy C, et al. (1977) The (14-C)deoxy glucose method for the measurement of local cerebral glucose utilisation: theory, procedure, and normal values in the conscious and anesthetized albino rat. J Neurochem 28:897–916
[33] Vaidyanathan G, Affleck DJ, Zalutsky MR (1995) Validation of 4-(fluorine-18) fluoro-3-iodobenzylguanidine as a positron-emitting analog of MIBG. J Nucl Med 36:644–650
[34] Wagner NH Jr, Burns HD, Dannals RF, et al. (1983) Imaging dopamine receptors in the human brain by positron emission tomography. Science 221:1264–1266
[35] Wahl RL, Hutchkins GD, Buchsbaum DJ, Liebert M, Grossman HB (1991) 18-F-2-deoxy-2-fluoro-deoxyglucose uptake into human tumor xenografts. Cancer 76:1544–1550
[36] Warburg O (1920) Über den Stoffwechsel der Carcinomzelle. Kolin Wochenschr Berl 4:534–536
[37] Warburg O (1931) The metabolism of tumors. Constable, London, pp 75–327
[38] Wieland DM, Wu JL, Brown LE, Mangner TJ, Swanson DP, Beierwaltes WM (1980) Radiolabeled adrenergic neuron blocking agents: adrenomedullary imaging with (131)iodobenzylguanidine. J Nucl Med 21:349–353

28 Breast cancer

N. Avril, K. Scheidhauer, W. Kuhn

28.1 Histopathology, incidence, and patient management

The mammary gland is composed of glandular tissue within a dense fibroareolar stroma. The glandular tissue consists of approximately 15 to 20 lobes, each of which include a series of branching ducts and lobules. Most breast cancers arise in the terminal duct lobular unit. Histological classification is divided into invasive and non-invasive carcinomas and subdivided into ductal and lobular types. The most common types, representing about 80% of invasive breast cancers, are ductal carcinomas. Invasive lobular carcinomas account for approximately 10% and medullary carcinomas for 5% of malignant breast tumors. The remaining tumors comprise a variety of histological types that are generally less malignant. Rare tumors include the usually benign phylloides tumors and occasionally soft tissue sarcomas and primary lymphomas. Noninvasive breast cancer consists of two histological and clinical subtypes, ductal (DCIS) and lobular (LCIS) in situ carcinomas. The carcinoma cells are confined within the terminal duct lobular unit and the adjacent ducts, but have not yet invaded through the basement membrane. Traditionally, they were regarded as an early detectable stage of malignant transformation but LCIS is increasingly considered as a risk factor for developing invasive breast cancer. The breast acini are distended by fairly uniform carcinoma cells which grow into the duct system or break through the basement membrane to become invasive carcinoma. Generally, LCIS does not present as a palpable tumor and is usually found incidentally in breast biopsies, often multifocal and bilateral. DCIS is increasingly diagnosed due to microcalcifications seen on mammograms and is more likely to be confined to one breast, even to one quadrant of the breast. Invasive breast cancer may present as a single tumor, multifocal if tumors are growing in the same quadrant of the breast and multicentric if they are detected in different quadrants. The disease can occur in any part of the breast but most frequently in the upper outer quadrant. Tumors are usually slow growing and tumor size is proportional to duration of disease.

Breast cancer is the most frequent malignant disease in women and the second leading cause of cancer death in the western countries. In the United States, more than 180 000 new cases are diagnosed annually and approximately 1 in 9 women develops breast cancer during her lifetime [27]. Breast cancer is uncommon below the age of 30 years; however, women with inherited specific genetic abnormalities, such as the BRCA gene, have a higher risk of developing breast cancer at young ages. In general, the risk increases with age, the maximum incidence being in the fifth and sixth decades. Infiltrating ductal carcinoma often present as a firm to hard lump. Lobular carcinomas are more difficult to detect since they are characterized by diffuse infiltration of the surrounding tissue and there is a 30% chance of a bilateral tumor arising in the contralateral breast. However, the majority of patients with breast cancer initially present with a breast lump. Therefore, a definitive diagnosis should be made on all breast lumps and it should not be assumed that a breast lump is benign in cases with inconclusive mammography and cytology. If the combination of clinical examination, mammography and fine needle cytology (triple approach) does not allow a definitive diagnosis to be made, the patients have to undergo invasive procedures. In the treatment of breast cancer, radical surgical procedures are increasingly replaced by breast conservation strategies. In many cases partial mastectomy or lumpectomy combined with radiation therapy have been proven to be as safe as mastectomy. Moreover, endocrine therapy and chemotherapy prior to (neoadjuvant) and following surgery (adjuvant) have additionally improved patient management.

28.2 Diagnosis of primary tumors

More than 80% of cancers are detected because of a suspicious mass, either by self-examination or by routine breast examination. Clinical signs are asymmetry of the breast contour, a protrusion, or a subtle dimpling of the skin (peau d'orange). Depending on the size of the breast and the density of breast tissue, most tumors are not palpable smaller than one centimeter in diameter. Breast carcinomas may be of almost any shape or consistency but they are most often described as irregularly shaped, firm or hard, painless nodules or masses. Physical examination typically does not allow an accurate differentiation between a malignant and non-malignant finding; therefore, imaging modalities are used to improve the diagnosis of breast cancer. Mammography localizes and assesses the extent of a lesion as well as identifying other suspicious masses. Two views of each breast are obtained, oblique and craniocaudal, during which the breast is compressed between two plates while the exposure is made. Abnormalities on the mammogram that suggest breast cancer include distinct, irregular, often crab-like densities, clusters of microcalcifications and distortion of normal breast architecture. Identification of microcalcifications and irregularly shaped breast masses provide high sensitivity and allow identification of 80–90% of patients with breast cancer. It is important to note that more than 80% of suspicious microcalcifications are benign resulting in low specificity of mammography. Only between 2 and 4 out of 10 patients with abnormal mammography who undergo surgery turn out to have breast cancer in histology. In addition, about 10% of breast carcinomas cannot be identified by mammography even when they are palpable. Therefore, the diagnosis must be established on morphological evidence using fine needle aspiration, core needle biopsy and often open biopsy.

Large series studies have shown that mammography allows detection of breast cancer in asymptomatic women. Moreover, mammography is capable of detecting pre-cancerous lesions and in situ carcinomas since certain types of DCIS are associated with characteristic microcalcifications. An ideal screening modality would permit highly sensitive detection of breast cancer, including pre-malignant conditions, and is generally available, noninvasive and easy to apply at reasonable cost. Mammography is the most useful screening modality for early detection of breast cancer and in women over the age of 50 years mortality has decreased by more than 30% (for an overview see Kopans [19]). Recommendations regarding the age of women to be screened and the frequency of screening vary widely. However, based on the available evidence, women aged 50 and over should undergo an annual screening examination including mammography and physical examination. Since the benefit of screening is proportional to the patient's risk of developing breast cancer, screening may be recommended in individual cases at younger ages.

Ultrasound allows immediate differentiation between cystic and solid lesions. Cystic lesions typically appear with smooth walls, sharp anterior and posterior borders and without internal echoes. Malignant tissue is typically characterized by irregularly shaped hypoechoic masses, posterior acoustical shadowing and ill-defined demarcation against surrounding breast tissue. For palpable breast masses, specificity seems to be superior to that of mammography but is still not sufficient to exclude breast cancer. Therefore, the number of unnecessary invasive procedures cannot be significantly reduced by means of ultrasonography. Recently, color Doppler has been shown to give additional information aiding the differentiation between benign and malignant masses by demonstrating malignant neovascularization. However, ultrasound can not detect microcalcifications, often the only indication of tumors and especially of small breast carcinomas. Moreover, the diagnostic accuracy of detecting breast cancer is greatly dependent on the experience of the observer. Currently, ultrasound provides additional diagnostic information about the internal composition of masses and can be used to guide cyst aspiration, fine needle aspiration, core needle biopsy and preoperative needle or wire localization.

Magnetic resonance (MR) imaging has several distinct advantages for breast imaging. These advantages include three-dimensional visualization of breast tissue with high spatial resolution, information about tissue vascularity and chest wall visualization. Moreover, MR imaging allows evaluation of dense breast parenchyma which often limits the detection of breast cancer in mammography. The use of paramagnetic contrast agents has been found to be essential in identifying breast masses (Fig. 28.1). Regional signal enhancement is a highly sensitive criterion for detecting breast cancer, in most stud-

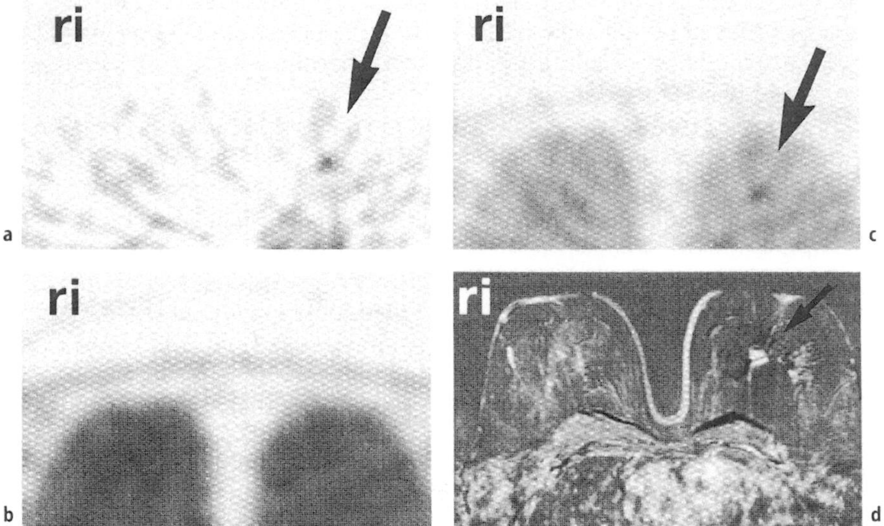

Fig. 28.1. Fifty-two year old woman with a breast carcinoma 0.8 cm in diameter in the left breast (see arrow). **a** Attentuation-corrected emission scan, **b** transmission scan, **c** image fusion of transmission and emission scan, **d** magnetic resonance imaging demonstrating focally increased signal intensity after administration of gadolinium-DTPA.

ies more than 90%, whereas specificity of MR imaging is reported to be less in comparison to mammography.

28.3 Staging

The staging system for carcinoma of the breast is the same for the American Joint Committee on Cancer (AJCC) and the Union Internationale Contre le Cancer (UICC)/TNM projects [32]. It applies to both invasive (infiltrating) and non-invasive (in situ) carcinomas. The pathological tumor size for classification is a measurement of only the invasive component. Microinvasion is the extension of cancer cells beyond the basement membrane into the adjacent tissues with no focus more than 0.1 cm in the greatest dimension. In case of multiple ipsilateral carcinomas the largest primary tumor is used to classify the T stage. In simultaneous bilateral breast carcinomas each carcinoma is staged separately. Inflammatory carcinoma is a clinicopathological entity characterized by diffuse brawny induration of the skin of the breast with an erysipeloid edge, usually without an underlying palpable mass. The tumor of inflammatory carcinoma is classified T4d. Table 28.1 summarizes pathological classification for primary tumors, regional lymph nodes and distant metastases. The degree of tubule formation by tumor cells, nuclear pleomorphism and mitotic counts is used for histopathological grading of inva-

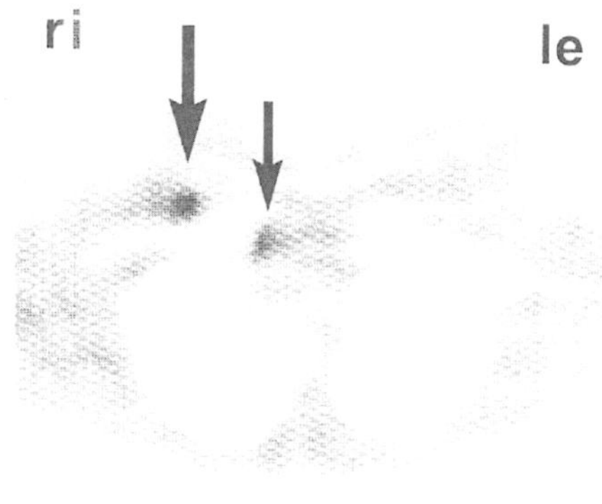

Fig. 28.2. Forty-seven year old woman with a breast carcinoma 1.5 cm in diameter in the right breast with a lesion in the arteria mammaria chain suspicious of lymph node metastasis.

Table 28.1. Pathologic TNM classification of breast cancer.

Primary tumor (T)	
Tx	Primary tumor cannot be assessed
T0	No evidence of primary tumor
Tis	Carcinoma in situ
T1	Tumor 2 cm or less in greatest dimension
T1mic	Microinvasion 0.1 cm or less in greatest dimension
T1a	Tumor more than 0.1 cm but not more than 0.5 cm in greatest dimension
T1b	Tumor more than 0.5 cm but not more than 1 cm in greatest dimension
T1c	Tumor more than 1 cm but not more than 2 in greatest dimension
T2	Tumor more than 2 cm but not more than 5 cm in greatest dimension
T3	Tumor more than 5 cm in greatest dimension
T4	Tumor of any size with direct extension to
T4a	– the chest wall (does not include the pectoral muscle)
T4b	– the skin
T4c	– the chest wall and the skin
T4d	Inflammatory carcinoma
Regional lymph nodes (N)	
Nx	Regional lymph nodes cannot be assessed
N0	No regional lymph node metastasis
N1	Metastasis to movable ipsilateral axillary lymph node(s)
N1a	Only micrometastases (none larger than 0.2 cm)
N1b	Metastasis to lymph node(s), any larger than 0.2 cm
N1bi	Metastasis in 1 to 3 lymph nodes, any more than 0.2 cm but less than 2 cm
N1bii	Metastasis to 4 or more lymph nodes, any more than 0.2 cm but less than 2 cm
N1biii	Extension beyond the capsule of a lymph node less than 2 cm in diameter
N1biv	Metastasis to a lymph node 2 cm or more in greatest dimension
N2	Metastasis to ipsilateral axillary lymph nodes that are fixed
N3	Metastasis to ipsilateral internal mammary lymph node(s)
Distant metastasis (M)	
Mx	Distant metastasis cannot be assessed
M0	No distant metastasis
M1	Distant metastasis *

* include metastasis to ipsilateral supraclavicular lymph nodes

sive breast cancer. G1 tumors are well differentiated, G2 moderately differentiated, G3 poorly differentiated and G4 undifferentiated.

28.4 PET imaging procedure and image analysis

To ensure a standardized metabolic state including low plasma glucose levels, it is necessary that oncology patients fast for at least 4 to 6 h prior to tracer injection. Moreover, insulin-mediated FDG uptake in normal tissue affects the arterial input function and may result in increased background activity. It is recommended that blood glucose is measured prior to administration of FDG as blood glucose level should not exceed 150 mg/100 ml. For imaging in 2D-mode, intravenous administration of about 300–400 MBq ($\sim$10 mCi) ^{18}F-FDG is used in most studies; however, Adler et al. reported a higher tumor detection rate using up to 750 MBq ($\sim$20 mCi) [1, 2]. To avoid artificial tracer retention in the axilla region, the tracer should be injected into an arm vein contralateral to the suspected tumor or into a foot vein. The influence of 3D-mode data acquisition on the results of breast imaging still needs to be studied. Imaging in the prone position with both arms at the side and the breast hanging free is recommended to avoid compression and deformation of the breast. Data acquisition should be started approximately 40–60 min after tracer injection and should last for at least 15 min. Recently, Börner et al. [11] showed increasing target-to-background ratios over time suggesting longer waiting periods between tracer injection and data acquisition; however, lower image quality, due to radionuclide decay, has to be taken into account. Attenuation correction is essential for optimal tumor localization as well as subsequent quantification of regional tracer uptake. Using iterative reconstruction algorithms result in better image quality; however, an increase in diagnostic accuracy has not yet been reported. Calculating standardized uptake values (SUV) by normalization to injected dose and body weight is the most common method for tumor quantification. Quantitative methods may be used to complement visual image analysis for differentiation between benign and malignant breast tumors, i.e., by using a SUV-normalized scale for image display [3]. In particular, SUV correction for partial volume effects and normalization to blood glucose has been shown to yield the highest diagnostic accuracy. Corresponding threshold values for optimal tumor characterization have been published for various quantification methods [3]. Dynamic data acquisition allows calculation of the tracer influx constant; however, this procedure is more complex and does not increase diagnostic accuracy. Visual image interpretation should include analysis of transaxial, coronal and sagittal views. Breast cancer typically presents with focally increased FDG uptake, whereas benign tumors are negative in PET imaging. Proliferative mammary dysplasia may result in moderately, but diffuse increased tracer uptake. Whole-body imaging, which is used for detection of distant metastases, can be improved by intravenous injection of furosemide

(20–40 mg) to reduce tracer retention in the urinary system and by scopolamine (20–40 mg) to reduce FDG uptake in the bowel.

28.5 PET imaging of the breast

The first FDG imaging in breast cancer patients was reported in 1989 by Minn and Soini [23]. They used a collimated gamma camera and successfully visualized 14 (82%) out of 17 primary breast carcinomas. Kubota et al. [20] first reported on PET imaging with FDG in one case with local recurrence, shortly afterwards. In a first series of 10 patients with extensive disease, Wahl et al. successfully identified all breast carcinomas [34]. In 28 patients, Adler et al. found a sensitivity of 96% for breast masses >1 cm in diameter [1]. Table 28.2 summarizes studies reported in the literature. Depending on criteria used for image interpretation, primary breast cancer was identified with a sensitivity ranging between 68% and 94% in our experience [4]. In a larger study of 185 breast tumors, we found an overall sensitivity of 64.4% for conservative image reading (CIR: regarding only definite FDG uptake as positive) and 80.3% for sensitive image reading (SIR: regarding definite and probable FDG uptake as positive) [6]. The increase in sensitivity resulted in a noticeable decrease in specificity, from 94.3% (CIR) to 75.5% (SIR). At stage pT1 (<2 cm), only 30 (68.2%) out of 44 breast carcinomas were detected, compared to 57 (91.9%) out of 62 at stage pT2 (2–5 cm).

Spatial resolution of the PET system, which is approximately 6–8 mm in most scanners that are currently used, significantly influences tumor detection. Partial volume effects cause a spread of the signal over an area larger than it actually occupies. This significantly underestimates radioactivity measurement in small tumors. In addition, the target-to-background ratio is an important factor in determining lesion detectability. Torizuka et al. [30] com-

Table 28.2. PET imaging of breast cancer.

Authors	Patients (n)	Breast Lesions (n)	Sensitivity (%)	Specificity (%)
Wahl et al. (1991)	10	10	100*	–
Tse et al. (1992)	10	14	86	100
Adler et al. (1993)	28	35	96	100
Hoh et al. (1993)	20	20	88	33**
Nieweg et al. (1993)	11	11	91	100
Bruce et al. (1995)	15	15	93	100
Avril et al. (1996)***	51	72	68–83	84–97
Scheidhauer et al. (1996)	30	30	91	86
Palmedo et al. (1997)	20	22	92	86
Avril et al. (2000)***	144	185	64–80	75.5–94

* The study was not designed to assess sensitivity; ** two out of three patients with benign tumors had false-positive results; *** results depend on criteria used for image analysis

pared the average FDG uptake in breast and lung cancer and found a significantly lower phosphorylation of FDG by hexokinase in breast cancer tissue. Moreover, FDG uptake in surrounding normal tissue is higher in the breast compared to the lung, resulting in decreased image contrast and detectability of tumors.

The histological tumor type plays an important role in the diagnostic accuracy of PET imaging. Crippa et al. [13] reported significantly lower SUV for lobular carcinomas compared to ductal carcinomas. In our experience, invasive lobular carcinomas accounted for a higher rate of false-negative results: 15 (65.2%) out of 23 invasive lobular carcinomas were false-negative compared to 23 (23.7%) out of 97 invasive ductal carcinomas [6]. This finding is of particular importance since this tumor type is more difficult to diagnose by means of imaging procedures. Lobular carcinomas are often difficult to detect mammographically, because of the diffuse growth pattern and tendency to form lesions with opacity equal to or less than surrounding parenchyma.

Identification of multifocal or multicentric breast cancer is an important factor in determining the possibility of breast-conserving surgery. However, since multifocal tumor sites are often small, the same limitations apply to PET imaging as discussed above. Even applying sensitive image reading, only 9 (50%) out of 18 patients presenting with multicentric or multifocal breast cancer were correctly identified [6]. It is important to note that PET imaging with FDG does not allow determination of the origin of malignant tumors. Breast sarcoma as well as malignant hematopoietic breast tumors are indistinguishable from breast carcinomas [8].

The diagnosis of in situ carcinomas has increased over the past decade, mainly due to increased use and technical improvement of mammography. There is little information available about the ability of PET imaging to detect noninvasive breast cancer. Tse et al. [31] studied 14 patients and found that 1 out of 2 false-negative cases had predominantly intraductal cancer with microscopic invasive foci. In our experience with 12 patients (10 DCIS and 2 LCIS), none out of six in situ carcinomas smaller than two centimeters could be identified. For larger tumors, 3 (50%) out of 6 displayed increased FDG uptake. Although the number of patients studied is small, these data suggest that detection of in situ carcinomas may not be improved by PET imaging.

Benign conditions of the breast are more common than breast cancer and are often difficult to differentiate from breast cancer. In general, benign breast masses display low FDG accumulation [1, 4, 6, 7, 28]. Scheidhauer et al. [28] studied seven patients with benign breast disease and found only one false-positive result. This patient showed focal inflammation at histology and had received local irradiation of a lymphoma one year prior to PET scanning. It is well known that cellular infiltrates of granulocytes and macrophages in abscesses, soft tissue infections, tuberculosis and sarcoidosis may result in increased glycolysis. However, inflammation of the breast does not represent a major diagnostic problem. We found only 3 out of 53 benign breast masses presenting with focally increased tracer uptake, including one rare case of a ductal adenoma, one case with dysplastic tissue and one fibroadenoma. Fibroadenomas are common benign tumors and only one out of nine displayed increased tracer uptake. Moreover, dysplastic tissue often accounts for false-positive results in MR imaging predominantly showing a diffuse pattern of little or only moderate FDG uptake.

28.6 Loco-regional staging of breast cancer patients

Identification of axillary lymph node metastases has been identified as the most important prognostic indicator, guiding decision making in adjuvant therapy. Patients diagnosed with breast cancer have to undergo axillary dissection for accurate staging since anatomically based imaging methods do not allow for accurate identification of loco-regional lymph metastases. Wahl et al. [34] studied 12 patients with PET and noted increased FDG uptake in axillary metastases. In 18 patients, Adler et al. [1] reported a sensitivity of 90% and a specificity of 100% for axillary PET imaging. Nine out of ten cases with positive results at axillary node dissection had positive PET scans. However, PET imaging did not determine the number of tumor-involved lymph nodes which is important for subsequent therapy recommendation. In a more recent study, the same authors reported on 50 breast cancer patients with 52 axillary lymph node dissections [2]. The sensitivity and negative predictive value were both 95%, and the overall accuracy was 77%. However, sensitive image reading resulted in 11 false-positive PET findings and a specificity of only 66%. Other studies also reported a considerable number of false-positive results without signs of inflammation which would be the most likely reason for false-positive FDG uptake in the axilla. We studied 51 patients and found an overall sensitivity of 79% for the detection of axillary lymph node metastases (corresponding specificity was 96%) [5]. When only patients with primary breast tumors >2 cm (>stage pT1) were considered, the sensitivity of axillary PET imaging increased to 94%, with no false-positive results. Lymph node metastases could not be identified in 4 of 6 patients with small primary breast cancers (stage pT1), resulting in a sensitivity of

Table 28.3. PET imaging of axillary lymph node metastases.

Authors	Patients (n)	Sensitivity (%)	Specificity (%)
Adler et al. (1993)	10	90	100
Avril et al. (1996)	51	79	96
Scheidhauer et al. (1996)	18	100	89
Utech et al. (1996)	124	100	75
Adler et al. (1996)	50	95	66
Crippa et al. (1998)	68	85	91
Smith et al. (1998)	50	90	97

only 33% in these patients. These results suggest that *detection of micrometastases and small tumor-infiltrated lymph nodes is limited by the currently achievable spatial resolution of PET imaging.* On the other hand, PET imaging provided additional information in 12 (29%) of 41 breast cancer patients demonstrating axillary involvement at level III (located medial to the border of the pectoralis minor muscle), periclavicular and retrosternal lymph node metastases as well as bone and lung metastases. Table 28.3 summarizes the findings of PET studies imaging axillary lymph node metastases.

28.7 Diagnosis of distant metastases and recurrent disease

Breast cancer may metastasize to almost any organ but most commonly to lymph nodes, lungs, liver and bones. In patients suspicious for tumor recurrence recommended work up usually includes chest x-ray, ultrasonography of the abdomen and bone scintigraphy. In addition, computed tomography and magnetic resonance imaging permit evaluation of suspected metastases in different organs.

The initial report from Minn and Soini [23] found not only increased FDG uptake in primary breast carcinomas and tumor-involved lymph nodes but also in pulmonary and liver metastases. As whole-body PET imaging became more available, several groups emphasized the potential role for accurate staging of breast cancer patients. Bender et al. [10] studied 75 patients with suspected recurrent or metastatic disease in order to compare the diagnostic accuracy of whole-body PET imaging with that of CT or MR imaging. PET imaging correctly identified 28 (97%) out of 29 patients with lymph node involvement, 15 (100%) out of 15 patients with bone metastases, 5 (83%) out of 6 with lung and 2 patients with liver metastases. Moreover, PET detected 8 lymph node and 7 bone metastases, which were not visualized by CT or magnetic resonance imaging. In another study Moon et al. [25] also found high diagnostic accuracy of whole-body PET imaging in patients with suspected recurrent or metastatic breast carcinoma. On a lesion basis, the sensitivity of PET imaging to detect distant metastases was 85% and specificity was 79%. On a patient basis, sensitivity and specificity were 93% and 79%, respectively. False-positive lesions were due to muscle uptake, inflammation, blood pool activity in the great vessels and bowel uptake. It is important to note that *bone metastases had a significantly larger proportion of false-negative lesions than other malignant sites.* This finding concurs with that of Minn and Soini who found a considerable variability of FDG uptake in bone metastases with osteolytic or mixed type lesions being better visualized than sclerotic lesions. Recently, Cook et al. [12] compared FDG-PET with conventional bone scintigraphy in 23 patients with skeletal metastases from breast cancer. PET detected more lesions than bone scintigraphy; however, in a subgroup of patients with osteoblastic disease, bone metastases were frequently undetectable by PET. Therefore, the clinical role of PET imaging compared to bone scintigraphy still needs to be determined. However, the advantage of whole-body PET imaging is its ability to detect soft tissue metastases in different sites and organs, and in the future it has the potential to replace the follow-up investigations currently employed.

Increasing application of breast conserving surgery requires close follow-up examinations for early detection of local recurrence. However, mammographical detection of recurrent breast cancer is often difficult, especially after breast augmentation mammoplasties. Wahl et al. [35] demonstrated the utility of PET to detect local recurrence in two women with silicone implants. PET clearly showed focal FDG accumulation in the suspicious breasts, corresponding to tumors of larger than 1.5 centimeter in diameter. In a larger series, Bender et al. [10] correctly diagnosed local recurrence in 16 (80%) out of 20 patients with PET, although MR imaging detected 14 (93%) out of 15 patients with a comparable specificity (96% for PET and 98% for MR imaging). All positive lesions showed intense FDG uptake, whereas false-negative results in PET imaging were found in patients presenting with small lesions (<7–10 mm).

28.8 Therapy monitoring

Recently, primary (neoadjuvant) chemotherapy has been introduced to improve the management of patients with locally advanced breast cancer as preoperative chemotherapy allows for a higher rate of breast conservation. Moreover, direct histopathological assessment of the response to chemotherapy offers the chance to apply alternative chemotherapeutic regimens if the first treatment is ineffective. In patients with locally advanced breast cancer, tumor response to chemotherapy has been identified as an important prognostic factor in predicting disease-free and overall survival [16, 21]. However, since clinical response does not necessarily reflect histopathological response, it is not possible to determine the effect of neoadjuvant chemotherapy until after definitive breast surgery. For distant metastases, therapy monitoring is more difficult since histopathological tissue examination is often not possible. Change in tumor size, assessed by anatomical imaging modalities, is the most important criterion, although, sequential measurement of tumor size frequently does not determine an early response or differentiate between viable tumor tissue and scar.

Studies reporting about therapy monitoring with PET have shown that quantification of tumor glucose metabolism is highly valuable for monitoring early effects of chemotherapy [9, 14, 17, 29, 36]. Wahl et al. [36] studied 11 women with newly diagnosed primary breast cancer undergoing chemo-hormonotherapy. There was a rapid and significant decrease in tumor glucose metabolism in responding patients and no significant decrease in non-responding patients. Bassa et al. [9] found a good correlation between the PET results and pathology findings at surgery as well as with the results of mammography and ultrasonography for residual disease. Jansson et al. [17] investigated [^{18}F]FDG and [^{11}C]methionine and concluded that therapy response could be determined earlier than with any other method of conventional therapy evaluation. Recently, Dehdashti et al. [14] studied whether increased FDG uptake in tumors, early after initiation of tamoxifen therapy, predicts a hormonally responsive breast cancer. None of the responders had a clinical flare reaction, but all demonstrated "metabolic flare". No evidence for flare was noted in the non-responders. It is not yet known if this highly interesting observation about an initial increase in glucose metabolism following hormone therapy can be directly translated to the effects of a more aggressive chemotherapy. In these patients, decrease of glucose metabolism after onset of therapy seems to be the more important criterion.

In our experience, FDG-PET can differentiate responder from non-responder early in the course of therapy [29]. We studied 22 patients with advanced breast cancer undergoing primary dose-intense chemotherapy. PET scans of the breast acquired after the first and second course of chemotherapy were compared with the baseline scan and quantification of regional FDG uptake was made for a total of 24 breast carcinomas. To evaluate the predictive value of PET imaging, histopathological response after completion of chemotherapy classified as gross residual disease (GRD) and minimal residual disease (MRD) served as the gold standard. With a change of tumor glucose metabolism during chemotherapy, significant ($p<0.05$) differences in tracer uptake between tumors with GRD compared to MRD were observed. PET differentiated between responding and non-responding tumors as early as after the first course of chemotherapy. After initiation of chemotherapy, tracer uptake showed little change in tumors with GRD found later in pathological analysis but decreased sharply to the background level in most tumors with MRD. After the first course, all responders were correctly identified (sensitivity 100%, specificity 85%) by a threshold defined as a decrease below 55% of the baseline scan. At this level, histopathological response could be predicted with an accuracy of 88% and 91% after the first and second course of therapy, respectively. We found that prediction of histopathological response provides prognostic information and may be helpful to improve patient management by avoiding ineffective chemotherapy and supporting the decision to continue dose-intensive preoperative chemotherapy in responding patients. These initial observations have to be confirmed in a larger series to more clearly define the clinical role of PET imaging for therapy monitoring.

28.9 Receptor imaging

The majority of breast cancers express estrogen (ER) and progesterone (PR) receptors. The ER receptor status provides important prognostic information since ER-positive tumors are generally less aggressive and often respond to hormone therapy. The hormone-receptor status is currently assessed from tumor tissue by in vitro assays. However, in vitro analysis provides little information about the functional status of the hormone receptors. Only about 60% of patients with positive ER expression respond to hormone therapy; on the other hand about 5–10% respond despite negative ER expression. Over the past few years a number of studies have reported on successful non-invasive imaging of hormone receptor expression by using appropriate radioligands. Various estrogen derivatives have been radiolabeled with positron and single photon emitters [18]. In vitro and in vivo studies have demonstrated high affinity to ER receptors by 16-[^{18}F]fluoro-17-estradiol (FES). FES has been synthesized with high specific activity providing successful imaging of ER-positive tumors [22, 24]. An excellent correlation between tumor uptake of FES and in vitro analysis of ER expression allows accurate determination of the ER status in breast cancer. Positive correlations have not only been found for primary tumors but also for metastastic lesions. Dehdashti et al. [15] studied 32 patients with primary breast masses and 21 patients with clinical evidence of recurrent or metastatic breast carcinoma, with both FES and FDG-PET. Good overall agreement (88%) was found between in vitro ER assays and FES-PET. However, there was no significant relationship between FDG uptake and ER status of the tumors, suggesting that glucose metabolism does not reflect the receptor status. When assessing the functional status of the hormone receptors, a decrease of FES uptake was found following initiation of tamoxifen therapy. These promising results suggest that using radiolabeled hormone receptor ligands for non-invasive prediction and monitoring of the response to antiestrogen therapy will be of value.

28.10 Summary

A considerable number of studies have shown the value of FDG-PET imaging in breast cancer patients. However, there are certain limitations that must be considered. The restricted sensitivity to detect small tumors does not allow the screening of asymptomatic women for breast cancer. Moreover, negative PET results in patients presenting with palpable breast masses or abnormal mammography do not exclude breast cancer. Therefore, PET imaging may not be used as a routine application for evaluation of primary breast tumors. A comparable diagnostic accuracy reported on scintimammography, which is far more widely available and less expensive, has also to be considered [26]. Nevertheless, PET represents a highly valuable method in clinically difficult cases. These include women with radiodense breast tissue, significant fibrocystic changes and fibrosis after radiotherapy. In our experience, PET imaging is especially helpful prior to surgery in patients with inconclusive results from MR imaging to identify the lesion which most likely represents breast cancer among contrast-enhancing tissue. However, due to the limitations discussed above, the number of unnecessary invasive procedures in benign breast masses may not be significantly reduced by currently available metabolic imaging techniques. On the other hand, the high positive predictive value to represent malignant tissue provided by increased metabolic activity allows one to preoperatively determine the extent of disease in patients presenting with advanced breast cancer. In this subgroup, PET imaging provides a high diagnostic accuracy for identification of loco-regional lymph node metastases. Detection of micrometastases and small, tumor-infiltrated lymph nodes is limited by the currently achievable spatial resolution of PET imaging. In these patients, application of the "sentinel lymph node concept" has been reported to predict the axillary lymph node status with high accuracy by identification and histological examination of the first lymph node receiving drainage from the primary tumor [33]. Therefore, both methods seem to be complementary for assessment of tumor spread to the axillary lymph nodes.

Whole-body PET imaging provides high diagnostic accuracy in detecting patients with recurrent or metastatic breast carcinoma. Further studies need to address whether or not various imaging procedures currently used for staging of breast cancer patients (chest x-ray, ultrasound, bone scintigraphy, CT and MR imaging) may be substituted by FDG-PET imaging in the near future. Since PET imaging seems to be highly useful for monitoring therapeutic effects, earlier than with any other imaging method currently available, identification of non-responders would greatly improve patient management by reducing the application of ineffective therapies. This would not only prevent patients from unnecessary side effects but also reduce costs significantly. Sequential PET scanning would not only allow monitoring of response to therapy but, in addition, PET could determine the extent of viable tumor tissue after completion of therapy. This would provide important prognostic information in patients with advanced disease. Moreover, in patients with residual tumor masses from anatomic imaging, PET may be very useful in differentiating between viable tumor tissue and scar. The use of radioligands allows non-invasive assessment of the hormone receptor status not only in primary tumors but also in metastatic tumor sites and provides important information about the functional status and biological availability of the receptors.

28.11 Recommendations for FDG-PET imaging

• Patient preparation	Fasted for >6 h
• Injection of FDG	300–400 MBq ($\sim$10 mCi), contralateral arm vein
• Scanning	45–60 min after tracer injection Patient in prone position, arms at the side, breasts hanging free
• Data acquisition	15–20 minutes emission scan, 2D mode, Transmission scan (1.5–3×10^6 counts/slice)

- Image reconstruction — Filtered back projection (e.g., Hanning 0.4–0.5 cycles per bin)
  Iterative reconstruction (e.g., OSEM, 4 subsets, 8 iterations)
- Image interpretation — Visual image analysis (focally increased FDG uptake)
  Quantification of regional tracer uptake
- Quantification — Calculation of SUV.

References

[1] Adler LP, Crowe JP, al-Kaisi NK, Sunshine JL (1993) Evaluation of breast masses and axillary lymph nodes with [F-18] 2-deoxy-2-fluoro-D-glucose PET. Radiology 187:743–750

[2] Adler LP, Faulhaber PF, Schnur KC, Al-Kasi NL, Shenk RR (1997) Axillary lymph node metastases: screening with [F-18]2-deoxy-2-fluoro-D-glucose (FDG) PET. Radiology 203:323–327

[3] Avril N, Bense S, Ziegler SI, Dose J, Weber W, Laubenbacher C, Römer W, Jänicke F, Schwaiger M (1997) Breast imaging with fluorine-18-FDG PET: quantitative image analysis. J Nucl Med 38:1186–1191

[4] Avril N, Dose J, Jänicke F, Bense S, Ziegler S, Laubenbacher C, Römer W, Pache H, Herz M, Allgayer B, Nathrath W, Graeff H, Schwaiger M (1996) Metabolic characterization of breast tumors with positron emission tomography using F-18 fluorodeoxyglucose. J Clin Oncol 14:1848–1857

[5] Avril N, Dose J, Jänicke F, Ziegler S, Römer W, Weber W, Herz M, Nathrath W, Graeff H, Schwaiger M (1996) Assessment of axillary lymph node involvement in breast cancer patients with positron emission tomography using radiolabeled 2-(fluorine-18)-fluoro-2-deoxy-D-glucose. J Natl Cancer Inst 88:1204–1209

[6] Avril N, Rose CA, Schelling M, Dose J, Kuhn W, Bense S, Weber W, Ziegler S, Graeff H, Schwaiger M (2000) Breast imaging with positron emission tomography and fluorine-18 fluorodeoxyglucose: use and limitations. (submitted)

[7] Avril N, Schelling M, Dose J, Weber W, Schwaiger M (1999) Utility of PET in breast cancer. Clin Pos Imag 2:261–271

[8] Bakheet SM, Powe J, Ezzat A, Al Suhaibani H, Tulbah A, Rostom A (1998) F-18 FDG whole-body positron emission tomography scan in primary breast sarcoma. Clin Nucl Med 23:604–608

[9] Bassa P, Kim EE, Inoue T, Wong FC, Korkmaz M, Yang DJ, Wong WH, Hicks KW, Buzdar AU, Podoloff DA (1996) Evaluation of preoperative chemotherapy using PET with fluorine-18-fluorodeoxyglucose in breast cancer. J Nucl Med 37:931–938

[10] Bender H, Kirst J, Palmedo H, Schomburg A, Wagner U, Ruhlmann J, Biersack HJ (1997) Value of 18 fluoro-deoxyglucose positron emission tomography in the staging of recurrent breast carcinoma. Anticancer Res 17:1687–1692

[11] Börner AR, Weckesser M, Herzog H, Schmitz T, Audretsch W, Nitz U, Bender HG, Müller-Gärtner HW (1999) Optimal scan time for fluorine-18 fluorodeoxyglucose positron emission tomography in breast cancer. Eur J Nucl Med 26:226–230

[12] Cook GJ, Houston S, Rubens R, Maisey MN, Fogelman I (1998) Detection of bone metastases in breast cancer by F-18 FDG PET: differing metabolic activity in osteoblastic and osteolytic lesions. J Clin Oncol 16:3375–3379

[13] Crippa F, Seregni E, Agresti R, Chiesa C, Pascali C, Bogni A, Decise D, De Sanctis V, Greco M, Daidone MG, Bombardieri E (1998) Association between F-18 fluorodeoxyglucose uptake and postoperative histopathology, hormone receptor status, thymidine

labelling index and p53 in primary breast cancer: a preliminary observation. Eur J Nucl Med 25:1429–1434

[14] Dehdashti F, Flanagan FL, Mortimer JE, Katzenellenbogen JA, Welch MJ, Siegel BA (1999) Positron emission tomographic assessment of "metabolic flare" to predict response of metastatic breast cancer to antiestrogen therapy. Eur J Nucl Med 26:51–56

[15] Dehdashti F, Mortimer JE, Siegel BA, Griffeth LK, Bonasera TJ, Fusselman MJ, Detert DD, Cutler PD, Katzenellenbogen JA, Welch MJ (1995) Positron tomographic assessment of estrogen receptors in breast cancer: comparison with FDG-PET and in vitro receptor assays. J Nucl Med 36:1766–1774

[16] Fisher B, Bryant J, Wolmark N, Mamounas E, Brown A, Fisher ER, Wickerham DL, Begovic M, DeCillis A, Robidoux A, Margolese RG, Cruz AB, Jr, Hoehn JL, Lees AW, Dimitrov NV, Bear HD (1998) Effect of preoperative chemotherapy on the outcome of women with operable breast cancer. J Clin Oncol 16:2672–2685

[17] Jansson T, Westlin JE, Ahlstrom H, Lilja A, Langstrom B, Bergh J (1995) Positron emission tomography studies in patients with locally advanced and/or metastatic breast cancer: a method for early therapy evaluation? J Clin Oncol 13:1470–1477

[18] Katzenellenbogen JA, Coleman RE, Hawkins RA, Krohn KA, Larson SM, Mendelsohn J, Osborne CK, Piwnica-Worms D, Reba RC, Siegel BA, Welch MJ, Shtern F (1995) Tumor receptor imaging: proceedings of the national cancer institute workshop, review of current work, and prospective for further investigations. Clin Cancer Res 1:921–932

[19] Kopans DB (1997) An overview of the breast cancer screening controversy. J Natl Cancer Inst Monogr 22:1–3

[20] Kubota K, Matsuzawa T, Amemiya A, Kondo M, Fujiwara T, Watanuki S, Ito M, Ido T (1989) Imaging of breast cancer with F-18 fluorodeoxyglucose and positron emission tomography. J Comput Assist Tomogr 13:1097–1098

[21] Kuerer HM, Newman LA, Smith TL, Ames FC, Hunt KK, Dhingra K, Theriault RL, Singh G, Binkley SM, Sneige N, Buchholz TA, Ross MI, McNeese MD, Buzdar AU, Hortobagyi GN, Singletary SE (1999) Clinical course of breast cancer patients with complete pathologic primary tumor and axillary lymph node response to doxorubicin-based neoadjuvant chemotherapy. J Clin Oncol 17:460–469

[22] McGuire AH, Dehdashti F, Siegel BA, Lyss AP, Brodack JW, Mathias CJ, Mintun MA, Katzenellenbogen JA, Welch MJ (1991) Positron tomographic assessment of 16 alpha-[18F] fluoro-17 beta-estradiol uptake in metastatic breast carcinoma. J Nucl Med 32:1526–1531

[23] Minn H, Soini I (1989) F-18 fluorodeoxyglucose scintigraphy in diagnosis and follow up of treatment in advanced breast cancer. Am J Clin Pathol 91:535–541

[24] Mintun MA, Welch MJ, Siegel BA, Mathias CJ, Brodack JW, McGuire AH, Katzenellenbogen JA (1988) Breast cancer: PET imaging of estrogen receptors. Br J Cancer 58:626–630

[25] Moon DH, Maddahi J, Silverman DH, Glaspy JA, Phelps ME, Hoh CK (1998) Accuracy of whole-body fluorine-18-FDG PET for the detection of recurrent or metastatic breast carcinoma. J Nucl Med 39:431–435

[26] Palmedo H, Bender H, Grunwald F, Mallmann P, Zamora P, Krebs D, Biersack HJ (1997) Comparison of fluorine-18 fluorodeoxyglucose positron emission tomography and technetium-99m methoxyisobutylisonitrile scintimammography in the detection of breast tumours. Eur J Nucl Med 24:1138–1145

[27] Parker SL, Tong T, Bolden S, Wingo PA (1996) Cancer statistics. CA Cancer J Clin 65:5–27

[28] Scheidhauer K, Scharl A, Pietrzyk U, Wagner R, Göhring UJ, Schomäcker K, Schicha H (1996) Qualitative F-18 FDG positron emission tomography in primary breast cancer: clinical relevance and practicability. Eur J Nucl Med 23:618–623

[29] Schelling M, Avril N, Nährig J, Kuhn W, Römer W, Sattler D, Wener W, Dose J, Jänicke F, Graeff H, Schwaiger M (2000) Positron emission tomography using F-18 fluorodeoxyglucose for monitoring primary chemotherapy in breast cancer. J Clin Oncol (in press)

[30] Torizuka T, Zasadny KR, Recker B, Wahl RL (1998) Untreated primary lung and breast cancers: correlation between F-18 FDG kinetic rate constants and findings of in vitro studies. Radiology 207:767–774

[31] Tse NY, Hoh CK, Hawkins RA, Zinner MJ, Dahlbom M, Choi Y, Maddahi J, Brunicardi FC, Phelps ME, Glaspy JA (1992) The application of positron emission tomographic imaging with fluorodeoxyglucose to the evaluation of breast disease. Ann Surg 216:27–34

[32] UICC (1997) TNM. Classification of Malignant Tumors. Wiley-Liss, New York

[33] Veronesi U, Paganelli G, Galimberti V, Viale G, Zurrida S, Bedoni M, Costa A, de Cicco C, Geraghty JG, Luini A, Sacchini V, Veronesi P (1997) Sentinel-node biopsy to avoid axillary dissection in breast cancer with clinically negative lymph-nodes. Lancet 349:1864–1867

[34] Wahl RL, Cody RL, Hutchins GD, Mudgett EE (1991) Primary and metastatic breast carcinoma: initial clinical evaluation with PET with the radiolabeled glucose analogue 2-[F-18]-fluoro-2-deoxy-D-glucose. Radiology 179:765–770

[35] Wahl RL, Helvie MA, Chang AE, Andersson I (1994) Detection of breast cancer in women after augmentation mammoplasty using fluorine-18-fluorodeoxyglucose-PET. J Nucl Med 35:872–875

[36] Wahl RL, Zasadny K, Helvie M, Hutchins GD, Weber B, Cody R (1993) Metabolic monitoring of breast cancer chemohormonotherapy using positron emission tomography: initial evaluation. J Clin Oncol 11:2101–2111

29 Ovarian cancer

F. Grünwald, B. Grünwald, G. Lucignani

29.1 Incidence, etiology, epidemiology

Ovarian cancer is the 5th frequent malignant tumor in women. Because of its overall poor prognosis at the time of detection, it is one of the most frequent causes of cancer-associated death in women. Epithelial ovarian cancers rank fifth of the overall mortality statistics in Western Europe and the United States. Only 20% of all ovarian cancers are classified as borderline tumors with low malignancy potential. The mean incidence of ovarian cancer is 13/100000 per year, showing a clear age dependency. In 40-year-old women the incidence is around 15/100000, whereas it is 55/100 000 in 75-year-old women. More than 90% of all ovarian tumors belong to the sporadic form with unknown etiology. In hereditary ovarian cancer at least two first-degree relatives are affected. It is important to differentiate between hereditary ovarian cancer and families with ovarian *and* breast cancer. The latter are associated in more than 90% with a mutation of the BRCA1 or BRCA2 gene. In addition to genetic risk factors, old age, early menarche, late menopause, nullipara and white race are associated with an increased risk for ovarian cancer. Births, breast feeding and the use of oral contraceptives are known to be protective with respect to ovarian cancer.

29.2 Histopathologic classification of malignant ovarian tumors [21, 22]

▸ A *epithelial tumors*
serous tumors
borderline tumors
cystadenoma
superficial papilloma
serous adenofibroma
malignant tumors
adenocarcinoma
papillary superficial carcinoma
serous malignant adenofibroma

mucinous tumors
borderline tumors
cystadenoma
mucinous adenofibroma
malignant tumors
adenocarcinoma
mucinous malignant adenofibroma
endometrioid malignant tumors
borderline tumors
adenoma
adenofibroma
malignant tumors
adenocarcinoma
malignant adenofibroma
endometrial stromal sarcoma
malignant mesodermal mixed tumor
clear cell tumors
borderline tumors
malignant tumors
clear cell carcinoma
clear cell adenocarcinoma
mixed cell epithelial tumors
borderline tumors
malignant tumors
Brenner's tumor
borderline tumors
malignant tumors
undifferentiated carcinoma
unclassified malignant epithelial tumor

► B *malignant germinal cord/stroma tumors*
malignant granulosa cell tumor
malignant thecoma
unclassified malignant germinal cord/stroma tumors

► C *steroid cell/lipid cell tumor*

► D *germ cell tumor*
dysgerminoma
yolk sac tumor
embryonal carcinoma
polyembryoma
chorionepithelioma
teratoma
immature teratoma
mature teratoma
malignant ovarian goitre

carcinoid
combined malignant germ cell tumors

- ▶ E *mixed germinal cord and germinal cell tumors*
- ▶ F *sarcoma without ovarian specificity*

29.3 Tumor extension staging, prognosis

29.3.1 Tumor extension and staging

In almost all cases malignant ovarian tumors initially spread to neighbor organs in the minor pelvis (e.g., uterus, fallopian tube). Peritoneal spreading with drop metastases (frequently localized in the Douglas pouch) occurs relatively early when the organ capsule has been penetrated, very frequently associated with ascites. Subsequently, metastases in the omentum and the subphrenic space develop via peritoneal spreading. The lymphogenic spreading occurs most frequently via pelvic, inguinal and paraaortal lymph nodes. This spreading route can be responsible for the expansion through the diaphragm with subsequent pleural effusion. Hematogenic metastases are relatively rare. TNM classification and FIGO/UICC guidelines are used for staging [20]. TNM classification and stages are presented in Table 29.1 and Table 29.2.

Table 29.1. TNM stage.

T	
T1	tumor limited to the ovaries
T1a	tumor limited to one ovary; capsule intact; no tumor tissue on the surface of the ovary; no malignant cells in ascites or in peritoneal lavage
T1b	tumor limited to both ovaries; capsule intact; no tumor tissue on the surface of the ovaries; no malignant cells in ascites or in peritoneal lavage
T1c	tumor limited to the ovaries; capsule ruptured or tumor on the surface of the ovaries or malignant cells in ascites or in peritoneal lavage
T2	tumor spread to the pelvis
T2a	spreading/implants at uterus/fallopian tube; no malignant cells in ascites or in peritoneal lavage
T2b	spreading to other organs of the pelvis; no malignant cells in ascites or in peritoneal lavage
T2c	spreading to pelvis organs; malignant cells in ascites or in peritoneal lavage
T3	peritoneal metastases outside the pelvis
T3a	microscopic peritoneal metastases outside the pelvis
T3b	macroscopic peritoneal metastases outside the pelvis ($\leq$ 2 cm)
T3c	macroscopic peritoneal metastases outside the pelvis (> 2 cm)
N	
N0	no lymph node metastases
N1	regional lymph node metastases
M	
M0	no distant metastases
M1	distant metastases

Table 29.2. FIGO/UICC staging.

Stage IA	T1a	N0	M0
Stage IB	T1b	N0	M0
Stage IC	T1c	N0	M0
Stage IIA	T2a	N0	M0
Stage IIB	T2b	N0	M0
Stage IIC	T2c	N0	M0
Stage IIIA	T3a	N0	M0
Stage IIIB	T3b	N0	M0
Stage IIIC	T3c	N0	M0
	each T	N1	M0
Stage IV	each T	each N	M1

29.3.2 Prognosis

Compared to other tumors, the overall prognosis of ovarian cancer is poor, mainly because these tumors become symptomatic in a late stage in most cases. In only 35% of the patients is the malignant ovarian tumor detected in FIGO stage I or II. Borderline tumors are one exception, their prognosis is mainly determined by the degree of ploidy and S-phase. In borderline tumors, the 10-year-survival rate is about 75%. Tumor stage, residual tumor mass after initial surgery, histologic type, degree of ploidy, S-phase, oncogen expression and CA 125 course (CA 19-9 in mucinous carcinoma) determine mainly the prognosis of patients with malignant tumors. The overall mean 5-year survival rate ranges between 30% and 40%. It is nearly 90% in stage I and less than 15% in stage IV [18].

29.4 Clinical signs and diagnostic procedures

29.4.1 Screening

Because of the lack of sufficient diagnostic procedures no screening programs for early detection of ovarian cancer are available [10]. Sometimes ovarian cancer is detected incidentally in a relatively early stage during the ultrasound, done because of complains not related to ovarian tumors or during a general check-up. BRCA1-positive patients are particularly controlled with care since these women have a risk up to 80% to be affected by ovarian cancer [3]. In this patient group, screening with frequently performed ultrasound will play a major role in the future.

29.4.2 Clinical signs

In most cases ovarian cancer becomes clinically evident by signs of advanced tumor progression because early symptoms are rare. In addition to "unspecific" abdominal pain, pollakisuria, uterine bleeding abnormalities and subsequently weight loss, ascites and symptoms of ileus are observed. Yolk sac tumors can become symptomatic by rupture, torsion or bleeding.

29.4.3 Preoperative diagnostic procedures

In addition to clinical history and physical examination detailed ultrasound (abdominal and vaginal), cystoscopy, rectoscopy, barium enema, chest X-ray and tumor marker measurement (CA 125, CA 19-9, CA 74-9, AFP, HCG) are essential preoperative diagnostic procedures. A puncture of the pleural cavity is necessary in cases with pleural effusion. Computed tomography and magnetic resonance imaging are helpful prior to surgery with respect to a detailed planning of the operation. An excretion urography should be included in cases with suspicious results of the ultrasound of the kidneys.

29.5 Therapy

Staging is based on the situs obtained during surgery and histology as well as cytology of intraoperatively taken samples. Therefore, extended surgery is essential not only with respect to total tumor resection or substantial debulking, but also with respect to a correct staging. In general, a laparatomy is performed. If the diagnosis "ovarian cancer" is obtained incidentally during laparascopy, an extension of the procedure becomes necessary. In addition to tumor resection, surgical procedures can include lavage, hysterectomy with adnectomy, infracolic omentectomy, resection of affected gut, diaphragm exploration or lymph node dissection (pelvic/paraaortal) in epithelial tumors. The removal of all malignant cells is the predominant aim of primary therapy in cases with confirmed stage I. In contrast, the surgical treatment of patients with stage II to IV is focused mainly on tumor debulking. Surgical therapy planning in cases with recurrence is not standardized and has to be decided individually. The success of preoperative chemotherapy depends mainly on the tumor cell mass. No adjuvant therapy is necessary in stage 1A, whereas it is used routinely in stage IC and is under discussion in stage IB (grade 3 tumors).

Most epithelial tumors are initially chemosensitive [16] but rapidly develop resistance against several cytostatic agents. During the past, in stage II to IV a combination of two chemotherapeutics was used, one agent being carboplatin or cisplatin, the other frequently cyclophosphamide or (recently) taxol. Current multicenter trials deal with the question, whether a combination of three agents is superior (epirubicine or adriamycin in addition). Treosulfan, ifosfamid and topotecan are second-line therapeutics. Particularly patients with a poor prognosis (FIGO III C and IV) were treated with gemcitabine as a second-line substance with promising results. Mitoxantrone, mitomycine and cisplatin can be used for palliative intraperitoneal chemotherapy. The indication for radiotherapy (mainly whole abdomen radiation) is controversially discussed. In general, survival rates seem to be improved by radiotherapy, particularly by the combination of fractionated radiation with chemotherapy. In the majority of patients with recurrence, symptoms are reduced by targeted radiation. In cases with recurrent ascites, radionuclides have been applied successfully by intraperitoneal instillation.

Unilateral adnectomy is performed in stage 1A borderline tumors, in some cases completed by a wedge resection of the contralateral ovary, an omentectomy or lymph node resection. In progressive disease, the indication for a second surgical therapy is established more frequently than in patients suffering from malignant tumors since the chance to cure the disease is significantly higher. Chemotherapy is applied in borderline tumors stage II B to IV, whereas it is discussed controversially in stage I C and II A – in contrast to malignant tumors.

29.6 Follow-up

In addition to anamnesis and physical examination, follow-up includes tumor marker measurement (CA 125 only, if this marker was increased preoperatively) and ultrasonography of the abdomen, kidneys and minor pelvis. Follow-up examinations are performed monthly during the first year, in the second and third year every three months and after three years every six months.

29.7 PET imaging

The importance of PET imaging in patients with suspected or confirmed ovarian cancer is determined by the late detection of the tumor and therefore relatively poor prognosis in most cases at the moment of establishing the final diagnosis. If possible, PET imaging should be performed in a whole-body technique. Because of the frequent occurrence of peritoneal and inguinal lymph node metastases, at least the region between the diaphragm and the proximal thigh has to be included. A catheterization of the bladder is recommended in addition to a sufficient hydration to improve image quality. Table 29.3 shows which examinations should be done prior to PET and which data have to be known for an optimal reading of FDG-PET.

Table 29.3. Results that should be known for carrying-out and reading of FDG-PET in ovarian cancer

Obligatory	tumor markers CA 125 (in recurrence only in cases of preoperatively informative levels) CA 19-9 in mucinous tumors AFP in endodermal tumors HCG in chorioncarcinoma ultrasound abdomen pelvis liver kidneys X-ray thorax
Optional	computed tomography pelvis abdomen liver magnetic resonance imaging pelvis abdomen liver X-ray excretion urography

29.7.1 Primary tumor

During the German consensus conference in Ulm in 1997 [12] this indication was classified as IIb (not yet evaluatable). Nevertheless, several studies have been published, dealing with PET imaging in primary tumor detection with FDG or ^{11}C-methionine [4, 5, 8, 14, 17, 23]. The reason why these studies have been carried out is probably the relatively clear design of such studies and the expected high specificity and sensitivity, since these studies were performed in patients with large tumors and advanced stages in the majority of the cases because of the usually late clinical manifestation of ovarian cancer. The typical pattern is a distinct increase of FDG uptake in solid/viable parts of the tumor with additional "cold" regions in cystic/necrotic parts. Sensitivity ranged between 50% and 90% in these studies; the specificity was between 60% and 80%. One study, performed by Hübner et al. [8], which also included dynamic acquisitions, was done in 51 patients and gave a positive predictive value of 86% and a negative predictive value of 76%. The detection of borderline tumors is more difficult since FDG uptake correlates with the grade of malignancy [17, 23]. Inflammatory processes can show up with an increased FDG uptake as well; therefore, the value of FDG-PET in the differential diagnosis between malignant and inflammatory alterations of the ovary is limited [17]. Tubo-ovarian abscesses, corpus luteum cysts and particularly Schwannomas can show increased FDG uptake. In addition, the intestinal activity can cause false-positive results and can especially be misinterpreted as peritoneal carcinosis. Relatively longitudinal areas of FDG uptake, particularly following the colon, are "unspecific" in most cases, whereas isolated, circumscribed lesions should be read as tumor. A direct comparison with MRI improves the diagnostic accuracy significantly with respect to areas of unspecific tracer uptake. Fenchel et al. [5] studied a group of 85 asymptomatic patients with ultrasound suspicious adnexal masses. They found a sensitivity of only 50% and a specificity of 78% in this group, in which 8 patients suffered from malignancy. The reason for the relatively low sensitivity is probably the high rate of borderline tumors and early stages of malignancies in this group because symptomatic cases were excluded. Since in stage 1 early tumor detection can particularly result in a significant improvement of the outcome, the clinical impact of PET should be evaluated in such patient groups with a high rate of benign masses (>90%) or very small malignancies. In general, the clinical significance of primary tumor detection will remain questionable in the future, even if high sensitivity and specificity values will be proven in large patient groups because in all cases of suspected ovarian cancer a laparatomy will be performed even if a completely negative PET result is obtained. In asymptomatic patients with suspicious adnexal masses, which is the most common clinical setting in which a malignant primary ovarian tumor has to be excluded, FDG-PET can not be recommended as a routine procedure.

29.7.2 Spreading

Prior to a – possibly curative – operation a detailed surgical planning is necessary to detect all sites of malignant tissue with high sensitivity and specificity. FDG-PET can give important clinical information in addition to ultrasound, computed tomography and magnetic resonance imaging since small lymph node metastases (5–10 mm diameter) can be evaluated with a higher specificity than using morphological procedures and a peritoneal carcinosis can be detected. During lymph node evaluation, special attention has to be paid to the pelvine, inguinal, paraaortal and (later) diaphragma-adjacent lymph node spreading. The detection of a peritoneal carcinosis is known to be very difficult using computed tomography. In FDG-PET studies, peritoneal carcinosis appears as large areas of increased tracer uptake (Fig. 29.1), often associated with additional circumscribed foci in the pelvis, abdomen and on the liver surface. Zimny et al. [23] reported a sensitivity of 72% and a specificity of 93%. In their study, the sensitivity regarding lymph node staging was only 50%, probably because of limitations in spatial resolution in patients with very small lymph nodes. Nevertheless, the specificity for lymph node evaluation was 95% in this study [23]. In spite of high expectations regarding immunoscintigraphy, this technique has not been sufficiently convincing in the first few years of clinical use. Extremely varying sensitivity and specificity values were reported [6, 13]. Immunoscintigraphy is not included in clinical programs for primary tumor diagnostic or staging and will not be competitive to FDG-PET imaging in the future.

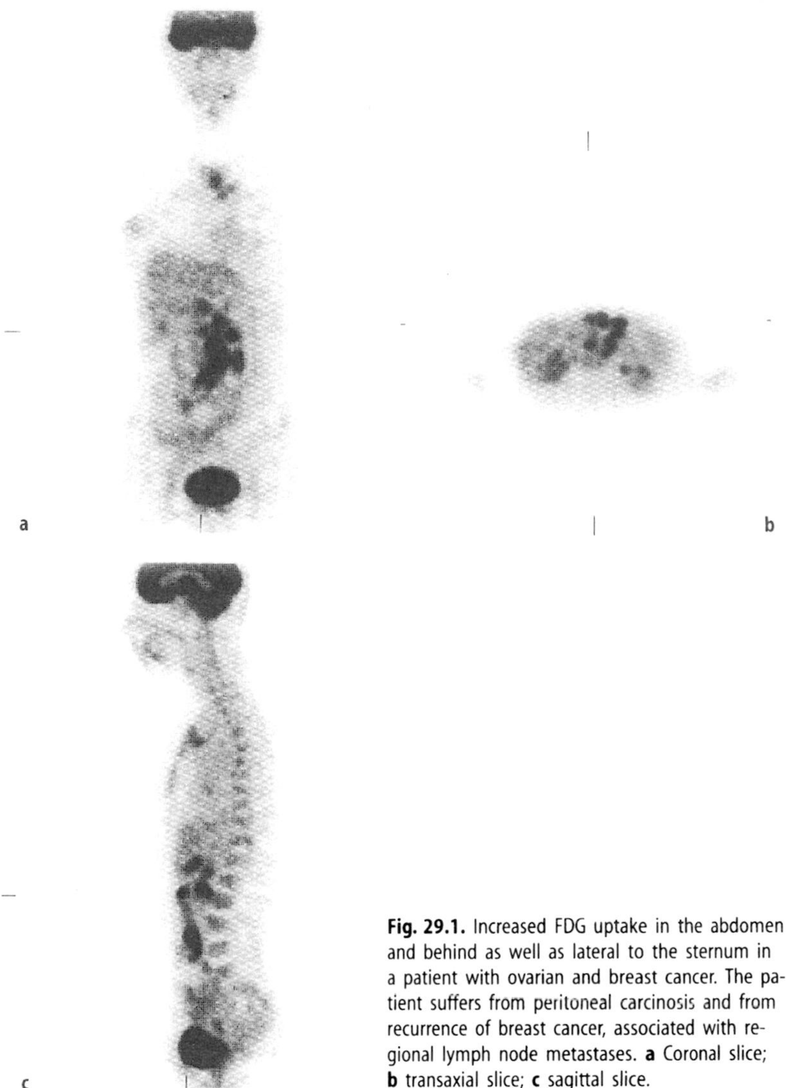

Fig. 29.1. Increased FDG uptake in the abdomen and behind as well as lateral to the sternum in a patient with ovarian and breast cancer. The patient suffers from peritoneal carcinosis and from recurrence of breast cancer, associated with regional lymph node metastases. **a** Coronal slice; **b** transaxial slice; **c** sagittal slice.

29.7.3 Recurrence/restaging

Because of the poor prognosis of patients suffering from recurrence, therapeutic consequences of extended diagnostic procedures are limited. Therefore, the relevance of imaging techniques (including FDG-PET) for tumor localization is questionable in cases with proven recurrence with respect to a significant improvement of survival rates. Nevertheless, uncertainty regarding recurrence is a common problem during follow-up, particularly because of the known limitations of morphologic techniques – due to scars. Especially in cases with tumor marker values that were not increased preoperatively, the tumor marker levels during follow-up are of limited use and therefore sensitive and specific methods are required. Recurrence can occur at all sites where the primary tumor spread initially and is frequently observed in the Douglas pouch and near the bladder. Studies on larger patient groups dealing with the use of PET imaging in ovarian cancer recurrence have not yet been published. Karlan et al. [11] observed microscopic tumor tissue in 5 out of 6 patients in spite of negative FDG-PET results. In contrast, all macroscopic tumor sites in patients highly suspicious for recurrence showed up with an increased FDG uptake. Holdeman et al. [7] reported a lower sensitivity of FDG-PET in small foci, particularly in cases without significant tumor marker increase. Baum et al. [2] found a superior sensitivity of FDG-PET comparing this method with computed tomography and immunoscintigraphy in a well-defined patient group.

29.7.4 Therapy control

One major application of PET imaging (particularly with FDG) in ovarian cancer is a short-term control of therapeutic interventions (chemotherapy in most cases), although larger studies have not yet been published. In contrast, computed tomography, magnetic resonance imaging and ultrasound have the disadvantage that changes of viability are initially not detectable since these are not associated with a change of tumor size during the first weeks. Therefore, the classification of therapy control in ovarian cancer as IIb in the German consensus conference [12] (evaluation not yet possible) is justified.

29.8 Outlook

Within the next few years a more exact evaluation of FDG-PET in staging and therapy control of ovarian cancer in larger patient groups is necessary to confirm current opinions based on only a few hard data. Well-defined aims would improve the significance of prospective studies dealing with the clinical use of FDG-PET during follow-up and restaging of patients with proven recurrence. Evaluation of new therapeutic strategies in ovarian cancer (particularly gene therapy) will play a major role in PET imaging, with respect to new chemotherapeutic agents as well as new tracers [1, 9]. In contrast to ultrasound, CT, and MRI, PET imaging allows a rapid evaluation of the success of new therapeutic strategies, which is particularly important, if these are associated with severe side effects. FDG-PET might be included into screening programs in high-risk women (e.g., BRCA1/BRCA2-positive women) for early detection of primary tumors. During a whole-body FDG-PET acquisition, the ovaries and breasts can be screened in one study. In addition, the development of new tracers can be expected within the next few years. With respect to ovarian cancer, tumor-seeking agents (particularly labeled with ^{11}C [14, 15]), hypoxia markers and labeled chemotherapeutics will probably play a major role in research projects.

29.9 Practical guide for performing and reading of FDG-PET in suspected or proven ovarian cancer

In general, acquisition and interpretation should follow the "procedure guideline for tumor imaging using fluorine-18-FDG", published by Schelbert et al. [19]:

- patient preparation:
  fasted for > 6 h, blood glucose < 100 mg/dl; hydration, forced diuresis (500 ml, 0.3 mg furosemide/kg body weight); bladder catheterization
- data acquisition:
  whole-body acquisition (if possible); emission scan after 45 min p.i.
- attenuation correction:
  using transmission scan, if possible; this is particularly important during control studies with respect to quantification
- reconstruction:
  filtered back projection; if available, using iterative algorithms, especially important for the evaluation of regions near the bladder
- interpretation:
  if possible, image fusion with CT or MRI
  visual: comparison of the maximum of FDG uptake with the liver; if FDG uptake ≥ liver: glucose utilization increased, typical for malignancy, although inflammation cannot be completely excluded;
  quantitative: SUV cut-off: 5.0 (note: as with visual interpretation no clear differentiation between tumors (particularly borderline tumors) and inflammation is possible using quantitative evaluation).

References

[1] Bauknecht T (1998) Neue therapeutische Ansätze inklusive Gentherapie. Onkologe 4:1159–1167

[2] Baum RP, Niesen A, Schröder O, Adams S, Hertel A, Osterloh M, Hör G (1998) A prospective evaluation of whole-body FDG-PET, CT scan, and immunoscintigraphy in the detection of ovarian carcinoma recurrence. Eur J Nucl Med 25:942 (abstr.)

[3] Burke W, Daly M, Garber J, Botkin J, Kahn MJE, Lynch P, McTiernan A, Offit K, Perlman J, Petersen G, Thomson E, Varricchio C (1997) Recommendations for follow-up care of individuals with an inherited predisposition to cancer. JAMA 277:997–1003

[4] Casey MJ, Gupta NC, Muths CK (1994) Experience with positron emission tomography (PET) scans in patients with ovarian cancer. Gynecol Oncol 53:331–338

[5] Fenchel S, Kotzerke J, Stöhr I, Grab D, Nüssle K, Rieber A, Kreienberg R, Brambs HJ, Reske SN (1999) Preoperative assessment of asymptomatic adnexal masses by positron emission tomography and F-18-fluorodeoxyglucose. Nuklearmedizin 38:101–107

[6] Granowska M, Mather SJ, Britton KE (1991) Diagnostic evaluation of 111In and 99mTc radiolabeled monoclonal antibodies in ovarian and colorectal cancer: correlations with surgery. Nucl Med Biol 18:413–424
[7] Holdeman KP, McIntosh DG, Smith ML, Matamoros A, Sunderland J, Harrison KA, Dalrymple GV (1994) PET imaging of ovarian cancer prior to second look laparatomy. J Nucl Med 35:117P (abstr)
[8] Hübner KF, McDonald TW, Niethammer JG, Smith GT, Gould HR, Buonocore E (1993) Assessment of primary and metastatic ovarian cancer by positron emission tomography (PET using 2-[18F]deoxyglucose (2-[18F]FDG). Gynecol Oncol 51:197–204
[9] Juweid M, Sharkey RM, Alavi A, Swayne LC, Herskovic T, Hanley D, Rubin AD, Pereira M, Goldenberg DM (1997) Regression of advanced refractory ovarian cancer treated with iodine-131-labeled anti-CEA monoclonal antibody. J Nucl Med 38:257–260
[10] Karlan BY (1995) Screening for ovarian cancer: what are the optimal surrogate endpoints for clinical trials? J Cell Biochem Suppl 23:227–232
[11] Karlan BY, Hawkins R, Hoh C, Lee M, Tse N, Cane P, Glaspy J (1993) Whole-body positron emission tomography with 2-[18F]-fluoro-2-deoxy-D-glucose can detect recurrent ovarian carcinoma. Gynecol Oncol 51:175–181
[12] Konsensus - Onko-PET (1997) Ergebnisse der 2. interdisziplinären Konsensuskonferenz im Ulm, 12.9.97; veröffentlicht in Nuklearmedizin 36:45–46
[13] Krag DN (1993) Clinical utility of immunoscintigraphy in managing ovarian cancer. J Nucl Med 34:545–548
[14] Lapela M, Leskinen-Kallio S, Varpula M, Grenman S, Salmi T, Alanen K, Nagren K, Lehikoinen P, Ruotsalainen U, Teras M, Joensuu H (1995) Metabolic imaging of ovarian tumors with carbon-11-methionine: a PET study. J Nucl Med 36:2196–2200
[15] Liu RS, Yuan CC, Chang CP, Chou KL, Chang CW, Ng HT, Yeh SH (1998) Positron emission tomography (PET) with [C-11] acetate (ACE) in detecting malignant gynecologic tumors. Eur J Nucl Med 25:963 (abstr)
[16] Meerpohl HG, du Bois A (1998) Primäre Chemotherapie. Onkologe 4:1131–1139
[17] Römer W, Avril N, Dode J, Ziegler S, Kuhn W, Herz M, Janicke F, Schwaiger M (1997) Metabolische Charakterisierung von Ovarialtumoren mit der Positronen-Emissions-Tomographie und F-18-Fluorodeoxyglukose. Fortschr Geb Röntgenstr Neuen Bildgeb Verfahr 166:62–68
[18] Runnebaum IB, Mollenkopf A, Kreienberg R, Meerpohl HG (1998) Epidemiologische und molekulargenetische Risikofaktoren beim Ovarialkarzinom. Onkologe 4:1096–1100
[19] Schelbert HR, Hoh CK, Royal HD, Brown M, Dahlbom MN, Dehdashti F, Wahl RL (1998) Procedure guideline for tumor imaging using fluorine-18-FDG. J Nucl Med 39:1302–1305
[20] UICC: TNM-Klassifikation maligner Tumoren, 4. Aufl., 2. Revision 1992. Springer-Verlag, Berlin Heidelberg, 1993
[21] Wagner G, Hermanek P (1995) Organspezifische Tumordokumentation, Prinzipien und Verschlüsselungsanweisungen für Klinik und Praxis. Springer-Verlag, Berlin Heidelberg
[22] World Health Organization: International histological classification of tumors, histological typing of ovarian tumors. Genf 1973
[23] Zimny M, Schröder W, Wolters S, Cremerius U, Rath W, Büll U (1997) 18F-Fluorodeoxyglukose PET beim Ovarialkarzinom: Methodik und erste Ergebnisse. Nuklearmedizin 36:228–233

30 Pitfalls in the interpretation of PET studies

L. G. Strauss

30.1 Introduction

Positron emission tomography (PET) has found widespread use in several countries due to the availability of new whole-body tomographs. Particularly in oncology, PET is being used for tumor diagnosis. The currently available PET systems provide an axial field-of-view exceeding 15 cm, which is helpful for partial or whole-body PET studies using multiple bed positions. Besides whole-body imaging, cross-sectional imaging is used for both qualitative and quantitative analysis of PET studies. Dependent on the PET system used, up to 63 slices for one frame (covering the axial field-of-view) are reconstructed.

The rapid technical progress in the development of PET systems as well as in the availability of suitable radiopharmaceuticals are prerequisites for the routine use of PET. The most commonly used PET radiopharmaceutical is [^{18}F]fluoro-deoxyglucose (FDG), due to the availability of standard synthesis procedures. The half-life of approximately two hours enables the transport of FDG from the production site to external PET centers. FDG had been used for tumor diagnosis for more than 10 years and was found to be useful, e.g., for the detection of recurrent tumors [30, 32]. The radiopharmaceutical FDG is transported like glucose and phosphorylated, but then more than 90% is trapped in the phosphorylated form. Due to the slow dephosphorylation of the tracer, in most of the studies a time window of 30–120 min following tracer injection can be used to acquire PET data. Several experimental studies have shown that the transport of FDG parallels the transport of glucose. An increase in the expression of the glucose transporter GLUT1 is associated with an increased FDG accumulation in most of the tumors [26]. The phosphorylation via hexokinase is an important step for the trapping of the radiopharmaceutical. It is still an open question if increased expression of hexokinase is associated with increased FDG accumulation. We noted increased enzyme activity in only two of 40 patients in our studies of squamous cell carcinoma of the head and neck [26].

It must be considered that FDG does not represent only a pure tumor-specific radiopharmaceutical but it is general opinion that FDG reflects the viability of structures and is associated with the number of living cells [16]. While malignant processes, in particular before therapeutic interventions, demonstrate a clear metabolic increase and thus a trapping of FDG, the FDG accumulation in most normal structures is clearly lower and shows a smaller dispersion. Problems with the evaluation of PET examinations can have very different causes. The most important factors include

- *image reconstruction artifacts*
- *visual evaluation*
- *falsely positive/negative results due to the tracer characteristics.*

30.2 Image reconstruction

Usually the reconstruction of PET images takes place via the system software, which generally provides filtered backprojection as the method of choice. This reconstruction procedure has the advantage of very fast image calculation. However, star-shaped artifacts are frequently observed, for example, due to high, local activity in the renal system or in the bladder (Fig. 30.1). A substantially better image quality is achieved using iterative im-

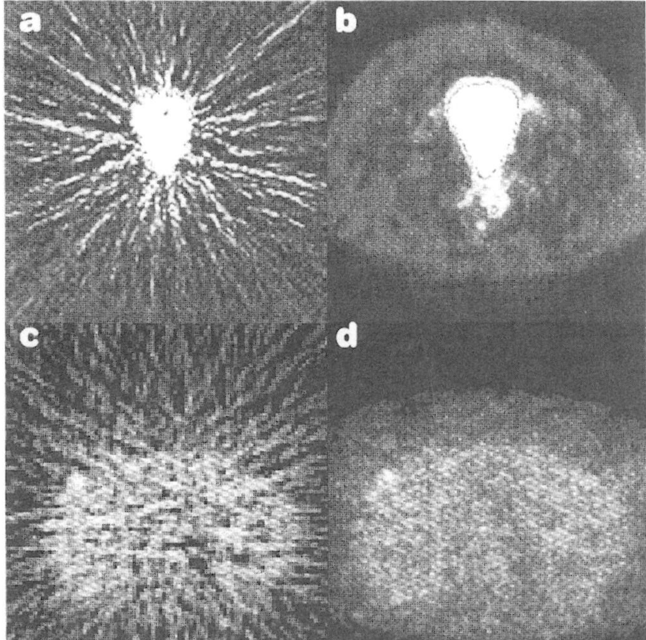

Fig. 30.1. Comparison of filtered backprojection (**a, c**) and iterative image reconstruction (**b, d**). High tracer concentrations in the bladder due to excreted FDG raise star-shaped artifacts with the conventional image reconstruction and limit the diagnostic evaluation (**a**). In contrast, the iterative reconstruction algorithm provides a substantially better image quality and permits the detection of a small recurrent tumor dorsal of the bladder (**b**). A small liver metastasis is better delineated with the use of the iterative reconstruction program (**c**, filtered backprojection; **d**, iterative reconstruction).

age reconstruction. This method produces images in several intermediate steps, which are corrected and optimized by comparison with the measured projections. The relatively high computational effort required in the past is reduced by suitable quasi-parallel reconstruction procedures taking only a few seconds per image [19].

Corrections are basically important to achieve an exact representation of the regional activity distribution of a radiopharmaceutical. In contrast to conventional single photon scintigraphy, the scatter fraction is smaller due to the high energy of 511 keV and amounts to only about 10–15% when 2D acquisition is used. Even of greater importance is the correction of the attenuation, which substantially reduces the usable signal even at 511 keV. During PET investigations a measurement of the transmission usually takes place via one or several external sources prior to the emission acquisition. Transmission correction files are then calculated from the transmission data, which serve for the correction of the emission data. Again, the use of the iterative reconstruction procedure for the calculation of the μ-map, the correction matrix for the emission measurements, is of major importance for the image quality of the emission images.

30.3 Visual evaluation

In the context of tumor staging, PET investigations are preferentially made using the whole-body mode, because a large field of view can be acquired and evaluated. This is particularly important regarding N- and M-staging. While the whole-body technique was originally executed in the pure emission mode without transmission correction, now the use of transmission-corrected scans is increasingly discussed.

The visual evaluation provides information about the relative accumulation of the radiopharmaceutical. Nonspecific accumulations, e.g., from repair processes, can contribute to false-positive results. Apart from surgically induced effects on tracer uptake, repair processes can also be observed after chemotherapy or radiotherapy and may contribute to the FDG accumulation (Fig. 30.2). Quantitative analysis is helpful for the differentiation of lesions. The calculation of dimensionless distribution values, for which we introduced the designation "standardized uptake value, SUV", can help to compare quantitative data from follow-up PET studies as well as for the comparison of PET results from different patients [31, 32]:

SUV = tracer concentration in the target area (Bq/ml)/(injected dose (Bq)/distribution volume (ml))

Usually the distribution volume is approximated by body weight. The resulting SUVs are distribution values, which represent a measure for the more or less accumulation of a pharmacon in relation to a uniform distribution (equivalent to SUV = 1.0). The example in Fig. 30.2 shows visually an in-

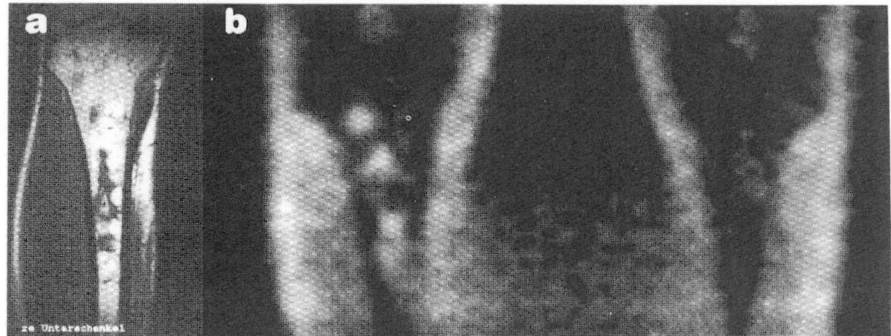

Fig. 30.2. MRI (**a**) and PET with FDG (**b**) of a young patient following chemotherapy due to a non-Hodgkin's lymphoma of the bone marrow. The lesions visible in the MRI correlate with circumscribed lesions in PET, associated with a higher FDG accumulation visually in comparison to the normal bone marrow. However, the quantitative evaluation demonstrated 0.8 SUV for the accumulating lesions in the bone marrow (normal opposite side: 0.5 SUV). Therefore, repair processes are likely to be the reason. The PET diagnosis of tissue repair was confirmed by histology.

creased accumulation of the tracer; however, the low, quantitative value (0.8 SUV) and the comparable accumulation on the healthy opposite side (0.5 SUV) does not support the diagnosis of a malignant process. Therefore, cellular repair after chemotherapy is the most likely reason for the FDG accumulation. This result was confirmed in the clinical follow-up by histology, based on biopsy.

Local tracer accumulations, which are visually as well as quantitatively in the pathological range, usually represent no major problem if they can be clearly assigned to normal, morphologic structures. Due to the elimination of FDG via the kidneys, focal activities in the renal system are frequently noted. More difficult may be the delineation of masses near the ureter, e.g., when a retroperitoneal space occupying lesion and/or lymph nodes are to be detected. In this situation, dynamic data acquisition can be favorable, since the change of the tracer accumulation in relation to the acquisition time is analyzed and can be diagnostically helpful.

30.4 Tracer characteristics

FDG represents a sensitive marker for the metabolism; however, due to the relative low specificity, tracer accumulation may be caused not only by tumors but also by benign processes, which may exhibit increased glucose transport and/or an increased metabolic rate for glucose. Substantial FDG uptake in inflammatory processes occurs in granulocytes [21, 22]. If PET with FDG is used in patients with questionable inflammatory processes, it can contribute to the diagnosis and/or search of a cause [18, 25, 29, 36]. Guhlmann et al. used PET with FDG in 31 patients with supposed osteomyelitis [14]. Regarding the recognition of osteomyelitis lesions, a high accuracy of 97% (sensitivity 100%, specificity 92%) resulted. Apart from chronically inflammatory changes, acute inflammatory processes also usually have an increased FDG accumulation, which may mimic malignant lesions [1, 35]. Thus regarding the differential diagnosis, the specificity of the method is limited. Abdel Nabi et al. examined patients with questionable colorectal tumors and found a sensitivity of 100% and a specificity of 43% for PET with FDG [1]. Fischbein et al. reported a sensitivity of 100% and specificity of 64% in 44 patients with head and neck tumors and/or recurrent lesions [10]. The reduced specificity was due to inflammatory changes [10]. Similar results are also expected for other kinds of tumors. In general, differential-diagnostic considerations should include the discussion of false-positive results due to questionable inflammatory processes.

The results show that among other aspects appropriate clinical information is also important, in order to avoid an incorrect classification. In individual cases, multi-tracer investigations can improve the differential diagnosis. According to our own experiences, [^{11}C]aminoisobutyric acid (AIB), a transportation marker for the alanine-like amino acid transport, does not show an accumulation in inflammatory processes contrary to malignant lesions [33]. This is particularly helpful for the differentiation of recurrent tumor vs. postoperative changes (Fig. 30.3). Our recent results show that AIB can provide additional information, if non-malignant processes are possible [34]. One limitation is the lower AIB accumulation as compared to FDG, because AIB is a pure transport marker, which is not trapped.

Low FDG accumulations are frequently observed following chemotherapy [7]. Besides AIB, the use of tracers for specific metabolic pathways in tumors may be considered in order to avoid false-positive results with FDG. An accumulation of tyrosine and dihydroxyphenylalanine (DOPA) is possible in

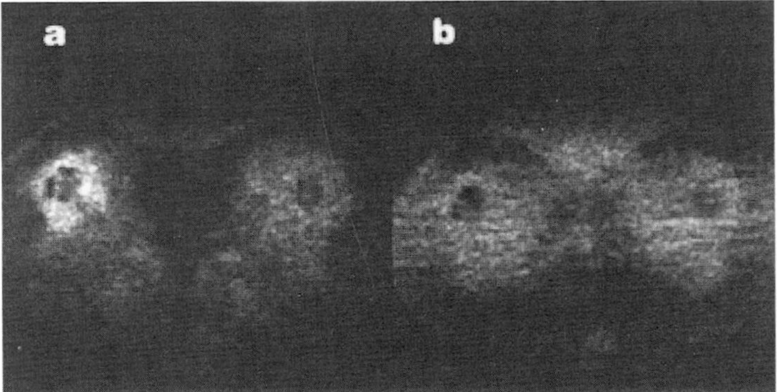

Fig. 30.3. PET with FDG (**a**) and AIB (**b**) in a patient with questionable recurrent soft tissue sarcoma and a fibula transplant. Significant increase of the FDG uptake offers differential-diagnostic difficulties. However, the missing AIB accumulation does not confirm the diagnosis of a recurrent tumor. The PET result was confirmed by clinical follow-up. The FDG accumulation is assigned to the normal healing process.

malignant melanoma, because both substances are part of the melanine synthesis pathway. Initial results with [^{18}F]DOPA resulted in a sensitivity of 77% for the detection of metastatic lesions in malignant melanoma [6]. Besides malignant melanomas, DOPA demonstrated a retention in patients with carcinoid when the FDG scan was negative (Fig. 30.4). DOPA may be considered in order to gain additional specific, diagnostic information.

A nonspecific increase in metabolism is usually observed following radiotherapy. PET studies in colorectal tumors prior to and after radiotherapy generally resulted in a decreasing FDG accumulation in the tumor area. However, a differentiation of residual tumor tissue and therapy-induced tissue alterations is usually not possible only on the basis of FDG uptake measurements [8, 15, 17]. This diagnostic problem is usually of minor importance immediately after radiotherapy, because in most patients the therapy will not be changed during this treatment interval. However, it must be emphasized that according to our experiences on follow-up studies in patients with colorectal carcinomas, an increase of the nonspecific metabolic uptake may be observed even after more than six months following radiotherapy. This applies in particular to combined photon/neutron therapy. Comparable results are also well known from the literature for other tumors. Fischman et al. report a case of increased FDG uptake in a patient 16 months after proton therapy of a meningeoma [11]. After surgical intervention the histological investigation resulted in only reactive changes and necroses. Ricci et al. found a sensitivity of 86% and specificity of 22% for PET with FDG based on the

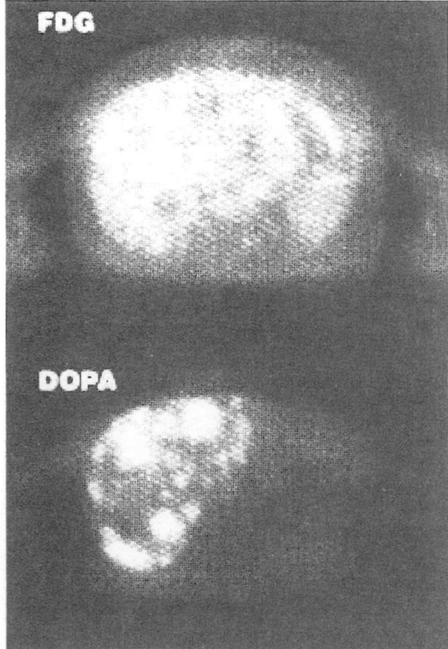

Fig. 30.4. FDG and [^{18}F]DOPA PET study in a patient with metastastic carcinoid. The metastases are hypometabolic in the FDG scan, while an increased tracer accumulation was observed following [^{18}F]DOPA injection.

evaluation of 84 patients with questionable recurrent brain tumors [27]. The low specificity of FDG is mainly due to the poor differentiation of radiation necrosis and recurrent tumor. Therefore, it appears that PET with FDG is not very helpful for therapeutic decisions in this situation and other tracers should be investigated. Contrary to brain tumors, better results are reported for the diagnosis of recurrent larynx carcinomas [13]. Greven et al. noted a sensitivity of 80% and specificity of 81%, while computed tomography had a sensitivity of only 58% and specificity of 100% [13].

PET with FDG is generally accepted as a sensitive method for the recognition of recurrent tumors after surgical interventions. Initial examinations with PET and FDG were made in patients with colorectal recurrencies and demonstrated high sensitivity [30]. The selection of patients was based on previous CT examinations, which showed a suspicious lesion with a diameter exceeding 1.5 cm [30]. Apart from the lesion size, which represents a substantial selection criterion for PET in principle, inflammatory processes, fis-

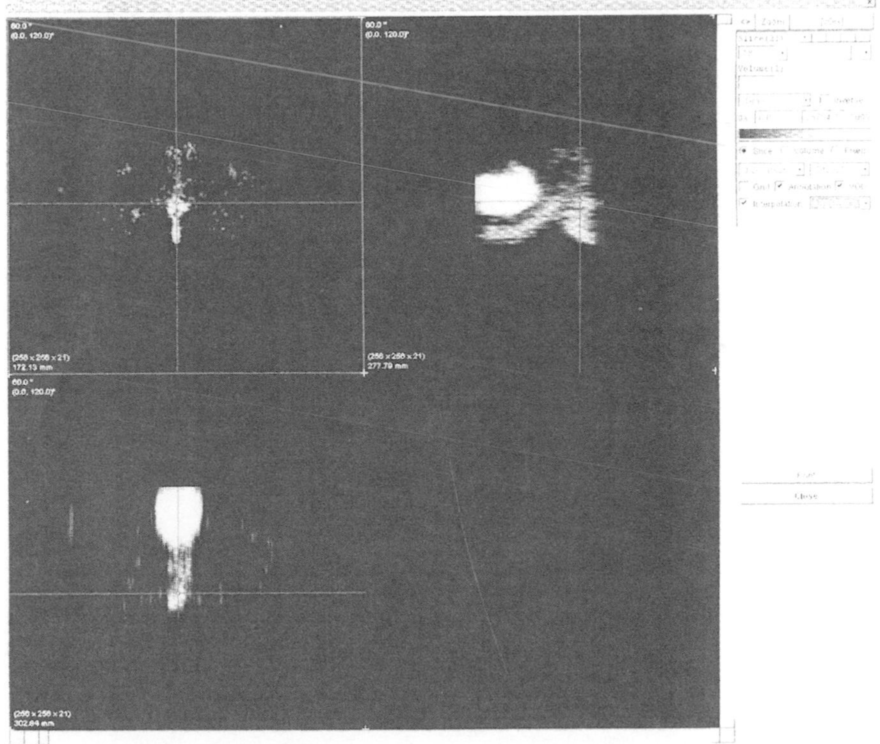

Fig. 30.5. Parametric image of the FDG distribution (transverse, sagittal, coronal) in a patient with a recurrent anal carcinoma and an abscess with fistula. Increased FDG uptake is observed in a structure dorsal to the bladder in the sagittal slice (on the top right), which corresponds according to morphology and clinical data to the fistula. The recurrent tumor (histologically confirmed) is delineated caudal to it with similar FDG uptake.

tulas, etc. should clinically be excluded prior to PET. The situation is difficult, if both inflammatory procedures and tumor tissue are present (Fig. 30.5). Clear differentiation is nearly impossible in these cases.

Apart from purely benign processes, such as inflammation, benign tumors may also offer differential-diagnostic problems. Thus, several space-demanding processes of the skeleton accumulated FDG and may obscure the detection of malignant lesions. Osteochondromas usually show a peripheral, low FDG accumulation and are rather differentiable in combination with a conventional radiographic image and/or CT. In contrast, eosinophilic granulomas, as are frequently observed in the context of histiozytosis X, show a clear FDG uptake, originating from the bone marrow and increasing at the periphery of the lesion (Fig. 30.6). The diagnostic situation often remains unclear and demands biopsy, because especially in young people the radiologic differential diagnosis includes an Ewing sarcoma due to the periosteal reactions [28].

Several malignant tumors frequently exhibit a low FDG metabolism, which may lead to false-negative results. Thus, well-differentiated, hepatocellular carcinomas show a FDG metabolism equivalent to the normal liver parenchyma and are, therefore, often difficult to delineate [5]. The use of other tracers may be helpful, e.g., [^{18}F]galactose, although this tracer has been examined so far only in individual cases. Preliminary data demonstrate that well-differentiated primary liver tumors are visible even in the early phase about 5 min post injection of [^{18}F]galactose, while in the late phase the tumors are usually hypometabolic as compared to the normal liver parenchyma [12]. It

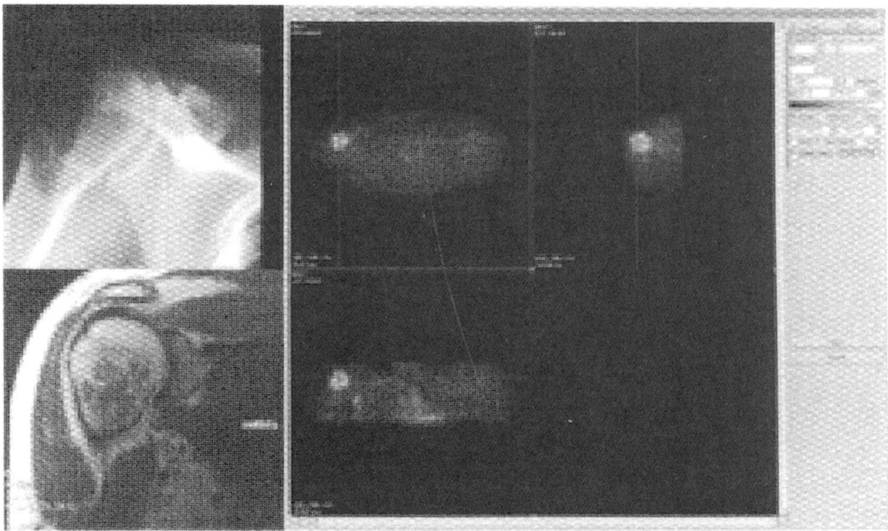

Fig. 30.6. Conventional X-ray (top left), MRI (bottom left) and PET with FDG (right) in a young patient with histologically proven, eosinophilic granuloma of the right humerus. The large, lytic lesion appearing in the X-ray clearly shows increased FDG uptake (3.1 SUV 60 min p.i.) in the dynamic series.

is assumed that the accumulation of galactose is associated with the degree of tumor differentiation.

An association of FDG uptake and tumor differentiation is also reported for other tumors. Thus, according to our experience soft tissue sarcomas in the G1 stage show low FDG accumulation. Nieweg et al. examined 18 patients with soft tissue sarcomas, whereby all tumors showed a positive FDG accumulation [24]. In this patient collective, a correlation between grading and the regional glucose metabolism (Patlak procedure) was found [24]. In a study of 41 patients with thyroid tumors Feine et al. reported a relation between FDG uptake and tumor differentiation [9]. Malignant, space-occupying lesions that possess still some aspects of the originating tissue seem to have a low FDG metabolism. Furthermore, hypernephromas and prostate carcinomas as well as highly differentiated teratomas can show low FDG accumulation and may lead to false-negative results. Therefore, the primary value of PET is not the T-staging but the improved N- and M-staging of these tumors [3]. Controversial data are reported for bladder carcinomas. Bachor et al. obtained a sensitivity of 85% for the detection of the primary tumor with PET and FDG [2]. In contrast, Kosuda reports a sensitivity of 66.7% despite the use of retrograde bladder flushing to minimize image artifacts [20]. Our own results refer to an improved diagnosis of the N-staging, while the primary tumors are frequently not detectable with FDG.

The increasing use of FDG in oncology for the diagnosis and staging of tumors also demonstrates the limitations, which are associated with the PET-FDG procedure. An optimization of the image quality by iterative reconstruction and attenuation correction is an important condition to avoid artifact-related false diagnoses. Suitable iterative reconstruction programs as well as evaluation programs on dedicated PC systems permit a flexible, quick and optimized evaluation [4, 19, 23]. Detailed knowledge of the biology of the different tumors as well as the FDG pharmacokinetics is important, in order to limit false-negative results and to detect possible false-positive findings in benign lesions.

References

[1] Abdel-Nabi H, Doerr RJ, Lamonica DM, Cronin VR, Galantowicz RJ, Carbone GM, Spaulding MB (1998) Staging of primary colorectal carcinomas with fluorine-18 fluorodeoxyglucose whole-body PET: correlation with histopathologic and CT findings. Radiology 206:755–760

[2] Bachor R, Kocher F, Gropengiesser F, Reske SN, Hautmann RE (1995) Positronenemissionstomographie. Einführung eines neuen Verfahrens in die Diagnostik urologischer Tumoren und erste klinische Ergebnisse. Urologe 34:138–142

[3] Bender H, Schomburg A, Albers P, Ruhlmann J, Biersack HJ (1997) Possible role of FDG-PET in the evaluation of urologic malignancies. Anticancer Res 17:1655–1660

[4] Burger C, Buck A (1997) Requirements and implementation of a flexible kinetic modeling tool. J Nucl Med 38:1818–1823

[5] Dimitrakopoulou-Strauss A, Gutzler F, Strauss LG, Irngartinger G, Oberdorfer F, Doll J, Stremmel W, van Kaick G (1996) PET-Studien mit C-11-Äthanol bei der intratumoralen Therapie von hepatozellulären Karzinomen. Radiologe 36:744–749

[6] Dimitrakopoulou-Strauss A, Schadendorf D, Naeher H, Mantaka P, Oberdorfer F, Strauss LG (1998) FDG and F-18-dihydroxyphenylalanine in patients with metastatic melanomas. Eur J Nucl Med 25:953 (abstr)

[7] Eil A, Dimitrakopoulou-Strauss A, Tilgen W, Oberdorfer F, Doll J, Strauss LG (1996) Functional imaging with positron emission tomography in patients with malignant melanoma. Onkologie 19:253–259

[8] Engenhart R, Kimmig B, Hover KH, Strauss LG, Lorenz WJ, Wannenmacher M (1990) Photon-neutron therapy for recurrent colorectal cancer – follow up and preliminary results. Strahlenther Onkol 166:95–98

[9] Feine U, Lietzenmayer R, Handke JP, Held J, Wohrle H, Mueller-Schauenburg W (1996) Fluorine-18-FDG and iodine-131-iodide uptake in thyroid cancer. J Nucl Med 37:1468–1472

[10] Fischbein NJ, Assar OS, Caputo GR, Kaplan MJ, Singer MI, Price DC, Dillon WP, Hawkins RA (1998) Clinical utility of positron emission tomography with ^{18}F-fluorodeoxyglucose in detecting residual/recurrent squamous cell carcinoma of the head and neck. Am J Neuroradiol 19:1189–1196

[11] Fischman AJ, Thornton AF, Frosch MP, Swearinger B, Gonzalez RG, Alpert NM (1997) FDG hypermetabolism associated with inflammatory necrotic changes following radiation of meningioma. J Nucl Med 38:1027–1029

[12] Fukuda H, Yamaguchi K, Matsuzawa T, Abe Y, Yamada K, Yoshioka S, Ito M, Fujiwara T, Tada M, Watanuki S, Ido T (1985) Imaging of hepatoma with 2-deoxy-2-[18F]fluoro-D-galactose by positron emission tomography. In: Matsuzawa T (ed) Proceedings of the International Symposium on Current and Future Aspects of Cancer Diagnosis with Positron Emission Tomography (PET 85). Tohoku University, Sendai, pp 24–27

[13] Greven KM, Williams DW 3rd, Keyes JW Jr, McGuirt WF, Watson NE Jr, Case LD (1997) Can positron emission tomography distinguish tumor recurrence from irradiation sequelae in patients treated for larynx cancer? Cancer J Sci Am 3:353–357

[14] Guhlmann A, Brecht-Kraus D, Suger G, Glatting G, Kotzerke J, Kinzl L, Reske SN (1998) Chronic osteomyelitis detection with FDG PET and correlation with histopathologic findings. Radiology 206:749–754

[15] Haberkorn U, Strauss LG, Dimitrakopoulou A, Engenhart R, Oberdorfer F, Ostertag H, Romahn J, van Kaick G (1991) PET studies of fluoro-deoxyglucose metabolism in patients with recurrent colorectal tumors receiving radiotherapy. J Nucl Med 32:1485–1490

[16] Higashi K, Clavo AC, Wahl RL (1993a) Does FDG uptake measure proliferative activity of human cancer cells? In vitro comparison with DNA flow cytometry and tritiated thymidine uptake. J Nucl Med 34:414–419

[17] Higashi K, Clavo AC, Wahl RL (1993b) In vitro assessment of 2-fluoro-2-deoxy-D-glucose, L-methionine and thymidine as agents to monitor the early response of a human adenocarcinoma cell line to radiotherapy. J Nucl Med 34:2278–2280

[18] Ichiya Y, Kuwabara Y, Sasaki M, Yoshida T, Akashi Y, Murayama S, Nakamura K, Fukumura T, Masuda K (1996) FDG-PET in infectious lesions: the detection and assessment of lesion activity. Ann Nucl Med 10:185–191

[19] Kontaxakis G, Strauss LG, van Kaick G, Sakas G, Pavlopoulos S (1998) Ordered-subsets acceleration of the ISRA, WLS and SAGE image reconstruction methods for emission tomography. Eur J Nucl Med 25:948 (abstr)

[20] Kosuda S, Kison PV, Greenough R, Grossman HB, Wahl RL (1997) Preliminary assessment of fluorine-18 fluorodeoxyglucose positron emission tomography in patients with bladder cancer. Eur J Nucl Med 24:615–620

[21] Kubota R, Yamada S, Kubota K, Ishiwata K, Tamahashi N, Ido T (1992) Intratumoral distribution of fluorine-18-fluorodeoxyglucose in vivo: high accumulation in macrophages and granulation tissues studied by microautoradiography. J Nucl Med 33:1972–1980

[22] Kubota R, Kubota K, Yamada S, Tada M, Ido T, Tamahashi N (1994) Microautoradiographic study for the differentiation of intratumoral macrophages, granulation tissues and cancer cells by the dynamics of fluorine-18-fluorodeoxyglucose uptake. J Nucl Med 35:104–112

[23] Mikolajczyk K, Szabatin M, Rudnicki P, Grodzki M, Burger C (1998) A JAVA environment for medical image data analysis: initial application for brain PET quantification. Med Inf 23:207–214
[24] Nieweg OE, Pruim J, van Ginkel RJ, Hoekstra HJ, Paans AM, Molenaar WM, Koops HS, Vaalburg W (1996) Fluorine-18-fluorodeoxyglucose PET imaging of soft-tissue sarcoma. J Nucl Med 37:257–261
[25] Palmer WE, Rosenthal DI, Schoenberg OI, Fischman AJ, Simon LS, Rubin RH, Polisson RP (1995) Quantification of inflammation in the wrist with gadolinium-enhanced MR imaging and PET with 2-[F-18]-fluoro-2-deoxy-D-glucose. Radiology 196:647–655
[26] Reißer C (1994) Maligne Tumoren im Kopf-Hals-Bereich: Bedeutung des Glukosestoffwechsels für die Diagnostik und das Therapiemanagement. Habilitation, Ruprecht-Karls-Universität Heidelberg
[27] Ricci PE, Karis JP, Heiserman JE, Fram EK, Bice AN, Drayer BP (1998) Differentiating recurrent tumor from radiation necrosis: time for re-evaluation of positron emission tomography? Am J Neuroradiol 19:407–413
[28] Rogers LF (1987) The osseous system: miscellaneous conditions. In: Juhl JH, Crummy AB (eds) Essentials of Radiologic Imaging. J.B. Lippincott Company, Philadelphia, pp 248–254
[29] Shreve PD (1998) Focal fluorine-18 fluorodeoxyglucose accumulation in inflammatory pancreatic disease. Eur J Nucl Med 25:259–264
[30] Strauss LG, Clorius JH, Schlag P, Lehner B, Kimmig B, Engenhart R, Marin-Grez M, Helus F, Oberdorfer F, Schmidlin P, van Kaick G (1989) Recurrence of colorectal tumors: PET evaluation. Radiology 170:329–332
[31] Strauss LG, Tilgen W, Haberkorn U, Knopp MV, Dimitrakopoulou A, Helus F, van Kaick G (1990) PET studies with F-18-deoxyglucose in metastatic melanoma. Radiology 177(P):199
[32] Strauss LG, Conti PS (1991) The applications of PET in clinical oncology. J Nucl Med 32:623–648
[33] Strauss LG (1996) Fluorine-18 deoxyglucose and false-positive results: a major problem in the diagnostics of oncological patients. Eur J Nucl Med 23:1409–1415
[34] Strauss LG (1997) Positron emission tomography: current role for diagnosis and therapy monitoring in oncology. Oncologist 2:381–388
[35] Tahara T, Ichiya Y, Kuwabara Y, Otsuka M, Miyake Y, Gunasekera R, Masuda K (1989) High [18F]-fluorodeoxyglucose uptake in abdominal abscesses: a PET study. J Comput Assist Tomogr 13:829–831
[36] Yamada S, Kubota K, Kubota R, Ido T, Tamahashi N (1995) High accumulation of fluorine-18-fluorodeoxyglucose in terpentine-induced inflammatory tissue. J Nucl Med 36:1301–1306

31 Monitoring of gene therapy with PET

U. Haberkorn

31.1 Suicide gene therapy of cancer

The transfer and expression of suicide genes into malignant tumor cells represents an attractive approach for human gene therapy. Suicide genes typically code for non-mammalian enzymes which convert nontoxic prodrugs into highly toxic metabolites. Therefore, systemic application of the nontoxic prodrug results in the production of the active drug at the tumor site. Although a broad range of suicide principles has been described, two suicide systems are applied in most studies: the cytosine deaminase (CD) and herpes simplex virus thymidine kinase (HSV-tk).

Cytosine deaminase, which is expressed in yeasts and bacteria, but not in mammalian organisms converts the antifungal agent 5-fluorocytosine (5-FC) to the highly toxic 5-fluorouracil (5-FU). In mammalian cells no anabolic pathway is known which leads to incorporation of 5-FC into the nucleic acid fraction. Therefore pharmacological effects are moderate and allow the application of high therapeutic doses [29, 43, 48]. 5-FU exerts its toxic effect by interfering with DNA and protein synthesis due to substitution of uracil by 5-FU in RNA and inhibition of thymidilate synthetase by 5-fluorodeoxyuridine monophosphate resulting in impaired DNA biosynthesis [39]. Nishiyama et al. [40] implanted CD-containing capsules into rat gliomas and subsequently treated the animals by systemic application of 5-FC. They observed significant amounts of 5-FU in the tumors as well as a decrease in tumor growth rate and systemic cytotoxicity. This approach for local chemotherapy was expanded by Wallace et al. [56] for the application in patients with disseminated tumor disease. They used monoclonal antibody (mAb)-enzyme conjugates to achieve a selective activation of 5-FC thereby obtaining a 7-fold higher level of 5-FU in the tumor after administration of mAb-CD and 5-FC compared to the systemic application of 5-FU.

Gene therapy with herpes simplex virus thymidine kinase as the suicide gene has been performed in a variety of tumor models in vitro as well as in vivo [3, 7, 8, 9, 12, 36, 41, 45]. In contrast to human thymidine kinase HSVtk is less specific and also phosphorylates nucleoside analogs such as acyclovir and ganciclovir (GCV) to their monophosphate metabolites [28]. These monophosphates are subsequently phosphorylated by cellular kinases to the di- and triphosphates. After integration of the triphosphate metabolites into DNA, chain termination occurs, followed by cell death. Encouraging results have been initially obtained in rat gliomas using a retroviral vector system for transfer and expression of the HSVtk gene [12, 45]. Recently, in vitro and in vivo studies have further demonstrated the potency of the CD suicide system. Tumor cells which had been infected with a retrovirus carrying the cytosine deaminase gene showed a strict correlation between 5-FC sensitivity and CD enzyme activity [26, 37, 38]. However, although not all of the tumor cells have to be infected to obtain a sufficient therapeutic response, repeated injections of the recombinant retroviruses may be necessary to reach a therapeutic level of enzyme activity in the tumor. Therefore a prerequisite for gene therapy using a suicide system is monitoring of suicide gene expression in the tumor for two reasons: to decide if repeated gene transductions of the tumor are necessary and to find a therapeutic window of maximum gene expression and consecutive prodrug administration [23]. Since 5-FC as well as GCV can be labeled with ^{18}F with sufficient in vivo stability [35, 54], positron emission tomography (PET) may be applied to assess the enzyme activity in vivo. Moreover, the measurement of therapeutic effects on the tumor metabolism may be useful for the prediction of therapeutic outcome at an early stage of the treatment. Positron emission tomography (PET) using tracers of tumor metabolism has been applied for the evaluation of treatment response in a variety of tumors and therapeutic regimens [4, 22, 25, 46], indicating that these tracers deliver useful parameters for the early assessment of therapeutic efficacy.

31.2 Monitoring of gene therapy by the assessment of metabolic effects

Monitoring of gene therapy using imaging procedures for the assessment of morphological changes has been performed with magnetic resonance imaging techniques in rats bearing C6 rat glioblastomas and also in patients with glioblastoma [27, 33, 51]. In these studies, either marked tumor necrosis after interleukin-2 gene transfer or regression after induction of HSVtk expression and GCV application were observed. Maron et al. [33] found an initial response to GCV treatment in 90% of the animals and a complete regression in two-thirds of the treated rats. Also, tumor recurrence could be observed. However, in these studies the therapeutic efficacy was evaluated using changes in tumor volume with examination intervals of two months between the end of the treatment and the first follow-up examination [27].

The measurement of metabolic changes after therapeutic intervention has proven to be superior to morphological procedures for the assessment of early therapy effects. In this respect, the FDG uptake has demonstrated to be a useful parameter for the evaluation of glucose metabolism [18, 25, 46, 55]. Since the HSVtk/GCV system induces DNA to chain termination, we also expect changes in thymidine incorporation into tumor cell DNA occur. This may be assessed using [^{11}C]thymidine which has been applied to determine DNA synthesis *in vivo* [10, 49].

We transfected a rat hepatoma cell line (Morris hepatoma MH3924A) with a retroviral vector containing the HSVtk gene [16, 17]. Thereafter, uptake measurements using thymidine (TdR), fluorodeoxyglucose (FDG), 3-O-methylglucose, AIB and methionine were performed in the presence of different concentrations of ganciclovir (GCV). In the HSVtk-expressing cell line an increased (up to 250%) thymidine uptake in the acid-soluble fraction and a decrease to 5.5% in the acid-insoluble fraction was found. The decrease of radioactivity in the nucleic acid fraction occurs early (4 h) after exposure of the cells to GCV and represents DNA chain termination induced by the HSVtk-ganciclovir system (Fig. 31.1). The phenomenon of a posttherapeutic increase of TdR or its metabolites in the acid-soluble fraction was observed in former studies after chemotherapy [22]. This effect may be explained by an increase in the activity of salvage pathway enzymes, e.g., of host thymidine kinase activity during repair of cell damage. Therefore, PET measurements with ^{11}C-TdR may be used to assess the effects of the HSVtk-GCV system on DNA synthesis if quantitation is based on a modeling approach.

During GCV treatment the uptake for FDG and 3-O-methylglucose increases up to 195% after 24 hours incubation with GCV. HPLC analysis revealed a decline of the FDG 6-phosphate fraction after 48 hours incubation with GCV. Consequently, a normalization of FDG uptake was observed after this incubation period (Fig. 31.2), whereas the 3-O-methylglucose uptake was still increased. Experiments performed with different amounts of HSVtk-expressing cells and control cells showed that these effects are dependent on the percent-

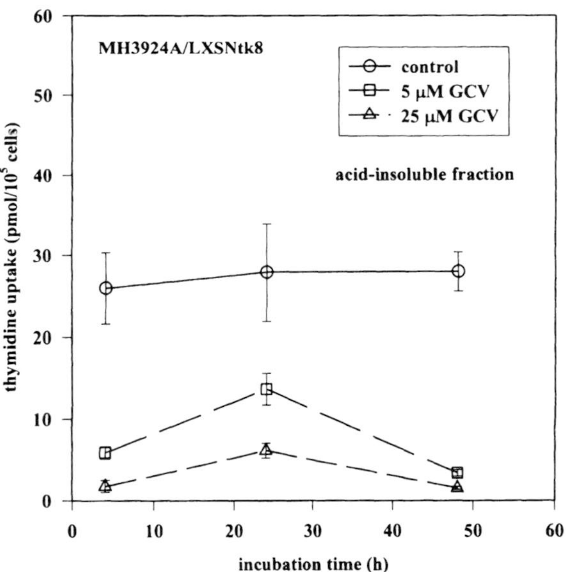

Fig. 31.1. Thymidine incorporation in HSVtk-expressing Morris hepatoma cells: uptake of [^{3}H]TdR in the acid-insoluble fraction in cells with or without treatment with ganciclovir (GCV).

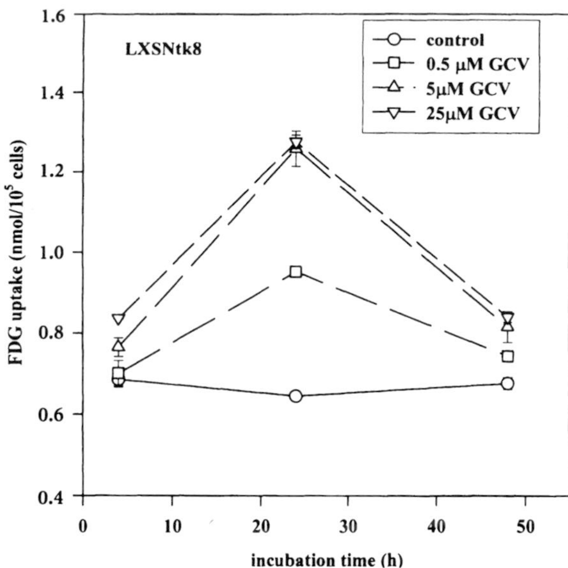

Fig. 31.2. FDG uptake (nmol/10^5 cells) in HSVtk-expressing cells after different incubation periods with 0.5, 5 and 25 μM ganciclovir (GCV).

age of HSVtk-expressing cells [17]. The AIB uptake decreased to 47%, while the methionine uptake in the acid-insoluble fraction decreased to 17%.

In clinical and experimental studies an increase of FDG uptake early after treatment of malignant tumors has been described [18, 21, 24, 46]. Cell culture experiments with rat adenocarcinoma cells under chemotherapy revealed that this effect is predominantly caused by an enhanced glucose transport [21]. As an underlying mechanism, the redistribution of the glucose transport protein from intracellular pools to the plasma membrane may be considered and is observed in cell culture studies as a general reaction to cellular stress [11, 42, 57, 59]. Since prodrug activation by the HSVtk leads to DNA chain termination and cell damage, the same reactions may also occur in tumor cells under gene therapy with this suicide system. Translocation of glucose transport proteins to the plasma membrane as a first reaction to cellular stress may cause enhancement of glucose transport and represents a short-term regulatory mechanism which acts independent of protein synthesis. However, an uncoupling of transport and phosphorylation was observed after 48 hour incubation. The amino acid uptake experiments are evidence of an inhibition of protein synthesis as well as of the neutral amino acid transport.

The same HSVtk-expressing Morris hepatoma cells were transplanted into ACI rats and dynamic PET measurements of [^{18}F]FDG uptake were performed in animals two days (n=7) and four days (n=5) after the onset of therapy with 100 mg GCV/kg body weight as well as after administration of sodium chloride (n=8). The arterial FDG plasma concentration was measured dynamically in an extracorporeal loop and the rate constants for FDG transport (k_1, k_2) and FDG phosphorylation (k_3) were calculated using a three-compartment model modified for heterogeneous tissues. Furthermore,

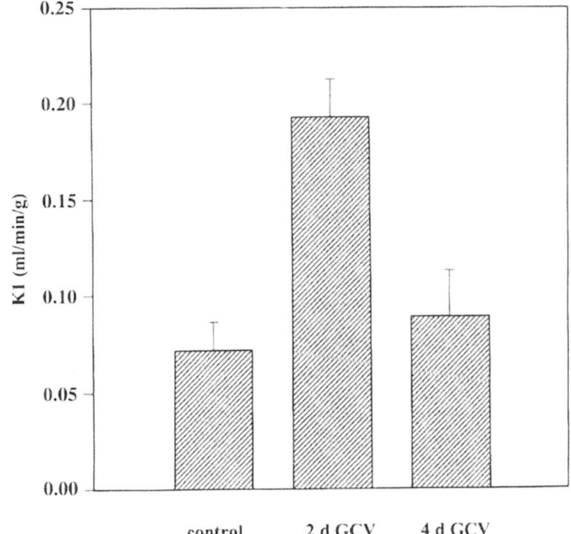

Fig. 31.3. FDG transport in untreated tumors (n=8) and in tumors after 2 days (n=7) or 4 days (n=5) treatment with 100 mg GCV/kg body weight.

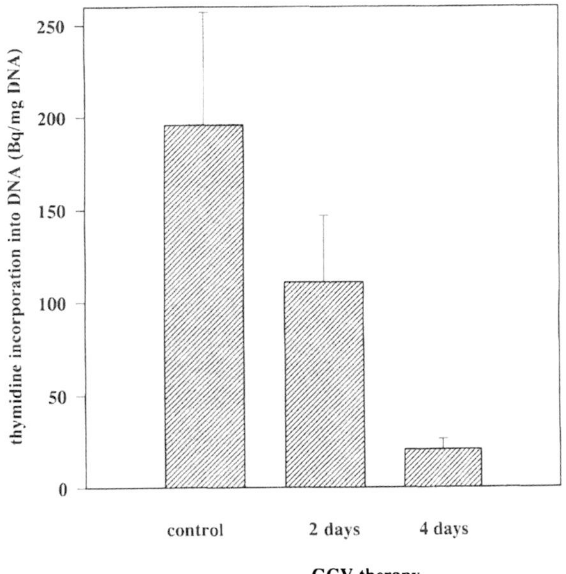

Fig. 31.4. Thymidine incorporation into the DNA of HSVtk-expressing Morris hepatomas after treatment with sodium chloride (controls) or after two and four days therapy with 100 mg ganciclovir/kg body weight.

the TdR incorporation into the tumor DNA was determined after i.v. administration of [^{3}H]TdR. An uncoupling of FDG transport and phosphorylation was found with enhanced k_1 (Fig. 31.3) and k_2 values and a normal k_3 value after two days of GCV treatment [19]. The increase in FDG transport normalized after four days whereas the phosphorylation rate increased. The TdR incorporation into the DNA of the tumors declined to 25% of the controls after 4 days of GCV treatment (Fig. 31.4). These data indicate that PET with [^{18}F]FDG and [^{11}C]TdR may be applied for monitoring of gene therapy with the HSVtk/GCV suicide system. Increased transport rates are evidence of stress reactions early after therapy. The measurement of TdR incorporation into the tumor DNA can be used as an indicator of therapy efficacy. The question of the time period between the onset of prodrug administration and the follow-up PET studies has to be answered in clinical studies.

31.3 Monitoring of gene therapy by the uptake of specific substrates

In the rat hepatoma model [16, 17] uptake measurements were performed for up to 48 hours in a HSVtk-expressing cell line and in a control cell line bearing the empty vector using 5-iodo-2′-fluoro-2′-deoxy-1-b-D-arabinofuranosyluracil (FIAU), fluorodeoxycystidine (FCdR) and ganciclovir.

The FCdR uptake was higher in the HSVtk-expressing cells with a maximum after 4 hours (12-fold and 3-fold higher in the acid-insoluble and acid-soluble fraction, respectively). After longer incubation periods the FCdR uptake declined. HPLC analysis showed a rapid and almost complete metabolization and degradation in both cell lines [16], which might be due to dehalogenation or the action of nucleosidases. The GCV uptake showed a time-dependent increase in HSVtk-expressing cells and a plateau in control cells. The HPLC analysis revealed unmetabolized GCV in control cells and a time-dependent shift of GCV to its phosphorylated metabolite in HSVtk-expressing cells [16]. Furthermore, the ganciclovir as well as the FIAU uptake were highly correlated to the percentage of HSVtk-expressing cells and to the growth inhibition as measured in bystander experiments ([16], Figs. 31.5 and 31.6). Similar results were obtained with genetically modified MCF7 human mammary carcinoma cells [20]. However, the rat Morris hepatoma cells revealed a much higher difference in GCV uptake than MCF7 cells, between HSVtk-expressing cells and control cells [16]. We also found that MCF7 cells are not as sensitive to the HSVtk/GCV system as Morris hepatoma cells. This difference in the amount of tracer accumulation and sensitivity may be explained by the slower rate of growth of MCF7 cells (doubling time: 23.72 ± 2.4 h) as compared to Morris hepatoma cells (doubling time: 16.8 ± 0.7 h).

To further elucidate the transport mechanism of ganciclovir, inhibition/competition experiments were performed. The nucleoside transport in mammalian cells is known to be heterogeneous with two classes of nucleoside transporters: the equilibrative, facilitated diffusion systems and the concentrative, sodium-dependent systems. In our experiments competition for all concentrative nucleoside transport systems and inhibition of the ganciclovir transport by the equilibrative transport systems were observed (Fig. 31.7), whereas the pyrimidine nucleobase system showed no contribution to the

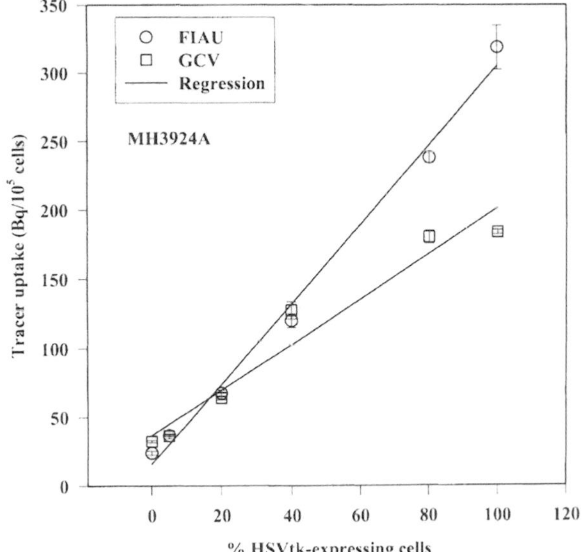

Fig. 31.5. GCV and FIAU uptake in different mixtures of control cells and HSVtk-expressing Morris hepatoma cells after 4 h incubation. The tracer uptake and the amount of HSVtk-expressing cells were correlated with r = 0.97 and r = 0.99, respectively.

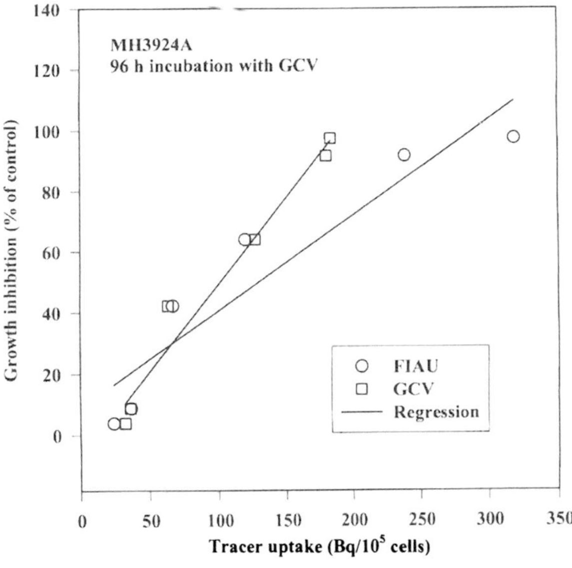

Fig. 31.6. Relation of total GCV and FIAU uptake after 4h incubation and the growth inhibition after 24 hours and 48 hours exposure to 5 μM GCV. The tracer uptake and the growth inhibition in HSVtk-expressing Morris hepatoma cells were correlated with r = 0.98 and r = 0.94, respectively,

ganciclovir uptake [16, 20]. In human erythrocytes acyclovir has been shown to be transported mainly by the purine nucleobase carrier [31]. Due to a hydroxymethyl group on its side chain, ganciclovir has a stronger similarity to nucleosides and, therefore, may be transported also by a nucleoside transporter. Moreover, the 3′-hydroxyl moiety of nucleosides was shown to be important for their interaction with the nucleoside transporter [14].

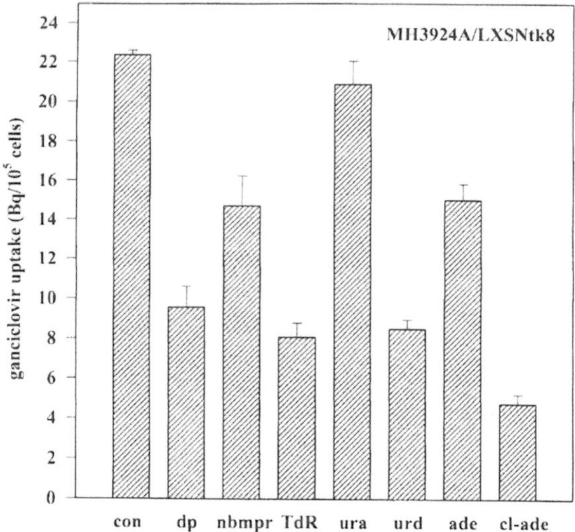

Fig. 31.7. Ganciclovir uptake in HSVtk-expressing hepatoma cells after 10 min incubation without and in the presence of dipyridamole (dp), nitrobenzyl-thioinosine (nbmpr), thymidine (TdR) or ganciclovir (GCV), uracil (ura), uridine (urd), adenine (ade) and 2-chloroadenosine (cl-ade). Mean and standard deviations (n= 3).

In rat hepatoma cells as well as in human mammary carcinoma cells the GCV uptake was shown to be much lower than the thymidine uptake [16, 20]. Therefore, in addition to low infection efficiency of the current viral delivery systems slow transport of the substrate and also its slow conversion into the phosphorylated metabolite is limiting for the therapeutic success of the HSVtk/GCV system. Cotransfection with nucleoside transporters or the use of other substrates for HSVtk with higher affinities for nucleoside transport and phosphorylation by HSVtk may improve therapy outcome.

The principle of in vivo HSVtk imaging was first demonstrated by Price et al. and Saito et al. for the visualization of HSV encephalitis [44, 47]. Recently in vivo studies have been done by several groups using different tracers [1, 2, 13, 34, 52, 53, 60]. Gambhir et al. used 8-[^{18}F]fluoroganciclovir (FGCV) for the imaging of adenovirus-directed hepatic expression of the HSV1-tk reporter gene in living mice [13]. There was a significant positive correlation between the percent-injected dose of FGCV retained per gram of liver and the levels of hepatic HSV1-tk reporter gene expression. Over a similar range of HSV1-tk expression in vivo, the percent injected dose retained per gram of liver was 0–23% for ganciclovir and 0–3% for FGCV. Alauddin et al. [1, 2] used of 9-(4-[^{18}F]fluoro-3-hydroxymethylbutyl)-guanine ([^{18}F]FHBG) and 9-[(3-[^{18}F]fluoro-1-hydroxy-2-propoxy)methyl]-guanine ([^{18}F]FHPG) for combined in vitro/in vivo studies with HT-29 human colon cancer cells, transduced with a retroviral vector and also found a significant higher uptake in transduced cells as compared with the controls. In vivo studies in tumor-bearing nude mice demonstrated that the tumor uptake of the radiotracer is 3- and 6-fold higher at 2 and 5 h, respectively, in transduced cells compared with the control cells. Others used radioiodinated nucleoside analogues as (E)-5-(2-iodovinyl)-2′-fluoro-2′-deoxyuridine (IVFRU) and 5-iodo-2′-fluoro-

2′-deoxy-1-b-D-arabinofuranosyluracil (FIAU) to visualize HSVtk expression [34, 52, 53, 60]. Tjuvajev et al. [52, 53] injected [^{131}I]- or [^{124}I]-labeled FIAU in brain and mammary tumors. Autoradiography as well as the SPECT and PET images revealed highly specific localization of the tracer to areas of HSV1-tk gene expression at 24, 36, and 48 h after i.v. administration. The amount of tracer uptake in the tumors was correlated to the in vitro ganciclovir sensitivity of the cell lines which were transplanted in these animals [52, 53]. Wiebe et al. [34, 60] report that IVFRU becomes metabolically trapped in tumor cells transduced with the HSVtk gene on a retroviral vector. Selective phosphorylation of radiolabeled IVFRU by HSVtk results in elevated radioactivity in HSVtk-expressing tumor cells in vitro and in vivo relative to cells lacking the HSVtk gene. Due to low non-target tissue uptake, unambiguous imaging of HSVtk-expressing tumors in mice is possible with labeled IVFRU. The advantage of iodinated tracers like FIAU may be that delayed imaging is possible. Since ^{18}F-labeled compounds allow only imaging early after administration of the tracer these iodinated compounds may prove to be more sensitive in vivo. However, quantification with iodine isotopes may be a problem either with ^{131}I, a γ- and β^- emitter with high radiation dose, or with the corresponding positron emitter ^{124}I, which shows only 23% β^+ radiation with high energy particles, multiple γ rays of high energy and leads to a high radiation dose.

In human glioblastoma cells, cytosine deaminase (CD) was evaluated. A human glioblastoma cell line was stably transfected with the E. coli CD gene [23] and experiments with [^{3}H]FC were performed. [^{3}H]5-FU was produced in CD-expressing cells, whereas in the control cells only [^{3}H]5-FC was detected [23]. Moreover, significant amounts of 5-FU were found in the medium of cultured cells, which may account for the bystander effect observed in previous experiments. However, uptake studies revealed a moderate and nonsaturable accumulation of radioactivity in the tumor cells suggesting that 5-FC enters the cells only via diffusion [23]. Although a significant difference in 5-FC uptake was seen between CD-positive cells and controls after 48 hour incubation, no difference was observed after a 2 hour incubation. Furthermore, a rapid efflux could be demonstrated. Therefore, 5-FC transport may be a limiting factor for this therapeutic procedure and quantitation with PET has to rely rather on dynamic studies and modeling, including HPLC analysis of the plasma, than on nonmodeling approaches [23]. To evaluate the 5-FC uptake in vivo, we transfected a rat prostate adenocarcinoma cell line with a retroviral vector bearing the E. coli CD gene. The cells were found to be sensitive to 5-FC exposure, but lost this sensitivity with time. This may be due to inactivation of the viral promoter (CMV) used in this vector. In vivo studies with PET and FC showed no preferential accumulation of the tracer in CD-expressing tumors although HPLC analysis revealed a production of 5-fluorouracil which was detectable in tumor lysates as well as in the blood of the animals [15].

31.4 Non-suicide reporter gene approaches

The dopamine D2 receptor gene has also been used as a reporter gene [30]. This gene represents an endogenous gene which is not likely to invoke an immune response. Furthermore, the corresponding tracer 3-(2′-[^{18}F]fluoroethyl)spiperone (FESP) rapidly crosses the blood-brain barrier, can be produced at high specific activity and is currently used in patients. As a SPECT tracer [^{123}I]iodobenzamine is available. MacLaren et al. used this system in nude mice with an adenoviral-directed hepatic gene delivery system and also in stably transfected tumor cells which were transplanted in animals. The tracer uptake in these animals was proportional to in vitro data of hepatic FESP accumulation, dopamine receptor ligand binding and the D2 receptor mRNA. Also tumors modified to express the D2 receptor retained significantly more FESP than wild-type tumors.

Another approach is based on the in vivo transchelation of oxotechnetate to a polypeptide motif from a biocompatible complex with a higher dissociation constant than that of a diglysilcysteine complex. It has been shown that synthetic peptides and recombinant proteins like the modified green fluorescence protein (gfp) can bind oxotechnetate with high efficiency [5, 6]. In these experiments rats were injected i.m. with synthetic peptides bearing a GGC motif. One hour later [^{99m}Tc]glucoheptonate was applied i.v. and the accumulation was measured by scintigraphy. The peptides with three metal-binding GGC motifs showed a threefold higher accumulation as compared to the controls. This principle can also be applied to recombinant proteins which appear at the plasma membrane. These genes can be cloned into bicistronic vectors which allow for the co-expression of therapeutic genes and in vivo reporter genes. Thereafter, radionuclide imaging may be used to detect gene expression.

Tyrosinase catalyzes the hydroxylation of tyrosine to DOPA and the oxidation of DOPA to DOPA-quinone which after cyclization and polymerization results in melanin production. Melanins are scavengers of metal ions as iron and indium through ionic binding. Tyrosinase transfer leads to the production of melanins in a variety of cells. This may be used for imaging with NMR or with ^{111}In and a gamma camera. Cells transfected with the tyrosinase gene stained positively for melanin and had a higher ^{111}In-binding capacity than the wild-type cells [58]. In transfection experiments a dependence of tracer accumulation on the amount of the vector used could be observed. The problems of this approach are possible low tyrosinase induction with low amounts of melanin and the cytotoxicity of melanin. These problems may be encountered by the construction of chimeric tyrosinase proteins and by positioning of the enzyme at the outer side of the membrane.

Recently the rat sodium/iodide symporter gene (rNIS) was cloned into a retroviral vector for transfer into melanoma cells [32]. In vitro iodide transport experiments revealed that the symporter functions similarly in rNIS-transduced tumor cells as in rat thyroid follicular cells. rNIS-transduced and wild-type human A375 melanoma xenografts transplanted into nude mice were imaged using a gamma camera after i.p. injections of ^{123}I and were visually distinguishable from and accumulate significantly more radionuclides than wild-type tumors.

31.5 Future studies

Future studies will be influenced by the development of new viral vectors which have to be more efficient in terms of infection rate and tissue specificity. Furthermore, the use of mutants of HSVtk may result in better imaging characteristics. Transfer of nucleoside transporters can be used to enhance the tracer influx into the genetically modified cells and thereby increase suicide enzyme detection as well as therapeutic efficiency. Receptor genes with a lower background as the dopamine D4 receptor or genes which allow the use of commercially available ligands as the somatostatin receptor subtype 2 may be evaluated for their use as in vivo reporter genes or even for therapeutic purposes.

References

[1] Alauddin MM, Conti PS (1998) Synthesis and preliminary evaluation of 9-(4-[18F]-fluoro-3-hydroxymethylbutyl)guanine ([18F]FHBG): a new potential imaging agent for viral infection and gene therapy using PET. Nucl Med Biol 25:175–180

[2] Alauddin MM, Shahinian A, Kundu RK, Gordon EM, Conti PS (1999) Evaluation of 9-[(3-18F-fluoro-1-hydroxy-2-propoxy)methyl]guanine ([18F]-FHPG) in vitro and in vivo as a probe for PET imaging of gene incorporation and expression in tumors. Nucl Med Biol 26:371–376

[3] Barba D, Hardin J, Sadelain M, Gage FH (1994) Development of anti-tumor immunity following thymidine kinase-mediated killing of experimental brain tumors. Proc Natl Acad Sci USA 91:4348–4352

[4] Bergstrom M, Muhr C, Lundberg PO, Bergstrom K, Gee AD, Fasth KJ, Langstrom B (1987) Rapid decrease in amino acid metabolism in prolactin-secreting pituitary adenomas after bromocriptine treatment: a PET study. J Comput Assist Tomogr 11:815–819

[5] Bogdanov A, Petherick P, Marecos E, Weissleder R (1997) In vivo localization of diglycylcysteine-bearing synthetic peptides by nuclear imaging of oxotechnetate transchelation. Nucl Med Biol 24:739–742

[6] Bogdanov A, Simonova M, Weissleder R (1998) Design of metal-binding green fluorescent protein variants. Biochim Biophys Acta 1397:56–64

[7] Borrelli E, Heyman R, Hsi M, Evans RM (1988) Targeting of an inducible toxic phenotype in animal cells. Proc Natl Acad Sci USA 85:7572–7576

[8] Caruso M, Panis Y, Gagandeep S, Houssin D, Salzmann JL, Klatzman D (1993) Regression of established macroscopic liver metastases after in situ transduction of a suicide gene. Proc Natl Acad Sci USA 90:7024–7028

[9] Chen SH, Shine HD, Goodman JC, Grossman RG, Woo SLC (1994) Gene therapy for brain tumors: regression of experimental gliomas by adenovirus-mediated gene transfer in vivo. Proc Natl Acad Sci USA 91:3054–3057

[10] Christman D, Crawford EJ, Friedkin M, Wolf AP (1972) Detection of DNA synthesis in intact organisms with positron-emitting (methyl-^{11}C)thymidine. Proc Natl Acad Sci USA 69:988–992

[11] Clancy BM, Czech MP (1990) Hexose transport stimulation and membrane redistribution of glucose transporter isoforms in response to cholera toxin, dibutyryl cyclic AMP, and insulin in 3T3 adipocytes. J Biol Chem 265:12434–12443
[12] Culver KW, Ram Z, Walbridge S et al. (1992) In vivo gene transfer with retroviral vector-producer cells for treatment of experimental brain tumors. Science 256:1550–1552
[13] Gambhir SS, Barrio JR, Phelps ME, Iyer M, Namavari M, Satyamurthy N, Wu L, Green LA, Bauer E, MacLaren DC, Nguyen K, Berk AJ, Cherry SR, Herschman HR (1999) Imaging adenoviral-directed reporter gene expression in living animals with positron emission tomography. Proc Natl Acad Sci USA 96:2333–2338
[14] Gati WP, Misra HK, Knaus EE, Wiebe LI (1984) Structural modifications at the 2′ and 3′ positions of some pyrimidine nucleosides as determinants of their interaction with the mouse erythrocyte nucleoside transporter. Biochem Pharmacol 33:3325–3331
[15] Haberkorn U (1999) Monitoring of gene transfer for cancer therapy with radioactive isotopes. Ann Nucl Med 13:369–377
[16] Haberkorn U, Altmann A, Morr I et al. (1997) Gene therapy with herpes simplex virus thymidine kinase in hepatoma cells: uptake of specific substrates. J Nucl Med 38:287–294
[17] Haberkorn U, Altmann A, Morr I, Germann C, Oberdorfer F, Kaick G van (1997) Multi tracer studies during gene therapy of hepatoma cells with HSV thymidine kinase and ganciclovir. J Nucl Med 38:1048–1054
[18] Haberkorn U, Bellemann ME, Altmann A, Gerlach L, Morr I, Oberdorfer F, Brix G, Doll J, Blatter J, Kaick G van (1997) F-18-fluoro-2-deoxyglucose uptake in rat prostate adenocarcinoma during chemotherapy with 2′,2′-difluoro-2′-deoxycytidine. J Nucl Med 38:1215–1221
[19] Haberkorn U, Bellemann ME, Gerlach L, Morr I, Trojan H, Brix G, Altmann A, Doll J, Kaick G van (1998) Uncoupling of 2-fluoro-2-deoxyglucose transport and phosphorylation in rat hepatoma during gene therapy with HSV thymidine kinase. Gene Ther 5:880–887
[20] Haberkorn U, Khazaie K, Morr I, Altmann A, Müller M, Kaick G van (1998) Ganciclovir uptake in human mammary carcinoma cells expressing Herpes Simplex Virus thymidine kinase. Nucl Med Biol 25:367–373
[21] Haberkorn U, Morr I, Oberdorfer F et al. (1994) Fluorodeoxyglucose uptake in vitro: aspects of method and effects of treatment with gemcitabine. J Nucl Med 35:1842–1850
[22] Haberkorn U, Oberdorfer F, Klenner T et al. (1994) Metabolic and transcriptional changes in osteosarcoma cells treated with chemotherapeutic drugs. Nucl Med Biol 21:835–845
[23] Haberkorn U, Oberdorfer F, Gebert J et al. (1996) Monitoring of gene therapy with cytosine deaminase: in vitro studies using ^{3}H-5-fluorocytosine. J Nucl Med 37:87–94
[24] Haberkorn U, Reinhardt M, Strauss LG et al. (1992) Metabolic design of combination therapy: use of enhanced fluorodeoxyglucose uptake caused by chemotherapy. J Nucl Med 33:1981–1987
[25] Haberkorn U, Strauss LG, Dimitrakopoulou A et al. (1993) Fluorodeoxyglucose imaging of advanced head and neck cancer after chemotherapy. J Nucl Med 34:12–17
[26] Huber BE, Austin EA, Good SS, Knick VC, Tibbels S, Richards CA (1993) In vivo antitumor activity of 5-fluorocytosine on human colorectal carcinoma cells genetically modified to express cytosine deaminase. Cancer Res 53:4619–4626
[27] Izquierdo M et al. (1995) Long-term rat survival after malignant brain tumour regression by retroviral gene therapy. Gene Ther 2:66–69
[28] Keller PM, Fyfe JA, Beauchamp L et al. (1981) Enzymatic phosphorylation of acyclic nucleoside analogs and correlations with antiherpetic activities. Biochem Pharmacol 30:3071–3077
[29] Koechlin BA, Rubio F, Palmer S, Gabriel T, Duschinsky R (1966) The metabolism of 5-fluorocytosine-2-^{14}C and of cytosine-1-^{14}C in the rat and the disposition of 5-fluorocytosine-2-^{14}C in man. Biochem Pharmac 15:435–446

[30] MacLaren DC, Gambhir SS, Satyamurthy N et al. (1999) Repetitive non-invasive imaging of the dopamine D2 receptor as a reporter gene in living animals. Gene Ther 6:785–791

[31] Mahony WB, Domin BA, McConnel RT, Zimmerman TP (1988) Acyclovir transport into human erythrocytes. J Biol Chem 263:9285–9291

[32] Mandell RB, Mandell LZ, Link CJ Jr (1999) Radioisotope concentrator gene therapy using the sodium/iodide symporter gene. Cancer Res 59:661–668

[33] Maron A et al. (1996) Gene therapy of rat C6 glioma using adenovirus-mediated transfer of the herpes simplex virus thymidine kinase gene: long-term follow up by magnetic resonance imaging. Gene Ther 3:315–322

[34] Morin KW, Knaus EE, Wiebe LI (1997) Non-invasive scintigraphic monitoring of gene expression in a HSV-1 thymidine kinase gene therapy model. Nucl Med Commun 18:599–605

[35] Monclus M, Luxen A, Van Naemen J et al. (1995) Development of PET radiopharmaceuticals for gene therapy: synthesis of 9-((1-(^{18}F)fluoro-3-hydroxy-2-propoxy)methyl)guanine. J Label Comp Radiopharm 37:193–195

[36] Moolten FL, Wells JM (1990) Curability of tumors bearing Herpes thymidine kinase genes transferred by retroviral vectors. J Natl Cancer Inst 82:297–300

[37] Mullen CA, Coale MM, Lowe R, Blaese RM (1994) Tumors expressing the cytosine deaminase suicide gene can be eliminated in vivo with 5-fluorocytosine and induce protective immunity to wild type tumor. Cancer Res 54:1503–1506

[38] Mullen CA, Kilstrup M, Blaese M (1992) Transfer of the bacterial gene for cytosine deaminase to mammalian cells confers lethal sensitivity to 5-fluorocytosine: a negative selection system. Proc Natl Acad Sci USA 89:33–37

[39] Myers CE (1981) The pharmacology of the fluoropyrimidines. Pharmacological Reviews 33:1–15

[40] Nishiyama T, Kawamura Y, Kawamoto K, Matsumura H, Yamamoto N, Ito T, Ohyama A, Katsuragi T, Sakai T (1985) Antineoplastic effects of 5-fluorocytosine in combination with cytosine deaminase capsules. Cancer Res 45:1753–1761

[41] Oldfield EH, Ram Z, Culver KW, Blaese RM, DeVroom HL, Anderson WF (1993) Gene therapy for the treatment of brain tumors using intra-tumoral transduction with the thymidine kinase gene and intravenous ganciclovir. Hum Gene Ther 1:39–69

[42] Pasternak CA, Aiyathurai JEJ, Makinde V et al. (1991) Regulation of glucose uptake by stressed cells. J Cell Physiol 149:324–331

[43] Polak A, Eschenhof E, Fernex M, Scholer HJ (1976) Metabolic studies with 5-fluorocytosine-6-^{14}C in mouse, rat, rabbit, dog and man. Chemotherapy 22:137–153

[44] Price R, Cardle K, Watanabe K (1983) The use of antiviral drugs to image herpes encephalitis. Cancer Res 43:3619–3627

[45] Ram Z, Culver WK, Walbridge S et al. (1993) In situ retroviral-mediated gene transfer for the treatment of brain tumors in rats. Cancer Res 53:83–88

[46] Rozenthal JM, Levine RL, Nickles RJ, Dobkin JA (1989) Glucose uptake by gliomas after treatment. Arch Neurol 46:1302–1307

[47] Saito Y, Price R, Rottenberg DA, Fox JJ, Su TL, Watanabe KA, Philipps FA (1982) Quantitative autoradiographic mapping of herpes simplex virus encephalitis with radiolabeled antiviral drug. Science 217:1151–1153

[48] Scholer HJ (1980) Flucytosine. In: Speller DCE (ed) *Antifungal Chemotherapy.* John Wiley & Sons, Chichester New York, pp 35–106

[49] Shields AF et al. (1990) Utilization of labeled thymidine in DNA synthesis: studies for PET. J Nucl Med 31:337–342

[50] Shields AF, Grierson JR, Dohmen BM et al. (1998) Imaging proliferation in vivo with (F-18)FLT and positron emission tomography. Nature Med 4:1334–1336

[51] Sobol RE et al. (1995) Interleukin-2 gene therapy in a patient with glioblastoma. Gene Ther 2:164–167

[52] Tjuvajev JG, Avril N, Oku T et al. (1998) Imaging herpes virus thymidine kinase gene transfer and expression by positron emission tomography. Cancer Res 58:4333–4341

[53] Tjuvajev JG, Stockhammer G, Desai R, Uehara H, Watanabe K, Gansbacher B, Blasberg RG (1995) Imaging the expression of transfected genes in vivo. Cancer Res 55:6126–6132

[54] Visser GWM, Boele S, Knops GHJN, Herscheid JDM, Hoekstra A (1985) Synthesis and biodistribution of (^{18}F)-5-fluorocytosine. Nucl Med Comm 6:455–459

[55] Wahl RL et al. (1993) Metabolic monitoring of breast cancer chemohormonotherapy using positron emission tomography: initial evaluation. J Clin Oncol 11:2101–2111

[56] Wallace PM, MacMaster JF, Smith VF, Kerr DE, Senter PD, Cosand WL (1994) Intratumoral generation of 5-fluorouracil mediated by an antibody-cytosine deaminase conjugate in combination with 5-fluorocytosine. Cancer Res 54:2719–2723

[57] Wertheimer E, Sasson S, Cerasi E, Ben-Neriah Y (1991) The ubiquitous glucose transporter GLUT-1 belongs to the glucose-regulated protein family of stress-inducible proteins. Proc Natl Acad Sci USA 88:2525–2529

[58] Weissleder R, Simonova M, Bogdanova A et al. (1997) MR imaging and scintigraphy of gene expression through melanin induction. Radiology 204:425–429

[59] Widnell CC, Baldwin SA, Davies A, Martin S, Pasternak CA (1990) Cellular stress induces a redistribution of the glucose transporter. FASEB J 4:1634–1637

[60] Wiebe LI, Morin KW, Knaus EE (1997) Radiopharmaceuticals to monitor gene transfer. Q J Nucl Med 41:79–89

List of Radiopharmaceuticals

5-iodo-2′-fluoro-2′deoxy-1-β-D-arabinofuranosyluracil (FIAU)
^{11}C
- [^{11}C]acetate
-[^{11}C]aminoisobutyric acid
- [^{11}C]aminocyclobutancarboxylic acid (ACBC)
- [^{11}C]bromocriptin
- [^{11}C]butanol
- [^{11}C]choline
- [^{11}C]carbondioxide CO2
[^{11}C]ethanol
- [^{11}C]hydroxytryptophan (HTP)
- [^{11}C]hydroxyephedrin
- L-[^{11}C]deprenyl
- L-[^{11}C]DOPA
- [^{11}C]methionine
- [^{11}C]methyl-D-glucose
- (N-[^{11}C]methyl)spiperone
- [^{11}C]putrescine
- [^{11}C]raclopride
- [^{11}C]somatostatin
- [^{11}C]thymidine
[^{14}C]deoxyglucose
13N
- [^{13}N]glutamate
- [^{13}N]NH_3
^{15}O
- [^{15}O]CO_2
- [^{15}O]H_2O
^{18}F
- 2-[^{18}F]AFDG
- 2-[^{18}F]fluoro-l-tyrosine
- 2-[^{18}F]fluoro-2-deoxy-D-glucose, see[^{18}F]FDG
- 2-[^{18}F]fluoro-2-deoxyarabinose-derivate
- 2-hydroxy-3-([^{18}F]fluoro-propan)-2-nitroimidazol ([^{18}F]FMISO)
- 3-[^{18}F]FDG
- 3-[^{18}F]fluoro-a-methyl-L-tyrosine
- 3-[^{18}F]fluoro-3′-derivative
- 3′-deoxy-3′-[^{18}F] fluorthymidine ([^{18}F]FLT)
- 4-(2-[^{18}F]fluorethylamino)-derivative
- 4-[^{18}F]fluoro-l-phenylalanin
- 4-[^{18}F]fluoro-L-proline
- 5-[^{18}F]fluorouracil
- 5-[^{18}F]fluoruridine
- 5′-deoxy-5′-[^{18}F]fluoro-thymidine
- 16-a-[^{18}F]fluoro-17β-estradiol
- [^{18}F]aciclovir
- [^{18}F]androgen receptor ligands
- [^{18}F]DOPA
- [^{18}F]FDG
- [^{18}F]fluoro-adenosine
- [^{18}F]fluoroiodo-benzylguanine
- [^{18}F]fluoro-ethanidazole
- [^{18}F]fluoropropyl-DPhe^{1}-octreotide
- [^{18}F]galactose
- [^{18}F]ganciclovir
- [^{18}F]penciclovir
- [^{18}F]progestinanalogue
- [^{18}F]sodiumfluoride
- O-(2-[^{18}F]fluoroethyl)-L-tyrosine
[^{62}Cu]ATSM
[^{62}Cu]PTSM
[^{67}Ga]scintigraphy
^{68}Ge/^{68}Ga
^{82}Rb
^{99m}Tc
[^{99m}Tc]DMSA
[^{99m}Tc]furifosmin
[^{99m}Tc]MDP
[^{99m}Tc]MIBI
[^{99m}Tc]tetrofosmin
[^{111}In]pentetreotide
^{123}I
[^{123}I]a-methyl-tyrosine
[^{123}I]MIBG
^{131}I
[^{131}I]lipidol
^{137}Cs
^{201}Tl

Subject Index

Appendix

Results of the German Consensus Conference "PET in Oncology" Ulm, Sept. 12, 1997

(see: Reske SN (1998) Positronen-Emissionstomographie in der Onkologie. Dtsch. Ärzteblatt 95: C 1370–1372).

Clinical value of PET

Category Ia – adequate, appropriate
Category Ib – acceptable
Category IIa – helpful
Category IIb – evaluation not yet possible
Category III – not useful

Category Ia – Indications

Differentiated thyroid cancer	– recurrence expected or metastases (TG elevation or pathological morphological imaging and negative iodine-scan)
Brain tumors	– diagnostics of recurrence in high-grade gliomas (FDG), diagnostics of recurrence in low-grade gliomas ([^{11}C]methionine) – detection of a malignant dedifferentiation of a glioma recurrence (FDG) – localization of the best biopsy area in pts. with glioma
Colorectal cancer	– restaging (local recurrence, lymph node metastases, distant metastases) in pts. with strong suspicion of disease (e.g., elevation of tumor markers or positive morphological imaging)

Head and neck cancer	– CUP syndrome (carcinoma of unknown primary) in pts. with negative morphological imaging and known histology
Malignant melanomas	– stage II and III: staging of lymph nodes and distant metastases
Non-small cell lung cancer (NSCLC)	– solitary pulmonary nodules in pts. at risk to have cancer – local recurrence – lymph node staging
Pancreatic cancer	– primary staging/differential diagnostics

Category Ib – Indications

Differentiated thyroid cancer	– in pts. with proven iodine positive recurrence/distant metastases for the detection of further tumor sites, if an influence on therapy can be expected
Brain tumors	– biological aggressiveness of gliomas – diagnostics of gliomas ([^{11}C]methionine or [^{18}F]tyrosine)
Colorectal cancer	– therapy control: after chemotherapy
head and neck cancer	– lymph node staging (primary resectable)
Malignant lymphomas	– residual tumor after therapy, primary staging
Testicular cancer, non-seminomas	– therapy control, apart from differentiated teratoma
Pancreatic cancer	– local recurrence, only in existence of a therapeutic option

Category IIa – Indications

Bladder cancer	– lymph node staging
Brain tumors	– preoperative functional diagnostics, therapy control
Colorectal cancer	– therapy control (radiation therapy)
Head and neck cancer	– local recurrence (more than three months after radiation therapy)
Malignant lymphomas	– restaging – diagnostics of recurrence

Breast cancer	- primary staging - local recurrence - lymph node staging - distant metastases in high-risk patients - therapy control
Non-small cell lung cancer (NSCLC)	- therapy control
Testicular cancer, non-seminomas	- lymph node staging - restaging
Ovarian cancer	- recurrence - restaging

Category IIb – Indications

Bladder cancer	- local recurrence (not of relevance because of poor prognosis) - distant metastases - therapy control
Differentiated thyroid cancer	- lymph nodes staging - therapy control
Endocrine/neuroendocrine tumors	- all questions
gynecologic tumors	- (vulva, endometrium, vagina, cervix) all questions
Colorectal cancer	- preoperative primary staging (if CEA >30 ng/ml and negative imaging concerning distant metastases)
Head and neck cancer	- lymph node staging (non-resectable primary tumor) - second cancer - therapy control
Malignant lymphomas	- early therapy control (later than six weeks after therapy): response during therapy
Malignant melanomas	- therapy control
Breast cancer	- distant metastases, except in high-risk patients
Non-small cell lung cancer (NSCLC)	- distant metastases
Testicular cancer, non-seminomas	- teratoma
Renal cell carcinoma	- local recurrence - distant metastases
Ovarian cancer	- primary tumor - distant metastases - peritoneal carcinomatosis - therapy control
Pancreatic cancer	- lymph node staging

	– distant metastases (problem: peritoneal carcinomatosis)
Prostate carcinoma	– local recurrence
Seminoma	– lymph node staging
	– therapy control

Special notes

Malignant lymphomas	– residual tumor after therapy and primary staging: category IIa
Breast cancer	– lymph node staging: category IIb
Testicular cancer, non-seminomas	– therapy control: category IIa
Ovarian cancer	– recurrence/restaging: category Ib

Category III – Indications (not clinically useful)

Bladder cancer	– primary diagnostics
Chronic lymphemia	– all diagnostics questions
Differentiated thyroid cancer	– primary diagnostics
Colorectal cancer	– primary staging preoperative (except CEA >30 ng/ml without known metastases)
Head and neck cancer	– primary diagnostics (except: see Ia – indications)
Malignant melanoma	– primary diagnostics, local recurrence, lymph node staging and staging of distant metastases in stage I tumors
Testicular cancer, non-seminomas	– primary diagnostics
	– local recurrence
Renal cell carcinoma	– lymph node staging
	– therapy control
Ovarian cancer	– local recurrence without therapeutical option therapy control
Prostate carcinoma	– primary diagnostics
	– lymph node staging
	– distant metastases
	– therapy control